ANNALS OF THE NEW YORK ACADEMY OF SCIENCES

Volume 853

The New York Academy of Sciences
2 East 63rd Street
New York, New York 10021

CARDIAC SARCOPLASMIC RETICULUM FUNCTION AND REGULATION OF CONTRACTILITY

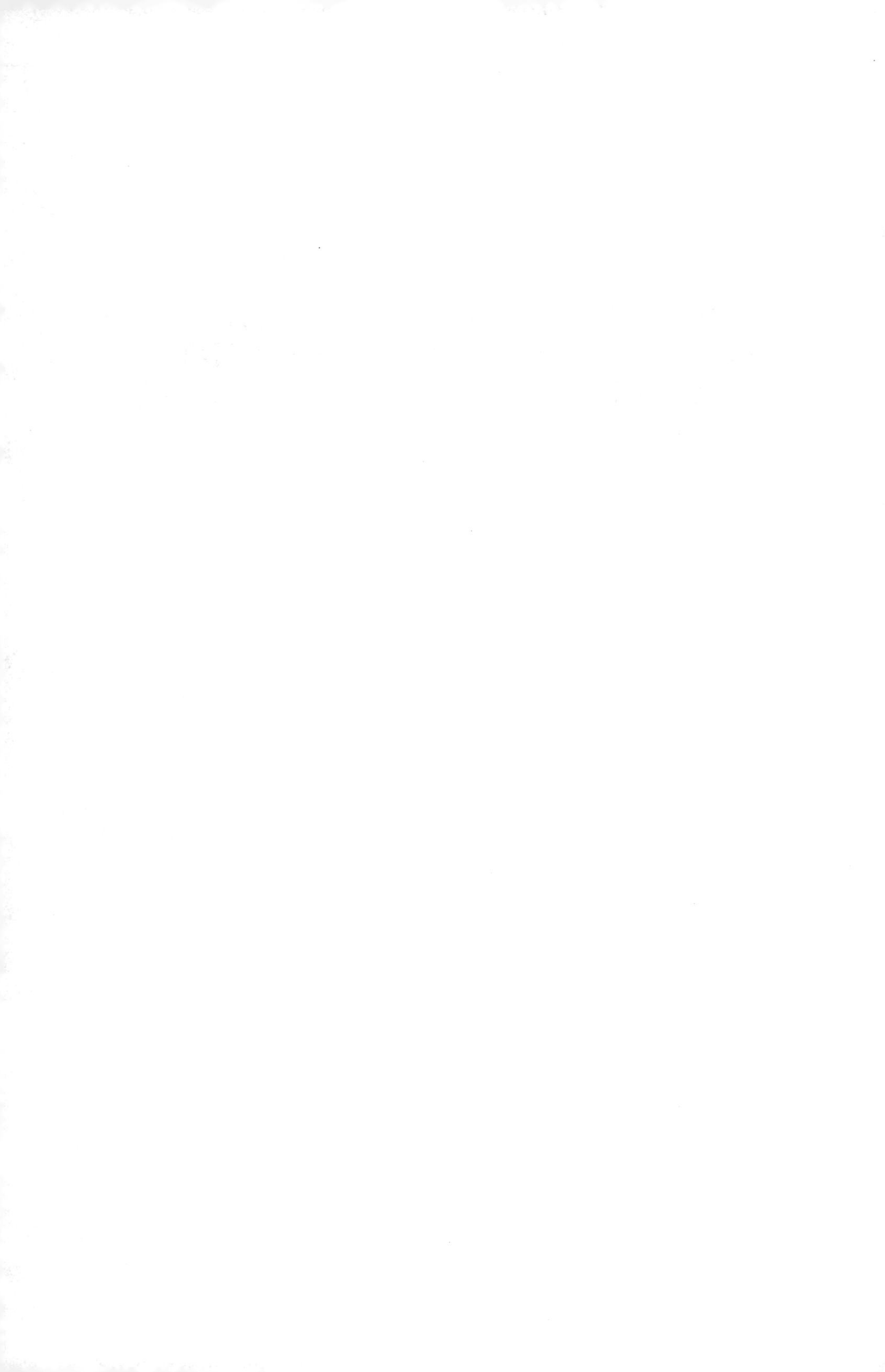

ANNALS OF THE NEW YORK ACADEMY OF SCIENCES

Volume 853

CARDIAC SARCOPLASMIC RETICULUM FUNCTION AND REGULATION OF CONTRACTILITY

Edited by Robert G. Johnson, Jr. and Evangelia G. Kranias

The New York Academy of Sciences
New York, New York
1998

Library of Congress Cataloging-in-Publication Data

Cardiac sarcoplasmic reticulum function and regulation of contractility / edited by Robert G. Johnson, Jr., and Evangelia G. Kranias.
p. cm.—(Annals of the New York Academy of Sciences, ISSN 0077-8923 ; v. 853)
Includes index.
ISBN 1-57331-129-4 (cloth : alk. paper).—ISBN 1-57331-130-8 (pbk. : alk. paper)
1. Heart—Contraction—Regulation—Congresses. 2. Sarcoplasmic reticulum—Congresses. 3. Heart cells—Congresses. I. Johnson, Robert G. (Robert Gahagen), 1952– . II. Kranias, Evangelia G. III. New York Academy of Sciences. IV. Series.
[DNLM: 1. Sarcoplasmic Reticulum—physiology congresses. 2. Myocardial Contraction—physiology congresses. 3. Contractile Proteins congresses. W1 AN626YL v.853 1998]
Q11.N5 vol. 853
[QP113.2]
500 s—dc21
[612.1'71]
DNLM/DLC
for Library of Congress 98-23010
CIP

ComCom/RRD
Printed in the United States of America
ISBN 1-57331-129-4 (cloth)
ISBN 1-57331-130-8 (paper)
ISSN 0077-8923

ANNALS OF THE NEW YORK ACADEMY OF SCIENCES

Volume 853
September 16, 1998

CARDIAC SARCOPLASMIC RETICULUM FUNCTION AND REGULATION OF CONTRACTILITY[a]

Editors and Conference Chairs
ROBERT G. JOHNSON, JR. AND EVANGELIA G. KRANIAS

Honorary Chair
WILHELM HASSELBACH

Scientific Advisory Board
GERD HASENFUSS, ARNOLD M. KATZ, DAVID H. MACLENNAN, KETTY SCHWARTZ, AND MICHIHIKO TADA

CONTENTS

[a] This volume is the result of a conference entitled **Cardiac Sarcoplasmic Reticulum Function and Regulation of Contractility** held by the New York Academy of Sciences on September 27–30, 1997 in Washington, D.C.

Part V. The Role of Sarcoplasmic Reticulum Proteins in Heart Disease

Part VI. Poster Papers

Financial assistance was received from:

Supporters
- BYK GULDEN
- JAPAN HEART FOUNDATION
- MERCK RESEARCH LABORATORIES
- MERCK & CO., INC., HUMAN HEALTH DIVISION
- PROCTOR & GAMBLE PHARMACEUTICALS

Contributors
- AMERICAN HEART ASSOCIATION
- AXON INSTRUMENTS
- BAYER, AG
- BERLIN-CHEMIE AG
- ELI LILLY AND CO., CARDIOVASCULAR RESEARCH DIVISION
- GENENTECH, INC.
- HOECHST MARION ROUSSEL
- ORION PHARMA
- PFIZER INC
- PHOTON TECHNOLOGY INTERNATIONAL
- SCHERING-PLOUGH RESEARCH INSTITUTE
- SMITHKLINE BEECHAM PHARMACEUTICALS
- THOMAE
- WYETH-AYERST RESEARCH

Introduction

This volume of the *Annals of the New York Academy of Sciences,* entitled *Cardiac Sarcoplasmic Reticulum Function and Regulation of Contractility,* contains state-of-the-art summaries of recent work and the current understanding on the structure, function, and regulation of the cardiac sarcoplasmic reticulum proteins, presented at the New York Academy of Sciences–sponsored meeting held in late September of 1997 in Washington, D.C. and attended by over two hundred scientists.

The cardiac sarcoplasmic reticulum (SR) is a dense intracellular membranous network in muscle cells that plays a key role in excitation-contraction coupling by its ability to regulate the intracellular calcium. Relaxation within cardiac muscle is mediated by a specific ATPase in the SR membrane, which sequesters calcium from the cytosol into the SR lumen, thereby removing it from the calcium-sensitive proteins of the myofilaments. The calcium stored within the SR lumen during cardiac muscle relaxation is released into the cytosol through a specialized ion channel, the calcium release channel, and this initiates contraction. In cardiac, but not skeletal muscle, the calcium ATPase is under regulation by an integral membrane protein called phospholamban (PLB). PLB in its dephosphorylated state is an inhibitor of the SR calcium ATPase activity, and phosphorylation of PLB by protein kinase A or calcium calmodulin-dependent kinase relieves this inhibition. Thus, the SR function tightly controls the beat-to-beat cardiac cycle: the rate and extent of myocardial relaxation is determined by the rate and extent of calcium uptake from the myoplasm into the SR, and the rate and extent of myocardial contraction is determined by the rate and extent of calcium release into the myoplasm. In addition, the degree of calcium ATPase regulation by PLB presents a fine-tuning mechanism for regulation of muscle relaxation and the graded response of the heart to increased work demand.

Until recently, the majority of investigative work covering calcium regulation within the heart focused primarily on the structure, function, and pathology of the myofilaments. However, the application of sophisticated molecular biological techniques and the generation of knockout and transgenic models over the past several years have made it possible to investigate the *ex vivo* and *in vivo* properties of the SR proteins and elucidate their role in cardiac contractility. For example, in-depth site-directed mutagenesis studies on the calcium ATPase and PLB have allowed important insights into the nature of the binding interaction of these two proteins; PLB can now be synthesized and highly purified in large quantities for structural studies; the calcium release channel can be investigated in a variety of preparations; and generation of transgenic animals with altered PLB and calcium ATPase expression levels have greatly advanced our understanding of the mechanisms involved in the regulation of SR transport and the overall regulation of myocardial contractility. Furthermore, recent evidence indicates that in heart failure there may be a mismatch of calcium ATPase to PLB. This mismatch may contribute to abnormal calcium handling, which has been observed in failed animal and human hearts, and, along with related disturbances in the SR calcium release channel, may explain the alterations in systolic and diastolic function associated with cardiac diseases.

The purpose of this conference was to bring together an interdisciplinary group of internationally recognized investigators in the field of cardiac SR proteins, ranging from molecular and structural biologists to clinical cardiologists and pharmacologists, to review the progress of the field, chart the unresolved questions, and discuss new insights into therapeutic approaches. Up to the time of this conference, despite the large number of meetings devoted to excitation-contraction coupling and muscle physiology, there had been no meeting devoted exclusively to the cardiac SR.

Many questions were asked and answered at the conference during the three days of presentations, posters, and discussions; several additional important and fundamental questions remain to be adequately and opportunely rejoined. A sampling of the critical issues is addressed below.

What are the functions of the cardiac SR proteins? As a result of several decades of research and the recent application of the powerful tools of molecular biology for deriving the sequence of the SR proteins and permitting transgenic manipulation, this question has been addressed for several proteins, as evidenced by the chapters in this volume. The focus has shifted towards understanding the molecular relationships between the proteins and their physiological regulation. Not to be lost sight of, however, is the continuing discussion over the magnitude of the contributions of the SR proteins in the abnormal calcium handling observed in nonphysiological (e.g., pathological) conditions, such as heart failure, and whether the contractile abnormalities can be traced entirely to defects in cardiac SR.

What are the structures of the cardiac SR proteins? This is particularly important in elucidating the nature of interaction between the calcium ATPase and PLB. Significant insight has been achieved through site-directed mutagenesis studies of the calcium ATPase and PLB, labeling studies, and electron image enhancement techniques. However, there is no high-resolution crystal structure of either protein, nor does high-resolution NMR data exist for the intact proteins (this is also true for the ryanodine receptor). Questions such as how phosphorylation of PLB influences its binding to the calcium ATPase are at best conjectural, and limit the ability to selectively target this low- molecular-weight protein. In addition, the functional implications of PLB as a pentamer have not been totally resolved: for example, does PLB form an ion channel? Finally, the lack of high-quality, high-resolution structural data for the cardiac SR proteins is one of the unfortunate, rate-limiting aspects of this entire scientific area; the existing data and inferences can only be described as tenebrous.

How are the cardiac SR proteins regulated? This was one of the central questions of the entire meeting. Now that the function of the proteins is recognized, their dynamic regulation by modification or changes in their levels of expression have reached the forefront of the inquiries.

Short-term regulation: Phosphorylation of PLB and the ryanodine receptor has been documented to occur over a short time scale, primarily under the control of beta-adrenergic stimulation. Phosphorylation of PLB has been clearly demonstrated to disinhibit the calcium ATPase and increase the affinity of this enzyme for calcium. But what is the purpose of phosphorylation of Thr17 in PLB? What is the proportion of PLB phosphorylated on Ser16, or Thr17, or Ser16Thr17 under different conditions? What is the proportion of PLB that must be phosphorylated to achieve maximum inotropic and lusitropic stimulation? The opening of the calcium release channel has also been postulated to be regulated by phosphorylation. However, the regulation of this channel in the context of excitation-contraction coupling (particularly the precise mechanism and the differences between skeletal and cardiac muscle) is not well understood; and whether the proper mechanism is violated in heart failure is not known.

Long-term regulation: Despite the localization of the calcium ATPase and PLB on different chromosomes, their expression levels appear to be tightly coordinated in the developing heart. However, inverse regulation is observed during thyroid states: in hyperthyroidism, the expression of the calcium pump increases and that of PLB decreases; while under hypothyroidism, the reverse occurs in the heart. Coordinate regulation of the calcium release channel in relationship to the calcium ATPase and PLB is not as well established. Unfortunately, a large percentage of the literature is based upon measurements of mRNA levels of these SR proteins; and these levels may not correlate with the actual protein levels. Thus, it is absolutely critical that high-quality data be obtained, especially in regard to clinical heart failure; and that samples be collected throughout the spectrum of failure development, from early stage to end stage, and normalized for the variety of etiologies.

What is the stoichiometry of the calcium ATPase, PLB, and the ryanodine receptor proteins under pathological conditions? This is an area of great promise but also many pitfalls. Data have been published suggesting that the output of the calcium pump may be diminished in heart failure and the expression of PLB also diminished, but less so, resulting in a relative overexpression of PLB (and therefore a relative increased inhibition of the pump). In addition, with down-regulation of the beta-adrenergic pathway, phosphorylation of PLB may be decreased under basal conditions. All of these factors could contribute to a relative increased inhibition of the pump. Unfortunately, many of the clinical samples examined are derived from end-stage heart failure; a major issue is whether similar findings are observed early in heart failure, and how they relate to clinical findings. Certainly, abnormalities in the expression of cardiac SR proteins resulting in sluggish calcium handling could very well explain many of the clinical abnormalities such as negative inotropy and lusitropy in the failing heart.

Is there a target within the cardiac SR that is appropriate for therapeutic intervention in heart failure? Will manipulation of this target have adverse effects? Will the intervention improve symptoms and mortality? Will the intervention prevent or retard the progression of heart failure? Reports in this book review the targets and the means available to hit the targets, including gene therapy to increase the calcium pump expression, interference with the calcium ATPase and PLB interaction using low-molecular-weight compounds, and modulation of the calcium release channel. In aggregate, the data suggest that modulation of several of the cardiac SR proteins by altering their regulatory effects or expression levels would support a positive inotropic and lusitropic activity. But the means to the ends, based upon current knowledge, will require a course around (not between) Scylla and Charybdis.

The organization of this volume follows the organization of the meeting into five sections. In the first section, the structure, function, and regulation of the cardiac SR calcium pump is reviewed. In the second section, the interaction of phospholamban with the calcium pump is explored along with the physiological role, structure, and phosphorylation states of phospholamban. The third section focuses on the calcium release channel, and the fourth section delves into the known pharmacology of each SR protein. The fifth and final section showcases what is known and postulated about the role of SR proteins in heart disease, building on the foundation of the other four sections.

A conference of this kind requires the assistance and support of many individuals and organizations. We were very fortunate to count on an outstanding scientific advisory board, including Drs. Gerd Hasenfuss, Arnold Katz, David MacLennan, Ketty Schwartz, and Michihiko Tada, all of whom provided valuable suggestions and contributions to the meeting. Special gratitude is extended to Dr. Katz for his encouragement and guidance during the early planning stages of the conference. We are also deeply indebted to Dr. Richard Walsh for his many contributions to this conference, including fund raising efforts, providing the closing summary, and organizing the premeeting workshop entitled "Regulation of Cardiac Function: Insights from a Clinical Point of View," which over 90% of the meeting participants attended on a glorious Sunday afternoon! Kudos to Drs. Katz, Morgan, and Walsh for their wonderful participation and leadership in this informal workshop, which set the clinical perspective for the basic science topics that followed. Additionally, a meeting of this kind and in this environment could not have been held without the generous financial support of those acknowledged separately in this volume. We would also like to thank and acknowledge Ms. Sherryl Greenberg of the Science and Techology Meetings Department of the New York Academy of Sciences for her administration of the meeting, and Mr. Richard Stiefel of the Editorial Department for the timely publication of this volume.

Finally, this volume is dedicated to two individuals, the honorary chairperson and the plenary speaker of the meeting. The honorary chairman made several original and fundamental observations that paved the way for the years of research that followed in the field. He was a unique asset and provided a historical perspective to the conference, which in today's scientific world is often lacking. The plenary speaker has provided unique and distinguished contributions into the structure and function of cardiac SR, which greatly advanced the cardiac muscle field. He has also been responsible for educating and training several generations of scientists and physicians in cardiac muscle physiology, and he was a vigorous intellectual contributor to the conference. Both individuals have defined and provided the fundamentals of the cardiac SR field, as the reader can observe in the first two chapters. Great accomplishments have been achieved by many of the scientists participating in this meeting, based upon extending several of the original observations by these two leaders. This volume is a compendium of how far the field has progressed, and presents a challenge to researchers (both in the field and peering in from the outside) to solve the remaining questions of the future. This volume is dedicated to Drs. Wilhelm Hasselbach and Arnold Katz.

—Robert G. Johnson, Jr. and Evangelia G. Kranias

The Ca^{2+}-ATPase of the Sarcoplasmic Reticulum in Skeletal and Cardiac Muscle

An Overview from the Very Beginning to More Recent Prospects

WILHELM HASSELBACH[a]

Max-Planck-Institut für Medizinische Forschung Heidelberg, Germany

ABSTRACT: The discovery of the ATP-driven calcium pump in the sarcoplasmic reticulum membranes reaches back to the postwar (World War II) years and would not be possible without the generous support by the American scientific community. It was this community that in pre- and postwar years gave shelter to many European scientists, which in return stimulated scientific development in the United States. These pre- and postwar relations helped to establish the calcium pump as a physiologically relevant mechanism in all kinds of cells. The pump and its counterpart, the calcium release channel, proved to be controlled by various intrinsic mechanisms. Rising hydrogen concentrations as occuring in ischemic muscles switch off pump activity and counteract allosterically caffeine-induced calcium release (CICR). Rising phosphate or the presence of other calcium-precipitating anions, on the other hand, prevents pump inhibition by intraluminal calcium precipitation, which, simultaneously, can increase the quantity of releasable calcium. The inactivation of CICR by removing medium chloride must be considered as a hint of additional mechanisms by which calcium-dependent activity regulation can be modified.

The discovery of the ATP-driven calcium pump in the sarcoplasmic reticulum (SR) membranes reaches back to the postwar (World War II) years and would not have been possible without the generous help of the American scientific community.[1] It was this community that 60 years ago granted shelter to many German and other European scientists in the time of terror in Germany and Europe. Later these refugees were among the first who helped reestablish human relations and scientific exchange. I think of, among others, Otto Meyerhof, Fritz Lipmann, David Nachmansohn, Ernst Fischer, and Emil Bozler. I also remember the two visits of the scientific commission sent by the Unitarian church and sponsored by the Overlander Trust to Tübingen, where I worked in the department of H. H. Weber. At the end of the forties and the beginning of the fifties these visits were of great psychological help, especially for the younger generation that had escaped the war. I still have some books on my shelf that were distributed during the second visit of the commission—among them a volume of the *Annals of the New York Academy of Sciences* from 1947 containing an article of Otto Meyerhof. In this article he mentioned three times studies performed in his institute in Heidelberg, which he was forced to leave in 1938.

I did not encounter the problem of cardiac contractility, the central topic of this volume, until 1954, when I came to Heidelberg with H. H. Weber, who took over Meyerhof's former department. Weber, whom I joined in 1949, was a physicochemically oriented physiologist.[2] He admired Otto Meyerhof, with whom he had collaborated for a short time in Berlin, where he had met David Nachmansohn and Fritz Lipmann. Al-

[a] Address for correspondence: Max-Planck-Institut für Medizinische Forschung, Jahnstrasse 29, D-69028 Heidelberg, Germany. Phone: 49-6221-486306; fax: 49-6221-486351.

ready in Heidelberg we had tried to understand the interaction between myosin, actin, and ATP, which at that time appeared to me an unsolvable problem. ATP hydrolysis as an energy-yielding reaction of muscle contraction had just before been established by Weber's group in Tübingen.[3] Weber's molecular approach in physiology, was an exception, at least in Germany. In Heidelberg we met the co-workers of Hermann Rein; Rein was Weber's immediate predecessor and in every respect an antagonist of him and his scientific approach. Rein was the main representative of German circulation research. Weber had become Rein's successor following his unexpected death, leaving behind a large group of enthusiastic young scientists. Their activity in preparing heart-lung preparations from dogs on a large scale impressed me very much. Experiments with warm-blooded animals were never done in Weber's department. Rein's group tried to understand the interaction of heart, liver, and spleen. Rein had previously gathered some evidence that the latter organs produce a substance that improve heart performance.[4] Richard Kuhn, who was the head of the chemistry department since its foundation, was enthusiastic about this prospect and delegated chemists to isolate the mysterious material from liver blood. We had endless discussions during tea time concerning the problem of cardiac efficiency and its possible modulation. It remained in my memory that the performance of dying hearts could for some moments be improved by perfusing them with solutions of elevated calcium concentration. They were always superior to fractions isolated by the chemists from liver blood. Finally, after six years of hard work, it had to be confessed that an effective spleen-liver substance did not exist. Although working over the years only with skeletal muscle preparations, I followed with great interest the increasing number of studies dealing with the peculiarities of heart muscle. I was deterred from working with it by the relatively low specific activity of the cardiac sarcoplasmic reticulum preparations and the low coupling ratios between calcium uptake and ATPase activity.

In 1962 I had the first opportunity to visit the United States. I am very grateful to John Gergely, who invited me to a muscle meeting in Dedham, near Boston. There I first presented our findings proving the existence of an ATP-driven calcium pump in the membranes of the sarcoplasmic reticulum.[5] These studies were pursued with the late M. Makinose, who had left Japan permanently in 1960. Initially—in the mid fifties—we were not aware of the membranous character of the material. Years in advance of us in one of his last studies, Meyerhof characterized the particulate material as an ATPase inhibited by calcium, which was in contrast to the activity of myosin.[6] It was quite difficult to extend this preconception in Weber's laboratory by an activating effect of calcium. Coming from Los Angeles in 1965, I could present quite a complete picture of the functioning of the pump at the the New York Academy of Sciences' meeting on biological membranes. My presentation was evidently an alien body in the program and therefore was placed at the end of the volume. I showed results, demonstrating that extra splitting and calcium uptake can be initiated not only by calcium addition, as usual, but also by late addition of oxalate.[7] This finding supported our concept of a mechanistic coupling between calcium uptake and ATP hydrolysis and disproved the result of a similar experiment intended to reject the coupling concept.[8] An experimental setup to determine in muscle homogenates not only the calcium uptake capacity of the reticulum but also its concentrating ability was also presented. It is rather interesting that under the experimental conditions—i.e., in the presence of oxalate—calcium concentrations much lower than those prevailing in the living muscle are maintained. The latter were not known with certainty at that time.

It took quite a long time until cardiologists or cardiophysiologists accepted the concept that the reticulum functions as an ATP -driven calcium pump in cardiac muscle. In fact, the objections based on the quite large quantities of calcium heart muscle has to handle, on the one hand, and the relative weak pump activity found in isolated material, on the other hand, were difficult to disprove. The development of elegant new optical techniques based on suitable calcium indicators in recent years has made it possible to functionally connect calcium release from the reticulum and its removal by the pump with muscle mechanics. A great gap in the concept that mechanical activity in skeletal and cardiac muscle is controlled by calcium release and removal from and by the reticulum was closed when the cisternal elements of the reticulum were discovered as specialized calcium releasing structures.[9–11] The key event was the finding that these structures could effectively and specifically be labeled under suitable conditions by ryanodine, which has been studied as a muscle poison for quite a long time without convincing results.[12] Instead of discussing nature's disturbing flexibility of inventing mechanisms for coordinating pump activity and channel function,[13–15] I want to focus on a few mechanisms as basic elements that affect simultaneously pump and channel activity. They concern the effect of hydrogen ions, phosphate ions, and in general anions. Hydrogen ions were quite early recognized as effective modulators of pump activity. We observed that calcium uptake and extra-ATPase activity steeply declined below pH 7.0, which has great physiological consequences since pH values in this range are commonly observed in ischemic heart or skeletal muscles.[16] The decline of both activities observed at high pH values is of minor pathophysiological relevance. Calcium transport is significantly more sensitive to alkalinization than ATP-splitting and phosphoprotein formation. The activity of the calcium release channel behaves analogously. Single-channel activity declines steeply between pH 7.0 and 6.0.[17] We found that ryanodine, which can be used as a functional probe of the channel,[18] only very slowly reacts with the isolated calcium release channel in heavy vesicular fractions at pH 6.2 and hyperbolically increases with rising hydroxyl-ion concentration, as shown in FIGURE 1. Yet, quite another profile characterizes caffeine-induced calcium release. Its steep rise between pH 6.5 and 7.0 is described by a Hill coefficient of 3.5, indicating a high degree of cooperativity of caffeine-induced channel opening.

As a second macromodulator, inorganic phosphate must be considered. In well-

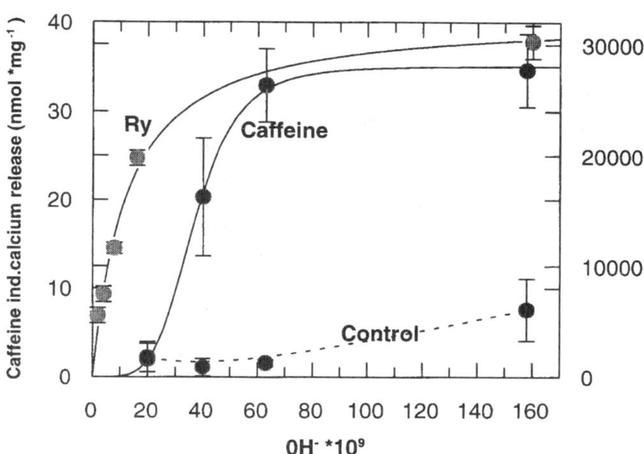

FIGURE 1. Dependence on OH– ion concentration of ryanodine binding to heavy sarcoplasmic reticulum vesicles and of caffeine-induced calcium release from actively loaded preparations. Ryanodine binding depends hyperpolocally on OH–concentration, while caffeine-induced calcium release reveals cooperativity.

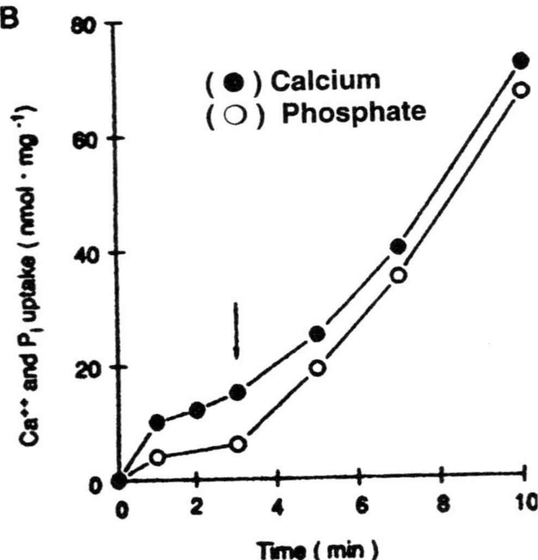

FIGURE 2. Co-uptake of calcium and endogenously produced phosphate by heavy sarcoplasmic reticulum vesicles. Uptake of calcium and phosphate were monitored in separate assays either supplemented with ^{45}Ca and cold ATP or with cold calcium and ^{32}P-ATP. ATP was regenerated from phosphoenolpyruvate.[21]

perfused and oxygenated muscles the concentration of total phosphate is quite low (1–2 mM) but easily rises beyond 20 mM under ischemic conditions. This rise interferes severely with tension development of skinned cardiac muscle fibers.[19] In the same concentration range, phosphate promotes calcium uptake of the pump.[20] In contrast to oxalate, phosphate is coaccumulated with calcium even at low concentrations as they arise from ATP-hydrolysis in media containing no additional phosphate[21] (FIG. 2). Most of the calcium stored is present as calcium phosphate. This is in line with Somlyo's finding on the location of these ions in contracting muscles.[22] The co-storage of phosphate like that of oxalate prevents pump inhibition by raising luminal calcium concentration. This is a very important safety device, on the one hand, and simultaneously can enlarge the amount of releasable calcium, on the other hand. We do not know how the co-transport of calcium and phosphate occurs. This problem is closely connected with the role of anions in calcium uptake and release, in general. Whatever may be the mechanism, phosphate and oxalate use the same pathway when calcium uptake is supported by oxalate as an effective calcium precipitant. This conclusion is based on the finding showing that phosphate excludes oxalate from being taken up and vice versa.[23] This exclusion becomes complete when the phosphate concentration is raised from 1 to 3 mM in the presence of 2 mM oxalate. To describe this exclusion a highly cooperative interaction between the anions and their pathway structures must be assumed. The effective competition between oxalate and phosphate indicates the involvement of an anion-specific pathway in the SR membranes. This concept is not restricted to the interaction of the pump with multivalent anions such as phosphate, pyrophosphate, or oxalate. Small anions, such as chloride, are also quite effective as they emerge from their inhibiting effect on oxalate-supported calcium uptake, as shown in FIGURE 3.[24] The assumption that we are dealing with competition between anions is supported by the finding that in the presence of phosphate or phosphate-plus-oxalate, chloride inhibition is considerably stronger than in the presence of oxalate alone. We do not know if this anion pathway modulating calcium uptake is similar to or identical with that involved in calcium release from the terminal cisternae. Yet, our finding showing that calcium-

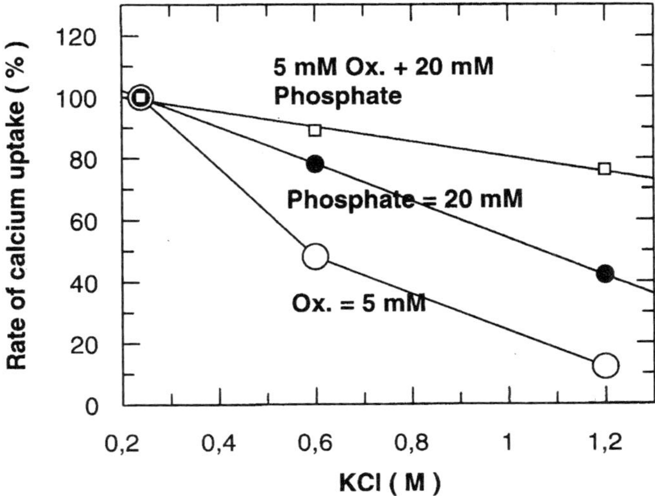

FIGURE 3. Inhibition of calcium uptake by chloride. Inhibition depends on the concentation of the precipitating anions: oxalate, phosphate, or oxalate + phosphate.[24]

induced calcium release from these actively loaded organelles does not occur in the absence of chloride ions underlines the role of anions also in the mechanism of calcium release through the physiological calcium release channel.[25–27] Anion specificity is further supported by the augmentation of calcium-induced calcium release when chloride is replaced by nitrate. The modification of calcium channel activity by ions also gov-

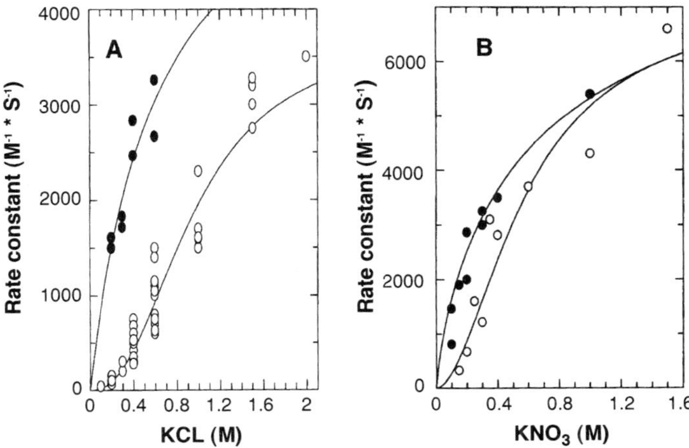

FIGURE 4. Activation of ryanodine binding by rising salt concentations. A. KCL, B. KNO_3. The presence of 1 mM ATP abolishes cooperativity (●); binding at low salt concentrations is enhanced.

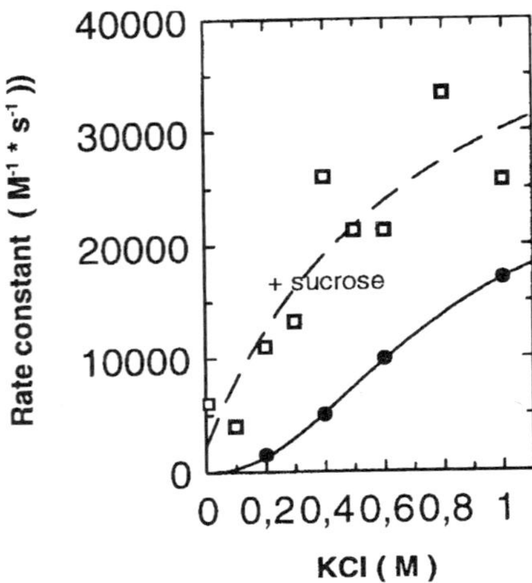

FIGURE 5. Activation of ryanodine binding by rising KCl concentration in absence and presence of sucrose. 1 M sucrose abolishes cooperativity.

erns the channel's reaction with its most potent inhibitor ryanodine. The activation of ryanodine binding by high salt concentrations is based on a highly cooperative interaction between salt and receptor. This concept emerges from the dependence of the rate of ryanodine binding on the concentrations of the activating salts (FIG. 4). Large differences in the effectiveness of various salts have been observed. The cooperative dependence of the reaction rate of ryanodine binding on salt concentration corresponds to the cooperative relations between the concentration of hydroxyl ions and ryanodine binding as well as caffeine-induced calcium release[28] (FIG. 1). These salt effects are distinctly affected by ATP and its analogs, which have long been known to be efficient modulators of calcium release.[29–31] The results included in FIGURE 4 show that ATP augments considerably the effect of lower salt concentrations and thereby abolishes the cooperative interaction of the salts with the ryanodine receptor. Most interestingly one does not need a highly charged ion species like ATP to diminish cooperativity. The same effect is obtained by the addition of 1 M sucrose to the ryanodine binding assay (FIG. 5). Thus we are confronted with a whole network of ionic and nonionic interactions between the various reactants that control calcium release and to a smaller extent also calcium uptake. This allows nature or the experimenter to manipulate the key reactions in muscle activation. Their apparent complexity is a great challenge in searching for a common link in the reactions leading to calcium release.

REFERENCES

1. HASSELBACH, W. & M. MAKINOSE. 1961. Die Calciumpumpe der Erschlaffungsgrane des Muskels und ihre Abhängigkeit von der ATP - Spaltung. Biochem. Z. **333:** 518–528
2. WEBER, H. H. 1953. Muskelkontraktion, Zellmotilität und ATP. Biochem. Biophys. Acta **12:** 150–162.
3. WEBER, H. H. 1934. Die Muskeleiweißkörper und der Feinbau des Skeletmuskels. Ergeb. Physiol. **34:** 110–150.
4. REIN, H. 1949. Über ein Regulationssystem ,, Milz-Leber ,, für den oxydaiven Stoffwechsel der Körpergewebe und besonders des Herzens. Naturwissenschaften **36:** 233–239
5. HASSELBACH, W. 1964. The calcium pump of the relaxing vesicles and the production of a relaxing factor. *In* Biochemistery of Muscle Contraction. J. Gergely, Ed.: 247–254. Little, Brown. New York.

6. Kielley, W. W. & O. Meyerhof. 1948. Studies on adenosinetriphosphatase on muscle. J. Biol. Chem. **176:** 591–601.
7. Hasselbach. W. 1966. Structural and enzymatic properties of the calcium transporting membranes of the sarcoplasmic reticulum. Ann. N.Y. Acad. Sci. **137:** 1041–1048.
8. Martonosi, A. & R. Ferretos. 1964. Sarcoplasmic reticulum. II. Correlation between adenosine triphosphatase activity and Ca^{++} uptake. J. Biol. Chem. **239:** 659–668.
9. Pessah, I. N., K. W. Anderson & J. E. Casida. 1986. Solubilisation and separation of Ca^{2+} -ATPase from the Ca^{2+} -ryanodine receptor complex. Biochem. Biophys. Res. Commun. **139:** 235–243.
10. Inui, M., A. Saito & S. Fleischer. 1987. Purification of the ryanodine receptor and identity with feet structures of junctional terminal cisternae of sarcoplasmic reticulum from fast skeletal muscle. J. Biol. Chem. **262:** 1740–1747.
11. Lai, F. A., H. P. Erickson, E. Rousseau, Q. Liu & G. Meissner. 1988. Purification and reconstitution of the calcium release channel from skeletal muscle. Nature **331:** 315–319.
12. Fairhurst, A. S. & W. Hasselbach. 1970. Calcium efflux from heavy sarcotubular fraction. Effect of ryanodine, caffeine and magnesium. Eur. J. Biochem. **13:** 504–509.
13. Kirchberger, A., M. Tada, D. I. Repke & A. Katz. 1972. Cyclic adenosine 3′5′ monophosphate–dependent protein kinase stimulation of calcium uptake by canine cardiac microsomes. J. Mol. Cell. Cardiol. **4:** 673–680.
14. Meissner, G. 1986. Evidence for a role of calmodulin in the regulation of calcium release from skeletal muscle sarcoplasmic reticulum. Biochemistry **25:** 244–251.
15. Timerman, A. P., E. Ogonbumni, E. Freud, G. Wiederrecht, A. R. Marks & S. Fleischer. 1993. The calcium release channel of sarcoplasmic reticulum is modulated by FK506-binding protein. J. Biol. Chem. **268:** 22992–22999.
16. Hasselbach, W. 1964. Relaxing factor and the relaxation of muscle. Prog. Biophys. **14:** 167–222.
17. Ma, J. & J. Zhao. 1994. Highly cooperative and hysteretic response of the skeletal muscle ryanodine receptor to changes in proton concentrations. Biophys. J. **67:** 626–633.
18. Meissner, G. & A. El-Hashem. 1992. Ryanodine as functional probe of skeletal muscle sarcoplasmic reticulum Ca2+ release channel. Mol. Cell. Biochem. **114:** 119–123.
19. Herzig, J. W. & J. C. Rüegg. 1977. Myocardial cross-bridge activity and its regulation by Ca^{++}, phosphate and stretch. *In* Myocardial Failure. G. Rieger, A. Weber & J. Goodwin, Eds.: 41–51. Springer Verlag, Berlin.
20. Hasselbach, W. & M. Makinose. 1963. Über den Mechanismus des Calciumtransportes durch die Membranen des sarcoplasmatischen Retikulums. Biochem. Zeitschr. **339:** 94–111.
21. Hasselbach, W. & A. Migala. 1992. Modulation by ryanodine of active calcium loading and caffeine induced calcium release of heavy sarcoplamic reticulum vesicles. Z. Naturforsch. **47c:** 429–439.
22. Somlyo, A. V., G. McCleelan, H. Gonzales-Serratos & A. P. Somlyo. 1985. Electron-probe X-ray analysis of post tetanic Ca and Mg movement across the sarcoplasmic reticulum in situ. J. Biol. Chem. **260:** 6801–6807.
23. Beil, F. U., D. von Chak, W. Hasselbach & H. H. Weber. 1977. Competition between oxalate and phosphate during active calcium accumulation by sarcoplasmic vesicles. Z. Naturforsch. **32c:** 281–287.
24. Barlogie, B. 1970. Die Calciumpermeabilität der Vesikel des saroplasmatischen Retikulums in Gegenwart von ATP. M.D. Thesis, Medical Faculty, University of Heidelberg, Germany.
25. Hasselbach, W. & A. Migala. 1992. Modulation by monovalent anions of calcium and caffeine induced calcium release from heavy sarcoplasmic reticulum vesicles. Z. Naturforsch. **47c:** 440–448.
26. Fruen, B. R., P. K. Kane, J. R. Mickelson & Ch. F. Louis. 1996. Chloride-dependent sarcoplasmic reticulum Ca^{2+} release correlates with increased Ca^{2+} activation of ryanodine receptor. Biophys. J. **71:** 2522–2530.
27. Meissner, G., E. Rios, A. Triphaty & D. A. Pasek. 1997. Regulation of skeletal muscle Ca2+-release channel (ryanodine receptor) by Ca^{2+} and monovalent cations and anions. J. Biol. Chem. **272:** 1628–1638.

28. HASSELBACH, W. & A. MIGALA. 1992. How many ryanodine binding sites are involved in caffeine induced calcium release from sarcoplasmic reticulum terminal cisternae vesicles. Z. Naturforsch. **47c:** 136–147.
29. MEISSNER, G. 1984. Adenine nucleotide stimulation of Ca2+ induced Ca2+-release in sarcoplasmic reticulum. **259:** 2365–2374.
30. SU, J. Y. & W. HASSELBACH, 1984. Caffeine-induced calcium release from isolated sarcpolasmic reticulum of rabbit skeletal muscle. Pflügers Arch. **400:** 14–21.
31. OGAWA, Y. & S. EBASHI. 1976. Calcium releasing action of β, γ-methylen adenosine triphospate on fragmented sarcoplasmic reticulum. J. Biochem. **80:** 1149–1157.

Discovery of Phospholamban

A Personal History

ARNOLD M. KATZ[a]

Cardiology Division, Department of Medicine, University of Connecticut Health Center, 263 Farmington Avenue, Farmington, Connecticut 06030-2249, USA

ABSTRACT: Early efforts to identify mechanisms by which sympathetic stimulation increases myocardial contractility led to studies of effects of β-adrenergic agonists and cyclic AMP on the cardiac contractile proteins and sarcoplasmic reticulum (SR); initial positive reports, however, could not be confirmed. The discovery that cyclic AMP-dependent protein kinases (PK-A) mediated intracellular actions of cyclic AMP led at least four groups to test the hypothesis that phosphorylation of the cardiac SR played a role in the actions of β-adrenergic agonists. Three of them (Wollenberger, Wray *et al.*, and LaRaia & Morkin) demonstrated that cardiac SR was a substrate for PK-A phosphorylation; however, the lability of the Ca^{2+} pump in these membranes made it difficult to demonstrate a functional significance of this finding. Our group, which had extensive experience in measuring SR Ca^{2+} transport, began by examining the ability of PK-A to activate the SR Ca^{2+} pump "poised" at half-saturating Ca^{2+} concentrations. Our initial positive result led to the discovery that a 22,000-dalton protein, named phospholamban by Phyllis B. Katz, mediated effects on Ca^{2+} transport by the SR that could explain both the inotropic and lusitropic effects of sympathetic stimulation.

More than 45 years ago, when I began my work in research, little was known of the mechanisms controlling cardiac contraction and relaxation. During the early 1950s, most cardiac physiologists believed that end-diastolic fiber length—Starling's Law of the Heart—was the major determinant of the work of the heart. While studies of the contractile proteins in skeletal muscle had been carried out in several laboratories around the world since the 19th century, this work was outside the mainstream of biochemistry because the actomyosins studied by muscle biochemists were messy insoluble protein aggregates, and so not suitable for the elegant crystallizations and kinetic studies then in vogue. As a result, almost nothing was known about the cellular mechanisms that mediate the physiological response of the heart to exercise, nor the actions of drugs and diseases that modified the capacity of the myocardium to perform work.

Yet a generation earlier, in 1922, a now-classical study of ventricular volume curves published by Carl J. Wiggers and my father, Louis N. Katz[1] showed not only a positive inotropic effect of epinephrine, but also that the increase in contractility is accompanied by a marked abbreviation of systole (FIG. 1). These findings, published less than a decade after Starling's classical papers, demonstrated not only that catecholamines—as well as increasing end-diastolic volume—could increase the force of the heart's contraction, but also that this inotropic effect is accompanied by a change in the lusitropic properties of the myocardium. However, these and other reports that catecholamines altered the intrinsic properties of the myocardium attracted little at-

[a] Phone: 860-679-2771; fax: 860-679-3346; e-mail: akatz@nso1.uchc.edu

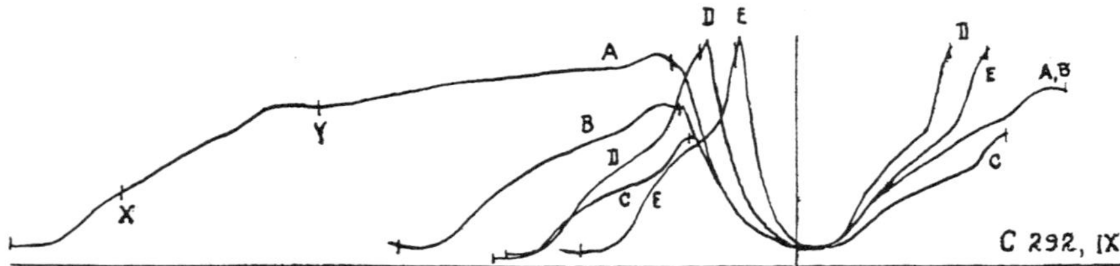

FIGURE 1. Series of volume curves (decreasing volume from top to bottom, time from left to right) showing effects of vagal slowing of heart rate **(Curves A–B)** compared to the control beat **(C)**. The latter also serves as the control for early **(Curve D)** and late **(Curve E)** beats after the administration of epinephrine, which show the effect of the β adrenergic agonist to increase stroke volume and abbreviate systole. (Reprinted with permission from Wiggers & Katz.[1])

tention until 1955, when Sarnoff's concept of the "family" of Starling curves[2] elegantly demonstrated the importance of changing myocardial contractility, and so effected a paradigm shift.[3]

Stimulated by efforts to explain changes in myocardial contractility, by the early 1960s efforts in this field began to integrate the paradigm of biochemistry and biophysics into cardiovascular research. Among the first questions to be addressed using this new paradigm was the mechanism by which catecholamines increase myocardial contractility.

EFFECTS ON ENERGY PRODUCTION

One of the first hypotheses as to the mechanism by which catecholamines increase myocardial contractility was that these agents augmented developed tension by increasing the production of high-energy phosphate compounds. Although it quickly became apparent that a cascade of reactions initiated by the catecholamines accelerates both glycolytic ATP production and lipolysis, these effects on cardiac energy production could not explain the ability of catecholamines to increase myocardial contractility.[4] The attractive hypothesis that enhanced energy production, the first clearly described biochemical response of the heart to catecholamines, is causally linked to the catecholamine-induced augmentation of the contractile response therefore had to be dismissed.

EFFECTS ON THE CONTRACTILE PROTEINS

The obvious question as to whether catecholamines exert their inotropic effects by a direct action on the contractile proteins was examined in a series of studies that initially yielded conflicting, but often positive results.[4] The discovery that cyclic AMP mediated the cellular responses to these neurotransmitters[5] then led to attempts to define a direct role for this second messenger in mediating the enhanced contractile response of the heart to β adrenergic agonists. Once again, early results were conflicting. As a research fellow at the University of California (Los Angeles) in the laboratory of Wilfried Mommaerts, who in the early 1960s had published[6] and then retracted[7] a claim that cyclic AMP modified the interactions between actin and myosin, I attempted to demonstrate an effect of cyclic AMP on the superprecipitation of actomyosins reconstituted from highly purified actin and myosin. However, I never found any effects on this system. I did not publish these negative data, but returned to this question a few years later after I took my first faculty position in physiology at Columbia University in New York. After an exhaustive study of highly purified cardiac contractile proteins, I concluded in 1967 that "the norepinephrine-induced increase of contractile activity in the intact heart is probably due to augmentation of the physiological stimulus delivered to activate the contractile proteins, rather than to a direct action of the sympathomimetic amines on the contractile proteins themselves."[8] Work in this area continued for almost a decade without any clear conclusion[4,9] until the discovery of the role of cyclic AMP–dependent protein kinase opened a new approach to this important question.

The discovery of the cyclic AMP–dependent protein kinases in the late 1960s[10,11] led several groups to test the hypothesis that one or more of the contractile proteins provided a substrate for cyclic AMP–induced phosphorylation. Once again, however, initial findings were conflicting. Most known contractile proteins were found by some to be phosphorylated by cyclic AMP–dependent protein kinases, but not all groups obtained the same results; more importantly, no clear functional changes were found to occur after the reported phosphorylations.[4]

Most of these ambiguities were resolved when it was recognized that even mild denaturation of these proteins exposed sites that were not phosphorylated in the native proteins, and that the proteins examined in the earlier studies could not be phosphorylated in the intact muscle.[12,13] This was followed by studies that demonstrated that cardiac troponin I was phosphorylated *in vivo* by agents that increase cyclic AMP levels in the heart.[14,15] However, the physiological consequence of this phosphorylation was not, as had been expected, an effect that would explain an increase in contractility. Instead, a decrease in the calcium sensitivity of actomyosin was found; this effect, by facilitating calcium *dissociation* from the contractile proteins,[16–20] favored relaxation instead of contraction. It is now clear that this lusitropic effect, which accompanies the more obvious inotropic effect of agents that increase cyclic AMP levels in the heart,[21] plays a key role in the accelerated relaxation observed more than 50 years before (FIG. 1).

EFFECTS ON THE SARCOPLASMIC RETICULUM

As had been seen in the early studies of the actions of catecholamines on the cardiac contractile proteins, the search for effects on the mechanisms that relax the heart initially yielded confusing, often inaccurate, results. Again, this work went through three phases: studies of direct effects of catecholamines, a search for direct effects of cyclic AMP, and finally studies of the effects of protein kinase–catalyzed phosphorylation. And once again, early reports that sarcoplasmic reticulum function could be modified by epinephrine and cyclic AMP turned out either to be artifactual, or due to unrecognized protein kinase–catalyzed phosphorylation.[4] The evolution of our knowledge of the effects of catecholamines on the sarcoplasmic reticulum, therefore, followed almost the same pattern as the research on the contractile proteins reviewed above.

In the early 1960s, before cardiac relaxation was understood to be due to calcium uptake by the sarcoplasmic reticulum, catecholamines had been reported to inhibit the effects of a cardiac "relaxing factor."[22,23] Subsequent studies, carried out after the discovery of the role of the calcium pump of the sarcoplasmic reticulum in the late 1960s, suggested that catecholamines stimulated calcium uptake by these membranes.[24–27]

However, other groups,[28–31] including mine,[32] failed to observe a direct effect of catecholamines on cardiac sarcoplasmic reticulum vesicles. An explanation for these discrepant findings was provided by our observation[33] that, because cardiac sarcoplasmic reticulum preparations contain both regulated adenylate cyclase and protein kinase activities, prolonged incubation of high concentrations of these membrane vesicles with epinephrine could accelerate calcium transport when endogenously produced cyclic AMP stimulated an endogenous cyclic AMP–dependent protein kinase that phosphorylated these membranes (see below).

As had occurred earlier in studies of the cardiac contractile proteins, discovery of the role of cyclic AMP as a second messenger led to a search for direct effects of this nucleotide. And once again, stimulation of calcium transport in cardiac sarcoplasmic reticulum vesicles by cyclic AMP was reported by several groups,[25,26,34,35] and once again, others[30,31,36,37] failed to observe this stimulatory effect. As already noted, although we were unable to find a direct effect of high cyclic AMP concentrations on calcium uptake,[32] prolonged incubation with high concentrations of sarcoplasmic reticulum vesicles allowed added cyclic AMP to stimulate the endogenous protein kinase activity and so to influence the behavior of these preparations.[33]

These controversies were resolved when cyclic AMP–dependent protein kinase was found to mediate the signal cascade initiated when β-adrenergic agonists bind to the membrane receptors. Four groups of investigators, including mine, independently tested the hypothesis that catecholamine effects on the myocardium occurred when cyclic AMP–dependent protein kinase catalyzed the phosphorylation of the sarcoplasmic reticulum. Our studies were stimulated by a casual conversation at the FASEB Meetings in Chicago in April, 1971 when Michihiko Tada, who was then a research fellow studying adenylyl cyclase in my laboratory at the Mount Sinai School of Medicine in New York, suggested that our negative findings with cyclic AMP[32] could have been due to the absence of the protein kinase in our experimental systems. This led Michi, aided by J. H. Helderman, then a medical student, and our expert technician Joanna Iorio Finegan, to spend several months working in the cold room to purify this enzyme from beef hearts. After obtaining excellent ^{32}P incorporation into histones, then the model substrate for cyclic AMP–dependent protein kinase, Michi began work on the effects of this enzyme on cardiac sarcoplasmic reticulum vesicles. Joined by Madeleine A. Kirchberger, we did our first experiments, but not in the most logical way, which would have been to determine whether membrane vesicles derived from the cardiac sarcoplasmic reticulum served as a substrate for this enzyme. There were two reasons that we did not use this approach. The first was that the very low yield of sarcoplasmic reticulum vesicles from the fresh canine hearts we had to use to obtain active preparations would have made it difficult to measure phosphorylation. More important was our recognition that the microsomal preparations then used by all workers in this field contained significant contamination from membranes other than the sarcoplasmic reticulum, which would have complicated interpretation of any ^{32}P incorporation. Because Doris Repke, my long-term associate, and I had mastered the measurement of oxalate-supported calcium uptake in both skeletal and cardiac sarcoplasmic reticulum preparations, we began instead by searching for a possible effect of cyclic AMP–dependent protein kinase on calcium transport rate. It should be noted that we had gained this expertise largely because, over the four years we had worked with the difficult system from heart muscle,[38] we had made virtually every mistake possible!

Our first experiment, carried out in April, 1972 and published in a short communication later that year,[39] showed a dramatic effect of the cyclic AMP–dependent protein kinase that Michi Tada had worked so hard to purify (FIG. 2). We immediately realized that these findings were to define our research directions for many years. On a personal

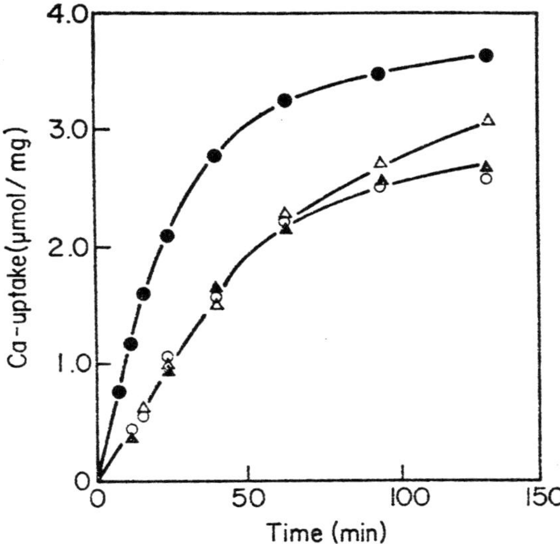

FIGURE 2. Effects of cyclic AMP alone *(solid triangles),* a cyclic AMP–dependent protein kinase *(open triangles),* and both together *(solid circles)* on oxalate-supported calcium uptake by cardiac sarcoplasmic reticulum. The control reaction is shown as the *open circles.* (Reprinted with permission from Kirchberger *et al.*[39])

note, I recall that my good friend and "competitor," Arnold Schwartz, who generally gave me a very difficult time when he reviewed my papers (as I did when I reviewed his), was instrumental in providing a rapid and fair review of this seminal paper.

As had happened to me once before, when in the early 1960s I thought I was alone in what appeared to be a new and empty field—in the earlier case the role of the regulatory proteins of the thin filament[40]—it quickly became clear that we were in a race. I have no doubt that this field had reached a point at which any perspicacious investigator could have seen the likelihood that the effects of catecholamines on the heart were mediated by cyclic AMP–dependent protein kinase, and that the cardiac sarcoplasmic reticulum was a logical substrate for this reaction. Thus, we should not have been surprised to learn that Wollenberger,[41] LaRaia and Morkin,[42] and Wray, Gray, and Olsson[43] had begun a similar line of study. These groups however, followed the most logical approach, which was first to determine whether the cardiac sarcoplasmic reticulum was a substrate for the protein kinase. And all three found that the cardiac sarcoplasmic reticulum was indeed a substrate for cyclic AMP–dependent phosphorylation. However, it turned out that our experience in the difficult measurement of calcium transport by these membranes had put us in a uniquely favorable position.

As already noted, the ability of cyclic AMP–dependent protein kinases to phosphorylate the cardiac sarcoplasmic reticulum was reported independently by three groups.[41–43] Wray, Gray, and Olsson also found that cardiac microsomal preparations enriched in sarcoplasmic reticulum vesicles contained a protein kinase that responded to a rise in cellular cyclic AMP by catalyzing the phosphorylation of the vesicles themselves.[43] Autophosphorylation of these membranes was described by LaRaia and Morkin[42] and later by Will *et al.*,[44] Fedelesová and Ziegelhöffer,[45] as well as ourselves.[39,46]

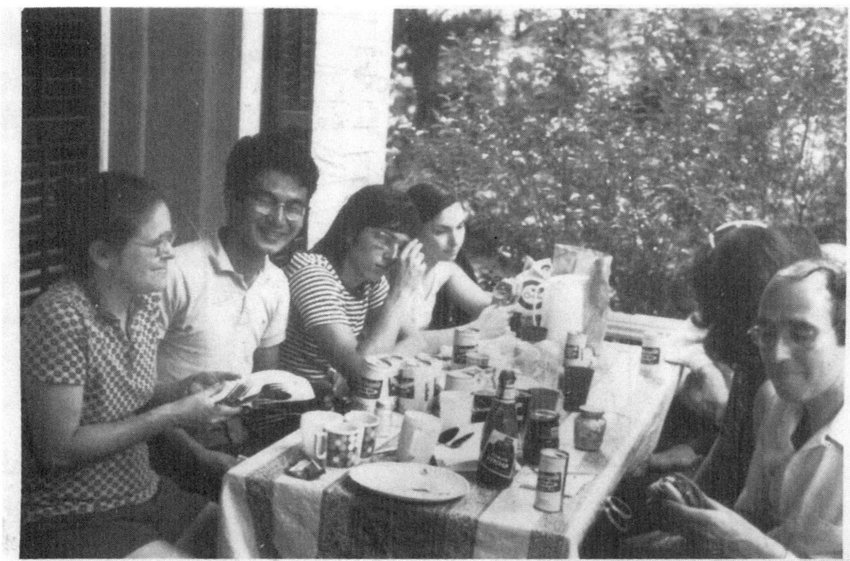

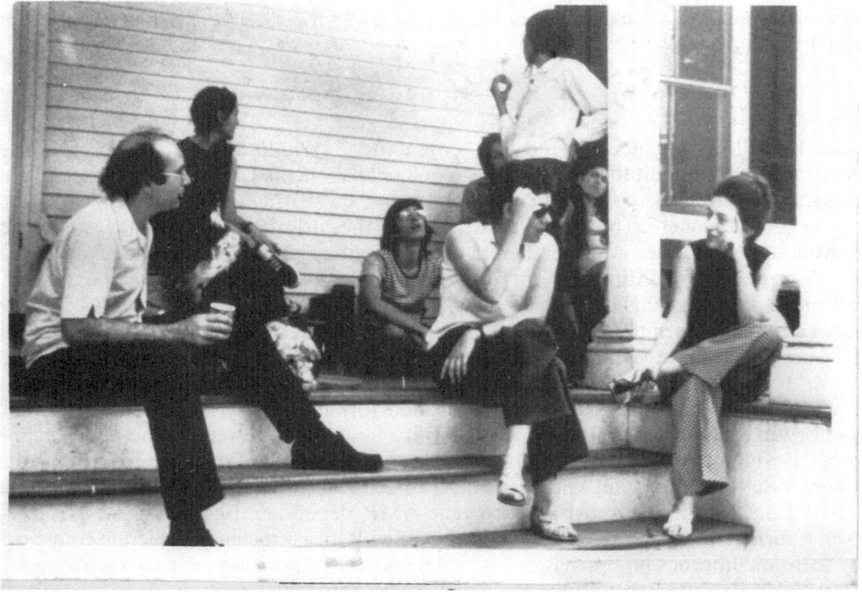

FIGURE 3. Photographs taken at the laboratory picnic in 1973 at which phospholamban was named. **Top:** At left in the foreground are Phyllis Katz and Michi Tada; the author is at the right. **Bottom:** From left to right along the top step are the author, Doris Repke, and Madeleine Kirchberger.

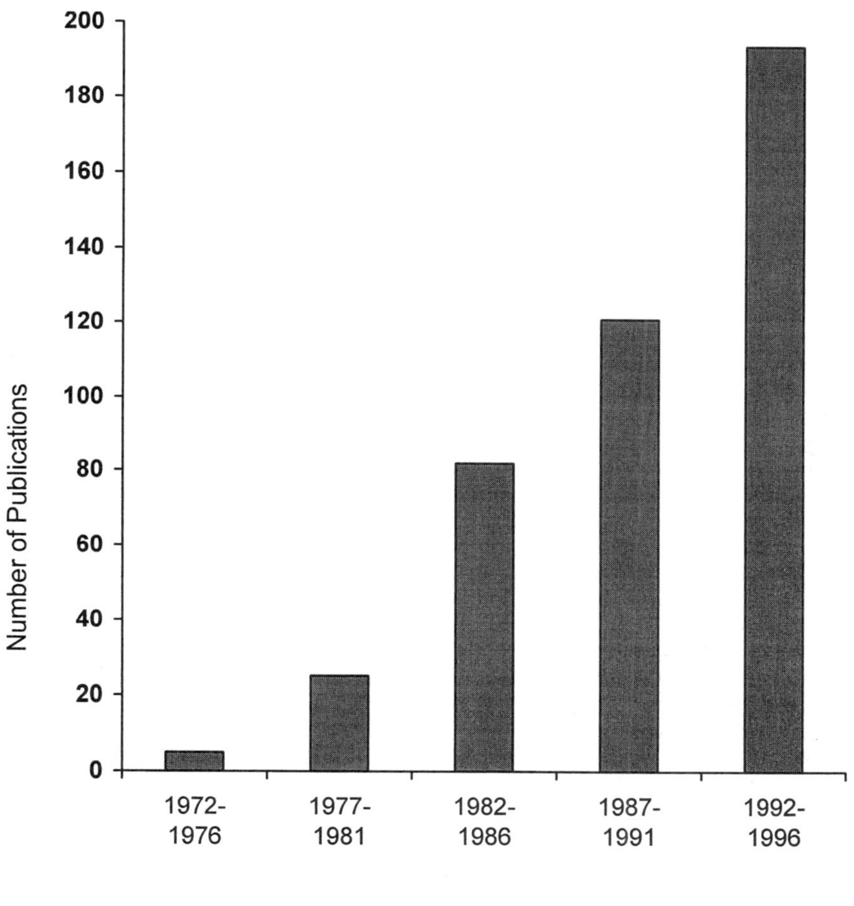

FIGURE 4. Articles citing phospholamban since the discovery of this protein.

This ability of an endogenous protein kinase to catalyze autophosphorylation of these membranes explained both earlier reports of others that prolonged incubation of cardiac sarcoplasmic reticulum vesicles with cyclic AMP could stimulate calcium transport (see above), and our initial observation that prolonged incubation with cyclic AMP accelerated calcium uptake (FIG. 2). We later found that although exogenous bovine cardiac protein kinase accelerated the rate of phosphorylation threefold, it did not increase the total amount of phosphorylation that could be catalyzed by the intrinsic protein kinase.[46]

An interesting aside is that several other groups attempted to repeat these studies using the more stable and abundant sarcoplasmic reticulum preparations from rabbit skeletal muscle, which at the time were used by most workers in this field. This led to considerable controversy because, as we later found,[4] the phospholamban system is absent in rabbit fast skeletal muscle. This fact became apparent after our finding that cyclic AMP–dependent protein kinase increased the calcium transport rate had been vehemently challenged at several national and international meetings! Looking back on all this, it is clear that we were fortunate in having had the solid experience with these systems needed to give us the confidence to work with the more difficult heart muscle preparations.

DISCOVERY OF PHOSPHOLAMBAN

Within two years after the initial studies of the effects of cyclic AMP–dependent protein kinase on these systems, the phosphate incorporated in the sarcoplasmic reticulum by this enzyme was found to be in the form of a phosphoester, mostly phosphoserine, rather than the acyl phosphate intermediate known to be formed by the calcium pump protein.[42,46] These findings led to an examination of the electrophoretic mobility of the phosphoprotein that regulated the calcium pump ATPase. At that time, it was known that the latter is a 100,000-dalton protein that forms the acyl phosphate intermediate involved in calcium transport.[47–50] It quickly became clear, however, that the substrate for protein kinase–catalyzed phosphorylation in the cardiac sarcoplasmic reticulum was a smaller protein having a molecular weight of 20,000 to 22,000,[42,51–55] rather than the 100,000-dalton calcium pump ATPase protein.

I had learned the importance of assigning names when, in 1965, I had discovered a protein fraction that sensitizes reconstituted actomyosin to calcium binding agents.[40] Because this regulatory protein was the second precipitate in a long and complex purification, I called this factor P_2 in my 1966 paper that detailed my discovery.[56] However, Setsuro Ebashi, in a preliminary report published in 1965 that described some biophysical properties but not the biological function of this protein,[57] had already named this factor *troponin.* Even if I had given my P_2 a more mellifluous name, however, it would have been Ebashi who deserved credit for the discovery of troponin.[40] In light of this experience, at our annual laboratory picnic in the summer of 1973 (FIG. 3), my wife Phyllis, who is a classicist, suggested the name *phospholamban* for the protein that regulated the cardiac sarcoplasmic reticulum. This term is derived from *phosphate* and the Greek word λαμβανειν, which means *to receive* or *to seize.* Although we first published this term in an abstract in 1973,[58] for reasons I still do not understand, we were not allowed to use this name in our full-length paper, published in the *Journal of Biological Chemistry* in 1975, which described the molecular weight and function of this regulatory protein.[52] However, we have had the "last word" because, since 1979, the *Journal of Biological Chemistry* has included *phospholamban* in its index! And since the discovery of phospholamban, this protein has been the subject of more than 400 papers (FIG. 4).

REFERENCES

1. WIGGERS, C. J. & L. N. KATZ. 1922. The contour of left ventricular volume curves under different conditions. Am. J. Physiol. **58:** 439–475.
2. SARNOFF, S. J. 1955. Myocardial contractility as described by ventricular function curves. Physiol. Rev. **35:** 107–122.
3. KATZ, A. M. 1988. Molecular biology in cardiology, a paradigmatic shift. J. Mol. Cell. Cardiol. **20:** 355–366.

4. KATZ, A. M. 1979. Role of the contractile proteins and sarcoplasmic reticulum in the response of the heart to catecholamines: An historical review. Adv. Cyclic Nucleotide Res. **11:** 303–343.
5. SUTHERLAND, E. W. & T. W. RALL. 1960. The relation of adenosine 3′,5′-phosphate and phosphorylase to the actions of catecholamines and other hormones. Pharmacol. Rev. **12:** 265–299.
6. UCHIDA, K. & W. F. H. M. MOMMAERTS. 1963. Modification of the contractile response of actomyosin by cyclic adenosine 3′,5′ phosphate. Biochem. Biophys. Res. Commun. **10:** 1–3.
7. MOMMAERTS, W. F. H. M., K. SERAYDARIAN & K. UCHIDA. 1963. On the relaxing substance of muscle. Biochem. Biophys. Res. Commun. **13:** 58–60.
8. KATZ, A. M. 1967. Absence of direct actions of norepinephrine on cardiac myosin and cardiac actomyosin. Am. J. Physiol. **212:** 39–42.
9. KATZ, A. M. 1970. Contractile proteins of the heart. Physiol. Rev. **50:** 63–158.
10. WALSH, D. A., J. P. PERKINS & E. G. KREBS. 1968. An adenosine 3′,5′-monophosphate–dependent protein kinase from rabbit skeletal muscle. J. Biol. Chem. **243:** 3763–3765.
11. MIYAMOTO, E., J. F. KUO & P. GREENGARD. 1969. Adenosine 3′,5′-monophosphate dependent protein kinase from brain. Science **165:** 64–65.
12. BYLUND, D. B. & E. G. KREBS. 1975. Effect of denaturation in the susceptibility of proteins to enzymic phosphorylation. J. Biol. Chem. **250:** 6355–6361.
13. STULL, J. T. 1975. Phosphorylation of skeletal muscle troponin in vivo. Pharmacologist **17:** 234.
14. ENGLAND, P. J. 1975. Correlation between contractions and phosphorylation of the inhibitory subunit of troponin in perfused rat heart. FEBS Lett. **50:** 57–60.
15. SOLARO, R. J., A. J. G. MOIR & S. V. PERRY. 1976. Phosphorylation of troponin I and the inotropic effect of adrenaline in the perfused rabbit heart. Nature **262:** 615–616.
16. RAY, K. P. & P. S. ENGLAND. 1976. Phosphorylation of the inhibitory subunit of troponin-I and its effect on the calcium dependence of cardiac myofibril ATPase. FEBS Lett. **70:** 11–16.
17. REDDY, Y. S. & L. E. WYBORNY. 1976. Phosphorylation of guinea pig actomyosin and its effect on ATPase activity. Biochem. Biophys. Res. Commun. **73:** 703–709.
18. BUSS, J. E. & J. T. STULL. 1977. Calcium binding to cardiac troponin and the effects of cyclic AMP–dependent protein kinase. FEBS Lett. **73:** 101–104.
19. MCCLELLAN, G. B. & S. WINEGRAD. 1977. Membrane control of cardiac contractility. Nature **268:** 261–263.
20. BAILIN, G. 1979. Phosphorylation of a bovine cardiac actin complex. Am. J. Physiol. **236:** C41–C46.
21. KATZ, A. M. 1983. Cyclic AMP effects on the myocardium: A man who blows hot and cold with one breath. J. Am. Coll. Cardiol. **2:** 143–149.
22. HONIG, C. R., A. C. STAM & P. MAHAN. 1962. Calcium and cardiac relaxing substance: Significance for excitation and inotropy. Am. J. Physiol. **203:** 137–140.
23. STAM, A. C., JR. & C. R. HONIG. 1962. Interaction of catecholamines and cardiac relaxing substance. Biochim. Biophys. Acta **58:** 139–140.
24. SHINEBOURNE, E. A., M. L. HESS, R. S. WHITE & J. HAMER. 1969. The effect of noradrenaline on the calcium uptake of the sarcoplasmic reticulum. Cardiovasc. Res. **3:** 113–117.
25. ENTMAN, M. L., G. S. LEVEY & S. E. EPSTEIN. 1969. Mechanism of action of epinephrine and glucagon on the canine heart. Evidence for increase in sarcotubular calcium stores mediated by cyclic 3′,5′-AMP. Circ. Res. **25:** 429–438.
26. EPSTEIN, S. E., G. S. LEVEY & C. L. SKELTON. 1971. Adenyl cyclase and cyclic AMP. Biochemical links in the regulation of myocardial contractility. Circulation **43:** 437–450.
27. GILLIBRAND, I. M. & R. WYSE. 1971. Uptake of calcium ions and the β-adrenergic receptor site in cardiac muscle. Proc. Biochem. Soc. **125:** 105P–106P.
28. CHIMOSKEY, J. F. & J. GERGELY. 1968. Effect of norepinephrine, ouabain, and pH on cardiac sarcoplasmic reticulum. Arch. Int. Pharmacodyn. Ther. **176:** 289–297.
29. YU, D. H. & S. TRIESTER. 1969. Effect of catecholamines on Ca^{2+} uptake by dog heart sarcoplasmic reticulum fractions. Fed. Proc. **28:** 542.

30. SABATINI-SMITH, S. 1971. The effects of prostaglandins E_1 and $F_{2\alpha}$, norepinephrine, and 3′-5′ adenosine monophosphate on calcium transport in electrically stimulated cardiac sarcoplasmic reticulum. Fed. Proc. **30:** 625.
31. DHALLA, N. S., P. V. SULAKHE & D. B. MCNAMARA. 1973. Studies on the relationship between adenylate cyclase activity and calcium transport by cardiac sarcotubular membranes. Biochim. Biophys. Acta **323:** 276–284.
32. KATZ, A. M. & D. I. REPKE. 1973. Calcium-membrane interactions in the myocardium: Effects of ouabain, epinephrine and 3′,5′-cyclic adenosine monophosphate. Am. J. Cardiol. **31:** 193–201.
33. KATZ, A. M., M. A. KIRCHBERGER, M. TADA & D. I. REPKE. 1973. Epinephrine-induced enhancement of myocardial contractility: Possible mediation by β-receptor: adenylate cyclase: adenosine 3′,5′-monophosphate-dependent protein kinase: calcium transport system located on the sarcoplasmic reticulum. J. Clin. Invest. **52:** 46a.
34. SHINEBOURNE, E. & R. WHITE. 1970. Cyclic AMP and calcium uptake of the sarcoplasmic reticulum in relation to increased rate of relaxation under the influence of catecholamines. Cardiovasc. Res. **4:** 194–200.
35. GERTZ, E. W., E. H. SONNENBLICK & P. J. LARAIA. 1971. Cyclic AMP and cardiac sarcoplasmic reticulum. Circulation (Suppl. II) **43:** 131a.
36. SULAKHE, P. V. & N. S. DHALLA. 1972. Excitation-contraction coupling in heart. 3. Evidence against the involvement of adenosine cyclic 3′,5′-monophosphate in calcium transport by sarcotubular vesicles of canine myocardium. Mol. Pharmacol. **6:** 659–666.
37. NAMM, D. H., E. L. WOODS & J. L. ZUCKER. 1972. Incorporation of the terminal phosphate of ATP into membranal protein of rabbit cardiac sarcoplasmic reticulum. Circ. Res. **31:** 308–316.
38. KATZ, A. M. & D. I. REPKE. 1967. Quantitative aspects of dog cardiac microsomal calcium binding and calcium uptake. Circulation Res. **21:** 153–162.
39. KIRCHBERGER, M. A. M. TADA, D. I. REPKE & A. M. KATZ. 1972. Cyclic adenosine 3′,5′-monophosphate–dependent protein kinase stimulation of calcium uptake by canine cardiac microsomes. J. Mol. Cell. Cardiol. **4:** 673–680.
40. KATZ, A. M. 1995. Discovery of the myofibrillar regulatory proteins: Tropomyosin and the troponin complex. Cardioscience **6:** 1–11.
41. WOLLENBERGER, A. 1972. Cyclic nucleotides and the regulation of heart beat. Abstracts of the Fifth International Congress of Pharmacology: 231–233.
42. LARAIA, P. J. & E. MORKIN. 1974. Adenosine 3′,5′-monophosphate dependent membrane phosphorylation; a possible mechanism for the control of microsomal calcium transport in heart muscle. Circ. Res. **35:** 298–306.
43. WRAY, H. L., R. R. GRAY & R. A. OLSSON. 1973. Cyclic adenosine 3′,5′-monophosphate–stimulated protein kinase and a substrate associated with cardiac sacroplasmic reticulum. J. Biol. Chem. **248:** 1496–1498.
44. WILL, H., B. SCHIRPKE & A. WOLLENBERGER. 1976. Stimulation of Ca^{2+} uptake by cyclic AMP and protein kinase in sarcoplasmic reticulum-rich and sarcolemma-rich microsomal fractions from rabbit heart. Acta Biol. Med. Ger. **35:** 529–541.
45. FEDELESOVÁ, M. & A. ZIEGELHÖFFER. 1975. Enhanced calcium accumulation related to increased protein phosphorylation in cardiac sarcoplasmic reticulum induced by cyclic 3′,5′-AMP or isoproterenol. Experientia **31:** 518–520.
46. KIRCHBERGER, M. A., M. TADA & A. M. KATZ. 1974. Adenosine 3′,5′-monophosphate-dependent protein kinase-catalyzed phosphorylation reaction and its relationship to calcium transport in cardiac sarcoplasmic reticulum. J. Biol. Chem. **249:** 6166–6173.
47. MACLENNAN, D. H. & P. C. HOLLAND. 1975. Calcium transport in sarcoplasmic reticulum. Annu. Rev. Biophys. Bioeng. **4:** 377–404.
48. TADA, M., T. YAMAMOTO & Y. TONOMURA. 1978. Molecular mechanism of active calcium transport by sarcoplasmic reticulum. Physiol. Rev. **58:** 1–79.
49. SUKO, J. & W. HASSELBACH. 1976. Characterization of cardiac sarcoplasmic reticulum ATP-ADP phosphate exchange and phosphorylation of the calcium transport adenosine triphosphatase. Eur. J. Biochem. **64:** 123–130.

50. LEVITSKY, D. O., M. K. ALIEV, A. L. KUZMIN, T. S. LEVCHENKO, V. N. SMIRNOV & E. I. CHAZOV. 1976. Isolation of calcium pump system and purification of calcium ion-dependent ATPase from heart muscle. Biochim. Biophys. Acta **443:** 468–484.
51. SCHWARTZ, A., M. L. ENTMAN, K. KANIIKE, L. K. LANE, W. B. VAN WINKLE & E. P. BORNET. 1976. The rate of calcium uptake in sarcoplasmic reticulum of cardiac muscle and skeletal muscle. Effects of cyclic AMP–dependent protein kinase and phosphorylase b kinase. Biochim. Biophys. Acta **426:** 57–72.
52. M., TADA, M., A. KIRCHBERGER & A. M. KATZ. 1975. Phosphorylation of a 22,000-dalton component of the cardiac sarcoplasmic reticulum by adenosine 3′,5′-monophosphate dependent protein kinase. J. Biol. Chem. **250:** 2640–2647.
53. WRAY, H. L. & R. R. GRAY. 1977. Cyclic AMP stimulation of membrane phosphorylation and Ca^{2+}-activated, Mg^{2+}-dependent ATPase in cardiac sarcoplasmic reticulum. Biochim. Biophys. Acta **461:** 441–459.
54. WILL, H., T. S. LEVCHENKO, D. O. LEVITSKY, V. N. SMIRNOV & A. WOLLENBERGER. 1979. Partial characterization of protein kinase–catalyzed phosphorylation of low molecular weight proteins in purified preparations of pigeon heart sarcolemma and sarcoplasmic reticulum. Biochim. Biophys. Acta **543:** 175–193.
55. LOUIS, C. F. & A. M. KATZ. 1977. Lactoperoxidase coupled iodination of cardiac sarcoplasmic reticulum proteins. Biochim. Biophys. Acta **494:** 255–265.
56. KATZ, A. M. 1966. Purification and properties of a tropomyosin-containing protein fraction that sensitizes reconstituted actomyosin to calcium-binding agents. J. Biol. Chem. **241:** 1522–1529.
57. EBASHI, S. & A. KODAMA. 1965. A new protein factor promoting aggregation of tropomyosin. J. Biochem. (Tokyo) **58:** 107–108.
58. TADA, M., M. A. KIRCHBERGER, J. A. IORIO & A. M. KATZ. 1973. Phosphorylation of a low molecular weight component (phospholamban) in cardiac sarcoplasmic reticulum catalyzed by a cyclic AMP–dependent protein kinase. Circulation **48** (Suppl IV): 25.

Comparative Ultrastructure of Ca^{2+} Release Units in Skeletal and Cardiac Muscle

CLARA FRANZINI-ARMSTRONG,[a,b] FELICIANO PROTASI,[a,c] AND VENKAT RAMESH[d]

[a]*Department of Cell and Developmental Biology, School of Medicine, University of Pennsylvania, Philadelphia, Pennsylvania 19104-6058, USA*

[d]*Department of Cardiology, Children's Hospital of Philadelphia, Philadelphia, Pennsylvania 19104, USA*

ABSTRACT: The sarcoplasmic reticulum (SR) of striated muscle fibers interacts with exterior membranes (surface membrane and transverse tubules) to form junctions that are involved in the internal release of calcium during excitation-contraction coupling. Release of calcium through the ryanodine receptors (RyRs) or calcium release channels of the SR is under the control of the L type calcium channels or dihydropyridine receptors (DHPRs) of exterior membranes. Interacting clusters of the two proteins constitute calcium release units. The cytoplasmic domains of RyRs are visible as large electron-dense structures (the feet) with four identical subunits in the junctional gap separating SR from exterior membranes. In freeze-fracture replicas of skeletal muscle, large intramembrane particles are grouped into clusters of tetrads in the exterior membranes, and the tetrads are located in correspondence of the four subunits of the feet. Lack of tetrads in dysgenic muscle fibers with a null mutation for DHPRs and appearance of the tetrads after transfection with cDNA for DHPR indicate identity of tetrads with four DHPRs. In cardiac muscle, DHPRs are located at the sites of SR-surface junctions, but they are not grouped into tetrads. This is consistent with a possible direct DHPR-RyR interaction in skeletal but not in cardiac muscle. The size and distribution of SR-surface junctions in skeletal and cardiac muscles provide further clues to their function.

A key event in excitation contraction (e-c) coupling of skeletal and cardiac muscles is the rapid release of Ca^{2+} from the internal membrane-limited system, the sarcoplasmic reticulum (SR), under the control of the exterior membranes (surface membrane and transverse, T tubules). Functional interaction between external and interior membrane systems involves two Ca^{2+} permeant channels: the dihydropyridine receptor (DHPR, or L type Ca^{2+} channel) of exterior membranes and the ryanodine receptor (RyR) or Ca^{2+} release channel of the SR. Understanding the topology and geometry of muscle membranes and the spatial relationship between the key molecules is essential to unraveling the mechanism of regulated Ca^{2+} release during activation of muscle contraction. Important clues are provided by functional and structural similarities as well as differences between skeletal and cardiac muscle. This review gives a brief comparative description of the e-c coupling apparatus in skeletal and cardiac muscle, giving particular attention to the comparative size and distribution the essential elements involved.

[b] Address for correspondence: Clara Franzini-Armstrong, B1 Anatomy-Chemistry Building, Department of Cell and Developmental Biology, School of Medicine, University of Pennsylvania, Philadelphia, Pennsylvania 19104-6058.

[c] Current address: Department of Anesthesiology, Brigham and Women's Hospital, 75 Francis Street, Boston, Massachusetts 02115.

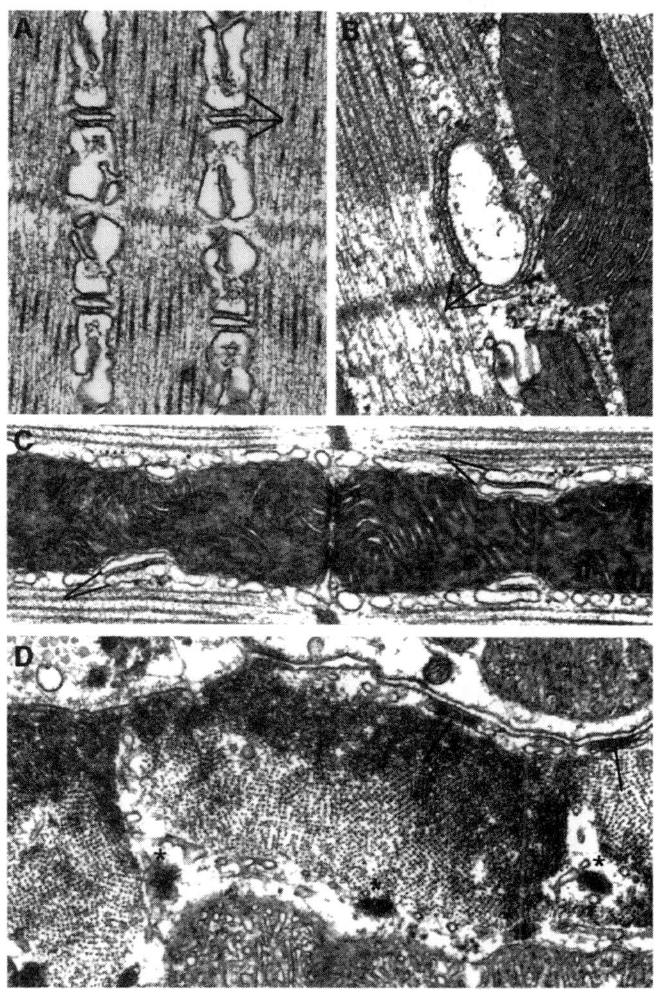

FIGURE 1. Examples of junctions between the sarcoplasmic reticulum and exterior membranes with a variety of geometries. Triads (three lines) are junctions between two SR elements and one segment of the T tubule network. **A.** Four triads in a skeletal muscle fiber from the toadfish swimbladder. The transverse tubules are flat ribbons with two narrow surfaces facing wide SR cisternae. The junctional surfaces are oriented transversely to the direction of the filaments. **B.** A triad in a cardiac muscle cell from the mouse left ventricle. The T tubule has a large diameter, and two flat SR cisternae surround it. The junctional surfaces are oriented longitudinally, or parallel to the direction of the filaments. **C.** Dyads (two lines) in the flight muscle of the dragonfly, located between the mitochondria and the myofibrils. The junctional surfaces are oriented longitudinally. **D.** Peripheral couplings (single lines), or junctions between the SR and the surface membrane in a cardiac cell from the chicken left ventricle. Other SR elements in the fiber interior *(asterisks)* have junctional components (feet and calsequestrin) but are not associated with exterior membranes. These are called corbular and/or extended junctional SR. Magnification: 50,000×.

SR and exterior membranes interact with each other at intracellular junctions, named triads, dyads and peripheral couplings on the basis of their geometry (FIG. 1). The Ca^{2+} release channels of the SR, also called ryanodine receptors, are located at the junctional sites and are visible as feet in the electron microscope (FIGS. 2A, B, D). In cardiac muscle, a special SR arrangement, containing the feet, but not forming junc-

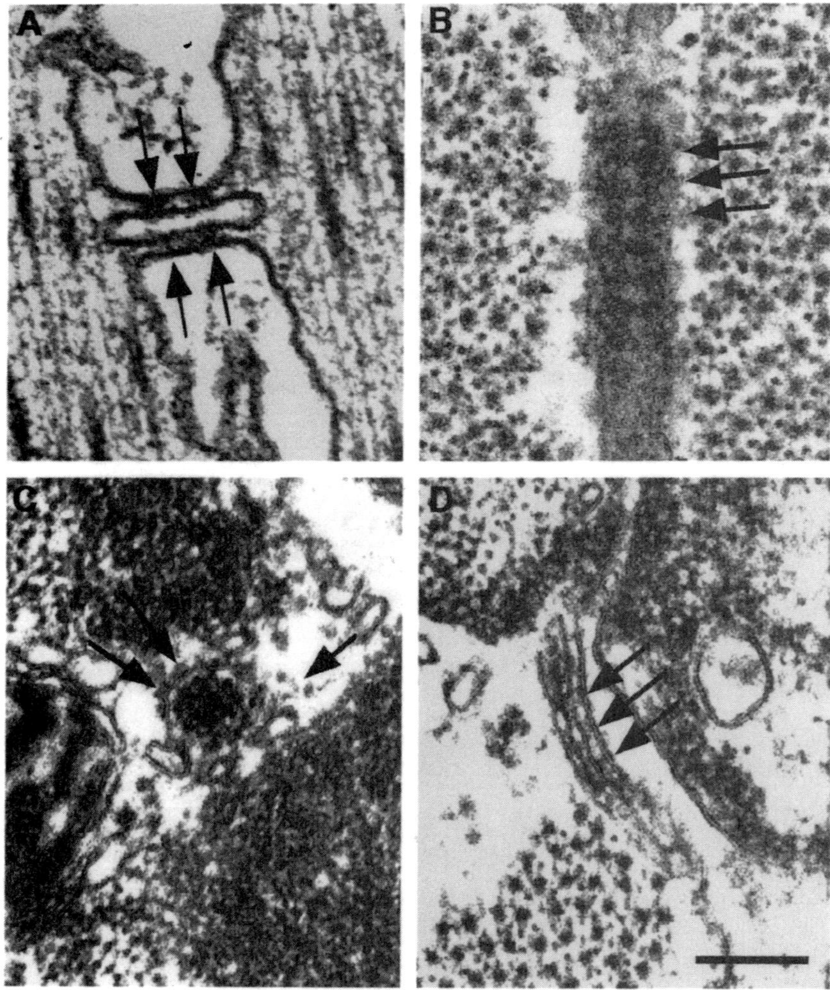

FIGURE 2. All SR elements participating in junctions (**A,B,** and **D**), and those forming the corbular SR (**C**) have feet (ryanodine receptors) associated with the junctional membrane. **A** and **B:** sections across and tangent to triads in the toadfish swimbladder. *Arrows* point to feet forming two rows within the junctional gap separating SR and T tubule membranes. **C** and **D:** corbular SR and a peripheral coupling from chick myocardium, showing periodically disposed feet *(arrows)*. The dense content of the SR is calsequestrin. Magnification: 133,000×, *bar* = 0.1 μm.

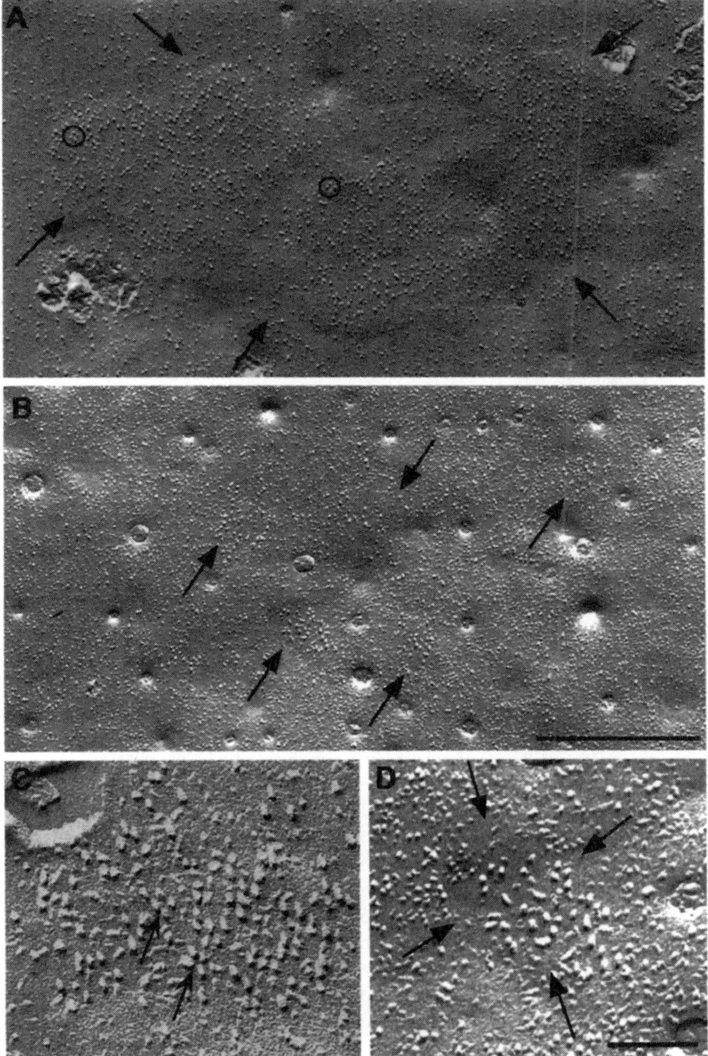

FIGURE 3. Dihydropyridine receptors (DHPRs) are detectable as tall intramembranous particles of large diameter in freeze-fracture replicas. Clusters of DHPRs are illustrated on the surface membrane of BC3H1, a cell line of skeletal muscle origin (**A,** between *arrows*); on the surface of chick ventricular myocardium (**B,** at *arrows;* **D** between *arrows*); and developing mouse skeletal muscle *in vivo* (**C**). DHPRs are clustered in both skeletal and cardiac muscle, but in a different manner. In skeletal muscle, DHPRs form arrays of tetrads (**C,** *arrows* point to individual tetrads), while in cardiac muscle DHPRs are randomly disposed. Magnification: **A,B:** 51,000×, *bar* = 0.5 µm; **C,D:** 135,000×, *bar* = 0.1 µm.

tions with the surface membrane (the corbular or extended junctional SR, EjSR), is also present (FIG. 2C). The T tubules and surface membrane participating in the junctions contain clusters of L-type Ca^{2+} channels or dihydropyridine receptors (FIGS. 3A and B). RyRs and DHPRs are located in correspondence to each other in discrete junctional domains of SR and exterior membranes, forming functional units named e-c coupling units or Ca^{2+} release units.[1,2] The junctional domains constituting Ca^{2+} release units are in turn separated from each other by nonjunctional domains of the two membranes, which contain a different complement of proteins. Thus the units are arranged in focal spots along the continuous exterior membranes. Modeling indicates that this discrete structural arrangement may result in the concerted action of several Ca^{2+} release channels within functional units, called couplons.[3]

GEOMETRICAL DIFFERENCES BETWEEN CARDIAC AND SKELETAL Ca^{2+} RELEASE UNITS

The Ca^{2+} release units in skeletal and cardiac muscle and the muscles of invertebrates have different geometries. In adult skeletal muscle of most vertebrates, transversely arranged T tubule networks prevail and the usual junction is a triad, with a transverse orientation and two or at most three elongated rows of feet (FIGS. 2A and B). During skeletal muscle differentiation, in the period between the initial formation of myofibrils and T tubule development, peripheral couplings are the only type of junction present. As soon as T tubules develop, however, longitudinally and, later, transversely arranged triads and dyads appear, and peripheral couplings become rare. A few fiber types, such as frog slow tonic fibers, maintain a high frequency of peripheral couplings. In muscles of arthropods, the junctions are mostly triad or dyads with a longitudinal orientation (FIG. 1C), and feet are arranged in a round plaque. Peripheral couplings may also be frequent. In cardiac muscle, T tubules have a much larger diameter than in skeletal muscle, and the most common junctions are in the form of dyads formed by the close apposition of a flat SR cisterna, which contacts the T tubule over a wide area. Occasionally a triad is present (FIG. 1B), but it has a different appearance from the skeletal muscle triad, due to the wider lumen of the T tubule. Peripheral couplings (FIGS. 1D and 2D) are often present in parallel with internal junctions. All myocardial cells in avian and frog hearts and in the atria of other vertebrates, lack T tubules and have frequent peripheral couplings. In addition, avian muscles are particularly rich in extended junctional SR, the avian equivalent of the mammalian corbular SR (FIGS. 1D, 2C).

These variations in the geometry of junctions affect the location, distribution, and overall quantity of the Ca^{2+} release channels within the muscle fiber. However, the specific mechanism by which Ca^{2+} release is initiated is not likely to differ between triads, dyads, and peripheral couplings within the same muscle type. EjSR, on the other hand, must be considered separately.

THE FUNCTIONAL IMPLICATIONS OF SIMILARITIES AND DIFFERENCES IN THE RELATIVE POSITIONS OF DHPR AND RYRS IN SKELETAL AND CARDIAC Ca^{2+} RELEASE UNITS

All Ca^{2+} release units have feet disposed in highly ordered arrangements, with very similar spacings. Minor differences in the orientation of feet have been detected between vertebrate and arthropod muscles, and it is not known whether the disposition is exactly the same in cardiac and skeletal muscles. These minor differences may not affect the function of the channels.

The disposition of DHPRs, on the other hand, is significantly different in cardiac muscle and muscles of invertebrates on the one hand, and in skeletal muscle on the other. In skeletal muscles, DHPRs are grouped into tetrads, or clusters of four DHPRs, located at the corners of small squares. The tetrads in turn are disposed in larger ordered arrays, so that the four components of the tetrads are located in correspondence of the four subunits of the feet.[4,5] This location is present only in skeletal muscles, and it constitutes the structural basis for a unique direct molecular interaction that allows the voltage sensor of e-c coupling (the DHPR[6,7]) to directly affect the permeability of the SR Ca^{2+} release channel (the RyR or foot), in the so-called mechanical model of e-c coupling.[8] The four components of the tetrads may act in concert.[9] Neither cardiac DHPR nor RyR can substitute for their skeletal isoforms in establishing a direct molecular interaction with their skeletal counterpart.[10,11] Direct confirmation that DHPRs and RyRs are functionally coupled in skeletal muscle come from the demonstration that a retrograde signal from RyRs is necessary for full functioning of DHPRs.[12]

In cardiac muscles, DHPRs are also clustered in close proximity to RyRs,[13] but they do not form tetrads and are not disposed in a detectable ordered arrangement and therefore are not likely to establish a link to the RyRs.[14,15] DHPR-RyR interaction in these muscles is dependent on extracellular Ca^{2+} and on Ca^{2+} current through the DHPRs, and so it is thought to be indirectly mediated by Ca^{2+}. The close DHPR-RyR proximity in cardiac muscle is appropriate if RyR opening is regulated by the Ca^{2+} current flowing through the DHPRs, perhaps through Ca^{2+} ions.

The disposition of DHPRs in muscles of arthropods is similar to that of cardiac muscle,[16] and this also is in keeping with the fact that e-c coupling in these muscles may be mediated by Ca^{2+}-activated Ca^{2+} release.[17,18]

An additional difference between cardiac and skeletal muscle is that while in the former all assemblies of feet are associated with DHPR-bearing membranes, in the latter the feet can also be independently located in clusters (within corbular and EjSR), which are located deep within the muscle fiber, at relatively large distances from either the surface of the cell or the T tubules.[19,20] These internal Ca^{2+} release units have the same RyR isoform as the peripheral couplings.[21] Thus, while in skeletal muscle a command from DHPRs may be the only means of initiating a Ca^{2+} release response from a cluster of feet, in cardiac muscle a Ca^{2+} release unit may be activated without intervention of DHPRs.

THE SPACING BETWEEN Ca^{2+} RELEASE UNITS

In cardiac muscles that lack T tubules, activation of the internal Ca^{2+} release units is necessarily dependent on diffusion of a messenger, presumably Ca^{2+}, from one unit to the other. Modeling of this interaction is critically dependent on knowing the distance between one unit and its immediate neighbor.[22] In avian myocardium, we compared the minimum distance separating peripheral couplings at the fiber surface from each other to the minimum distance between EjSR elements located within a narrow transverse layer at the level of the Z line. The minimum distance between adjacent peripheral couplings, 472 ± 5 nm (mean $\pm$ 1 SEM, $n = 340$), is significantly larger than the average distance for EjSR, 135 ± 15 nm ($n = 263$). Interestingly, the minimum distance between adjacent Ca^{2+} release units (triads) along the T tubules of three representative skeletal muscle fibers—fast twitch fibers from frog semitendinosus and ileofibularis and from male toadfish swimbladder muscle—are quite small (101 ± 2 nm, $n = 225$ for both frog muscle and 107 ± 2 nm, $n = 358$ for the toadfish).

A comparative look at skeletal muscle shows that the distances between Ca^{2+} release units vary depending on fiber types within the same animal. The units in fast twitch

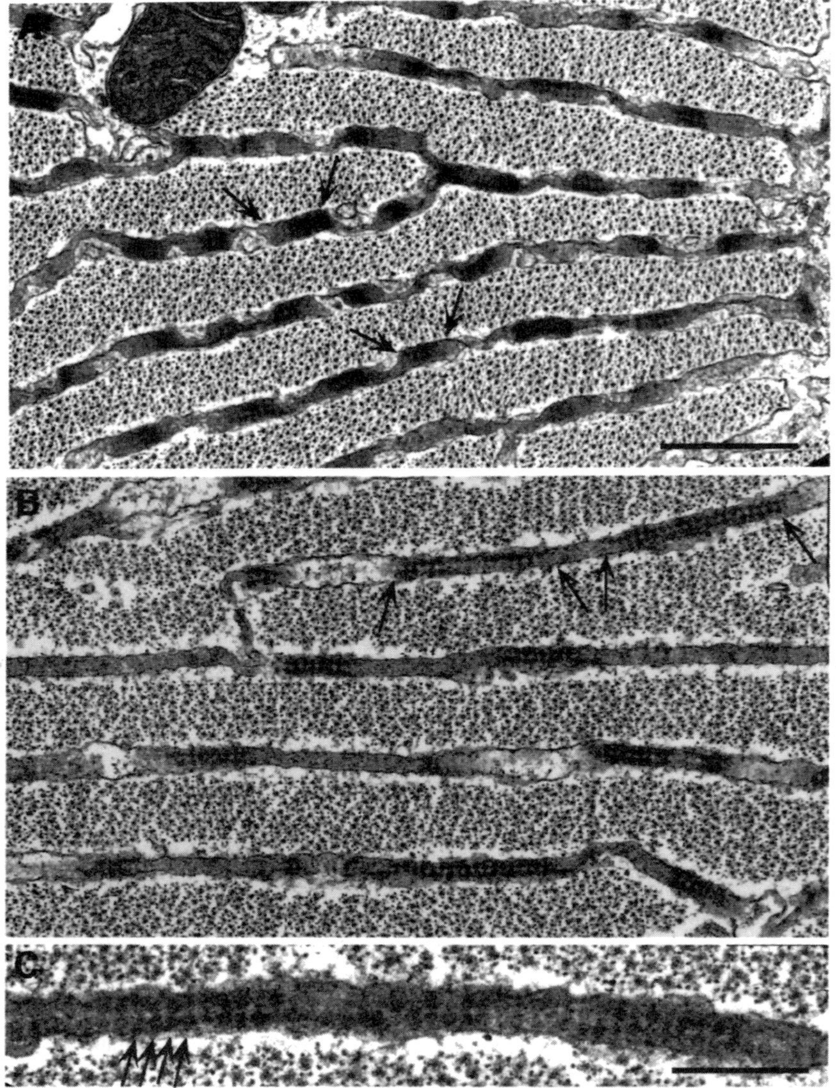

FIGURE 4. The size of calcium release units varies greatly in skeletal muscles, depending on the length of the T tubule segment that is engaged in association with the SR. In general, the size of the release units is related to the fiber type: fast muscle fibers have larger calcium release units (see text). The superfast toadfish swimbladder muscle, illustrated here, is an exception, because the muscle in the male swimbladder has short junctions (**A,** between *arrows*), while the junctions in the same muscle from the female has longer junctions (**B,** between *arrows;* **C,** *arrows* point to couples of feet). In the male, short junctions bear at most 24 feet on either side of the T tubule, while in the female an individual junction may contain as many as 115 feet on one side. Magnification: **A,B:** 35,000×, *bar* = 0.5 μm; **C,** 70,000×, *bar* = 0.25 μm.

fibers are separated by very short stretches of nonjunctional T tubules (see above), while in slow twitch and even more so in slow tonic fibers the distances can be very large.[23–25] One of the direct results of large spacings between Ca^{2+} release units is of course the fact that the total concentration of feet is smaller, and thus e-c coupling results in a smaller Ca^{2+} release. In the fast muscle of the toadfish swimbladder, where Ca^{2+} release units are very close to each other and thus the overall density of feet in the fiber is large (FIG. 4), the Ca^{2+} transients are very fast and very large.[26]

IS THERE A FUNCTIONAL SIGNIFICANCE TO THE SIZE OF Ca^{2+} RELEASE UNITS?

In skeletal muscle fibers of different types, Ca^{2+} release units are not only spaced at variable intervals along the T tubules, but also have variable sizes. In general, the faster the muscle, the larger the e-c coupling unit, and thus the larger the content of feet and DHPRs. The average number of feet per unit (or, in this case, triad) varies between 112 for the superfast toadfish swimbladder muscle, and 20 for the frog slow tonic fiber. Units in guinea pig fast twitch oxidative, fast twitch oxidative-glycolytic, and slow twitch fibers average 68, 48, and 34 feet each, and the frog twitch fibers of somewhat mixed character have 72 (iloeofibularis) and 58 (semitendinosus) feet/triad. One notable exception in the trend for larger units in faster muscles, is the superfast male toadfish swimbladder muscle, in which triads have 36 feet on the average, a number similar to that in the much slower tonic fibers of the frog.

In cardiac muscle, the size of Ca^{2+} release units may also vary, from 29–30 feet per unit in chick myocardium, to 150–200 feet/unit in mouse and rat left ventricle. Thus some Ca^{2+} release units in cardiac muscle have a larger content of feet than the units in very fast skeletal muscles, despite the slower rate of activity of the muscle fibers. One possible explanation for this unexpected observation may be that the apparently single, large units in cardiac muscle may in reality be an aggregate of smaller, closely spaced units.

Ca^{2+} RELEASE UNITS AND SPARKS

The qualitative and quantitative data given above are relevant to modeling the events that lead to Ca^{2+} release in cardiac and skeletal muscle and are particularly important in the understanding of small events in Ca^{2+} release activity or "sparks."

We can derive the following considerations from our data. The diffusion distances between EjSR, in cardiac muscles lacking T tubules, are quite short, particularly in the fast-acting fibers of the finch.[27] This is consistent with a possible saltatory conduction involving diffusion of calcium, as proposed.[27] Peripheral couplings (PCs), on the other hand, are activated by events that involve DHPRs and thus depend on membrane depolarization. Each PC, we would expect, is independently activated by its own DHPRs and does not need to be closely positioned relative to the others. Indeed, this is what we observe.

In view of the above arguments, some skeletal muscles with very short distances between Ca^{2+} release units provide a puzzle. If these units have the same properties as the EjSR, we would expect spread of Ca^{2+} release activation. However, it is known that Ca^{2+} release from SR does not spread independently from the T tubule depolarization in skeletal muscle.[28,29] Hence, Ca^{2+} release units in skeletal muscle would seem to be more refractory to activation by Ca^{2+} than the cardiac ones. A model of interactions within the units in skeletal muscle that do not lead to overall spread has been recently published.[3]

The size of Ca^{2+} release units is appropriately related to fiber properties within the skeletal muscles. However, when the cardiac muscles are considered, the trend breaks down. Mouse and rat left ventricles have units that contain 2–5 times as many feet as the superfast fibers in female toadfish swimbladder and 8–14 times those in the male. This means that either the units may behave in a fundamentally different way in the two types of muscles, or that the size of the units is important only in that it allows more feet to be packed along the same length of T tubule. In this respect, note that the small units in slow muscles are separated by large distances, but those in the fast toadfish muscle from the male are very closely spaced.

Finally, we ask what is the relationship between Ca^{2+} release units and sparks? The term refers to small, individual Ca^{2+} release events detectable in both cardiac and skeletal muscle under either rest or submaximal stimulation conditions.[30,31] The volume occupied by a detectable spark may contain 3–10 Ca^{2+} release units, but under the conditions for spark detection, it is debated whether more than one unit may contribute to an individual spark. As regards the contribution of the feet within a single unit to the detected spark, there are three possibilities: (1) A spark detects a unitary Ca^{2+} release event due to the opening of a single RyR acting independently of other channels in the unit.[30,32,33] In this case, variations in the apparent size of the release event are due to geometrical factors (position of the release site relative to the confocal plane of focus) and the duration of the opening state of the channel. (2) A spark may be due to the opening of either a single or no more than a few neighboring channels that are perhaps functionally linked.[34] It is tempting to assume that in skeletal muscle the alternate RyR channels that are not associated with tetrads may thus be activated. If this is the case, sparks that vary by a factor of 2–3 should be detectable. (3) Finally, a spark may be due to the simultaneous activity of many if not all the channels within a Ca^{2+} release unit.[35] This would be the case if activity of one channel would strongly affect the open probability of its neighbors within the same unit. In cardiac muscles this may be expected, since it is assumed that calcium released from one Ca^{2+} release unit may activate the neighboring units. If that is the case, one would also expect that calcium released from one channel within a unit should be able to activate neighboring channels within the same unit, unless complex inhibitory effects come into play (see Ref. 36). Considering that a cardiac Ca^{2+} release unit may contain 100 or more channels, an event involving most of a unit would be very large relative to an event involving a single channel. Currently, most Ca release events detected as sparks are interpreted on the basis of the activity of very few RyRs.

REFERENCES

1. Franzini-Armstrong, C. & A. O. Jorgenson. 1994. Structure and development of e-c coupling units in skeletal muscle. Annu. Rev. Physiol. **56:** 509–534.
2. Flucher, B. E. & C. Franzini-Armstrong. 1996. Formation of junctions involved in excitation-contraction coupling in skeletal and cardiac muscle. Proc. Natl. Acad. Sci. USA **93:** 265–278.
3. Stern, M. D., P. Gonzalo & E. Rios. 1997. A local control model of excitation-contraction coupling in skeletal muscle. J. Gen. Physiol. **110:** 1–26.
4. Franzini-Armstrong, C. & C. W. Kish. 1995. Alternate disposition of tetrads in peripheral couplings of skeletal muscle. J. Muscle Res. Cell Motil. **16:** 19–324.
5. Protasi, F., C. Franzini-Armstrong & B. Flucher. 1997. Coordinated incorporation of skeletal muscle dihydropyridine receptors and ryanodine receptors in peripheral couplings of BC3H1 cells. J. Cell Biol. **137:** 859–870.
6. Rios, E. & G. Brum. 1987. Involvement of dihydropyridine receptors in excitation- contraction coupling in skeletal muscle. Nature **325:** 717–720.
7. Tanabe, T. *et al.* 1988. Restoration of excitation-contraction coupling and slow calcium

current in dysgenic muscle by dihydropyridine receptor complementary DNA. Nature **346:** 567–569.
8. SCHNEIDER, M. F. & W. K. CHANDLER. 1973. Voltage dependent charge movement of skeletal muscle: A possible step in excitation-contraction coupling. Nature **242:** 244–246.
9. JONG, D. S., P. C. PAPE & K. W. CHANDLER. 1995. Effect of sarcoplasmic reticulum calcium depletion on intramembranous charge movement in frog cut muscle fibers. J. Gen. Physiol. **106:** 659–704.
10. TANABE, T. *et al.* 1990. Cardiac-type excitation-contraction coupling in dysgenic skeletal muscle injected with cardiac dihydropyridine receptor cDNA. Nature **344:** 451–453.
11. NAKAI, J. *et al.* 1997. Functional non-equality of the cardiac and skeletal ryanodine receptors. Proc. Natl. Acad. Sci. USA **94:** 1019–1022.
12. NAKAI, T. J. *et al.* 1996. Enhanced dihydropyridine receptor channel activity in the presence of ryanodine receptor. Nature **380:** 72–75.
13. CARL, S. L. *et al.* 1995. Immunolocalization of sarcolemmal dihydropyridine receptor and sarcoplasmic reticular triadin and ryanodine receptor in rabbit ventricle and atrium. J. Cell Biol. **129:** 672–682.
14. PROTASI, F., X.-H. SUN & C. FRANZINI-ARMSTRONG. 1996. Formation and maturation of calcium release units in developing and adult avian myocardium. Dev. Biol. **173:** 265–278.
15. SUN, X.-H. *et al.* 1995. Molecular architecture of membranes involved in excitation-contraction coupling of cardiac muscle. J. Cell Biol. **129:** 659–673.
16. EASTWOOD, A. B., C. FRANZINI-ARMSTRONG & C. PERACCHIA. 1982. Structure of membranes in crayfish muscle: Comparison of phasic and tonic fibers. J. Muscle Res. Cell Motil. **3:** 273–294.
17. PALADE, P. & S. GYORKE. 1993. Excitation-contraction coupling in crustacea: Do studies on these primitive creatures offer insights about EC coupling more generally? J Muscle Res. Cell Motil. **14:** 283–287.
18. GYORKE, S. & P. PALADE. 1993. Role of local Ca^{2+} domains in activation of Ca^{2+} induced Ca^{2+} release in crayfish muscle fibers. Am. J. Phys. **264:** C1505–1512.
19. JEWETT, P. H., S. D. LEONARD & J. R. SOMMER. 1973. Chicken cardiac muscle: Its elusive extended junctional sarcoplasmic reticulum and sarcoplasmic reticulum fenestrations. J. Cell Biol. **56:** 595–600.
20. SOMMER, J. R. 1995. Comparative anatomy: In praise of a powerful approach to elucidate mechanisms translating cardiac excitation into purposeful contraction. J. Mol. Cell. Cardiol. **27:** 19–35.
21. JUNKER, J., J. R. SOMMER & G. MEISSNER. 1994. Extended junctional sarcoplasmic reticulum of avian cardiac muscle contains functional ryanodine receptors. J. Biol. Chem. **269:** 1627–1634.
22. STERN, M. D. 1992. Theory of excitation-contraction coupling in cardiac muscle. Biophys. S. J. **63:** 497–517.
23. FRANZINI-ARMSTRONG, C., C. CHAMP & D. G. FERGUSON. 1988. Discrimination between fast and slow twitch fibres of guinea pig skeletal muscle using the relative surface density of junctional transverse tubule membrane. J. Muscle Res. Cell Motil. **9:** 403–414.
24. APPELT, D. *et al.* 1989. Quantitation of feet content in two types of muscle fibers from hind limb of the rat. Tissue & Cell **21:** 783–794.
25. APPELT, D., V. SHEN & C. FRANZINI-ARMSTRONG. 1991. Quantitation of Ca ATPase, feet and mitochondria in super fast muscle fibres from the toadfish, Opsanus tau. J. Muscle Res. Cell Motil. **12:** 543–552.
26. ROME, L. C. *et al.* 1996. The whistle and the rattle: The design of sound producing muscles. Proc. Natl. Acad. Sci. USA **93:** 8095–8100.
27. SOMMER, J. R., T. HIGH & I. TAYLOR. 1997. The geometry of the EJSR Z-rete in avian cardiac muscle. Proceedings of the 55th Annual Meeting of the Microscopy Society of America. G. W. Bailey & A. J. Garratt-Reed, Eds.: 940–941. San Francisco Press. San Francisco.
28. HUXLEY, A. F. & R. E. TAYLOR. 1958. Local activation of skeletal muscle fibers. J. Physiol. (Lond.) **144:** 426–441.
29. PAPE, P. C., D. S. JONG & K. W. CHANDLER. 1995. Calcium release and its voltage dependence in frog cut muscle fibers equilibrated with 20 mM EGTA. J. Gen. Physiol. **106:** 259–336.

30. CHENG, H., W. J. LEDERER & M. B. CANNELL. 1993. Calcium sparks: Elementary events underlying excitation-contraction coupling in heart muscle. Science **262:** 740–744.
31. LOPEZ-LOPEZ, J. R. *et al.* 1994. Local, stochastic release of Ca^{2+} in voltage-clamped rat heart cells: Visualization with confocal microscopy. J. Physiol. **480:** 21–29.
32. CHENG, H., M. B. CANNELL & W. J. LEDERER. 1995. $[Ca^{2+}]i$ during excitation-contraction coupling in cardiac myocytes. Circ. Res. **76:** 236–241.
33. XIAO, R. P. *et al.* 1997. The immunophilin FK506-binding protein modulates Ca^{2+} release channel closure in rat heart. J. Physiol. **500:** 343–354.
34. TSUGORKA, A., E. RIOS & L. A. BLATTER. 1995. Imaging elementary events of calcium release in skeletal muscle cells. Science **269:** 1723–1726.
35. LIPP, P. & E. NIGGLI. 1996. Submicroscopic calcium signals as fundamental events of excitation-contraction coupling in guinea-pig cardiac myocytes. J. Physiol. **492:** 31–38.
36. GYORKE S. & P. PALADE. 1994. Ca^{2+} dependent negative control mechanism for Ca^{2+} induced Ca^{2+} release in crayfish muscle. J. Physiol. **476:** 315–322.

Sites of Regulatory Interaction between Calcium ATPases and Phospholamban[a]

DAVID H. MacLENNAN, YOSHIHIRO KIMURA, AND TOSHIHIKO TOYOFUKU

Banting and Best Department of Medical Research, University of Toronto, Charles H. Best Institute, 112 College Street, Toronto, Ontario, Canada M5G1L6

ABSTRACT: Phospholamban (PLN) is a 52–amino acid, integral membrane protein that interacts with and reversibly inhibits the activity of the cardiac sarcoplasmic reticulum Ca^{2+} ATPase (SERCA2a). We have used site-directed mutagenesis to analyze the sites of interaction between PLN and SERCA2a. First, we used chimera formation between SERCA2a and SERCA3 (which is weakly inhibited by PLN) to determine the interacting residues in cytoplasmic sequences of SERCA2 and PLN. Then, we expressed SERCA2a with the transmembrane sequence of PLN and demonstrated that the sites of inhibitory interaction are located in transmembrane sequences of the two proteins. We proposed that a four-base circuit involving noninhibitory cytoplasmic and inhibitory transmembrane sites in PLN and SERCA2a best describes the interaction. Recently, we have used alanine-scanning mutagenesis to show an asymmetric distribution of function in the transmembrane domain of PLN—one helical face interacts with PLN molecules in a pentamer, and the other interacts with SERCA2a. Gain of function by mutation of PLN-interacting residues indicates that the inhibitory species of PLN is a monomer. Thus regulatory steps include PLN dissociation, PLN/SERCA2a inhibitory association, and PLN/SERCA2a dissociation induced by phosphorylation of PLN (in the noninhibitory cytoplasmic domain) or by binding of Ca^{2+} by SERCA2a (in the inhibitory transmembrane domain).

Phospholamban (PLN), a pentameric protein made up of 6,000-Da subunits, is located in the sarcoplasmic reticulum of cardiac, slow-twitch, and smooth muscles. It contains 52 amino acids, which are organized into three physical and functional domains.[1–3] Domain Ia, consisting of residues 1–20, of which the first 16 are likely to be in an α-helical conformation,[4] and domain Ib, consisting of residues 21–30 and likely to be less structured, constitute the cytoplasmic sector. Domain Ia has a net positive charge, but, since Ser^{16} can be phosphorylated by protein kinase A and Thr^{17} can be phosphorylated by calmodulin kinase,[3] the net charge can be shifted from positive to neutral or even negative. Domain Ib is polar, positively charged, and rich in amidated residues. Domain II is the transmembrane domain, made up solely of uncharged residues, probably in an α-helical conformation.

[a] This work was supported, in part, by an International Human Frontier Science Program Organization grant to D.H.M. and, in part, by a grant from the Heart and Stroke Foundation of Ontario to D.H.M. Y.K. was supported by a postdoctoral fellowship from the Heart and Stroke Foundation of Canada, and T.T. was supported by a postdoctoral fellowship from the Medical Research Council of Canada.

BIOCHEMICAL ANALYSIS OF PLN/SERCA2a INTERACTIONS

James *et al.*[5] cross-linked Lys^3 of PLN to Lys^{397} or Lys^{400} of SERCA2 under conditions where SERCA2 was inhibited. Cross-linking did not occur in the presence of saturating levels of Ca^{2+} or when PLN was phosphorylated. These results suggested that there is a physical interaction between PLN and SERCA2 that inhibits the rate of Ca^{2+} transport and that this physical interaction is disrupted by the phosphorylation of PLN or by the availability to SERCA2 of higher levels of Ca^{2+}. An antibody against residues 7–16 of PLN mimics phosphorylation of PLN by activating the Ca^{2+} ATPase.[6]

Several investigators have attempted to study the interaction of PLN domains with SERCA2a by reconstitution of purified SERCA2 with high concentrations of purified PLN or PLN fragments.[7–14] In studies carried out by Sasaki *et al.*,[10] the addition of an excess of soluble, synthetic PLN^{1-31} suppressed V_{max} without affecting Ca^{2+} affinity of purified SERCA2a, while the *in vitro* reconstitution of purified SERCA2a with an unphysiological, 100-fold molar excess of synthetic PLN^{28-47} lowered the apparent Ca^{2+} affinity of SERCA2a. While some attempts to reproduce these experiments were successful,[11,12] others were not.[13,14] Reddy *et al.*[13] reported reconstitution with a 3:1 PLN/SERCA1 ratio, but found that the addition of excess PLN^{26-52} uncoupled Ca^{2+} transport from ATP hydrolysis. Thus these experiments did not provide very definitive evidence for separate cytoplasmic or transmembrane interaction sites between SERCA2a and PLN.

A major goal in our laboratory is to define the sites of molecular interaction between PLN and SERCA2 by coexpressing PLN and SERCA2 in a heterologous cell culture system.[15–19] We can reproduce the essential measures of PLN/SERCA2 interaction using microsomes from a transfected, heterologous cell culture system, thereby providing an excellent alternative to *in vitro* reconstitution systems.

SERCA CYTOPLASMIC INTERACTION SITES

When we coexpressed PLN with SERCA1 or SERCA2, we found that apparent Ca^{2+} affinity was lowered; but when we coexpressed PLN with SERCA3, we observed little effect on the naturally low apparent Ca^{2+} affinity of SERCA3.[20] We made chimeras between SERCA2 and SERCA3 and found that high apparent Ca^{2+} affinity required the inclusion of the nucleotide binding/hinge domain of SERCA2 in the chimeras.[17] We then coexpressed each of the 14 SERCA2/SERCA3 chimeras with PLN and found that PLN would interact functionally only with those chimeras that had both residues 467–762, constituting the nucleotide binding/hinge domain of SERCA2 (which conferred high Ca^{2+} affinity to the chimera), and residues 336–412 within the phosphorylation domain of SERCA2 (which apparently contained a PLN interaction site). These studies identified only a cytoplasmic interaction domain with PLN, but they did not rule out other interaction sites, since SERCA2a interaction sites would have to differ in the molecules making up the chimeras in order to be identified.

We mutated all of the charged residues and some of the uncharged residues in SERCA2 between Arg^{365} and Asp^{408}. Mutation affected functional interaction only for residues $KDDKPV^{402}$.[19] To prove that these were the essential interacting residues, we made a SERCA2 chimera containing the SERCA3 phosphorylation domain. This chimera did not interact functionally with PLN. If the SERCA3 sequence $QGEQLV^{402}$ were substituted with the SERCA2 sequence, $KDDKPV^{402}$, or with the SERCA1 sequence, $KGEKPV^{402}$, function was restored. These and other experiments demonstrated that the SERCA2 residues essential for PLN interaction are: at least one basic residue at positions 397 or 400; at least one acidic residue at positions 398 or 399; a Pro at position 401; and a long chain hydrophic residue at position 402.[19]

PLN CYTOPLASMIC INTERACTION SITES

We used our coexpression and alanine-scanning mutagenesis system to evaluate the roles of amino acids 1 to 30 in domains Ia and Ib of PLN in the PLN-SERCA2 interaction. We converted all domain Ia residues to the small, nonpolar amino acid, Ala, and we mutated Ala to Val. Loss of function occurred only with six amino acids, Glu^2, Val^4, Leu^7, Arg^9, Ile^{12} and Arg^{14} (FIG. 1).[18]

We also created a variety of other mutations relating function to alterations of charge and hydrophobicity. Net charge in residues 2–18 is an important element in the PLN/SERCA2a interaction. If residues 2 to 18 had a net charge of +1 or +2, the molecule was functional. If the net charge were 0, –2, –3, or +3, function was lost. Function was also lost if the long alkyl side chains of Val^4, Leu^7, or Ile^{12} were replaced by the methyl group of Ala. Thus both electrostatic and hydrophobic residues are critical in both SERCA2 and PLN interaction site sequences.

Alanine-scanning mutagenesis of domain Ib provided some surprising results.[21] While mutation to Ala of Arg^{25}, Gln^{26}, and Leu^{28} induced a partial loss of inhibitory function, mutation to Ala of Asn^{27}, Gln^{29}, and Asn^{30} induced a gain of inhibitory function (FIG. 1). Gain or loss of function is expressed as the shift in apparent K_{Ca} (the Ca^{2+} concentration that gives half-maximal Ca^{2+} transport activity for SERCA2a). In the mutant N27A, the gain of function, expressed as ΔK_{Ca}, was greater than –0.6 pCa units, compared to a shift of –0.35 pCa units for wild-type PLN. Losses in inhibitory function by mutation in domain Ib were relatively minor and did not warrant the assignment of any specific residues in this domain to PLN/SERCA2a interaction sites. While the gain of function mutants were intriguing, they could be explained only when inhibitory interactions occurring in domain II were understood.

PLN/SERCA2a TRANSMEMBRANE INTERACTION SITES

In order to evaluate the question of whether inhibitory interactions between PLN and SERCA2a occur in transmembrane sequences of the two molecules, we made new PLN constructs in which we either replaced domain I residues 1–27 with a single Met, removed domain Ib residues 21–29, or added different epitope tags (Myc, Flag, or HA) near the NH_2-terminus of PLN domain II.[22] We then coexpressed these constructs with SERCA isoforms to achieve *in vivo* reconstitution. PLN, when coexpressed with SERCA2a, normally shifts the curve of Ca^{2+}-dependence of Ca^{2+} uptake towards a lower apparent Ca^{2+} affinity. The shift in apparent K_{Ca} with PLN is normally –0.31 to –0.35 pCa units. Met-PLN^{28-52}, when coexpressed with SERCA2a, shifted K_{Ca} by –0.17 pCa units. The ΔK_{Ca} value for Myc-PLN^{30-52} was –0.34 pCa units; for Flag-PLN^{28-52}, –0.41 pCa units; and for HA-PLN^{28-52}, –0.63 pCa units, a "supershift." Our most effective inhibitor of SERCA2a, however, was the internally deleted mutant, PLN^{1-20}–PLN^{30-52}. When the ratio of PLN^{1-20}–PLN^{30-52} cDNA to SERCA2a cDNA in the cotransfection system was 1:2, the shift in apparent K_{Ca} was –0.87 pCa units, but when the transfection ratio was 1:1, the shift in K_{Ca} was more than –1 pCa unit.

The truncated PLN constructs also lowered apparent K_{Ca} for SERCA1a and SERCA3. This is consistent with the fact that all three SERCA molecules have conserved transmembrane sequences and, in particular, the Ca^{2+} binding helices M4, M5, and M6 are virtually identical among the three isoforms.[23] This finding highlights the

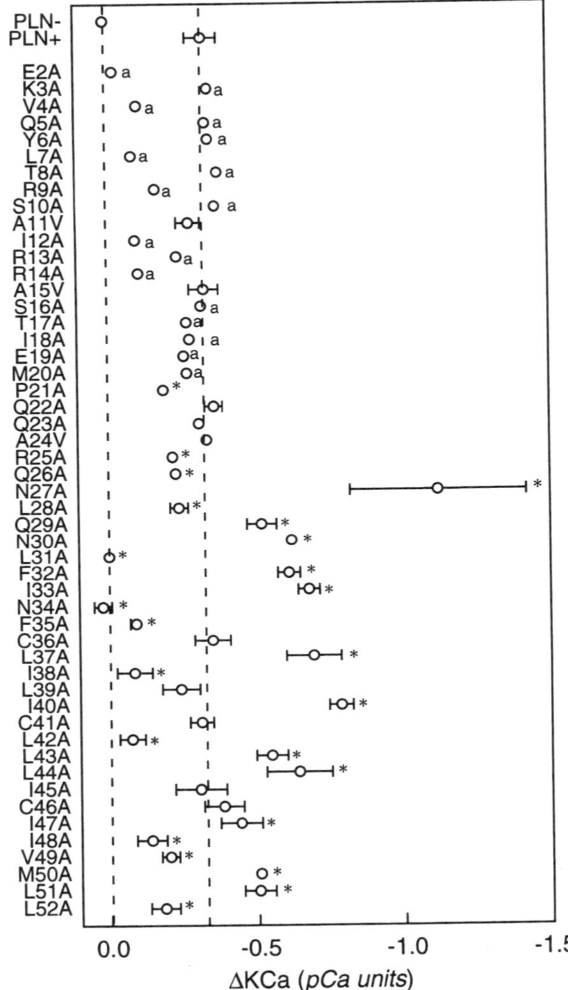

FIGURE 1. Effects of mutations in domains Ia, Ib, and II of PLN on the affinity of SERCA2a for Ca^{2+}. For each mutant, the normal amino acid residue is defined on the **left** in a *single-letter code,* its position in the sequence is identified by a *number,* and the newly introduced amino acid residue is defined on the **right** in a *single-letter code.* K_{Ca} is the Ca^{2+} concentration at which half-maximal Ca^{2+} uptake rates were observed. The *vertical dashed line* on the **left** represents the K_{Ca} value for SERCA2a expressed in the absence of PLN ($K_{Ca} = 6.55$), and the *vertical dashed line* on the **right** represents K_{Ca} in the presence of wild-type PLN ($K_{Ca} = 6.22$). The ΔK_{Ca} values on the *abscissa* are negative relative to the K_{Ca} for SERCA2a alone (the apparent affinity of SERCA2a for Ca^{2+} is decreased in the presence of PLN). Data are mean ± SD. **a** indicates results obtained from Ref. 19. * indicates $p < 0.05$ vs. –PLN, as judged by analysis of variance followed by the Scheffe F-test. (Adapted from Refs. 18 and 28 with permission.)

fact that the absence of the cytoplasmic interaction sequence in SERCA3 is of no significance if the cytoplasmic domain of PLN is stripped away, raising the possibility that the lack of a cytoplasmic interaction site in SERCA3 sterically inhibits PLN from forming inhibitory interactions in the transmembrane domain of SERCA3.

A monoclonal antibody against PLN domain Ia activated PLN^{1-20}–PLN^{30-52}–inhibited SERCA2a just as it does for PLN-inhibited SERCA2a.[6,24,25] An antibody against the Flag epitope also reversed the inhibition of SERCA2a by Flag-PLN^{28-52}. Thus the inhibition of SERCA2a, induced by truncated PLN constructs, could be reversed by modulation of the cytoplasmic domain of the chimeric PLN constructs, just as modulation of the cytoplasmic domain of intact PLN by phosphorylation or antibody interaction can modulate PLN inhibition of SERCA2a.

From these results, we proposed a model of PLN/SERCA2a interaction in which PLN interacts with SERCA2a in at least two sites, one in the cytoplasmic sequences of PLN and SERCA2a, and one within the transmembrane sequences of PLN and SERCA2a.[22] We proposed that the interaction between the transmembrance sequences of PLN and SERCA2a inhibits SERCA2a by altering its apparent Ca^{2+} affinity. We also proposed that interaction between PLN domain Ia and the cytoplasmic domain of SERCA2a is not, by itself, inhibitory, but can modulate the inhibitory interactions in the transmembrane domains through long-range coupling. If the cytoplasmic interaction were disrupted by PLN phosphorylation or binding of antibody, the inhibitory intramembrane interactions would also be disrupted. If the inhibitory transmembrane interaction sites were disrupted by Ca^{2+}, which at effective concentrations could bind only to the high-affinity Ca^{2+} binding and translocation sites in the transmembrane domain of SERCA molecules,[26] then the noninhibitory cytoplasmic interaction sites would also be disrupted.

In a striking analogy, long-range interactions between the catalytic ATP hydrolytic site in the cytoplasmic headpiece domain of SERCA1 and the Ca^{2+} binding and translocation sites in the transmembrane domain, mediated through a stalk sector, are an integral feature of Ca^{2+} transport by SERCA molecules.[27] PLN also has functional cytoplasmic (domain Ia) and transmembrane (domain II) domains, which are separated by a stalk sector (domain Ib) so that long-range interactions might occur between these functional domains. Long-range coupling might occur entirely within the PLN molecule, or be mediated by conduction through the SERCA2a molecule from its cytoplasmic to its transmembrane sites of interaction with PLN. In this case, a four-site regulatory circuit, possibly involving the catalytic site in the cytoplasmic domain of SERCA2a and the Ca^{2+} binding and translocation sites in the transmembrane domain of SERCA2a, might best describe the interactions between SERCA2a and PLN.[22]

AMINO ACIDS IN PLN TRANSMEMBRANE INTERACTION SITE

Having identified the transmembrane sequences of PLN and SERCa2a as inhibitory interaction sites,[22] we used alanine-scanning mutagenesis to define the residues in PLN that are involved in these interactions.[28] We mutated each of PLN transmembrane (domain II) amino acids, Leu^{31} through Leu^{52}, to Ala and coexpressed the mutant PLN cDNAs with SERCA2a cDNA. PLN mutants L31A, N34A, F35A, I38A, L42A, I48A, V49A, and L52A had diminished inhibitory function relative to PLN, as indicated by ΔK_{Ca} values between 0 and about –0.2 pCa units (FIG. 1). PLN mutants F32A, I33A, L37A, I40A, L43A, L44A, I47A, M50A, and L51A gained inhibitory function relative to PLN, as indicated by ΔK_{Ca} values between about –0.43 and –0.8 pCa units (FIG. 1). Autry and Jones,[29] in independent experiments, also found that the mutant L37A increased PLN inhibitory function.

When plotted on a helical wheel, loss and gain of function of the PLN mutants was seen to be cyclical and progressive, repeating every three or four residues, as would be expected if loss of function were associated with mutations on one face of the PLN domain II helix and gain of function were associated with mutations on the opposite face.

Wild-type PLN is at least 75% pentameric in SDS-PAGE, but is dissociated to a monomer by boiling in SDS under reducing or nonreducing conditions.[30] Scanning mutagenesis has shown that mutants of Leu[37], Ile[40], Leu[44], and Ile[47] are monomeric without boiling, as suggested by their mobility in SDS-PAGE.[31,32] These studies have led to structural models in which these residues lie on one face of the PLN domain II helix and play a role in pentamer formation.[32,33]

When we used SDS-PAGE to analyze the pentamer stability of unboiled samples of PLN and each of the 22 PLN mutants, the mutants could be divided into four classes on the basis of estimates of the percent monomer in each mutant protein (TABLE 1). Class 1 had the same or less monomer than wild-type PLN; class 2 had roughly twice as much monomer as PLN; class 3 had roughly three times as much monomer as PLN; and class 4 had roughly four times as much monomer as PLN, being virtually 100%

TABLE 1. Relationship between Monomer Content and Inhibitory Function for PLN and PLN Mutants

Class	Mutants	% Monomer (Mean ± SEM)	*n*	Function
	Wild type	26 ± 3	7	N
1	N34A	18 ± 6	5	L
	I38A	24 ± 10	4	L
	I45A	13 ± 7	6	N
	V49A	11 ± 3	5	L
	L52A	17 ± 6	5	L
2	L31A	54 ± 9	6	L
	F35A	33 ± 13	4	L
	C36A	50 ± 13	4	N
	L39A	39 ± 10	4	N
	L42A	40 ± 11	7	L
	C46A	51 ± 13	7	N
	I48A	38 ± 15	4	L
3	F32A	69 ± 13	6	G
	I33A	71 ± 15	5	G
	C41A	74 ± 10	7	N
	L43A	78 ± 7	8	G
	M50A	65 ± 5	4	G
	L51A	85 ± 4	6	G
4	L37A	94 ± 1	4	G
	I40A	100 ± 3	4	G
	L44A	97 ± 3	4	G
	I47A	95 ± 2	4	G

NOTE: Monomer % was determined by scanning densitometry of individual lanes from SDS-PAGE gels, which were transferred to 0.05 μ nitrocellulose membranes and immunoblotted with antibody 1D11 against the PLN cytoplasmic domain. Antibody binding to pentameric and monomeric bands in the same lane was measured by chemiluminescence. Inhibitory function is indicated: N, normal; L, loss of inhibitory function; G, gain of inhibitory function. (Adapted from Ref. 28 with permission.)

monomer. Loss and conservation of pentamer stability, like loss and gain of function, was cyclical and progressive, repeating every three or four residues, as would be expected if loss of stability were associated with mutations on one face of the PLN domain II helix. The cyclical changes of loss and gain of function and of pentamer stability were clearly in phase.[28]

When the location of each mutated amino acid was plotted on a helical wheel representing the PLN domain II helix (Fig. 2), loss-of-function mutants were located on one face of the helix (the proposed exterior face of each helix in a PLN pentamer,[32,33] and measurement of percent monomer placed all of these residues in classes 1 or 2. Gain-of-function mutants were located on the opposite face of the helix (the proposed interior face of each helix in a PLN pentamer[32,33]), and measurement of percent monomer placed all of these mutants in classes 3 or 4.[28]

We proposed that the loss of function that occurred with each of the eight mutants, L31A, N34A, F35A, I38A, L42A, I48A, V49A, and L52A, on the exterior face of the

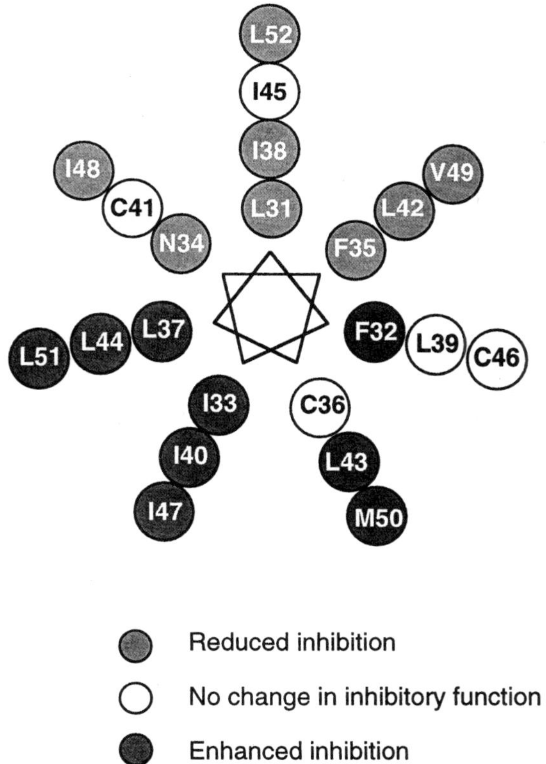

FIGURE 2. A helical wheel model of PLN domains Ib and II with 3.5 residues/turn. *Darkly shaded circles* represent mutations that enhanced the inhibitory function of PLN and enhanced monomer formation. *Lightly shaded circles* represent mutations that reduced inhibitory function. *Unshaded circles* represent mutations in which function was unaltered. (Adapted from Ref. 28 with permission.)

helix reflects the fact that each of these residues is normally involved with the formation of inhibitory interactions with complementary amino acids in the hydrophobic, transmembrane helices in SERCA2a.

We proposed that gain of function in the nine Class 3 and 4 mutants, I33A, F32A, L37A, I40A, L43A, L44A, I47A, M50A, and L51A, lying on the interior face of the helix, was a direct consequence of enhanced monomer formation. The 2.5–fold increase in inhibitory function that accompanied the 3- to 4-fold enhancement of monomer formation provided kinetic evidence that PLN monomers are the active inhibitory form, while PLN pentamers represent a noninhibitory or less-inhibitory reservoir. In chemical terms, an increase in the concentration of PLN monomers, a function of the dissociation constant of the PLN pentamer, would increase the concentration of the inhibited PLN monomer/SERCA2a complex through mass action (FIG. 3).

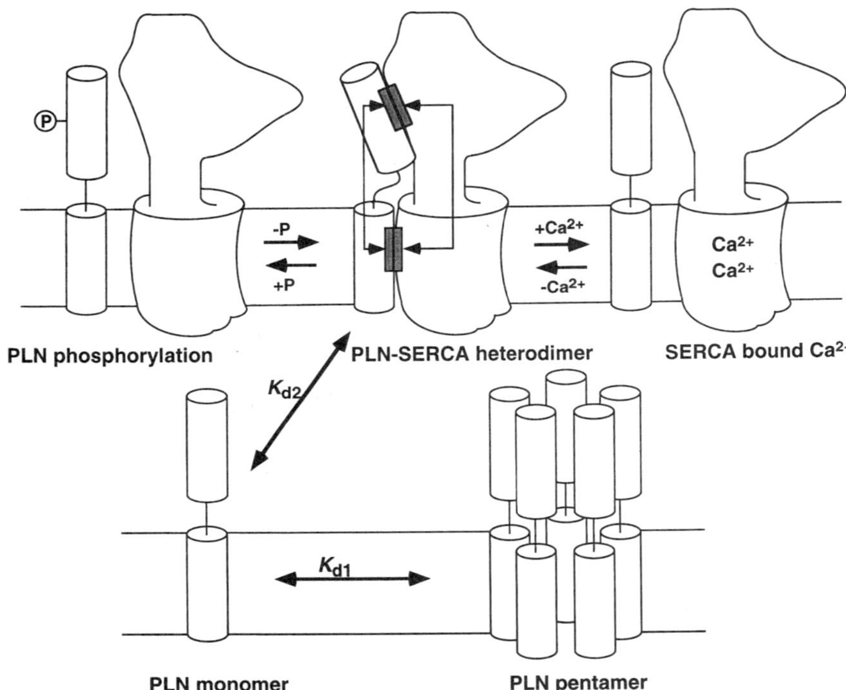

FIGURE 3. A model for the reversible inhibition of SERCA2a activity by PLN. Reversible inhibition is proposed to involve dissociation of the PLN pentamer (mutation-sensitive), formation of the inhibited PLN/SERCA2a heterodimer (mutation-sensitive), and dissociation of the heterodimer. Interactions involving the transmembrane domain of PLN (PLN domain II) inhibit SERCA2a activity and are disrupted by the binding of Ca^{2+} to the transmembrane sequences of SERCA2a. Cytoplasmic interactions involving PLN domain Ia are not inhibitory, but their disruption by phosphorylation and alteration in the net charge of PLN domain Ia also disrupts the intramembrane inhibitory interactions through long-range interactions within both PLN and SERCA2a. These internal regulatory interactions are represented by *arrows* connecting the four sites of inhibitory interaction *(shaded)*. Phosphorylation of the pentamer is not ruled out in this model. (Adapted from Ref. 28 with permission.)

We tested the hypothesis that gain-of-function mutants are activated by an increase in their monomer concentration, while loss-of-function PLN mutants have nonfunctional substitutions at sites that are essential for interaction with SERCA2a, by making double mutants containing either N34A or F35A (loss of function, pentameric) and either L37A or I40A (gain of function, monomeric). The double mutants N34A/I40A and F35A/L37A were inactive, even though they were both monomeric.[28] The fact that loss-of-function mutants were dominant over gain-of-function mutants suggests that these mutants could form monomers and, possibly, PLN monomer/SERCA2a complexes, but they could not form inhibitory interactions.

MODEL FOR PLN/SERCA2a INTERACTIONS

FIGURE 3 illustrates our model for PLN interaction with SERCA2a. We deduce that PLN monomers (M) are the active species and that their dissociation from pentamers (P) is an essential step in SERCA2a (S) inhibition by PLN. The fact that PLN is up to 25% depolymerized under normal conditions,[28,34] implies that PLN monomers are normally in relatively abundant supply. The dissociation constants for both the PLN pentamer (K_{d1}) and the PLN monomer/SERCA2a heterodimer (K_{d2}) will control both the PLN monomer concentration [M] and the concentration of the monomer-inhibited form of SERCA2a [MS], as defined below:

$$P \overset{K_{d1}}{\leftrightarrow} 5M \qquad (K_{d1} = [P] / [M]^5)$$

$$M + S \overset{K_{d2}}{\leftrightarrow} MS \quad (K_{d2} = [MS] / [M]\,[S])$$

The baseline of inhibition of wild-type SERCA2a by wild-type PLN will be proportional to [MS], but [MS] can be altered by mutations or by physiological perturbations. Mutations that enhance PLN monomer formation will alter K_{d1}, increasing [M] and, through mass action, [MS]. Mutations that increase the affinity of the interaction between M and S will alter K_{d2} and increase [MS], while mutations that decrease the affinity between M and S will decrease [MS]. Binding of Ca^{2+} to the transmembrane helices of SERCA2a[35] and phosphorylation of the cytoplasmic domain of PLN[1,3,5] alter K_{d2}, enhancing PLN/SERCA2a heterodimer dissociation and activating SERCA2a.

DOMAIN IB MUTANTS AFFECT K_{d2}

Our postulate that dissociation of the PNL/SERCA2a complex is a second determinant of PLN inhibitory function is relevant to our findings with the domain Ib mutants.[21] They form pentamers that dissociate into the normal proportion of monomers, indicating that K_{d1} is not altered. However, they could affect dissociation of the PLN/SERCA2a complex, thereby leading to a more stable form of the inhibited PLN/SERCA2a complex and manifesting as a gain of inhibitory function by the mutant. As a test of the hypothesis that the domain Ib mutants increase the stability of the PLN/SERCA2a complex, we combined a domain II mutant, which was devoid of function, presumably because mutation had diminished its affinity for interacting residues in the transmembrane domain of SERCA2a, with the strong gain-of-function mutant, N27A, which should have an enhanced affinity for an interaction site at the membrane interface in the structure of SERCA2a. In line with our hypothesis, we recovered partial inhibitory function for the double mutant N27A/N34A.

A further test of the hypothesis that domain Ib and domain II mutants increase PLN inhibitory function by different mechanisms involved combining two strong inhibitory mutations, one from domain Ib and one from domain II. The gain of function for the double mutant N30A/I40A was nearly the sum of the gain of function for the N30A mutant plus the gain of function for the I40A mutant, in line with our view that these two mutations lead to different mechanisms of inhibition, the effects of which are likely to be additive. The results of analysis of double mutants are, therefore, fully consistent with the postulate that mutant N30A affects PLN/SERCA2a dissociation, while I40A affects PLN pentamer dissociation.

FIGURE I highlights the fact that gain of function accompanies mutations in domain Ib and in domain II. Different explanations are required for the gain of function that follows mutation of specific residues in domain II and for the gain of function that follows mutation of specific residues in domain Ib. We propose that the gain of function mutants result in higher concentrations of the inhibited PLN/SERCA2a complex, but through at least two different mechanisms—enhanced formation of monomers in the case of the domain II mutants, and enhanced stabilization of PLN/SERCA2a interactions in the case of the domain Ib mutants.

MEDICAL RELEVANCE OF PLN/SERCA2a INTERACTION SITES

Our observations have important physiological and medical relevance. If mutations of Phe^{32}, Ile^{33}, Leu^{37}, Ile^{40}, Leu^{43}, Leu^{44}, Ile^{47}, Met^{50}, and Leu^{51} were to occur naturally, we predict that they would increase [MS] to levels that would inhibit Ca^{2+} removal from the cytoplasm of myocardial cells. Although other Ca^{2+} removal systems might compensate,[36] we predict that the resulting disruption in Ca^{2+} regulation would lead to inherited cardiomyopathies. We also predict that mutations such as the N27A mutation in the domain Ib loop (FIG. 1), or elsewhere in PLN or SERCA2a, which would increase the affinity between M and S, would also increase [MS], leading to gain of PLN inhibitory function and, potentially, to inherited cardiomyopathies.

In the context of this symposium, it is apparent that the ability to manipulate the interaction between PLN and SERCA2a through drug therapy would have the potential for improvement of function in a failing heart. It is our hope that understanding of the mechanism of interaction between PLN and SERCA2a will contribute to the eventual development of useful therapies for failing cardiac function.

ACKNOWLEDGMENTS

We gratefully acknowledge the contributions of Drs. Michihiko Tada, Junichi Fujii, N. Michael Green, and Robert G. Johnson during the course of the work described in this review, and the technical assistance of Kazimierz Kurzydlowski, Vijay. K. Khanna, and Stella de Leon.

REFERENCES

1. FUJII, J., M. KADOMA, M. TADA, H. TODA & F. SAKIYAMA. 1986. Biochem. Biophys. Res. Commun. **138:** 1044–1050.

2. Fujii, J., A. Ueno, K. Kitano, S. Tanaka, M. Kadoma & M. Tada. 1987. J. Clin. Invest. **79:** 301–304.
3. Simmerman, H. K., J. H. Collins, J. L. Theibert, A. D. Wegener & L. R. Jones. 1986. J. Biol. Chem. **261:** 13333–13341.
4. Mortishire-Smith, R. J., S. M. Pitzenberger, C. J. Burke, C. R. Middaugh, V. M. Garsky & R. G. Johnson. 1995. Biochemistry **34:** 7603–7613.
5. James, P., M. Inui, M. Tada, M. Chiesi & E. Carafoli. 1989. Nature **342:** 90–92.
6. Suzuki, T. & J. H. Wang. 1986. J. Biol. Chem. **261:** 7018–7023.
7. Inui, M., B. K. Chamberlain, A. Saito & S. Fleischer. 1986. J. Biol. Chem. **261:** 1794–1800.
8. Kim, H. W., N. A. Steenaart, D. G. Ferguson & E. G. Kranias. 1990. J. Biol. Chem. **265:** 1702–1709.
9. Sasaki, T., M. Inui, Y. Kimura, T. Kuzuya & M. Tada. 1992. J. Biol. Chem. **267:** 1674–1679.
10. Szymanska, G., H. W. Kim, J. Cuppoletti & E. G. Kranias. 1992. Mol. Cell. Biochem. **114:** 65–71.
11. Hughes, G., J. M. East & A. G. Lee. 1994. Biochem. J. **303:** 511–516.
12. Hughes, G., A. P. Starling, R. P. Sharma, J. M. East & A. G. Lee. 1996. Biochem. J. **318:** 973–979.
13. Reddy, L. G., L. R. Jones, S. E. Cala, J. J. O'Brian, S. A. Tatulian & D. L. Stokes. 1995. J. Biol. Chem. **270:** 9390–9397.
14. Jones, L. R. & L. J. Field. 1993. J. Biol. Chem. **268:** 11486–11488.
15. Fujii, J., K. Maruyama, M. Tada & D. H. MacLennan. 1989. J. Biol. Chem. **264:** 12950–12955.
16. Fujii, J., K. Maruyama, M. Tada & D. H. MacLennan. 1990. FEBS Lett. **273:** 232–234.
17. Toyofuku, T., K. Kurzydlowski, M. Tada & D. H. MacLennan. 1993. J. Biol. Chem. **268:** 2809–2815.
18. Toyofuku, T., K. Kurzydlowski, M. Tada & D. H. MacLennan. 1994. J. Biol. Chem. **269:** 3088–3094.
19. Toyofuku, T., K. Kurzydlowski, M. Tada & D. H. MacLennan. 1994. J. Biol. Chem. **269:** 22929–22932.
20. Toyofuku, T., K. Kurzydlowski, J. Lytton & D. H. MacLennan. 1992. J. Biol. Chem. **267:** 14490–14496.
21. Kimura, Y., K. Kurzydlowski, M. Tada & D. H. MacLennan. 1998. J. Biol. Chem. **273:** In press.
22. Kimura, Y., K. Kurzydlowski, M. Tada & D. H. MacLennan. 1996. J. Biol. Chem. **271:** 21726–21731.
23. Burk, S. E., J. Lytton, D. H. MacLennan & G. E. Shull. 1989. J. Biol. Chem. **264:** 18561–18568.
24. Morris, G. L., H. C. Cheng, J. Colyer & J. H. Wang. 1991. J. Biol. Chem. **266:** 11270–11275.
25. Briggs, F. N., K. F. Lee, A. W. Wechsler & L. R. Jones. 1992. J. Biol. Chem. **267:** 26056–26061.
26. Rice, W. J. & D. H. MacLennan. 1996. J. Biol. Chem. **271:** 31412–31419.
27. MacLennan, D. H., D. M. Clarke, T. W. Loo & I. S. Skerjanc. 1992. Acta Physiol. Scand. Suppl. **607:** 141–150.
28. Kimura, Y., K. Kurzydlowski, M. Tada & D. H. MacLennan. 1997. J. Biol. Chem. **272:** 15061–15064.
29. Autry, J. M. & L. R. Jones. 1997. J. Biol. Chem. **272:** 15872–15880.
30. Jones, L. R., H. K. Simmerman, W. W. Wilson, F. R. Gurd & A. D. Wegener. 1985. J. Biol. Chem. **260:** 7721–7730.
31. Arkin, I. T., P. D. Adams, K. R. MacKenzie, M. A. Lemmon, A. T. Brunger & D. M. Engelman. 1994. EMBO J. **13:** 4757–4764.
32. Simmerman, H. K. B., Y. M. Kobayashi, J. M. Autry & L. R. Jones. 1996. J. Biol. Chem. **271:** 5941–5946.
33. Adams, P. D., I. T. Arkin, D. M. Engelman & A. T. Brunger. 1995. Nature Struct. Biol. **2:** 154–162.

34. CORNEA, R. L., L. R. JONES, J. M. AUTRY & D. D. THOMAS. 1997. Biochemistry **36:** 2960–2967.
35. CLARKE, D. M., T. W. LOO, G. INESI & D. H. MACLENNAN. 1989. Nature **339:** 476–478.
36. ODERMATT, A., P. E. TASCHNER, V. K. KHANNA, H. F. BUSCH, G. KARPATI, C. K. JABLECKI, M. H. BREUNING & D. H. MACLENNAN. 1996. Nature Genet. **14:** 191–194.

Influences of Increased Expression of the Ca^{2+} ATPase of the Sarcoplasmic Reticulum by a Transgenic Approach on Cardiac Contractility

WOLFGANG H. DILLMANN[a]

Department of Medicine, University of California, San Diego, 9500 Gilman Drive, San Diego, California 92093-0618, USA

ABSTRACT: Congestive heart failure is a significant clinical problem and leads to abnormalities in Ca^{2+} transients and to decreases in the level of the Ca^{2+} ATPase of the sarcoplasmic reticulum according to reports to some investigators. The Ca^{2+} ATPase of the sarcoplasmic reticulum (SERCA2) contributes in an important manner to diastolic Ca^{2+} lowering and relaxation of the heart. To determine the contractile alterations resulting from increased SERCA2 expression, we generated transgenic mice overexpressing a rat SERCA2 transgene. In these mice, SERCA2 mRNA was increased 2.6-fold, the relative synthesis rate of SERCA2 protein 1.8-fold, and SERCA2 protein levels 1.2-fold. Functional analysis of Ca^{2+} handling and contractile parameters in isolated cardiac myocytes indicated that the intracellular Ca^{2+} decline and myocyte relengthening were each accelerated by 22–23%. In addition, studies in isolated papillary muscles showed that the time to half-maximal post-rest potentiation was significantly shorter, hinting at an increased Ca^{2+} loading of the sarcoplasmic reticulum. Furthermore, *in vivo* cardiac functional studies demonstrated a significant accelerated contraction and relaxation in SERCA2 transgenic mice. We also cloned a SERCA2 transgene and mutants of the phospholamban gene into E1 deleted replication-deficient human adenovirus 5 viral vectors and infected cardiac myocytes. In the cardiac myocytes, endogenous SERCA2 levels were decreased by PMA treatment. Infection of such myocytes with a SERCA2 expressing adenovirus could reconstitute the Ca^{2+} transient, and augmented oxalate facilitated SERCA2 Ca^{2+} uptake. In addition, phospholamban mutants with changes of basic to acidic amino acids in the cytoplasmic domain increased SERCA2 activity by 30–35%. These findings, therefore, suggest that increased SERCA2 activity can be achieved by increasing SERCA2 levels or by expressing phospholamban mutants. Increased SERCA2 activity can lead to significant enhancements of Ca^{2+} transients and myocardial contractility.

Congestive heart failure is a significant clinical problem in the United States, with the occurrence of congestive heart failure by clinical criteria in about 2% of the United States population leading to an overall mortality of 50% within five years.[1] About 40% of patients have diastolic heart failure. Abnormalities in the Ca^{2+} transient have been linked to cardiac hypertrophy and congestive heart failure.[2] Several reports indicate that a delayed decline of the free cytoplasmic Ca^{2+} concentration is linked to decreased levels of expression of the Ca^{2+} ATPase of the sarcoplasmic reticulum (SERCA2) in material obtained from patients with dilated cardiomyopathy.[3,4] Other investigators have not observed such a decrease in SERCA2 protein levels in failing human hearts.[5] Several recent reports have indicated that the Ca^{2+} pumping activity of SERCA2 is a major

[a] Phone: 619-534-9934; fax: 619-534-9932.

contributor to Ca^{2+} lowering. SERCA2 contributes 70–80% to total diastolic Ca^{2+} lowering, whereas the Na^+/Ca^{2+} exchanger contributes 10–15%; and the remainder of Ca^{2+} lowering is achieved by the Ca^{2+} ATPase of the sarcolemma.[6] SERCA2 is localized in the longitudinal part of the sarcoplasmic reticulum (SR) and pumps 2 mol of Ca^{2+} for 1 mol of ATP converted to ADP. SERCA2 activity is markedly inhibited by the unphosphorylated form of phospholamban, which lowers the Ca^{2+} affinity for the SERCA2 pump.[7]

Because of reports of decreased SERCA2 levels in failing hearts it would be desirable to have a transgenic animal model expressing a SERCA2 transgene in the heart. We wanted, therefore, to determine if a SERCA2 transgene can be expressed in cardiac myocytes of the mouse heart and what the biochemical and functional consequences of increased SERCA2 expression would be.

We, therefore, produced SERCA2 transgenic mice by a conventional approach.[8] A rat SERCA2 transgene was driven by a human cytomegalovirus enhancer chicken β-actin promoter.[9] The SERCA2 transgene included the first two introns of the rat SERCA2 gene, and the third exon was fused within the reading frame to the remainder of rat SERCA2 cDNA. The inclusion of intronic sequences enhances transgene expression in transgenic animals.[10] We obtained two transgenic lines that passed the transgene to their offspring. One of these lines, CJ5, was characterized in further detail. These animals were used in the heterozygous state. A second line, CJ2, showed an increase in SERCA2 expression in heterozygous animals, but at a lower level than that observed in the CJ5 animals; and these animals were bred to a homozygous status. Similar results related to effects of SERCA2 were obtained in the CJ5 and CJ2 lines; however, most of the results discussed in this report were derived from the CJ5 line. The animals were fully viable, and no difference in body weight, heart weight, heart weight/body weight ratio, heart rate, left ventricular systolic pressure, or left ventricular end diastolic pressure was noted between wild-type mice and SERCA2 transgenic mice.[8] On Northern blots, mRNA levels for several gene products involved in Ca^{2+} flux were characterized. In heterozygous CJ5 mice, the total amount of SERCA2 mRNA was 2.6 fold higher than in transgene-negative litter mates. In contrast, in heterozygous CJ2 mice, SERCA2 mRNA levels were increased by 1.5 fold. The level of mRNA coding for the ryanodine receptor and calsequestrin showed no significant difference in wild-type and transgenic mice. In contrast, the mRNA for phospholamban was increased by 43%, and the Na^+/Ca^{2+} exchanger mRNA was increased by 83% in SERCA2 transgenic mice. Protein levels were quantitated by Western blot analysis, and the increase in phospholamban mRNA and the Na^+/Ca^{2+} exchanger mRNA levels did not lead to an increase in the corresponding protein levels. In contrast, the increase in SERCA2 mRNA levels led to a 20% increase in SERCA2 protein levels when normalized either by phospholamban or β-actin proteins. A marked discrepancy between a much more significant increase in SERCA2 mRNA levels versus SERCA2 protein levels has, therefore, to be noted. To explore this discrepancy in further detail, the relative synthesis rate of SERCA2 protein was determined and was found to be increased by 82% in SERCA2-expressing mice versus wild-type mice. It, therefore, appears that the lower total amount of SERCA2 protein versus SERCA2 mRNA cannot result only from a decreased synthesis rate, but must be, in part, related to an increased turnover of the SERCA2 protein in the transgenic animals.

In order to determine if the increased SERCA2 expression resulted in functional alterations, we prepared adult cardiac myocytes and determined Ca^{2+} transients and contractile behavior in those myocytes.[8] We normalized Fura-2 obtained transients to the respective basal diastolic and peak systolic ratios. The transients declined more rapidly in SERCA2 transgenic mice than in control mice. The time to reach a 50% decline was 23% faster than in control myocytes. Contractile properties of cardiac myocytes were determined by a standard video camera interfaced with a video edge detector. The $T_{1/2}$ for 50% maximal relaxation was 22% faster in transgenic myocytes than in control myocytes. These functional parameters in isolated cardiac myocytes, therefore, corresponded to the 20% increase in SERCA2 protein levels. To investigate potential changes of intracellular Ca^{2+} handling and to get an indirect insight into Ca^{2+} loading of the SR, the contractile behavior of isolated papillary muscle was examined by post-rest potentiation studies. The stress of the post-rest contraction increased with the duration of the rest interval for muscles from transgene-negative litter mates and from SERCA2 transgenic animals. The time to half maximal potentiation was significantly shorter in muscle from SERCA2 transgenic mice than in control mice. These findings indirectly indicate that the SR was loaded by Ca^{2+} to a higher extent than the SR in transgene-negative mice. Preliminary results obtained in collaboration with Dr. Barry (Salt Lake City, UT) indicated that the Ca^{2+} loading of the SR in the transgenic mice was increased by 20%.

Cardiac function under *in vivo* conditions was evaluated by cardiac characterization. We found that the dP/dt_{max} was significantly more positive and the LV dP/dt_{min} was significantly more negative in SERCA2 transgenic mice in comparison to wild-type mice.[8] In addition, we calculated the preload independent isovolumic relaxation parameter tau. Tau was significantly shorter in SERCA2 transgenic mice by 20% in comparison to wild-type mice.

In summary, our results indicate that transgenic mice can be constructed that overexpress the rat SERCA2 transgene in cardiac myocytes. This leads to a marked increase in SERCA2 mRNA expression, but to a much lower level of SERCA2 protein expression. The reason for this lower SERCA2 protein expression is currently unclear, but one could speculate that the longitudinal SR has only limited additional incorporation sites for SERCA2 pumps. In addition, a 20% increase in SERCA2 protein expression from a SERCA2 transgene leads to corresponding accelerations of the downslope of the Ca^{2+} transient, resulting in an increased speed of shortening of isolated myocytes and to an increase of dP/dt_{max} and dP/dt_{min} under *in vivo* conditions. The increase in systolic parameters results, most likely, from the increased availability of Ca^{2+} for release from the SR during the contraction cycle.

In addition, we wanted to determine if the expression of a SERCA2 transgene can compensate for decreased expression of endogenous SERCA2 message. Attempts to down-regulate the endogenous SERCA2 gene in the mouse by introducing pressure overload using abdominal aortic constriction and salt loading did not result in significant lowering of SERCA2 mRNA. Preliminary results indicated that in such hearts cardiac hypertrophy developed, as evidenced by a 30% increase in the heart weight/body weight ratio and a significant increase in atrial naturetic factor (ANF) mRNA levels. As an alternate maneuver, we introduced hypothyroidism in wild-type and SERCA2 transgenic mice to lower endogenous SERCA2 gene expression. Previous work has indicated that thyroid hormone markedly up-regulates the endogenous SERCA2 gene.[11] Quantitating mRNA from myosin heavy chain (MHC) β and SERCA2 on Northern blots indicated that putting mice on a low-iodine diet and propylthiouracil (PTU) in their drinking water significantly increased MHCβ mRNA levels in the heart of hypothyroid mice. Previous work has indicated that MHCβ increases markedly with hypothyroidism.[12] In wild-type mice, SERCA2 mRNA levels decreased by 55%. In contrast, in transgenic mice made hypothyroid, SERCA2 mRNA levels were similar to those found in euthyroid control mice. Maintenance of SERCA2 mRNA levels in the hypothyroid transgenic mice also led to a corresponding compensation when force development and decline were measured in isolated papillary muscle from these different mice. These results showed that at a stimulation frequency of 2 Hz, the relaxation time to 90% of developed force RT 90 was 122% in SERCA2 hypothyroid mice, compared to the function in transgene-negative hypothyroid animals. This compensation occurred in spite of increasing phospholamban levels in hypothyroid animals.[13] These findings, therefore, indicate that a hypothyroidism-induced decrease in endogenous SERCA2 gene expression is more than adequately compensated for at the mRNA and functional level by the expression of a SERCA2 transgene.

It is of significant interest to determine if the pressure overload–induced decrease in SERCA2 protein levels and pumping activity and alterations in Ca^{2+} transients can be compensated by transgene expression. In order to address this question, we constructed in collaboration with Dr. Vetter and Dr. Ganten in Berlin SERCA2 transgenic rats using the same construct that was used to produce SERCA2 transgenic mice. Preliminary analysis of these animals indicates that SERCA2 mRNA levels are increased by 55% in SERCA2 transgenic rats. This results in a 26% increase of cardiac SR Ca^{2+} uptake measured by a Ca^{2+} oxalate binding assay in left ventricular homogenates from SERCA2 transgenic rats versus control rats. In future studies, pressure overload–induced decreases in endogenous SERCA2 expression will be induced, and compensatory effects of SERCA2 transgene expression will be examined. Previous studies from several groups[14,15] and preliminary data from our laboratory indicate that constriction of the ascending aorta in 120-g rats leads to a significant 40–50% lowering of SERCA2 mRNA levels 10 days after applying the aortic constriction.

An alternate approach to increasing SERCA2 transgene expression in cardiac myocytes is using viral vectors that encode the appropriate transgene to infect myocytes. We cloned a rat SERCA2 transgene into the E1 region of a human adenovirus 5 vector.[16] The resulting construct is replication deficient, but infects over 90% of neonatal or adult cardiac myocytes in cell culture. Adenoviral SERCA2 transgene expression leads to a very significant increase of SERCA2 mRNA and SERCA2 protein in cardiac myocytes. In order to determine if adenovirus-derived SERCA2 transgene products could compensate for decreases in endogenous SERCA2 level, we treated cultured neonatal myocytes with the phorbol ester phorbol myristate acetate (PMA), which leads to a significant decrease of endogenous SERCA2 expression.[17,18] PMA-treated neonatal myocytes had a 75% reduction in SERCA2 mRNA, which led to a 40% reduction in SERCA2 protein levels. SERCA2 adenovirus infection increased SERCA2 mRNA levels 2.5-fold over the control value and reconstituted SERCA2 protein levels in PMA-treated cells.[16] The increase in SERCA2 protein levels was associated with a 32% reduction in the time for decline of the IndoI Ca^{2+} transient to the half-maximal level. In addition, a 34% augmentation of oxalate-faciliated SR Ca^{2+} uptake was also occurring in SERCA2 adenovirus–infected neonatal myocytes. These results, therefore, show that adenovirus-mediated expression of a SERCA2 transgene can reconstitute the depressed endogenous SERCA2 levels induced by phorbol ester treatment. The restitution of protein levels are accompanied by corresponding changes in the shortening behavior and in augmented SR Ca^{2+} ATPase uptake. It is, therefore, conceivable that such an approach may be used in the future to normalize altered Ca^{2+} regulation in heart failure. However, it needs to be mentioned that currently gene therapy–based approaches for the cardiovascular system using currently existing viral vectors meet with relatively limited success. In our work injection of adenoviral vectors into the coronary artery of rabbits leads only to minimal infection of cardiac myocytes in the left ventricle. However, newer viral vectors may circumvent this problem.

Phospholamban in its unphosphorylated state markedly inhibits the SR Ca^{2+} ATPase pump.[7] We, therefore, wanted to determine if mutations of phospholamban in the cytoplasmic domain of the phospholamban protein, where it interacts with SERCA2,[19] could lead to increased SERCA2 activity in neonatal or adult cardiac myocytes. For this purpose, we cloned phospholamban in the antisense orientation into adenoviral vectors. In addition, mutants of rat phospholamban, generated by changing the 3rd amino acid, lysine, to glutamic acid and the 14th amino acid, arginine, to glutamic acid were cloned into adenoviral vectors. Western blot analysis of myocytes infected with these adenoviral vectors indicated that the antisense phospholamban significantly lowers phospholamban protein levels. The mutant phospholamban leads to a different migration behavior of the pentameric phospholamban. Functional effects were determined using a Ca^{2+} oxalate-facilitated uptake assay in neonatal cardiac myocytes.[16] Antisense phospholamban increased SERCA2 activity, as measured by the EC_{50} of the Ca^{2+} activity, by 35%; and the mutant phospholamban K3ER14E increased SERCA2 activity by 31%. In adult cardiac myocytes infected with adenoviral vectors expressing the antisense phospholamban, SERCA2 activity was increased by 27%, and the mutant phospholamban increased SERCA2 activity by 35%.

These findings indicate, therefore, that phospholamban mutants appropriately integrate into the SR membrane and compete with wild-type phospholamban for interaction with SERCA2 in cardiac myocytes. Future gene therapy–based approaches may, therefore, also take advantage of alterations in phospholamban-SERCA2 interaction.

Approaches directed at an improvement of contractile function of the failing heart by increasing SERCA2 activity have been briefly described in this report. It is currently unclear if the desired enhancement of the Ca^{2+} transients leads to an overall contractile improvement without less-desirable additional effects. For example, increased SERCA2 activity will lead to increased ATP consumption, which may be detrimental if the failing heart is starved for high-energy phosphates. In addition, increasing SERCA2 activity may increase the Ca^{2+} filling of the SR, which could result in an undesirable increased excitability of cardiac myocytes. Investigating transgenic animals and myocytes infected with viral vectors resulting in different alterations in proteins participating in Ca^{2+} handling will provide insights into this question.

REFERENCES

1. Lenfant, C. 1994. Report of the task force on research in heart failure. Circulation **90:** 1118–1123.
2. Gwathmey, J. K., L. Copelas, R. MacKinnon *et al.* 1987. Abnormal intracellular calcium handling in myocardium from patients with end-stage heart failure. Circ. Res. **61:** 70–76.
3. Meyer, M., W. Schillinger, B. Pieske *et al.* 1995. Alterations of sarcoplasmic reticulum proteins in failing human dilated cardiomyopathy. Circulation **92:** 778–784.
4. Arai, M., N. R. Alpert, D. H. MacLennan *et al.* 1993. Alterations in sarcoplasmic reticulum gene expression in human heart failure. Circ. Res. **72:** 463–469.
5. Movsesian, M. A., M. Karimi, K. Green & L. R. Jones. 1994. Ca^{2+}-transporting ATPase, phospholamban, and calsequestrin levels in nonfailing and failing human myocardium. Circulation **90:** 653–657.
6. Bassani, R. A., J. W. M. Bassani & D. M. Bers. 1992. Mitochondrial and sarcolemmal Ca^{2+} transport reduce $[Ca^{2+}]$ during caffeine contractures in rabbit cardiac myocytes. J. Physiol. **453:** 591–608.
7. Tada, M., M. Inui, M. Yamada *et al.* 1983. Effects of phospholamban phosphorylation catalyzed by adenosine 3′:5′-monophosphate and calmodulin-dependent protein kinases on calcium transport ATPase of cardiac sarcoplasmic reticulum. J. Mol. Cell. Cardiol. **15:** 335–346.
8. He, H., F. J. Giordano, R. Hilal-Dandan *et al.* 1997. Overexpression of the rat sarcoplasmic reticulum Ca^{2+} ATPase gene in the heart of transgenic mice accelerates calcium transients and cardiac relaxation. J. Clin. Invest. **100:** 380–389.
9. Niwa, H., K. I. Yamamura & J. I. Miyzaki. 1991. Efficient selection for high expression transfectants with a novel, eukaryotic vector. Gene **108:** 193–200.
10. Choi, T., M. Huang, C. Gorman & R. Jaenisch. 1991. A generic intron increases gene expression in transgenic mice. Mol. Cell. Biol. **11:** 3070–3074.

11. ROHRER, D. K., R. HARTONG & W. H. DILLMANN. 1990. Influence of thyroid hormone and retinoic acid on slow sarcoplasmic reticulum Ca^{2+} ATPase and myosin heavy chain α gene expression in cardiac myocytes. J. Biol. Chem. **266:** 8638–8646.
12. SINHA, A. M., P. K. UMEDA, C. J. KAVINSKY *et al.* 1982. Molecular cloning of mRNA sequences for cardiac alpha- and beta-form myosin heavy chains: Expression in ventricles of normal, hypothyroid, and thyrotoxic rabbits. Proc. Natl. Acad. Sci. USA **79:** 5847–5851.
13. KISS, E., G. JAKAB, E. G. KRANIAS & I. EDES. 1994. Thyroid hormone-induced alterations in phospholamban protein expression. Circ. Res. **75:** 245–251.
14. DE LA BASTIE, D., D. LEVITSKY, L. RAPPAPORT *et al.* 1990. Function of the sarcoplasmic reticulum and expression of its Ca^{2+} ATPase gene in pressure overload–induced cardiac hypertrophy in the rat. Circ. Res. **66:** 554–564.
15. KOMURO, I., M. KURABAYASHI, Y. SHIBAZAKI *et al.* 1989. Molecular cloning and characterization of a Ca^{2+} + Mg^{2+}–dependent adenosine triphosphatase from rat cardiac sarcoplasmic reticulum. J. Clin. Invest. **83:** 1102–1108.
16. GIORDANO, F., H. HE, P. MCDONOUGH *et al.* 1997 Adenovirus-mediated gene transfer reconstitutes depressed sarcoplasmic reticulum Ca^{2+} ATPase levels and shortens prolonged cardiac myocyte Ca^{2+} transients. Circulation **96:** 400–403.
17. HARTONG, R., F. J. VILLARREAL, F. GIORDANO *et al.* 1996. Phorbol myristate acetate induced hypertrophy of neonatal rat cardiac myocytes is associated with deceased sarcoplasmic reticulum Ca^{2+} ATPase (SERCA2) gene expression and calcium reuptake. J. Mol. Cell. Cardiol. **28:** 2467–2477.
18. QI, M., J. W. M. BASSANI, D. M. BERS & A. M. SAMAREL. 1996. Phorbol 12-myristate 13-acetate alters SR Ca^{2+} ATPase gene expression in cultured neonatal rat heart cells. Am. J. Physiol. **271:** H1031–H1039.
19. KIMURA, Y., K. KURZYDLOWSKI, M. TADA & D. H. MACLENNAN. 1997. Phospholamban inhibitory function is activated by depolymerization. J. Biol. Chem. **272:** 15061–15064.

Phospholamban Ablation and Compensatory Responses in the Mammalian Heart[a]

GUOXIANG CHU,[b] DONALD G. FERGUSON,[c] ISTVAN EDES,[d] EVA KISS,[e] YOJI SATO,[b] AND EVANGELIA G. KRANIAS[b,f]

[b]*Department of Pharmacology and Cell Biophysics, University of Cincinnati College of Medicine, Cincinnati, Ohio 45267-0575, USA*

[c]*Department of Anatomy, Case Western Reserve University, Cleveland, Ohio 44106, USA*

[d]*Department of Heart and Lung Diseases, University Medical School Debrecen, 4004 Debrecen, Hungary*

[e]*Division of Cardiology, 2nd Department of Medicine, Szent-Gyorgyi Medical University, H-6701 Szeged, Hungary*

ABSTRACT: Phospholamban is a low molecular weight phosphoprotein in cardiac sarcoplasmic reticulum. The regulatory role of phospholamban *in vivo* has recently been elucidated by targeting the gene of this protein in embryonic stem cells and generating phospholamban-deficient mice. The phospholamban knockout hearts exhibited significantly enhanced contractile parameters and attenuated responses to β-agonists. The hyperdynamic cardiac function of the phospholamban knockout mice was not accompanied by any cytoarchitectural abnormalities or alterations in the expression levels of the cardiac sarcoplasmic reticulum Ca^{2+}-ATPase, calsequestrin, Na^+-Ca^{2+} exchanger, or the contractile proteins. Furthermore, the attenuation of the cardiac responses to β-agonists was not due to alterations in the phosphorylation levels of the other key cardiac phosphoproteins in the phospholamban knockout hearts. However, ablation of phospholamban was associated with down-regulation of the ryanodine receptor, which suggests that a cross-talk between cardiac sarcoplasmic reticulum Ca^{2+} uptake and Ca^{2+} release occurred in an attempt to maintain Ca^{2+} homeostasis in these hyperdynamic phospholamban knockout hearts.

Phospholamban is a low molecular weight phosphoprotein, associated with cardiac sarcoplasmic reticulum (SR). The dephosphorylated form of phospholamban is an inhibitor of the SR Ca^{2+}-ATPase affinity for Ca^{2+}, and phosphorylation of phospholamban relieves its inhibitory effects.[1–3] *In vitro* studies have shown that phospholamban can become phosphorylated at Ser^{10} by protein kinase C, at Ser^{16} by cAMP-dependent protein kinase, and at Thr^{17} by Ca^{2+}-calmodulin–dependent protein kinase.[4,5] The stimulatory effects of the protein kinases can be reversed by an endogenous protein phosphatase activity.[6] Phospholamban is also phosphorylated in intact, beating hearts during isoproterenol stimulation.[7,8] The increases in phospholamban phosphorylation are associated with increases in SR Ca^{2+} uptake rates and increases in the rates of myocardial relaxation, observed during β-adrenergic stimulation of the heart.[7,9]

The role of phospholamban in the regulation of basal myocardial contractility has

[a] This work was supported by National Institutes of Health Grants HL26057, HL22619, HL07382, RR12358, and TW00861.

[f] Address for correspondence: Evangelia G. Kranias, Ph.D., Department of Pharmacology and Cell Biophysics, University of Cincinnati College of Medicine, 231 Bethesda Avenue, Cincinnati, Ohio 45267-0575. Phone: 513-558-2377; fax: 513-558-2269; e-mail: Kraniaeg@email.uc.edu

been recently elucidated through the development of a phospholamban knockout mouse.[10] These mice, created using gene-targeting methodology in embryonic stem cells, exhibited hyperdynamic cardiac function. The cardiac phenotype was analyzed utilizing an integrative approach and combining studies at the subcellular, organ, and whole animal levels.[10–12] The phospholamban knockout hearts exhibited significant increases in the SR Ca^{2+}-ATPase affinity for Ca^{2+} and in the basal contractile parameters compared with wild-type littermates. Furthermore, the inotropic and lusitropic effects of isoproterenol on cardiac function were significantly attenuated in phospholamban knockout mice compared with wild-type mice.[10–13] Collectively, these studies indicated that phospholamban is a critical inhibitor of basal cardiac function and a major regulator of the heart's responses to β-adrenergic agonists.

However, it is not presently clear whether cardiac compensatory mechanisms accompanied phospholamban ablation to accommodate the enhanced SR Ca^{2+}-ATPase activity and maintain Ca^{2+} homeostasis in the myocardium. It is often observed that in genetically modified mice, deletion of a specific gene leads to enhancement of the expression or function of other genes, and such underlying compensation may compromise or contribute to the observed phenotype.[14] Thus, it becomes important to examine whether such molecular cross-talk among genes occurred in the phospholamban knockout mouse to accommodate the functional consequences of phospholamban ablation. The primary candidate genes include those encoding for the SR Ca^{2+}-cycling proteins: the Ca^{2+}-ATPase, calsequestrin, and ryanodine receptor. Other important candidates in the regulation of Ca^{2+} homeostasis in the myocardium are the Na^+-Ca^{2+} exchanger and the contractile proteins. Furthermore, alterations in the major cardiac regulatory phosphoproteins to accommodate phospholamban ablation may be responsible for the attenuated β-adrenergic responses in the phospholamban knockout hearts. Thus, it is very important to investigate the contribution of possible compensatory mechanisms in the cardiac phenotype of the phospholamban knockout mouse and assess the extent to which such mechanisms compromise the biochemical and physiological effects of phospholamban ablation.

METHODS

Generation of Phospholamban Gene-Targeted Mice

The homozygous mutant mice deficient in phospholamban were generated by gene-targeting methodology in embryonic stem cells as previously described.[10] The phospholamban-targeting construct was generated from the mouse phospholamban gene. The embryonic stem cells containing the expected homologous recombination event were detected by polymerase chain reaction (PCR) and Southern blot analyses, microinjected into blastocysts, and implanted into pseudopregnant foster mothers. The heterozygous offspring harboring a targeted-phospholamban allele were bred to homozygosity. Wild-type littermates with identical mixed background were used as controls.

Electron Microscopic Studies

The mouse hearts were rapidly removed and perfused using a Langendorff apparatus. Following 5 minutes of equilibration with Kreb's solution, the hearts were perfused with fixative (2.5% glutaraldehyde buffered in 0.1 M Na-cacodylate) for 2 minutes. The papillary muscles were dissected from the left ventricles and fixed by immersion in buffered glutaraldehyde for an additional 90 minutes. The heart tissue was washed in 0.1 M Na-cacodylate, post-fixed in 1% osmium tetroxide for an hour, dehydrated through a graded series of ethanol, and embedded in Epon epoxy resin. Thin sections were cut using a Reichert Ultracut S and stained in uranyl acetate and lead citrate; electron micrographs were obtained using a JEOL 100C transmission electron microscope.

Heart Perfusions

Mouse hearts were perfused in a Langendorff mode as previously described.[13] Briefly, the heart was perfused with modified Krebs buffer solution (37 °C) saturated with 95% O_2 and 5% CO_2. A PE-50 catheter was inserted via a pulmonary vein into the left ventricle and forced through the ventricular apex. The catheter was attached to a pressure transducer to measure the contractile parameters, which was coupled with a computerized data acquisition system (MicroMed). The maximal rates of the intraventricular pressure development (+dP/dt) and decline (–dP/dt) were monitored as indices for contraction and relaxation. The time to peak pressure (TPP) and half–relaxation time (RT1/2) were also calculated from this pressure recording.

Northern and Dot Blot Analysis

Total RNA was prepared from whole hearts by the method of Chomczynski and Sacchi.[15] Total RNA was analyzed by either Northern blot or dot blot hybridization assays.[16] For Northern analysis, 10 µg total RNA was heated at 60 °C for 5 minutes, size-fractionated on 0.8% agarose gels containing 2.2 M formaldehyde, and transferred onto gene screen membranes. Northern blot analysis was used to confirm the specificities of the synthesized oligonucleotide and cDNA probes used in this study, and to determine the relative levels of the Na^+-Ca^{2+} exchanger mRNA. For dot blot analysis, two-fold serial dilutions of 10 µg total RNA were applied to gene screen membranes using a BIO-RAD dot blot filtration apparatus. The membranes were baked at 80 °C for 2 h under vacuum, prehybridized for 1–2 h at 42 °C, and then hybridized to specific oligonucleotide probes at 42 °C for 16 h. The probes were end-labeled using [γ-^{32}P]ATP and T_4 polynucleotide kinase. 18s mRNA was also used as an internal standard to correct for variations in RNA sample loading and blotting efficiency.

Western Blot Analysis

Quantitative immunoblotting of mouse cardiac homogenates was performed as previously described.[17] To determine protein levels of ryanodine receptor, the cardiac homogenates were separated by SDS-PAGE on 6% gels and transferred to 0.45 µm nitrocellulose membranes (BioRad Laboratories). Transfer was performed at 4 °C overnight at 253 mA in 192 mM glycine, 25 mM Tris, 0.0006% SDS, and 0.5% methanol with a buffer change after 4–5 hours. The membranes were incubated with an anti-ryanodine receptor monoclonal antibody (1:1000, Affinity Bioreagents Inc.). To determine the calsequestrin levels, the cardiac homogenates (50 µg) were electrophoretically separated on a 8% SDS-polyacrylamide gel. Immunoblotting was performed using a 1:100 dilution of a polyclonal rabbit antibody to canine cardiac calsequestrin as previously described.[18] The protein levels of the Na^+-Ca^{2+} exchanger were determined using quantitative immunoblotting in conjunction with the BioMax chemiluminescence detection system (Eastman Kodak Co.) according to manufacturer's instructions. To determine the protein levels of myosin, the homogenates (2–5 μg) were separated by SDS-PAGE on 8% gels and transferred to 0.22 μm nitrocellulose membranes; the membranes were incubated with a monoclonal antibody to cardiac myosin heavy chain (1:500 dilution, Accurate Chemical & Scientific Co.). For quantitative immunoblotting of actin, cardiac troponin T, and troponin I, the homogenates (10–50 μg) were separated by SDS-PAGE on 13% gels. The membranes were incubated with mouse monoclonal antibodies to actin (1:500 dilution, Accurate Chemical & Scientific Co.), cardiac troponin T, or cardiac troponin I (1:1000 dilution, Research Diagnostics, Inc.).

Radioligand Binding Assay

Whole cardiac homogenates were used for the ligand binding assays of ryanodine receptors as previously described,[19,20] with minor modifications. Radioligand binding assays were performed in the presence of the protease inhibitor cocktail containing 75 nM aprotinin, 0.23 μM phenylmethylsulfonyl fluoride, 0.83 mM benzamidine, 1 mM iodoacetimide, 1.1 μM leupeptin, and 0.7 μM pepstatin A. Twelve concentrations (0.1 to 40 nmol/L) of [^{3}H]-ryanodine (84 Ci/mmol, DuPont New Research Products) were assayed with and without unlabeled ryanodine (17 μM). Unlabeled ryanodine was used to displace [^{3}H]-ryanodine and allow measurement of specific ryanodine binding.

In Vivo *Phosphorylation*

The hearts were initially perfused as described above. The perfusion was then switched to a recirculating system containing 2 mCi [^{32}P]orthophosphate for 30 min. After this labeling period, the heart was stimulated with isoproterenol (0.15 μM) for 2 min. This isoproterenol concentration and the duration of stimulation were chosen because they have been previously shown to result in maximal inotropic responses.[10] The heart was then freeze-clamped, powdered, and homogenized for preparation of myofibrils and membrane vesicles. Microsomal preparations and the purification of myofibrils were carried out as previously described.[21,22] Polyacrylamide gel electrophoresis of ^{32}P-labeled proteins was performed according to Laemmli[23] with 7.5–20% gradient gels. The radioactive bands and ^{32}P incorporation into the various cardiac proteins was identified and determined using phosphorimager, autoradiography and liquid scintillation spectrometry. Data were expressed as pmoles ^{32}P/mg protein. The values were corrected with the specific activity of [γ-^{32}P]ATP, which was determined from the specific activity of [^{32}P]phosphocreatine in each perfused heart.[24]

RESULTS

Cardiac Remodeling by Phospholamban Deficiency

The phospholamban knockout mouse was generated by gene-targeting methodology in embryonic stem cells.[10] Phospholamban ablation was not associated with any phenotypic changes at the gross level. Examination of the hearts at the ultrastructural level revealed no cytoarchitectural disruption in the phospholamban knockout mice compared to age-matched wild-type mice (FIG. 1). The ultrastructure, location, and organization of the SR, the subcellular membrane system known to contain phospholamban, were identical in the cardiac tissue from wild-type (FIG. 1, A&B) and phos-

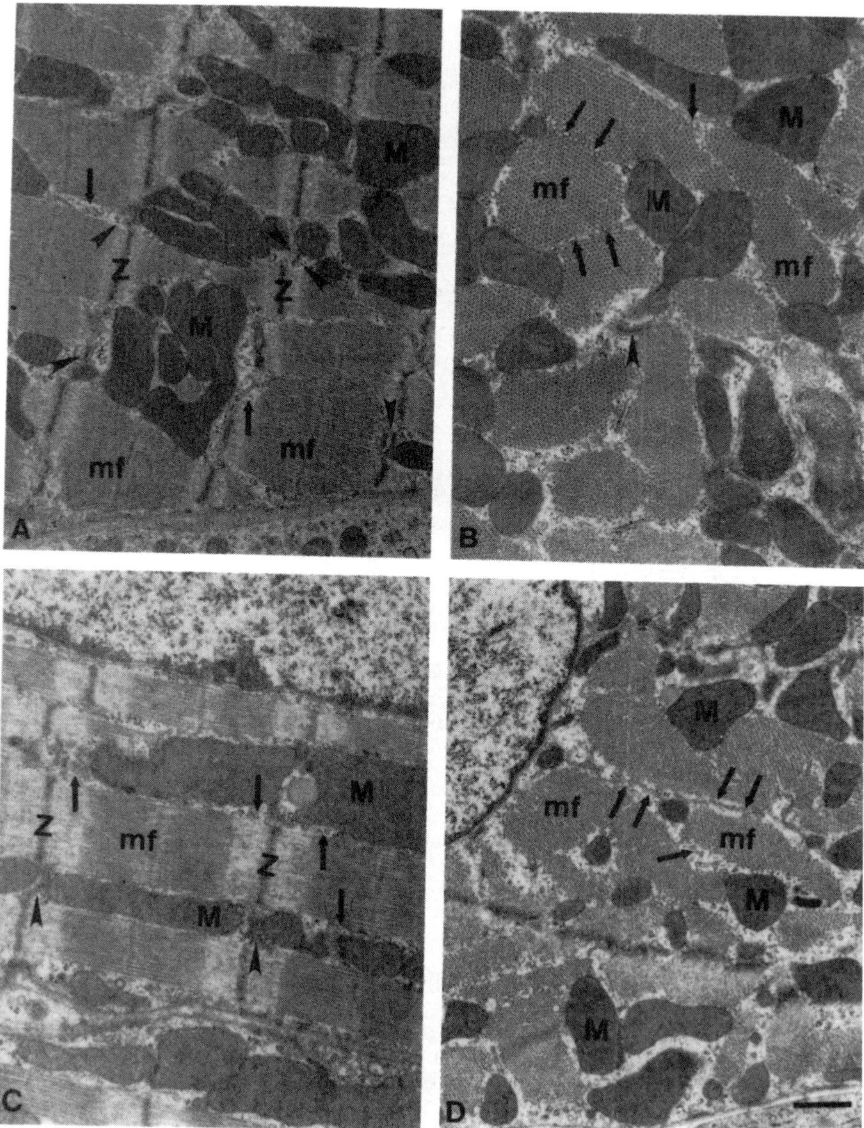

FIGURE 1. Ultrastructure of ventricular cells from wild-type and phospholamban-deficient mice. A comparison of electron micrographs obtained from longitudinal sections of wild-type **(A)** and phospholamban-deficient **(C)** mouse left ventricles demonstrates that the myofibrillar arrangements of the contractile apparatus (mf), the organization and distribution of the free sarcoplasmic reticulum *(arrows)*, the junctional SR *(arrowheads)*, and the distribution of the mitochondria (M) are unaltered by phospholamban ablation. This is confirmed in cross-sections of wild-type **(B)** and phospholamban-deficient **(D)** mouse ventricles. *Bar:* 595 nm **(A),** 475 nm **(B),** 550 nm **(C)** and 720 nm **(D).**

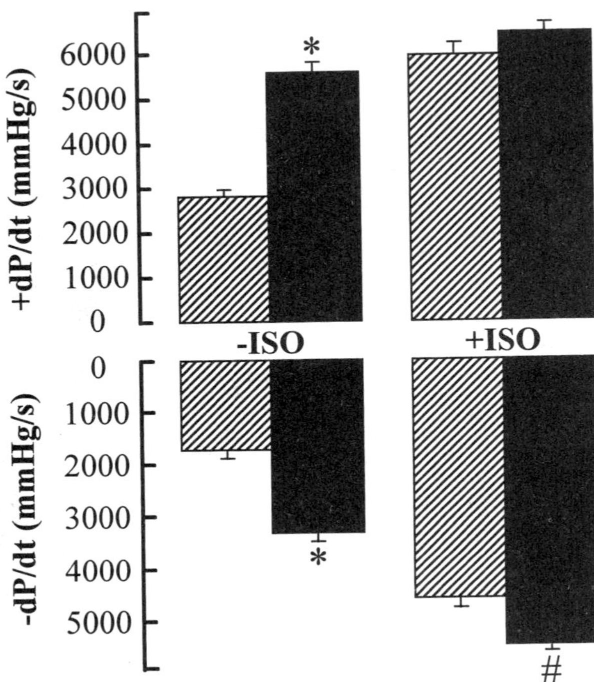

FIGURE 2. The maximal rates of contraction (+dP/dt) and relaxation (–dP/dt) of isolated heart preparations from phospholamban knockout (▆) and wild-type (▨) mice and the maximal effects of isoproterenol (ISO) on the contractile parameters. The wild-type and phospholamban knockout hearts were perfused in a Langendorff mode under identical loading conditions in the absence (–) or presence (+) of isoproterenol. Values are mean ± SEM of 6 hearts. $^*p < 0.05$ vs. wild-type and $^{\#}p < 0.05$ vs. basal values of phospholamban knockout hearts.

pholamban knockout (FIG. 1, C&D) mice. However, Langendorff perfusion of phospholamban knockout hearts indicated significant enhancement of the myocardial contractile parameters (FIG. 2) with no changes in the spontaneous heart rate. The time to peak pressure and half-relaxation time were also significantly shortened by phospholamban deficiency. Isoproterenol perfusion (0.15 μM) was associated with significant stimulation in the rates of contraction (+dP/dt: 208%) and relaxation (–dP/dt: 260%) in the wild-type hearts, whereas it stimulated the relaxation rate by only 35% in the phospholamban knockout hearts (FIG. 2).

Ca^{2+} Handling Proteins

To determine whether ablation of phospholamban and the accompanied enhancement of cardiac contractile parameters were associated with any alterations of the SR Ca^{2+}-ATPase, the activity of this enzyme was examined in Ca^{2+}-uptake experiments. The initial rates of SR Ca^{2+} uptake in cardiac homogenates were assessed as a function of

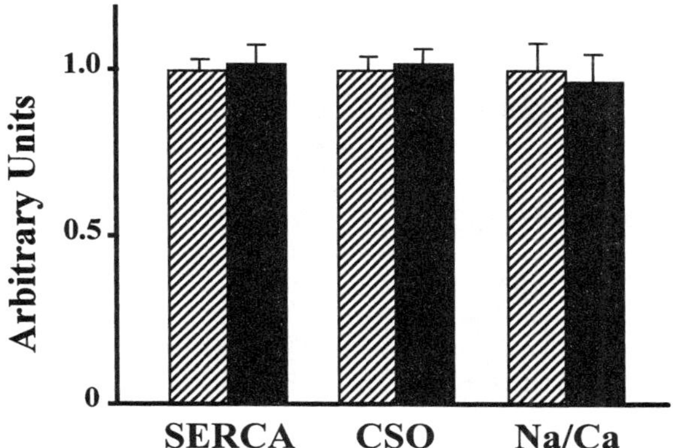

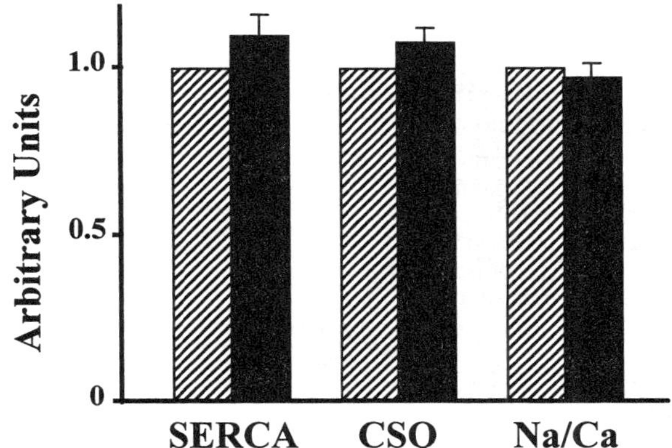

FIGURE 3. Relative expression levels of Ca^{2+}-cycling proteins at the mRNA **(A)** and protein **(B)** levels in hearts from phospholamban knockout (▆) compared to wild-type (▨) mice. Signals of the KO hearts were normalized to those of wild-types, which were set at 1.0. Values are mean ± SEM, $n = 5–7$. SERCA: SR Ca^{2+}-ATPase; CSQ: calsequestrin; Na/Ca: Na^{+}-Ca^{2+} exchanger.

[Ca^{2+}]. There was no alteration in the V_{max} of the SR Ca^{2+} transport system,[10] indicating that the expression levels and the activity of the SR Ca^{2+}-ATPase were not altered in the phospholamban knockout hearts. However, the affinity of the SR Ca^{2+}-ATPase for Ca^{2+}, a property modulated by phospholamban, was increased upon ablation of phospholamban. Furthermore, dot blot analysis and quantitative immunoblotting revealed no differences in either the transcript or the protein levels of the SR Ca^{2+}-ATPase between wild-type and phospholamban knockout hearts (FIG. 3, A&B).

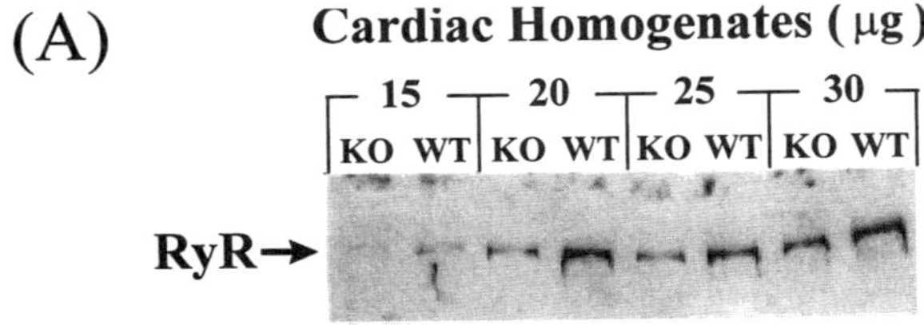

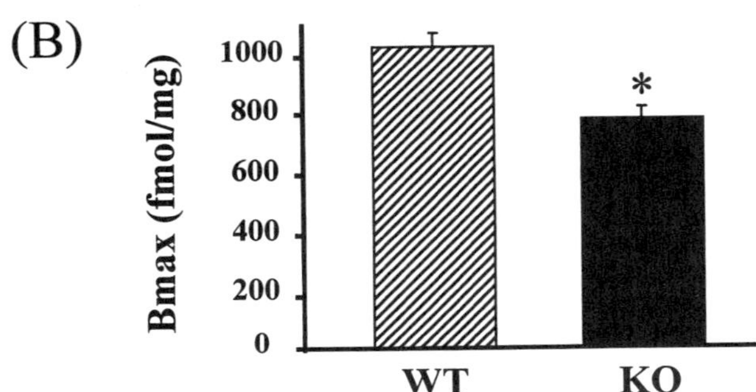

FIGURE 4. **(A)** Quantitative immunoblotting of the ryanodine receptor protein in cardiac homogenates from phospholamban knockout (KO) and wild-type (WT) mice. Cardiac homogenates (15, 20, 25, 30 μg) were separated by SDS-PAGE (6%), transferred to a nitrocellulose membrane, and incubated with an anti-ryanodine receptor monoclonal antibody. **(B)** Radioligand binding assay of ryanodine receptors in cardiac homogenates from phospholamban knockout (■) and wild-type (▨) mice. Data were fit with a single class of binding sites and analyzed by the radioligand binding analysis computer software. RyR: ryanodine receptor; Bmax: the maximal number of binding sites. Values are mean ± SEM, $n = 6$, $^*p < 0.05$ vs. WT.

Examination of the transcript or the protein levels of calsequestrin and the sarcolemmal Na^+-Ca^{2+} exchanger indicated no significant differences between phospholamban knockout and wild-type hearts either (FIG. 3, A&B). However, phospholamban deficiency was associated with a significant reduction (26%) in the levels of the ryanodine receptor protein (FIG. 4A). The reduction in protein levels was consistent with a 24% decrease in maximal ryanodine binding in phospholamban knockout hearts compared with wild-type hearts (FIG. 4B), while the ryanodine binding affinity was similar between phospholamban knockout and wild-type hearts (Kd: 10.4 ± 1.4 nM in phospholamban knockout vs. 12.3 ± 1.0 nM in wild-type, $n = 6$, $p > 0.05$).

Myofibrillar Proteins

The contractile proteins, myosin, actin, and troponins are known to play a major role in controlling the muscle contractile machinery. Thus, the transcript levels of these proteins were evaluated by dot blot analysis. There were no significant alterations in the mRNA levels of α-myosin heavy chain, α-cardiac actin, α-skeletal actin, or troponin I (FIG. 5A) between phospholamban knockout and wild-type hearts. Furthermore, there

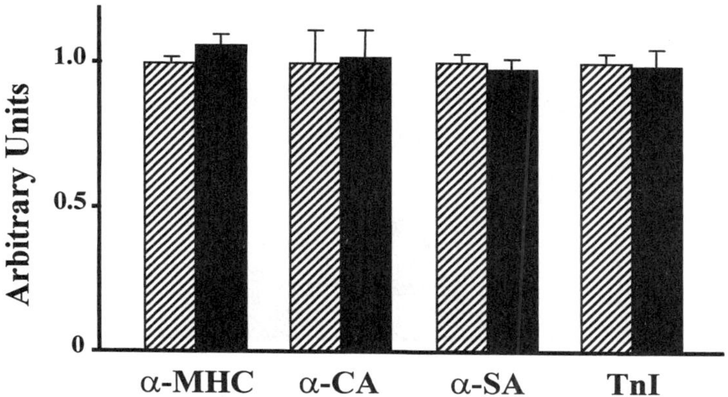

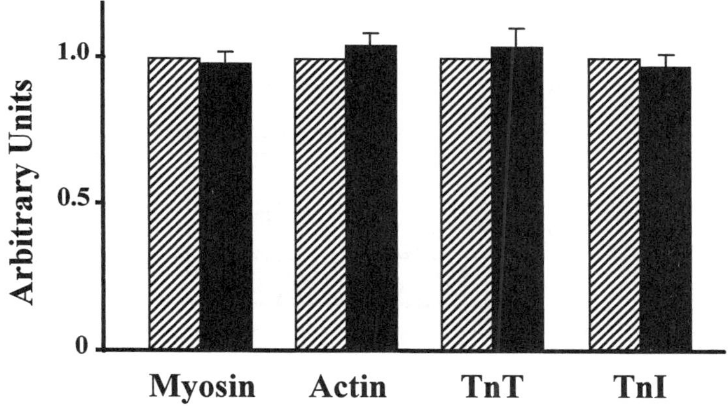

FIGURE 5. Relative expression levels of Ca^{2+}-cycling proteins at the mRNA **(A)** and protein **(B)** levels in hearts from phospholamban knockout (■) compared to wild-type (▨) mice. Signals of the phospholamban knockout hearts were normalized to those of wild-types, which were set at 1.0. Values are mean ± SEM, $n = 5–6$. α-MHC: α-myosin heavy chain; α-CA: α-cardiac actin; α-SA: α-skeletal actin; TnI: troponin I; TnT: troponin T.

were no alterations in the protein levels of myosin, actin, troponin T and troponin I (FIG. 5B). Examination of β-myosin heavy chain expression indicated that the transcript levels of this gene were undetectable in phospholamban knockout or wild-type hearts. Thus, phospholamban ablation did not trigger any transition between α- and β-myosin heavy chain proteins in an effort to accommodate the enhanced SR Ca^{2+}-ATPase activity and hyperdynamic cardiac function in the intact mouse heart.

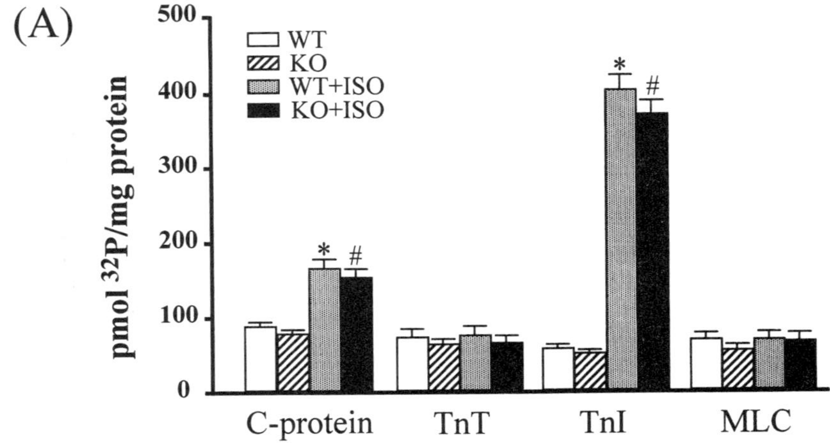

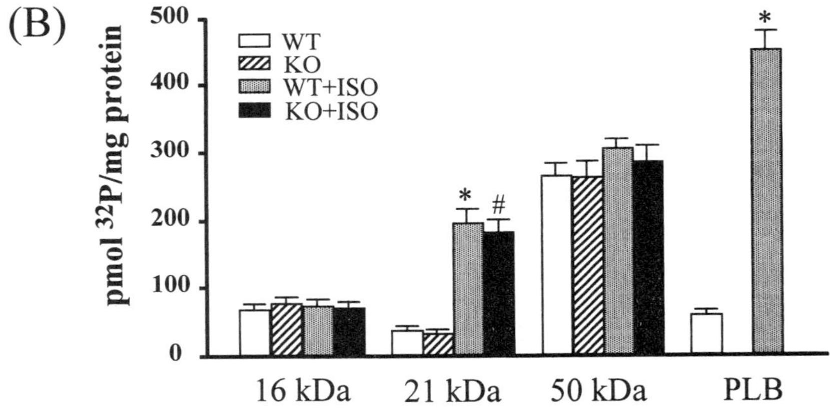

FIGURE 6. ^{32}P incorporation into myofibrillar proteins **(A)** and membrane proteins **(B)** isolated from phospholamban knockout (KO) and wild-type (WT) hearts perfused with [^{32}P]orthophosphate under basal and isoproterenol-stimulated (+ISO) conditions. TnT: troponin T; TnI: troponin I; MLC: myosin light chain; PLB: phospholamban. Values are mean ± SEM of 4 hearts in pmol ^{32}P/mg protein. $^{*}p < 0.05$ vs. WT and $^{\#}$ $p < 0.05$ vs. KO basal values.

β-*Adrenergic Receptor Signaling Pathway*

To elucidate whether the attenuation of β-adrenergic stimulation in phospholamban knockout hearts was due to alterations in the signal transduction pathway, the β-receptor density, adenylyl cyclase activity, and cAMP levels were assessed; there were no significant differences under basal or maximal isoproterenol-stimulated conditions between phospholamban knockout and wild-type hearts.[13] Furthermore, we examined whether phospholamban ablation was associated with any alterations in the phosphorylation patterns of the other key cardiac phosphoproteins. Thus, phospholamban knockout and wild-type hearts were perfused with ^{32}P-labeled Krebs buffer, and the degree of phosphorylation of the myofibrillar and SR proteins was examined in the absence or presence of isopreterenol. The degree of ^{32}P-incorporation into C-protein, troponin T, troponin I, and myosin light chain was similar between phospholamban knockout and wild-type hearts under basal conditions (FIG. 6A). Upon isoproterenol stimulation, the degree of ^{32}P-incorporation into C-protein and troponin I was significantly increased in both the phospholamban knockout and wild-type hearts compared with the nonstimulated hearts, and these increases were similar between the two animal groups. Assessment of phosphoproteins in the SR-enriched membrane preparations demonstrated that isoproterenol stimulation was associated with significant increases of ^{32}P-incorporation into phospholamban in the wild-type hearts and a 21-kDa protein in both wild-type and phospholamban knockout hearts (FIG. 6B). No significant change in the extent of phosphorylation of the 16-kDa and 50-kDa proteins was detected in either the nonstimulated or isoproterenol-stimulated phospholamban knockout hearts compared with wild-type hearts (FIG. 6B).

DISCUSSION

In the present studies, ultrastructural examination revealed no morphological defects in the phospholamban knockout mouse hearts, whereas Langendorff perfusion indicated significant enhancement of cardiac contractile parameters compared to age-matched wild-type hearts. The hyperdynamic cardiac function was not associated with any alteration in the SR Ca^{2+}-ATPase mRNA or protein levels, suggesting that phospholamban and the SR Ca^{2+}-ATPase gene expression levels are not coordinately regulated in the mammalian heart. Other changes at the SR level may involve the expression levels of calsequestrin, the protein that acts as a Ca^{2+} buffer or store in the SR lumen,[25] and the ryanodine receptor, which releases SR Ca^{2+} during contraction.[26] Ablation of phospholamban did not result in any alterations in the transcript or protein levels of calsequestrin, indicating that calsequestrin has a high buffering capacity for Ca^{2+} or that a sufficient number of spare calsequestrin molecules exist in wild-type hearts, which can be recruited to accommodate the increased Ca^{2+} taken up in the SR of the phospholamban knockout hearts. However, the ryanodine receptor levels were significantly reduced in the phospholamban knockout hearts. Furthermore, ryanodine binding assays revealed a similar degree of reduction in the maximal number of ryanodine receptors upon ablation of phospholamban. The down-regulation of this Ca^{2+}-release channel indicates a cross-talk between SR Ca^{2+}-uptake and Ca^{2+}-release, which may serve as an important compensatory mechanism in an attempt to maintain Ca^{2+} homeostasis in these hyperdynamic phospholamban knockout hearts.[27]

In addition to the SR Ca^{2+}-cycling proteins, the contractile proteins have been shown to play an important role in controlling myocardial contractility. Alterations in myosin heavy chain isoenzyme levels were associated with alterations in cardiac function,[28,29] while overexpression of α-skeletal actin resulted in increased contractility of mouse hearts.[30] However, there were no significant differences observed in the expression levels of myosin, actin, and troponin isoforms between phospholamban knockout and wild-type hearts. Thus, in the absence of any alterations in the major contractile proteins, the enhanced rates of cardiac relaxation in phospholamban knockout hearts are due mainly to the increases in the SR Ca^{2+} uptake rates.

Furthermore, phospholamban deficiency attenuated the cardiac stimulatory responses to β-adrenergic agonists. Thus, it was important to determine whether the observed attenuation was due to compensatory responses associated with alterations in the phosphorylation levels of the other key cardiac regulatory phosphoproteins. These phosphoproteins include troponin I and C-protein in the myofibrils[8,9] and phospholemman in the sarcolemmal membranes.[31] Phosphorylation of troponin I has been suggested to increase the rate of Ca^{2+} removal from troponin C,[9,32] while phosphorylation of C-protein was observed to lower the stimulation of actin-activated myosin ATPase activity.[33] Thus, phosphorylation of these proteins may be at least partially responsible for the increased rates of relaxation in isoproterenol-stimulated hearts. However, assessment of the degree of phosphorylation of the myofibrillar proteins, troponin I, and C-protein indicated no significant differences between phospholamban knockout and wild-type hearts under either basal or maximal isoproterenol-stimulated conditions. Examination of the membrane fractions from wild-type hearts revealed the presence of two proteins, phospholamban and a 21-kDa protein, whose degree of phosphorylation increased upon isoproterenol stimulation. Phospholamban was absent in the phospholamban knockout hearts, but the 21-kDa protein was present in both phospholamban knockout and wild-type hearts; and the magnitude of the increases in ^{32}P incorporation into this polypeptide upon isoproterenol stimulation was similar between the phospholamban knockout and wild-type hearts. These findings indicate that the phosphoprotein mediators of the β-adrenergic signaling system are similar under both basal and isoproterenol-stimulated conditions between the phospholamban knockout and wild-type hearts, suggesting that the attenuation of the isoproterenol-mediated lusitropic and inotropic effects in the phospholamban knockout hearts is not due to alterations in their β-adrenergic signal transduction pathway.

In summary, phospholamban deficiency was associated with significant enhancement of the rates of contraction and relaxation, as well as attenuation of responses to β-adrenergic stimulation in the mouse heart. The hyperdynamic cardiac function of the phospholamban knockout mice was not accompanied by any cytoarchitectural abnormalities or alterations in the expression levels of the SR Ca^{2+}-ATPase, calsequestrin, Na^{+}-Ca^{2+} exchanger, or the contractile proteins. However, ablation of phospholamban was associated with down-regulation of the ryanodine receptor, to compensate for the increased SR Ca^{2+} uptake in an attempt to maintain Ca^{2+} homeostasis in the myocardium. Furthermore, the attenuation of the contractile responses to β-agonists was not due to alterations in the phosphorylation levels of the other key cardiac phosphoproteins in the phospholamban knockout hearts. Thus, the augmentation of contractile parameters and the attenuation of β-adrenergic stimulation in the phospholamban knockout hearts are due mainly to the "uninhibited" SR Ca^{2+}-ATPase activity as a result of phospholamban ablation. It remains to be determined whether the observed phenotype of the phospholamban knockout hearts is preserved through aging, stress, and pathophysiological conditions.

REFERENCES

1. KOSS, K. L. & E. G. KRANIAS. 1996. Phospholamban: A prominent regulator of myocardial contractility. Circ. Res. **79:** 1059–1063.
2. KIM, H. W., N. A. STEENAART, D. G. FERGUSON & E. G. KRANIAS. 1990. Functional reconstitution of the cardiac sarcoplasmic reticulum Ca^{2+}-ATPase with phospholamban in phospholipid vesicles. J. Biol. Chem. **265:** 1702–1709.
3. HICKS, M. J., M. SHIGEKAWA & A. M. KATZ. 1979. Mechanism by which cyclic adenosine 3′5′-monophosphate–dependent protein kinase stimulates calcium transport in cardiac sarcoplasmic reticulum. Circ. Res. **44:** 384–391.
4. MOVSESIAN, M. A., M. NISHIKAWA & R. S. ADELSTEIN. 1984. Phosphorylation of phospholamban by calcium-activated phospholipid-dependent protein kinase. J. Biol. Chem. **259:** 8029–8032.
5. SIMMERMAN, H. K., J. H. COLLINS, J. L. THEIBERT, A. D. WEGENER & L. R. JONES. 1986. Se-

quence analysis of phospholamban: Identification of phosphorylation sites and two major structural domains. J. Biol. Chem. **261:** 13333–13341.
6. KRANIAS, E. G. 1985. Regulation of calcium transport by protein phosphatase activity associated with cardiac sarcoplasmic reticulum. J. Biol. Chem. **260:** 11006–11010.
7. WEGENER, A. D., H. K. SIMMERMAN, J. P. LINDEMANN & L. R. JONES. 1989. Phospholamban phosphorylation in intact ventricles: Phosphorylation of serine 16 and threonine 17 in response to beta-adrenergic stimulation. J. Biol. Chem. **264:** 11468–11474.
8. KRANIAS, E. G. & R. J. SOLARO. 1982. Phosphorylation of troponin I and phospholamban during catecholamine stimulation of rabbit heart. Nature **298:** 182–184.
9. KRANIAS, E. G., J. L. GARVEY, R. D. SRIVASTAVA & R. J. SOLARO. 1985. Phosphorylation and functional modifications of sarcoplasmic reticulum and myofibrils in isolated rabbit hearts stimulated with isoprenaline. Biochem. J. **226:** 113–121.
10. LUO, W., I. L. GRUPP, J. HARRER, S. PONNIAH, G. GRUPP, J. J. DUFFY, T. DOETSCHMAN & E. G. KRANIAS. 1994. Targeted ablation of the phospholamban gene is associated with markedly enhanced myocardial contractility and loss of β-agonist stimulation. Circ. Res. **75:** 401–409.
11. WOLSKA, B. M., M. O. STOJANOVIC, W. LUO, E. G. KRANIAS & R. J. SOLARO. 1996. Effect of ablation of phospholamban on dynamics of cardiac myocyte contraction and intracellular Ca^{2+}. Am. J. Physiol. **271:** C391–C397.
12. HOIT, B. D., S. F. KHOURY, E. G. KRANIAS, N. BALL & R. A. WALSH. 1995. In vivo echocardiographic detection of enhanced left ventricular function in gene-targeted mice with phospholamban deficiency. Circ. Res. **77:** 632–637.
13. KISS, E., I. EDES, Y. SATO, W. LUO, S. B. LIGGETT & E. G. KRANIAS. 1997. β-Adrenergic regulation of cAMP and protein phosphorylation in phospholamban-knockout mouse hearts. Am. J. Physiol. **272:** H785–H790.
14. SHASTRY, B. S. 1994. More to learn from gene knockouts. Mol. Cell. Biochem. **136:** 171–182.
15. CHOMCZYNSKI, P. & N. SACCHI. 1987. Single-step method of RNA isolation by acid guanidinium thiocyanate-phenol-chloroform extraction. Anal. Biochem. **162:** 156–159.
16. SAMBROOK, J., E. F. FRITSCH & T. MANIATIS. 1989. Molecular Cloning. Cold Spring Harbor Laboratory Press. New York.
17. HARRER, J. M., E. KISS & E. G. KRANIAS. 1995. Application of the immunoblot technique for quantitation of protein levels in cardiac homogenates. BioTechniques **18:** 995–997.
18. ROCKMAN, H. A., R. HAMILTON, L. R. JONES, C. A. MILANO, L. MAO & R. J. LEFKOWITZ. 1996. Enhanced myocardial relaxation *in vivo* in transgenic mice overexpressing the β_2-adrenergic receptor is associated with reduced phospholamban protein. J. Clin. Invest. **97:** 1618–1623.
19. BERS, D. M. & V. M. STIFFEL. 1993. Ratio of ryanodine to dehydropyridine receptors in cardiac and skeletal muscle and implications for E-C coupling. Am. J. Physiol. **264:** C1587–C1593.
20. VATNER, D. E., N. SATO, K. KIUCHI, R. P. SHANNON & S. F. VATNER. 1994. Decrease in myocardial ryanodine receptors and altered excitation-concentration coupling early in the development of heart failure. Circulation **90:** 1423–1430.
21. EDES, I. & E. G. KRANIAS. 1990. Phospholamban and troponin I are substrates for protein kinase C in vitro but not in intact beating guinea pig hearts. Circ. Res. **67:** 394–400.
22. SOLARO, R. J., D. C. PANG & F. N. BRIGGS. 1971. The purification of cardiac myofibrils with Triton X-100. Biochim. Biophys. Acta **245:** 259–262.
23. LAEMMLI, U. K. 1970. Cleavage of structural proteins during the assembly of the head of bacteriophage T_4. Nature **227:** 680–685.
24. KOPP, S. J. & M. BARANY. 1979. Phosphorylation of the 19,000 dalton light chain of myosin in perfused rat heart under the influence of negative and positive inotropic agents. J. Biol. Chem. **254:** 12007–12012.
25. MACLENNAN, D. H. & P. T. WONG. 1971. Isolation of a calcium-sequestering protein from sarcoplasmic reticulum. Proc. Natl. Acad. Sci. USA **68:** 1231–1235.
26. SORRENTINO, V. & P. VOLPE. 1993. Ryanodine receptors: How many, where and why? Trends Pharmacol. Sci. **14:** 98–103.
27. CHU, G., W. LUO, J. P. SLACK, C. TILGMANN, W. E. SWEET, M. SPINDLER, K. W. SAUPE, G. P. BOIVIN, C. S. MORAVEC, M. A. MATLIB, I. L. GRUPP, J. S. INGWALL & E. G. KRANIAS.

1996. Compensatory mechanisms associated with the hyperdynamic function of phospholamban-deficient mouse hearts. Circ. Res. **79:** 1064–1076.

28. Ng, W. A., I. L. Grupp, A. Subramaniam & J. Robbins. 1991. Cardiac myosin heavy chain mRNA expression and myocardial function in the mouse heart. Circ. Res. **69:** 1742–1750.
29. Boluyt, M. O., L. O'Neill, A. L. Meredith, O. H. L. Bing, W. W. Brooks, C. H. Conrad, M. T. Crow & E. G. Lakatta. 1994. Alterations in cardiac gene expression during the transition from stable hypertrophy to heart failure: Marked upregulation of genes encoding extracellular matrix components. Circ. Res. **75:** 23–32.
30. Hewett, T. E., I. L. Grupp, G. Grupp & J. Robbins. 1994. α-Skeletal actin is associated with increased contractility in the mouse heart. Circ. Res. **74:** 740–746.
31. Presti, C. F., L. R. Jones & J. P. Lindemann. 1985. Isoproterenol-induced phosphorylation of a 15-kilodalton sarcolemmal protein in intact myocardium. J. Biol. Chem. **260:** 3860–3867.
32. Robertson, S. P., J. D. Johnson, M. J. Holroyde, E. G. Kranias, J. D. Potter & R. J. Solaro. 1982. The effects of troponin I phosphorylation on the Ca^{2+}-binding properties of the Ca^{2+}-regulatory site of bovine cardiac troponin. J. Biol. Chem. **257:** 260–263.
33. Hartzell, H. C. 1985. Effects of phosphorylated and unphosphorylated C-protein on cardiac actomyosin ATPase. J. Mol. Biol. **186:** 185–195.

Structural Studies on Phospholamban and Implications for Regulation of the Ca^{2+}-ATPase

RUSSELL J. MORTISHIRE-SMITH,[a,b] HOWARD BROUGHTON,[b] VICTOR M. GARSKY,[c] ERNEST J. MAYER,[d] AND ROBERT G. JOHNSON, JR.[d]

[b]Merck Sharp and Dohme Research Laboratories, Neuroscience Research Centre, Terlings Park, Eastwick Road, Harlow, Essex CM20 2QR, United Kingdom
Departments of [c]Medicinal Chemistry and [d]Pharmacology, Merck Research Laboratories, WP44-L206, POB4, West Point, Pennsylvania 19486, USA

ABSTRACT: The cardiac sarcoplasmic reticulum (SR) protein phospholamban (PLB) is an endogenous inhibitor of the SR Ca^{2+}-ATPase. Phosphorylation of PLB relieves this inhibition and up-regulates calcium transport. PLB has proved remarkably difficult to study by conventional solution-state nuclear magnetic resonance (NMR) methods, due primarily to the extreme hydrophobic nature of the protein and its propensity to form pentamers. That the C-terminal domain of PLB is helical and membrane spanning is now well established; the structure of the cytoplasmic domain is relatively ill defined. In order to discern the effect of phosphorylation on the structure of the cytoplasmic domain, we have characterized a variety of model peptides in several structure-inducing and/or lipid-mimicking environments using circular dichroism and solution-state NMR. The resolution of peptide structures obtained in aqueous trifluoroethanol was markedly improved by the incorporation of ^{15}N labels into the peptide backbone, allowing a variety of isotope edited, filtered, and resolved techniques to be applied. Molecular dynamics simulations on the full-length protein were combined with an analysis of published data to suggest a revised model for the structure of PLB.

BACKGROUND

Phospholamban (PLB) is a relatively small membrane-associated protein localized within the sarcoplasmic reticulum of the cardiac myocyte,1 where it behaves as an endogenous inhibitor of the SR Ca2+-ATPase.2–4 Phosphorylation at either Ser-16 or Thr-17 markedly decreases the affinity of PLB for the Ca2+-ATPase, resulting in a concomitant apparent increase in the affinity of the Ca2+-ATPase for calcium. Discerning the nature of the structural change in PLB on phosphorylation is thus key to understanding its mechanism of action as a Ca2+-ATPase inhibitor.

Phospholamban is usefully divided into three regions (FIG. 1)—a transmembrane domain, and two cytoplasmic regions divided by a proline at position 21. Mutations to the first 18 residues (domain Ia) have a marked effect on the regulatory ability of phospholamban.[5] Unconservative mutations to the aspartamine and glutamine residues in domain 1b have no effect on pentamer formation, or on regulatory ability.[6] A variety of models have been proposed for the three-dimensional structure of phospholam-

[a] Corresponding author: Phone: 011-44-1279-440464; fax: 011-44-1279-440730; e-mail: russell__mortishire-smith@merck.com

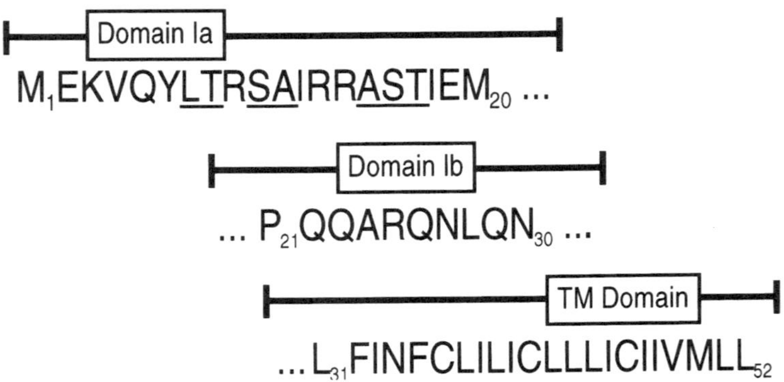

FIGURE 1. Primary sequence of phospholamban and proposed domain structure. In PLB(1–25), *underlined residues* were labeled with ^{15}N.

ban.[7–9] There is consensus within these models that the final 20 residues (domain II) comprise a transmembrane-spanning helix, and mutagenesis studies have shown that it is this region alone that is responsible for pentamer formation.[10] However, these proposed models differ in the length and position of helix formation within the cytoplasmic component; *in extremis,* it has been postulated that phospholamban contains only a short N-terminal helix,[5] or else is helical from residues 11 to 52.[11]

Biomolecular NMR is normally the method of choice to characterize the structure of small proteins such as PLB. However, phospholamban is extremely insoluble in the absence of lipids, and behaves as a pentamer in the presence of detergents and lipids.[12] This gives PLB an effective molecular weight of >30 kilodaltons, putting it outside the size range where conventional biomolecular NMR is useful. Since the cytoplasmic component of phospholamban is a key determinant of function and is accessible to synthesis and study, we chose to characterize this region of the protein and the effect of phosphorylation on structure.

METHODS

Synthesis of Phospholamban Peptides

Chemical synthesis and purification of the ^{15}N-labeled PLB(1–25) peptide was performed as previously described.[13]

Nuclear Magnetic Resonance Spectroscopy

NMR samples were prepared at concentrations varying between 1.8 and 4.0 mM in 90% H_2O/D_2O, 30% TFE-d_3/H_2O, or 90% H_2O/300 mM SDS-d_{25} (Promochem). The pH of all samples was adjusted to 3.0 or 4.2 (uncorrected for deuterium isotope effects) using microliter amounts of NaOH/HCl, in order to reduce amide exchange rates. Circular dichroism (CD) spectra obtained at pH 3.0 were identical to those acquired at pH 7.0. Spectra were acquired on a Bruker AMX-500 spectrometer operating at 500.13 MHz and were referenced to internal sodium trimethylsilylpropionate at 0.0 ppm. The following spectra were acquired in all three solvent systems: DQF-COSY,[14] TOCSY[15] (100-ms and 300-ms mixing times) and NOESY (100-ms, 200-ms, and 300-ms mixing times).[16] ^{1}H-^{15}N HMQC,[17] HMQC-TOCSY,[18] HMQC-NOESY,[19] and ^{15}N-edited and filtered NOESY[20,21] experiments were acquired using standard pulse sequences. Two-dimensional spectra were acquired in the phase-sensitive mode with quadrature detection in ω_1 using time-proportional phase incrementation.[22,23] Solvent signals were suppressed with selective presaturation. Data were processed with a Silicon Graphics Indigo-2 R10000 computer using Felix software (Biosym Technologies) and analyzed

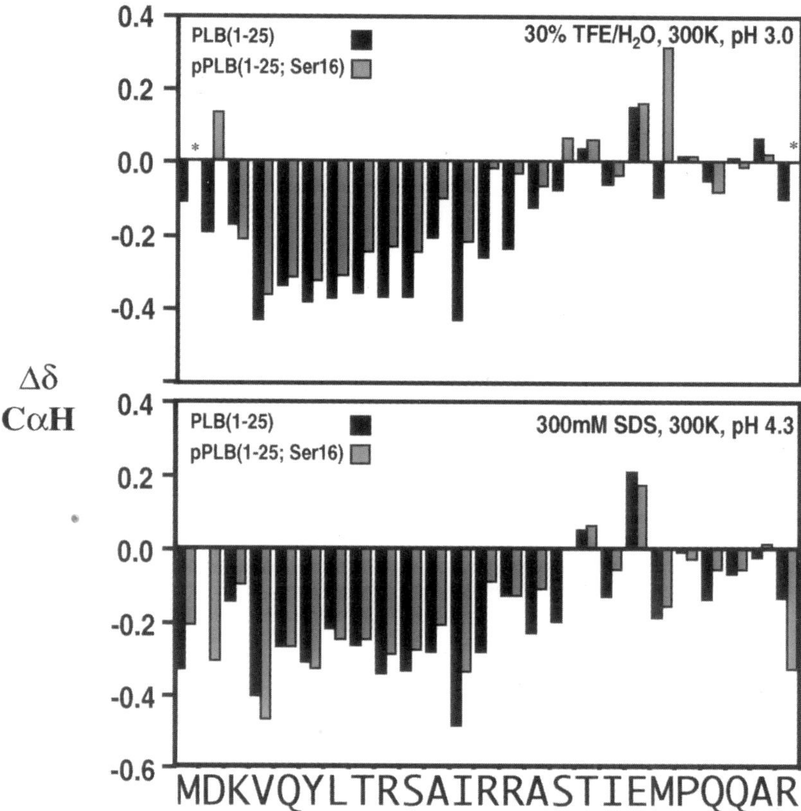

FIGURE 2. Comparison of C$^{\alpha}$H secondary shifts (vertical axis) by residue (horizontal axis) for PLB(1–25) *(dark bars)* and pPLB(1–25; Ser-16) *(light bars)* in aqueous TFE **(top)** and 300 mM SDS **(bottom).** *Starred bars* denote residues that could not be assigned due to resonance overlap.

using NMRVIEW.[24] Data sets were generally multiplied by squared sine-bell window functions and zero filled once in both dimensions before Fourier transformation. Final data set sizes were generally 4096 by 1024 real data points.

Structure Calculations

Structure calculations were performed with the distance geometry program DIANA[25,26] using a REDAC strategy.[27] NOE distance upper bounds were determined from cross peak intensities by calibration against known interproton distances in elements of regular secondary structure, and by reference to protons of fixed separation (geminal protons and aromatic protons of Tyr-6). Upper bounds were assigned as 2.5, 3.0, 3.7, and 4.5 Å for backbone-backbone NOEs and 3.0, 3.5, 4.2, and 5.0 Å for all other constraints from homonuclear NOESY spectra. Van der Waals lower bounds were used. Dihedral angle constraints were classified as $-90 < \phi < -40$ for $^3J_{Hn\alpha} \leq 5.5$ Hz, $-160 < \phi < -80$ for 8.5 Hz $< {}^3J_{HN\alpha} \leq$ 10.0 Hz and $-140 < \phi < -100$ for $^3J_{HN\alpha} \geq$ 10.0 Hz.[28]

Molecular Dynamics Simulations

Molecular dynamics (MD) simulations were performed on a Silicon Graphics Indigo2 with an R10000 processor, using SYBYL (Tripos Associates). Simulations were carried out starting from the human phospholamban sequence, or a variant in which Pro-21 was replaced by Ala, with the peptide sequence initialized to an ideal α-helical conformation (ϕ=–60, ψ=–40). Five independent MD simulations were performed over 250 ps each using a Kollman united atom force field, at a temperature of 300 K, with a dialectric constant $\varepsilon = 2$. Nonbonded interactions were truncated at 8 Å. The temperature was ramped to 300 K in 50-K increments lasting 5 ps each, after which velocity scaling was turned off. Fluctuations in the NH bond vector were analyzed by extracting the ϕ torsion angle for each residue at 250-fs intervals during the simulation, averaging these angles over the course of the simulation and calculating the rms deviation from the mean.

RESULTS AND DISCUSSION

It has previously been shown from both circular dichroism experiments and ^{1}H NMR studies that peptides derived from the cytoplasmic domain of phospholamban are largely unstructured in aqueous solution.[13,29,30] Using homonuclear NMR experiments, complete assignments were obtained for PLB(1–25) and pPLB(1–25; Ser-16) in mixtures of trifluoroethanol (TFE) and water, and in detergent micelles. An indicator of secondary structure in peptides is provided by the $C^\alpha H$ secondary shift value, defined as the difference between the observed chemical shift and the random coil chemical shift for each residue.[31] The calculated $C^\alpha H$ secondary shifts for PLB(1–25) and pPLB(1–25; Ser-16) in aqueous TFE and 300 mM sodium dodecyl sulfate (SDS) are shown in FIGURE 2, and indicate that PLB(1–25) folds to form a stable helix from residue 1 to residues 15/16. The stability of the helix is clearly affected by phosphorylation.

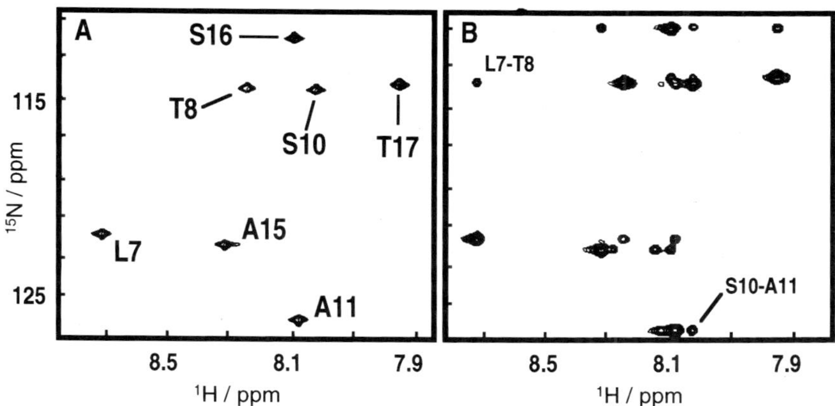

FIGURE 3. A. ^{1}H-^{15}N HMQC experiment on selectively ^{15}N labeled PLB(1–25) in 30% TFE/H_2O, 300 K, pH 3.05. **B.** Amide region of a ^{1}H-^{15}N HMQC-NOESY experiment acquired with a mixing time of 300 ms on selectively ^{15}N-labeled PLB(1–25) in 30% TFE/H_2O, 300K, pH 3.05. Selected NOEs are labeled with their assignment.

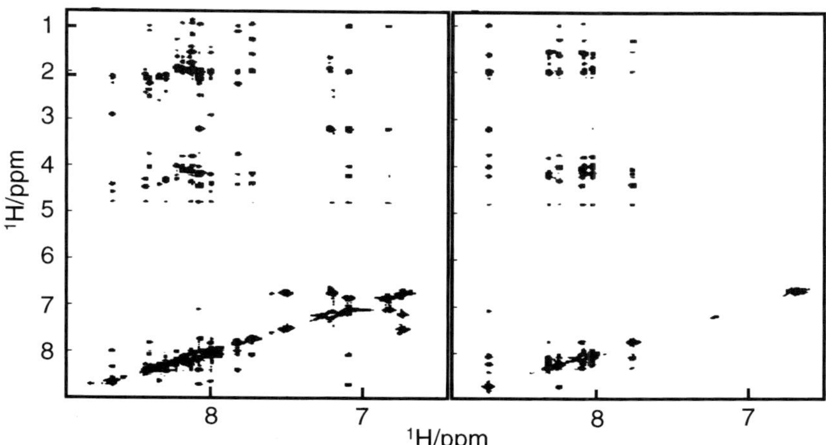

FIGURE 4. Selected regions from **(left)** ω_2 ^{15}N filtered experiment and **(right)** ω_2 ^{15}N selected experiment on selectively ^{15}N-labeled PLB(1–25) in 30% TFE/H_2O, 300K, pH 3.05.

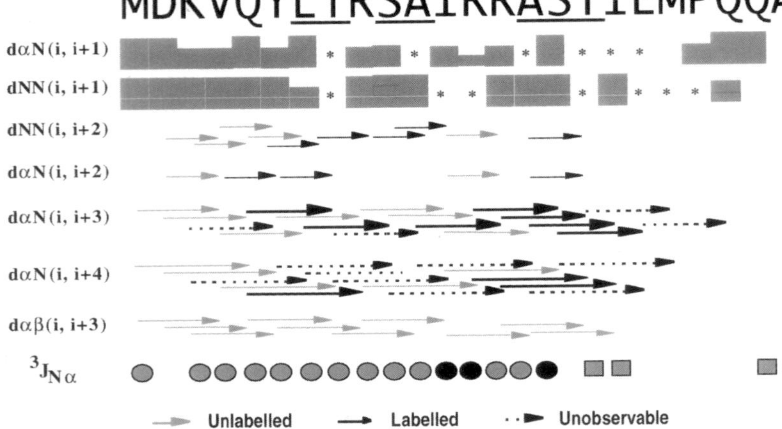

FIGURE 5. Summary of observed sequential and medium range NOE connectivities for selectively labelled PLB(1–25) in 30% TFE/H_2O, pH 3.05, 300 K. Sequential NOEs are represented by *shaded blocks;* the number of blocks is a qualitative measure of relative NOE intensity. Medium range NOEs are represented by *bars* connecting the appropriate residues. NOEs that could not be confidently assigned due to resonance degeneracy, but that would be expected in a region of regular helical secondary structure, are denoted by *dashed lines. Light circles* denote $^3J_{N\alpha}$ coupling constants smaller than 5.5 Hz, while *light boxes* denote values greater than 8.0 Hz. NOEs/couplings identified from homonuclear datasets only are depicted in *gray,* while the additional NOEs/couplings obtained from a variety of heteronuclear experiments are depicted in *black.*

The homonuclear NMR data obtained for PLB(1–25) have been used to calculate a formal solution conformation in aqueous TFE.[13] The resolution of solution structures obtained from distance geometry calculations using nuclear Overhauser effect (NOE) and torsion constraints is a direct function of the number of constraints that can be applied. For PLB(1–25), overlap between backbone amide resonances limits the number of NOEs that can confidently be assigned. This problem occurs to a much greater extent for pPLB(1–25; Ser-16) in aqueous TFE and detergent micelles. Consequently, to improve the quality of the PLB(1–25) solution structure, the peptide was synthetically labeled with ^{15}N at seven positions (FIG. 1), permitting the use of isotope resolved, edited and filtered experiments to resolve some of the ambiguities in resonance assignments that had previously limited structure calculations. FIGURE 3 shows both the ^1H-^{15}N HMQC experiment and the amide region of an HMQC-NOESY experiment. NOEs that are overlapped in the homonuclear spectra can be assigned in the latter experiment by virtue of the additional ^{15}N dimension. ω_2-edited and ω_2-selected NOESY and TOCSY experiments were also acquired on PLB(1–25) in 30% aqueous TFE (FIG. 4).

From these experiments, a further 25 distance constraints and three torsion constraints were obtained (FIG. 5) and used together with those obtained from homonuclear data as input to structure calculations. The results of these calculations are shown in FIGURE 6. The increased number of constraints leads to a root mean square devia-

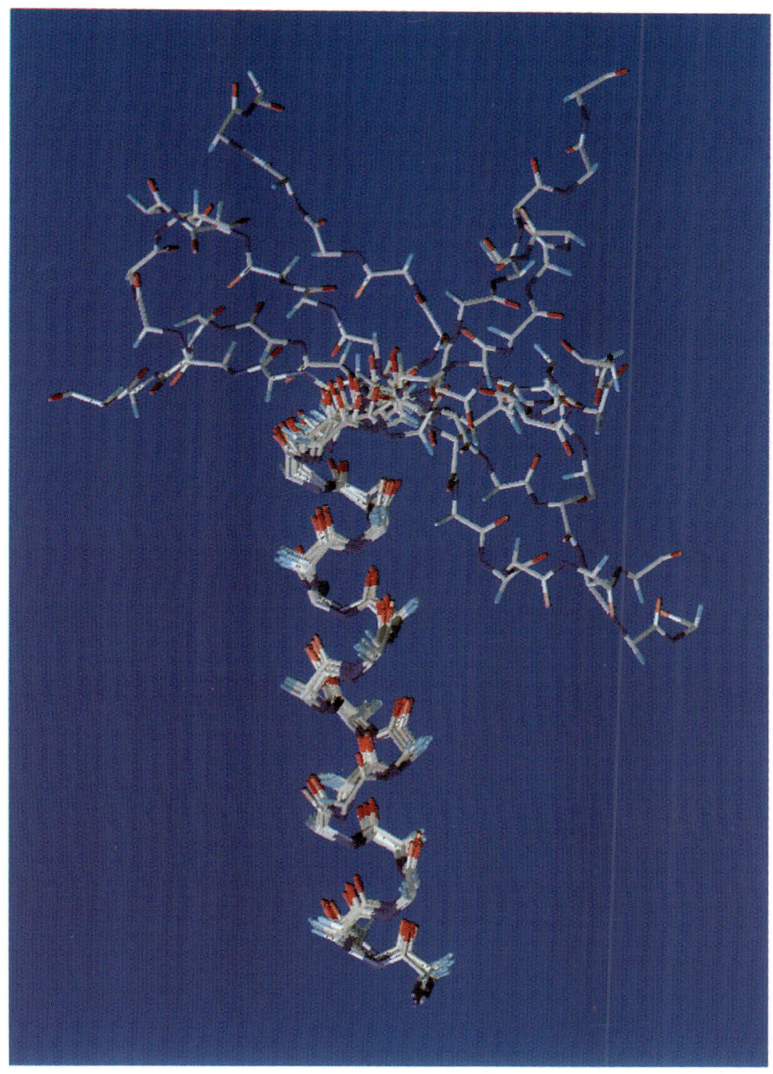

FIGURE 6. Backbone traces of the 10 lowest energy conformers of PLB(1–25) in 30% TFE/H_2O, pH 3.05, 300 K with residues 1–16 superposed. Conformers were calculated using constraints obtained from both homonuclear and heteronuclear experiments.

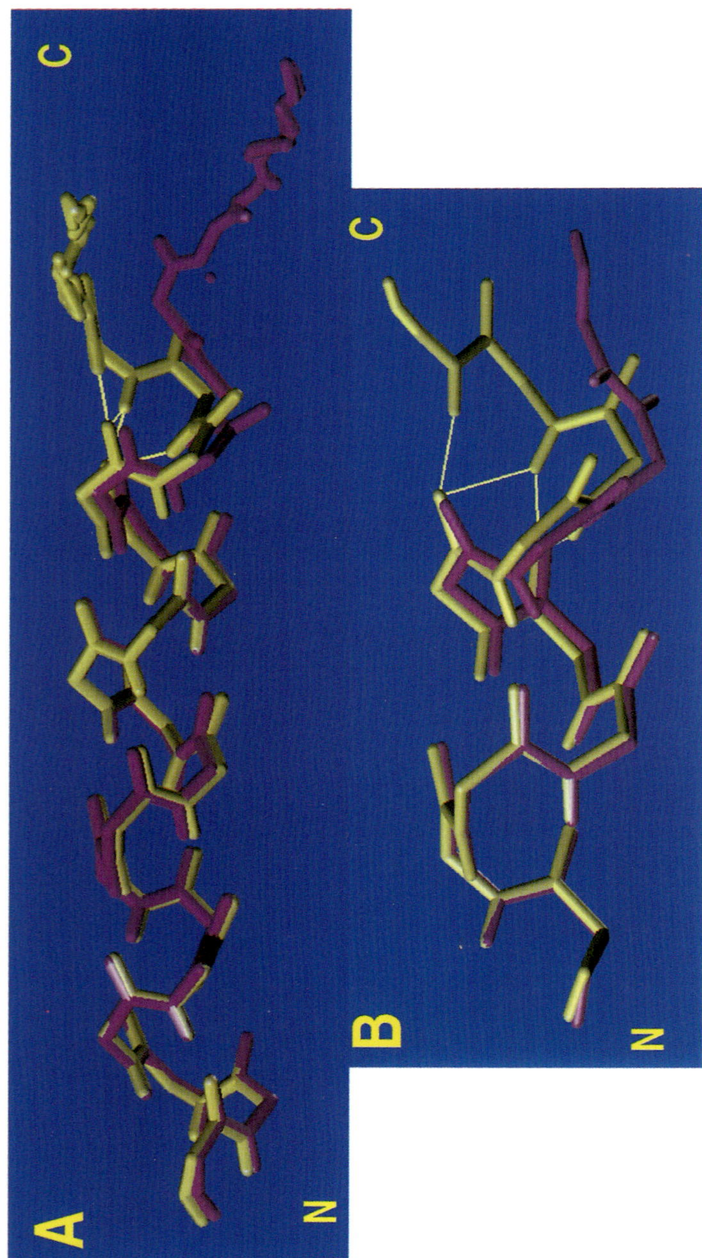

FIGURE 7. A. Comparison of structures obtained from homonuclear data alone[13] *(dark tubes)* and with heteronuclear data included *(light tubes)*. **B.** Detail of hydrogen bonding network at C-terminus of helix.

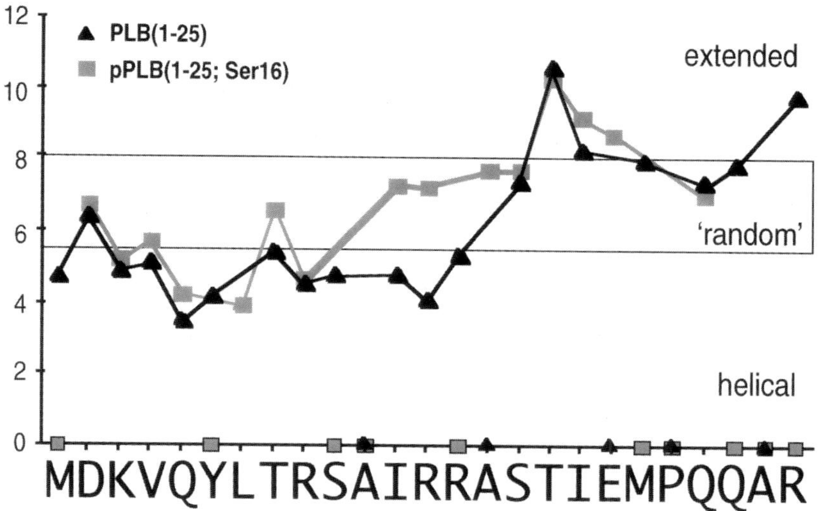

FIGURE 8. Backbone $C^{\alpha}H$-NH coupling constants determined for PLB(1–25) *(dark triangles)* and pPLB(1–25; Ser-16) *(light squares)* in 30% TFE/H_2O, pH 3.05, 300 K.

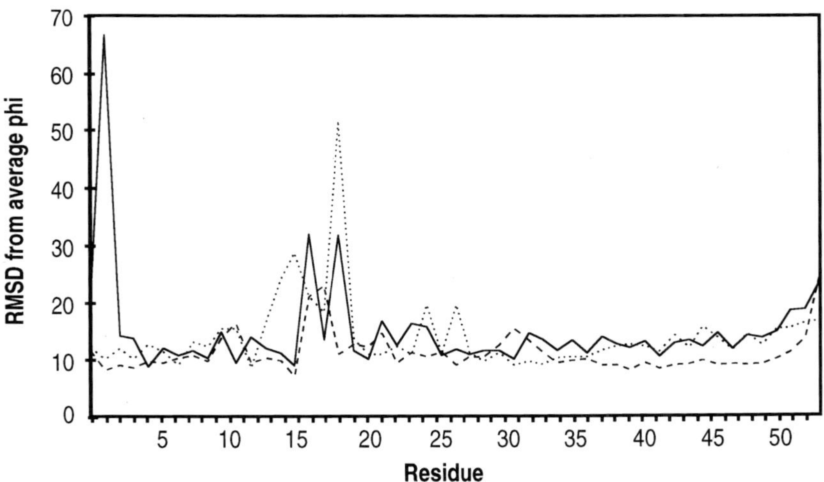

FIGURE 9. Root mean square deviations (RMSD) from mean ϕ during 250 ps of three separate molecular dynamics simulations on PLB(1–52).

tion (RMSD) from the mean of 0.44 Å for the backbone heavy atoms of the 10 lowest energy conformers. Furthermore, several NOEs could be assigned at the C-terminus of the helix that were previously unassignable, and these result in a lengthening of the helix at its C-terminus by approximately one half-turn (FIG. 7A). Thus, Thr -14 CO now forms a hydrogen bond to Ile-18 NH, and Ala-15 CO forms a hydrogen bond to Glu-19 (FIG. 7B).

Previously, we have shown that phosphorylation of PLB(1–25) at Ser-16 leads to a marked decrease in downfield secondary chemical shifts for residues 1–16, consistent with destabilization of the helix. This destabilization is also manifested in the $^3J_{HN\alpha}$ coupling constants. Additional (and otherwise inaccessible) NH-C$^\alpha$H coupling constants were obtained from ^{1}H-^{15}N HMQC experiments on both PLB(1–25) and pPLB(1–25, Ser-16) in aqueous trifluoroethanol (FIG. 8). Values for NH-C$^\alpha$H coupling constants greater than 8 Hz are associated with extended secondary structure, while values greater than 5.5 Hz are associated with helical secondary structure. For residues 1 to 11, there is an approximately 10% increase in $^3J_{HN\alpha}$ upon phosphorylation. However, for residues 12, 13, 15, and 16 in pPLB(1–25; Ser16) the $^3J_{HN\alpha}$ values are all in the random coil region of conformational space consistent once again with a disruption to the helix upon phosphorylation.

In these model systems, then, phosphorylation at Ser-16 has two effects. The α-helix is generally destabilized along its entire length, manifesting itself in a reduction of C$^\alpha$H secondary shifts; and there is a specific local effect at the C-terminus of the helix such that approximately the final 1.5 turns appear to unwind.

Molecular Dynamics Simulations

It has previously been shown that it is possible to predict major structural features in membrane proteins from molecular dynamics simulations.[32,33] In this methodology, a protein sequence is generated and given an idealized helical conformation, following which the protein is allowed to experience a period of unrestrained molecular dynamics in a continuum with a reduced dielectric constant, typically $\varepsilon = 2$. Over the course of the simulation, the fluctuations in backbone NH orientation are evaluated. Regions experiencing large fluctuations in backbone NH vectors are predicted to be mobile in a membrane environment. Experimental evidence for the validity of this approach is provided by the good agreement of predictions with NMR relaxation measurements, which are an indication of true mobility.[33]

The results of three separate simulations on unphosphorylated human PLB(1–52) are shown in FIGURE 9. While there are minor differences in the observed backbone fluctuations between each simulation, residues 14 to 19 generally experience a much greater degree of backbone mobility than does the remainder of the protein. As expected, the ends of the helix are also somewhat frayed. At first sight, the simplest explanation for the observed increase in mobility is that Pro-21 is simply acting as a helix-breaking residue, lacking the ability to form N-terminal hydrogen bonds. However, in simulations differing only in the replacement of Pro-21 by alanine (data not shown), the same local increase in mobility was observed. The observed mobility is more likely to derive from the two adjacent β-branched residues Thr-17–Ile18, which act as a helix-breaking signal.

The secondary structure of full-length phospholamban has been investigated in a single NMR study by Maslennikov and co-workers,[34] who solublized a monomeric mutant (C41F) in a 1:1 mixture of chloroform/methanol. Based on homo-

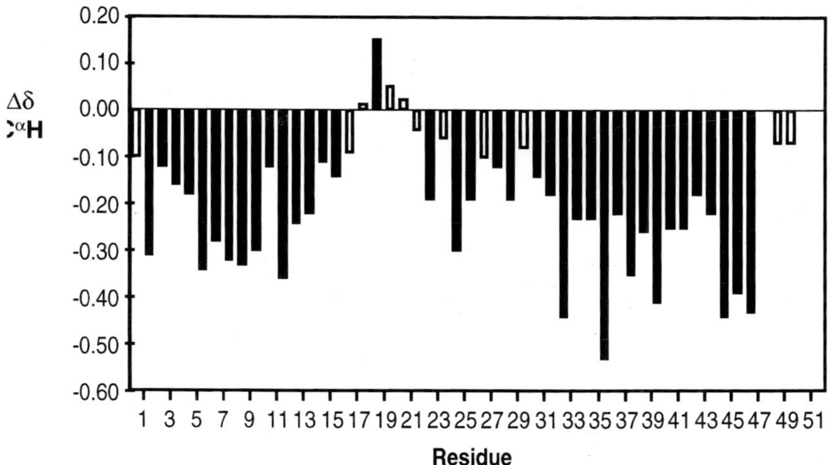

FIGURE 10. C$^{\alpha}$H secondary shifts for PLB(1–52; C41F) (vertical axis) by residue (horizontal axis). CaH chemical shifts were taken from Reference 34.

nuclear NMR data, a working model for the structure of PLB was proposed in which helices are formed by residues 1–20, and 22–52, with a flexible hinge formed by Pro-21. Extensive resonance degeneracy precluded structure generation from NOE distance constraints. The calculated C$^{\alpha}$H secondary shifts[31] for PLB(1–52; C41F) in 50% methanol/chloroform are shown in FIGURE 10. Using Wishart's criteria for stable secondary structure,[35] stable helices are formed by residues 2 to 16, and 31 to 52. Most interestingly, there is a distinct region of predicted random coil structure between residues 17 and 22. The secondary shifts for this NMR study of phospholamban were mapped onto the surface of a helical tube representing an idealized 52-residue helix (FIG. 11, top), such that the radius and color of the tube are proportional to backbone mobility, and are compared with the mean RMSD from the mean ϕ during 750 ps of molecular dynamics (MD) (FIG. 11, bottom). Residues predicted to be mobile from MD simulations correlate directly with apparent random coil structure in solution.[34]

MD simulations on PLB(1–52) phosphorylated at Ser-16 were performed in a manner identical to that previously described, and the results are shown in FIGURE 12. According to these simulations, phosphorylation is predicted to result in an increase in mobility that is N-terminally extended to residues 9–11, comparable with the unwinding observed in our model peptides. The driving force for this unwinding appears in the simulations to be the formation of charge-charge interactions between the phosphorylated side chain of Ser-16 and the guanidinium groups of either Arg-13 or Arg-14 (FIG. 13). Such an interaction between phospho-Ser-16 and Arg-14 has previously been observed for model peptides in aqueous solution.[36]

The simulations described here were of necessity performed with a monomeric model of PLB *in vacuo,* and it is possible that intermolecular interactions between monomers in the PLB pentamer may modify the behavior of PLB *in vivo.*

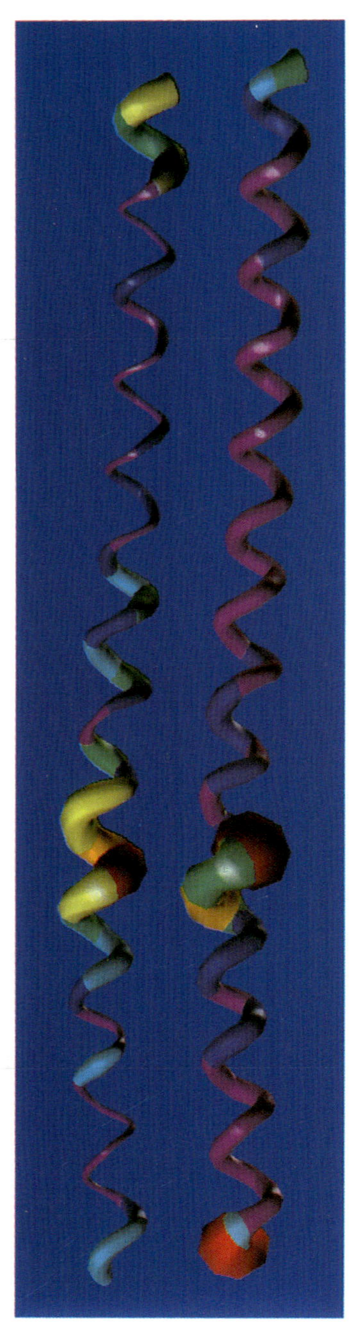

FIGURE 11. Comparison of **(top)** secondary $C^{\alpha}H$ shifts for PLB(1–52; C41F) in 50% $CDCl_3/CD_3OH$ with **(bottom)** average RMSD from mean ϕ for PLB(1–52). Tube diameters and hues are scaled according to **(top)** $\Delta\delta(C^{\alpha}H)$ and **(bottom)** average RMSD.

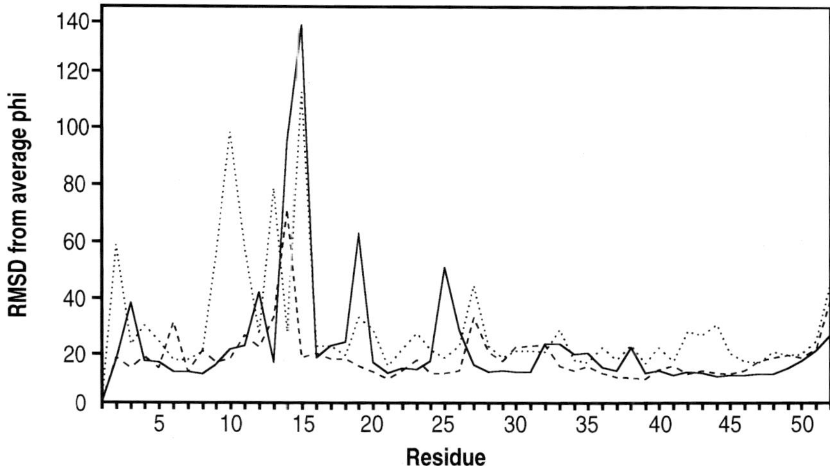

FIGURE 12. Root mean square deviations from mean ϕ during 250 ps of three separate molecular dynamics simulations on pPLB(1–52; Ser-16).

In these model systems phosphorylation appears to act as a conformational switch that specifically destabilizes the cytoplasmic helix, and by increasing the mobility of a relatively unstructured loop, uncouples domain Ia from the remainder of the protein. Thomas *et al.* have shown that phosphorylation has an effect on the exposure of PLB to lipids, reflecting a change in the structural relationship between PLB pentamer and bilayer.[37] Whether the conformational change in PLB as a result of phosphorylation that our model studies predict is a side effect of change in charge state from +3 to +1, or is directly responsible for disruption of molecular recognition between PLB and Ca^{2+}-ATPase remains to be defined.

ACKNOWLEDGMENTS

The authors are grateful to Stan Opella for advice on MD simulations.

[*Figure 13 is overleaf.*]

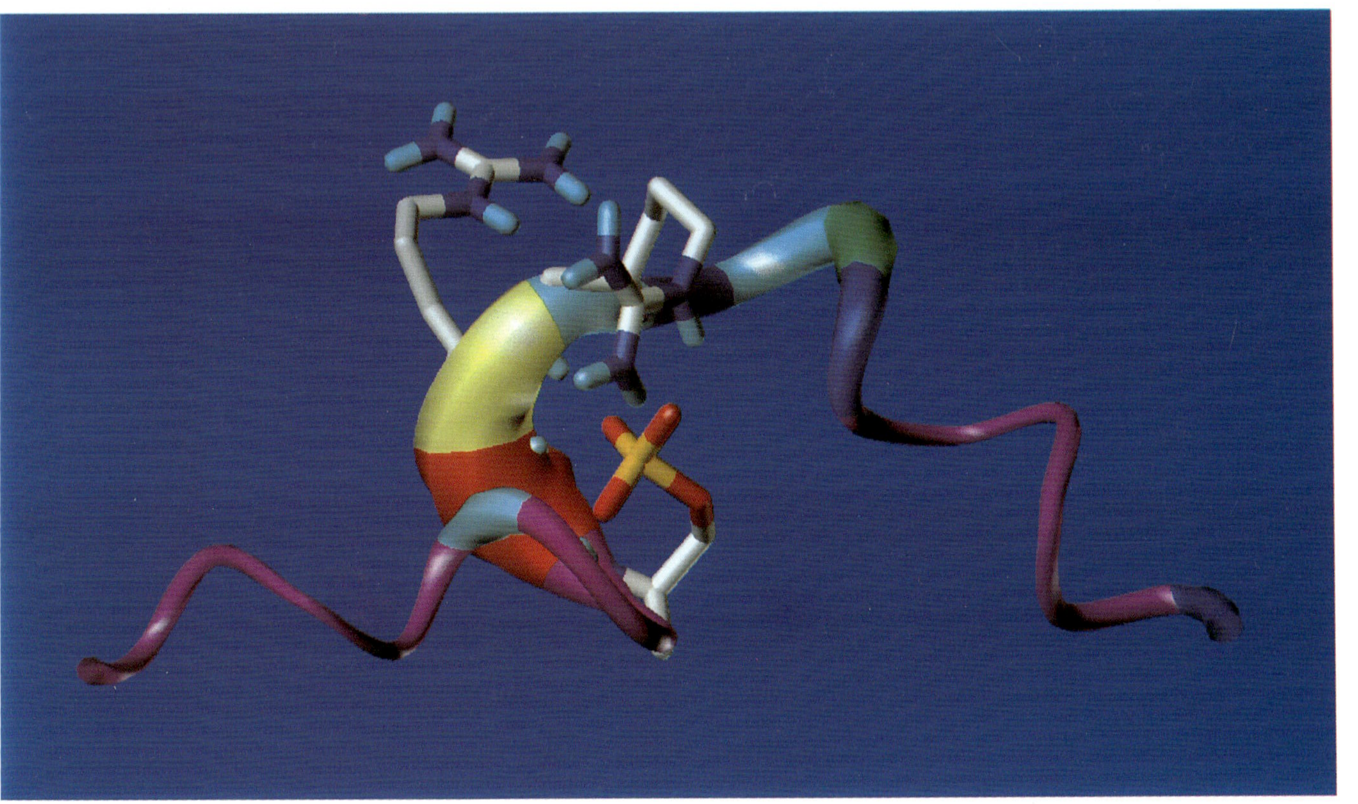

FIGURE 13. Representative final structure from MD simulations on pPLB(1–52; Ser-16) showing charge-charge interactions between the side chains of Arg-13 and phospho-Ser-16. The average backbone mobility during the simulations is mapped onto the backbone by tube diameter and hue.

REFERENCES

1. TADA, M. & A. M. KATZ. 1982. Phosphorylation of the sarcoplasmic reticulum and sarcolemma. Annu. Rev. Physiol. **44:** 401–423.
2. HICKS, M. J., M. SHIGEKAWA & A. M. KATZ. 1979. Mechanism by which cyclic adenosine 3′:5′-monophosphate-dependent protein kinase stimulates calcium transport in cardiac sarcoplasmic reticulum. Circ. Res., **44**(3): 384–391.
3. TADA, M., M. A. KIRCHBERGER, D. I. REPKE & A. M. KATZ. 1974. Effects of a cardiac cyclic AMP dependent protein kinase on the cardiac sarcoplasmic reticulum. II. Stimulation of calcium transport in cardiac sarcoplasmic reticulum by adenosine 3′,5′-monophosphate dependent protein kinase. J. Biol. Chem. **249**(19):6174–6180.
4. JAMES, P., M. INUI, M. TADA, M. CHIESI & E. CARAFOLI. 1989. Nature and site of phospholamban regulation of the calcium pump of sarcoplasmic reticulum. Nature (London) **342**(6245): 90–92.
5. TOYOFUKU, T., K. KURZYDLOWSKI, J. LYTTON & D. H. MACLENNAN. 1994. Amino acids Glu2 to Ile18 in the cytoplasmic domain of phospholamban are essential for functional association with the Ca^{2+}-ATPase of sarcoplasmic reticulum. J. Biol. Chem. **269:** 3088–3094.
6. FUJII, J., K. MARUYAMA, M. TADA & D. H. MACLENNAN. 1989. Expression and site-specific mutagenesis of phospholamban. Studies of residues involved in phosphorylation and pentamer formation. J. Biol. Chem. **264**(22): 12950–12955.
7. YOUNG, E. F., M. J. MCKEE, D. G. FERGUSON & E. G. KRANIAS. 1989. Structural characterization of phospholamban in cardiac sarcoplasmic reticulum membranes by cross-linking. Membr. Biochem. **8:** 95–106.
8. SIMMERMAN, H. K. B., D. E. LOVELACE & L. R. JONES. 1989. Secondary structure of detergent-solubilized phospholamban, a phosphorylatable, oligomeric protein of cardiac sarcoplasmic reticulum Biochim. Biophys. Acta **997:** 322–329.
9. ARKIN, I. T., M. ROTHMAN, C. F. C. LUDLAM, S. AIMOTO, D. M. ENGELMAN, K. J. ROTHSCHILD & S. O. SMITH. 1995. Structural model of the phospholamban ion channel complex in phospholipid membranes. J. Mol. Biol. **248**(4): 824–834.
10. KIMURA, Y., K. KURZYDLOWSKI, M. TADA & D. H. MACLENNAN. 1997. Phospholamban inhibitory function is activated by depolymerization. J. Biol. Chem. **272**(24): 15061–15064.
11. ARKIN, I. T., M. ROTHMAN, C. F. C LUDLAM, S. AIMOTO, D. M. ENGELMAN, K. J. ROTHSCHILD & S. O. SMITH. 1995. Structural model of the phospholamban ion channel complex in phospholipid membranes. J. Mol. Biol. **248**(4): 824–834.
12. IMAGAWA, T., T. WATANABE & T. NAKAMURA. 1986. Subunit structure and multiple phosphorylation sites of phospholamban. J. Biochem. (Tokyo) **99**(1): 41–53.
13. MORTISHIRE-SMITH, R. J., S. M. PITZENBERGER, C. J. BURKE, C. R. MIDDAUGH, V. M. GARSKY & R. G. JOHNSON. 1995. Solution structure of the cytoplasmic domain of phospholamban: phosphorylation leads to a local perturbation in secondary structure. Biochemistry **34**(23): 7603–7613.
14. RANCE, M., O. W. SOERENSEN, G. BODENHAUSEN, G. WAGNER, R. R. ERNST & K. WUETHRICH. 1983. Improved spectral resolution in COSY proton NMR spectra of proteins via double quantum filtering. Biochem. Biophys. Res. Commun. **117**(2): 479–485.
15. RANCE, M. 1987. Improved techniques for homonuclear rotating-frame and isotropic mixing experiments. J. Magn. Reson. **74**(3): 557–564.
16. JEENER, J., B. H. MEIER., P. BACHMANN & R. R. ERNST. 1979. Investigation of exchange processes by two-dimensional NMR spectroscopy. J. Chem. Phys. **71**(11): 4546–4553.
17. BAX, A., R. H. GRIFFEY & B. L. HAWKINS, 1983. Correlation of proton and nitrogen-15 chemical shifts by multiple quantum NMR. J. Magn. Reson. **55**(2): 301–315.
18. DAVIS, D. G. 1989. Enhanced correlations in proton-detected heteronuclear two-dimensional spectroscopy via spin-locked proton magnetization transfer. J. Magn. Reson. **84**(2): 417–424.
19. NORWOOD, T. J., J. BOYD, J. E. HERITAGE, N. SOFFE & I. D. CAMPBELL. 1990. Comparison of techniques for proton-detected heteronuclear proton-nitrogen-15 spectroscopy. J. Magn. Reson. **87**(3): 488–501.
20. GRIFFEY, R. H. & A. G. REDFIELD. 1987. Proton-detected heteronuclear edited and corre-

lated nuclear magnetic resonance and nuclear Overhauser effect in solution. Q. Rev. Biophys. **19**(1–2): 51–82.
21. GEMMECKER, G., E. T. OLEJNICZAK & S. W. FESIK. 1992. An improved method for selectivity observing protons attached to carbon-12 in the presence of proton-carbon-13 spin pairs. J. Magn. Reson. **96**(1): 199–204.
22. BODENHAUSEN, G., R. L. VOLD & R. R. VOLD. 1980. Multiple quantum spin-echo spectroscopy. J. Magn. Reson. **37**(1): 93–106.
23. MARION, D. & K. WUETHRICH. 1983. Application of phase sensitive two-dimensional correlated spectroscopy (COSY) for measurements of proton-proton spin-spin coupling constants in proteins. Biochem. Biophys. Res. Commun. **113**(3): 967–974.
24. JOHNSON, B. A. & R. A. BLEVINS. 1994. NMRView: A computer program for the visualization and analysis of NMR data. J. Biomol. NMR **4**(5): 603–614.
25. GUENTERT, P., Y. Q. QIAN, G. OTTING, M. MUELLER, W. GEHRING & K. WUETHRICH. 1991. Structure determination of the Antp(C39 $\rightarrow$ S) homeodomain from nuclear magnetic resonance data in solution using a novel strategy for the structure calculation with the programs DIANA, CALIBA, HABAS and GLOMSA. J. Mol. Biol. **217**(3): 531–540.
26. GUENTERT, P., W. BRAUN & K. WUETHRICH. 1991. Efficient computation of three-dimensional protein structures in solution from nuclear magnetic resonance data using the program DIANA and the supporting programs CALIBA, HABAS and GLOMSA. J. Mol. Biol., **217**(3): 517–530.
27. GUENTERT, P. & K. WUETHRICH. 1991. Improved efficiency of protein structure calculations from NMR data using the program DIANA with redundant dihedral angle constraints. J. Biomol. NMR **1**(4): 447–456.
28. PARDI, A., M. BILLETER & K. WUETHRICH. 1984. Calibration of the angular dependence of the amide proton-Cα proton coupling constants, 3JHNα, in a globular protein. Use of 3JHNα for identification of helical secondary structure. J. Mol. Biol. **180**(3): 741–751.
29. TERZI, E., L. POTEUR & E. TRIFILIEFF. 1992. Evidence for a phosphorylation-induced conformational change in phospholamban cytoplasmic domain by CD analysis. FEBS Lett. **309**(3): 413–416.
30. HUBBARD, J. A., L. K. MACLACHLAN, E. MEENAN, C. J. SALTER, D. G. REID, P. LAHOURATATE, J. HUMPHRIES, N. STEVENS. D. BELL *et al.* 1994. Conformation of the cytoplasmic domain of phospholamban by NMR and CD. Mol. Membr. Biol. **11**(4): 263–269.
31. WISHART, D. S., B. D. SYKES & F. M. RICHARDS. 1991. Relationship between nuclear magnetic resonance chemical shift and protein secondary structure. J. Mol. Biol. **222**(2): 311–333.
32. TOBIAS, D. J., J. GESELL, M. K. KLEIN & S. J. OPELLA. 1995. A simple protocol for the identification of helical and mobile residues in membrane proteins. J. Mol. Biol. **253:** 391–395.
33. TOBIAS, D. J., M. L. KLEIN & S. J. OPELLA. 1993. Molecular dynamics simulation of Pf1 coat protein. Biophys. J. **64**(3): 670–675.
34. MASLENNIKOV, I. V., A. G. SOBOL, J. ANAGLI, P. JAMES, T. VORHERR, A. S. ARSENIEV & E. CARAFOLI. 1995. The secondary structure of phospholamban: a two-dimensional NMR study. Biochem. Biophys. Res. Commun. **217**(3): 1200–1207.
35. WISHART, D. S., B. D. SYKES & F. M. RICHARDS. 1992. The chemical shift index: A fast and simple method for the assignment of protein secondary structure through NMR spectroscopy. Biochemistry **31**(6): 1647–1651.
36. QUIRK, P. G., V. B. PATCHELL, J. COLYER, G. A. DRAGO & Y. GAO. 1996. Conformational effects of serine phosphorylation in phospholamban peptides. Eur. J. Biochem. **236**(1): 85–91.
37. CORNEA, R. L., L. R. JONES, J. M. AUTRY & D. D. THOMAS. 1997. Mutation and phosphorylation change the oligomeric structure of phospholamban in lipid bilayers. Biochemistry **36**(10): 2960–2967.

Phosphorylation States of Phospholamban[a]

JOHN COLYER[b]

School of Biochemistry and Molecular Biology, University of Leeds, Leeds LS2 9JT, United Kingdom

ABSTRACT: Phospholamban is a small integral membrane protein of cardiac, smooth, and slow-twitch skeletal muscle sarcoplasmic reticulum that interacts with the Ca^{2+} pump of these organelles and inhibits Ca^{2+}-pump activity while in the dephosphorylated form. Three sites of Ser/Thr phosphorylation have been identified in the primary sequence of phospholamban, at Ser-10, Ser-16, and Thr-17. *In vitro* studies indicate that these residues are phosphorylated by PKC (Ser-10), PKA, PKG or PKC (Ser-16), and CaM kinase II (Thr-17). Phosphorylation of Ser-16 (or Thr-17) is accompanied by an increase in Ca^{2+} pump activity in direct proportion to the stoichiometry of phosphorylation. Dual phosphorylation of both Ser-16 and Thr-17 does not cause any further stimulation of pump function over that achieved by stoichiometric phosphorylation of a single site. Examination of the pattern of phosphorylation *in vivo* has been aided by the generation of polyclonal antibodies specific for the phosphorylated forms of phospholamban. β-Adrenergic stimulation of cardiac muscle results in phosphorylation of both Ser-16 and Thr-17. The time course of Ser-16 phosphorylation precedes Thr-17. The spatial distribution of Ser-16 and Thr-17 phosphorylated forms of phospholamban is not identical; phospholamban located in the nuclear membrane of a cardiac myocyte is phosphorylated exclusively on Ser-16, whereas phospholamban molecules in the SR membrane of the same cell are phosphorylated on Ser-16 and/or Thr-17. Finally, we have identified a novel stimulus for the phosphorylation of phospholamban. Ca^{2+} store depletion, achieved by exposure of myocytes to SERCA inhibitors, prompts the phosphorylation of phospholamban on Ser-16. This would be expected to increase Ca^{2+} uptake by the SR in an attempt to achieve the refilling of the SR.

Phospholamban is a membrane protein of 52 residues in length[1] that controls the cardiac sarcoplasmic reticulum (SR) Ca^{2+} pump by direct physical interaction.[2] This control arises from suppression of Ca^{2+} pump activity by dephosphorylated phospholamban, a situation that is reversed upon phosphorylation of phospholamban at one of at least two sites, Ser-16 and Thr-17. β-Adrenergic stimulation of cardiac muscle provokes stimulation of Ser-16 and Thr-17 phosphorylation of phospholamban, with the consequent acceleration of Ca^{2+} transport into the SR, which is believed to underlie the positive inotropic and positive lusitropic effects of β-agonists. In this article, I will describe the mode of interpretation of phospholamban phosphorylation by the Ca^{2+} pump, present evidence for the use of the two sites of phosphorylation of phospholamban in live cardiac myocytes, and describe a novel stimulus for phospholamban phosphorylation, the depletion of Ca^{2+} from the SR lumen.

[a] The financial support of the British Heart Foundation (BS/6, PG/92126, PG/95020, PG/96125, FS/92014 and FS/96068) and Medical Research Council (G9428756MA) is acknowledged with thanks.

[b] Phone: +44-113-233-3124; fax: +44-113-233-3167; e-mail: j.colyer@leeds.ac.uk

PHOSPHORYLATION OF PLB

The oligomeric assembly of phospholamban (PLB), which in the membrane is believed to be a dynamic equilibrium between monomer and pentamer,[3] is an interesting structure from the standpoint of the reaction mechanism of phosphorylation. It presents scope for a cooperative or processive reaction mechanism of phosphorylation when the appropriate kinase or phosphatase engages a pentameric substrate. Examination of this issue is possible by virtue of the discrete electrophoretic mobility change that accompanies phosphorylation of either Ser-16 or Thr-17 of PLB.[4,5] This change can be observed in SDS-PAGE format, where the monomeric unit of phospholamban exhibits an apparent increase in molecular weight upon Ser or Thr phosphorylation, and a second apparent increase in weight upon dual phosphorylation of both Ser and Thr. These properties are not confined to the monomer, but can be observed in the pentameric species of phospholamban, too. Here, the electrophoretic behavior of individual subunits within a pentamer retains a dependence on phosphorylation status, and contributes equally to the electrophoretic behavior of the pentamer as a whole.[4] Thus the electrophoretic mobility of an individual pentamer is the sum of the equal contributions from each of the five individual subunits. For instance, a pentamer with no subunits phosphorylated can be resolved from one with a single subunit phosphorylated on either Ser-16 or Thr-17. This discrete separation extends across the entire spectrum of phosphorylated species from no subunits phosphorylated (P_0) to all five subunits phosphorylated on both Ser-16 and Thr-17 (P_{10}).[5] An example of this is displayed in FIGURE 1. The pentamer with all subunits dephosphorylated exhibits the

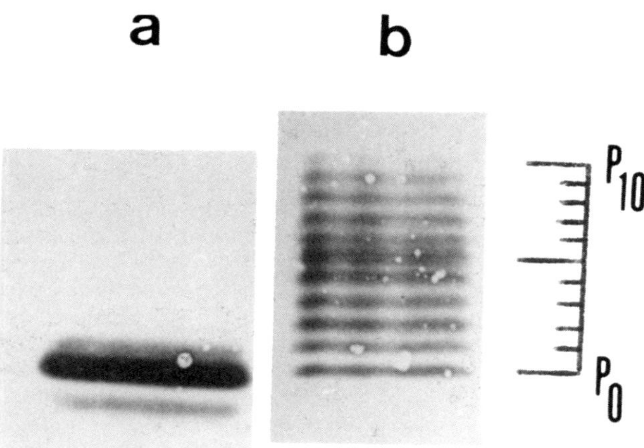

FIGURE 1. Electrophoretic resolution of the phosphorylation states of phospholamban. Three μg of canine cardiac SR proteins **(a)** dephosphorylated and **(b)** phosphorylated by PK-A and CaM kinase II were separated by SDS-PAGE (15% acrylamide) and transfered to PVDF membrane. Pentameric forms of phospholamban were detected using monoclonal antibody A1[6] as described in Ref. 4. P_0 represents pentamers with no subunits phosphorylated; P_{10} represents pentamers with all five subunits phosphorylated on Ser-16 and Thr-17. A continuum of species between these two extremes is evident in this sample, which was not phosphorylated to full stoichiometry.

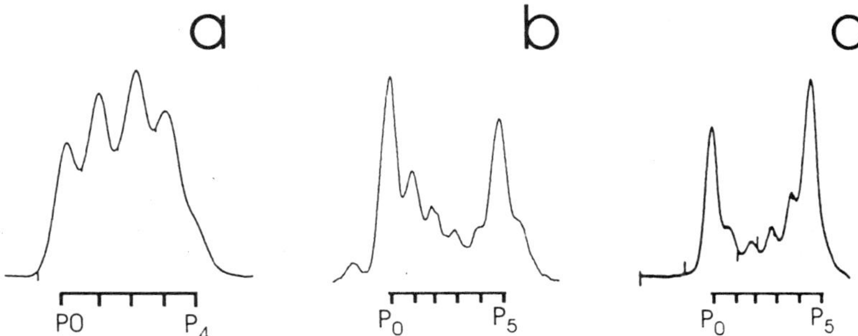

FIGURE 2. Reaction mechanism of phospholamban phosphorylation and dephosphorylation. Phospholamban in SR vesicles was phosphorylated by **(a)** PK-A (Ser-16) or **(b)** CaM Kinase II (Thr-17), or was dephosphorylated by **(c)** PP-1. Pentamers were resolved and detected as in FIGURE 1, and densitometric scans of the repertoire of phosphorylation species are displayed. At three similar stages of reaction (about 33% complete) two patterns of phosphorylation species are evident. PK-A phosphorylation **(a)** produces a spectrum of phosphorylation products predicted by the binomial equation[4] and is thus a random process. CaM kinase II phosphorylation **(b)** and dephosphorylation **(c)** utilize cooperative reaction mechanisms that result in high concentrations of P_0 and P_5, with little increase in any other form of phospholamban pentamer.

smallest M_r. The apparent weight increases in discrete increments with each subunit that becomes phosphorylated at the first site (species P_1 to P_5). A second round of apparent M_r increases accompanies phosphorylation of PLB subunits at a second site (P_6 to P_{10}). Thus the P_{10} form of the pentamer comprises a pentameric oligomer of phospholamban with all subunits phosphorylated at two positions (Ser-16 and Thr-17 in FIG. 1).

These electrophoretic properties have facilitated the detailed investigation of the mechanism of phosphorylation (random or cooperative) and the decoding of the response of SERCA activity to changes in the phosphorylation stoichiometry of PLB. FIGURE 2 summarizes the reaction mechanism of Ser-16 and Thr-17 phosphorylation. Quantitative immunoblotting using monoclonal antibody A1[6] was employed to identify the repertoire of phosphorylation species generated by cyclic AMP-dependent protein kinase (PKA), calmodulin-dependent kinase II (CaM KII) or during dephosphorylation by protein phosphatase–1 (PP-1), and to describe the relative concentration of each. A single experimental observation approximately one-third of the way through the process of phosphorylation (or dephosphorylation) has been displayed in each case (FIG. 2a–c). The frequency of species P_0 to P_5 differs considerably between samples phosphorylated on Ser-16 (PKA, FIG. 2a) and Thr-17 (CaM KII, FIG. 2b). This identifies a radically different mechanism of PLB phosphorylation by these two kinases, which can be described as a random process in the case of PKA (close correlation of experimental data with predictions of the binomial equation[4]) and a nonrandom process in the case of CaM KII (no correlation with binomial prediction[5]). Thr-17 phosphorylation by CaM KII occurs via a cooperative reaction mechanism,[5] as does dephosphorylation of either Ser-16[4] (FIG. 2c) or Thr-17.[7] The ability of CaM KII and PP-1 to utilize a cooperative reaction mechanism with PLB identifies the presence of an oligomeric assembly of phospholamban in the SR membrane, and suggests that the oligomeric assembly of PLB engaged by these enzymes is pentameric.[8]

RESPONSE OF SERCA TO PLB PHOSPHORYLATION

The control of SERCA Ca^{2+}-pump activity by PLB appears to be achieved by the physical association of phospholamban with the pump.[2] At least two sites of contact are proposed, one within the cytoplasmic domain of SERCA involving residues 397–402,[9] and a second site within the transmembrane domains.[10] The interaction of PLB with the pump at these sites results in a suppression of Ca^{2+}-pump function; V_{max} attenuated through the cytoplasmic domain interactions,[10,11] and K_{Ca} increased via the transmembrane contacts.[10] Phosphorylation of phospholamban relieves this inhibition most probably by altering one or both of these intereactions; however, the relationship between phosphorylation stoichiometry and pump activation is not transparent. It remains to be established whether the pentamer or monomer of PLB (or both) are able to interface with the pump and control SERCA activity. Recent evidence suggests that monomeric mutants of PLB are able to control pump function[12] and indeed may have increased inhibitory effects. The monomeric nature of most of these mutants has to date been described only in SDS, and thus it will be important to describe their oligomeric state in lipid bilayers as we attempt to resolve the inhibitory roles of pentameric and monomeric forms of PLB.

Early attempts to define the dependence of pump function on PLB phosphorylation noted that increases in phosphorylation were paralleled by increases in Ca^{2+}-pump activity.[13] However, these studies were not able to define phosphorylation in terms of molar stoichiometry. This was achieved most recently using the immunoquantitation of discrete phosphorylation species of phospholamban (as in FIG. 1) to calculate the molar phosphorylation stoichiometry.[5] Ca^{2+}-pump function responded to phosphory-

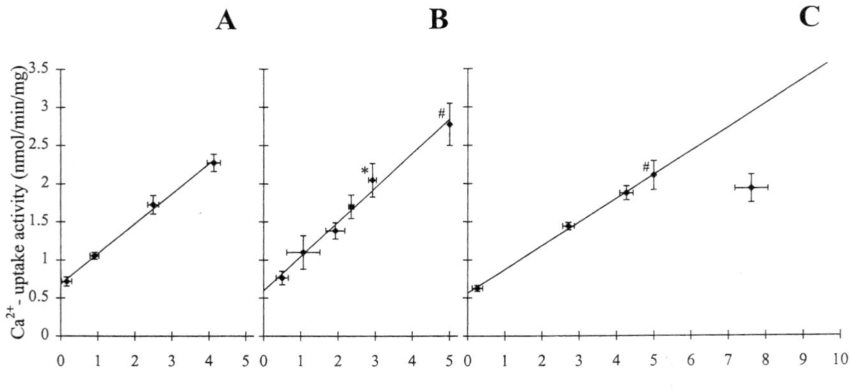

FIGURE 3. Translation of PLB phosphorylation into Ca^{2+}-pump stimulation. Ca^{2+} uptake into cardiac SR vesicles was determined using a Fluo-3 based assay[5] at pCa 7. Phosphorylation of phospholamban to defined stoichiometries was performed using **(A)** PK-A (Ser-16), **(B)** CaM kinase II (Thr-17), or **(C)** both enzymes. The stoichiometry of phosphorylation was measured in each sample as described in Ref. 5. Ser-16 phosphorylation produced a linear increase in Ca^{2+}-pump activity **(A).** Thr-17 phosphorylation also produced a linear increase in Ca^{2+}-pump function, of identical slope to that of Ser-16 (* in **B** denotes Ser-16 phosphorylated sample; # denotes maximal stimulation by monoclonal antibody A1[6]). Dual phosphorylation does not result in further stimulation of pump activity **(C).**

lation of phospholamban in direct proportion to the molar phosphorylation stoichiometry. This relationship was true for Ser-16 phosphorylation and Thr-17 phosphorylation, but not for the dual phosphorylated (Ser-16 and Thr-17) forms of PLB (FIG. 3).[7,14] Dual phosphorylation of a monomer of phospholamban does not lead to stimulation of pump function to a level in excess of that achieved by monophosphorylation of the same unit of phospholamban.[7,14]

PLB PHOSPHORYLATION *IN VIVO*

Aware of the relationship between pump function and phosphorylation status of phospholamban *in vitro,* we are able to examine SR Ca^{2+} transport and the regulation of this *in vivo* by the study of phosphorylation of phospholamban alone. This simplified view is largely accurate, although it must be recalled that dual phosphorylated forms of PLB break the simple relationship with pump function (pump function is proportional to phosphorylation stoichiometry) and complicate the issue somewhat.

The study of phospholamban phosphorylation *in vivo* has been successful using a number of approaches including radioactive labeling of ATP pools *in vivo*[15] and "back phosphorylation" *in vitro.*[16] We examined an alternative route of study potentially capable of accessing the information of these earlier studies and extending these to include the spatial refinement of phosphorylation signaling. We produced antibodies specific for the phosphorylated forms of phospholamban,[17] Ser-16 and Thr-17. Phosphorylation site–specific antibodies have now been generated to a variety of target proteins (comprehensively reviewed in Ref. 18), and are characterized as being specific for the protein of interest only when phosphorylated at a particular site. In some instances this can result in the recognition of two sites within the same protein, or two distinct proteins (e.g., DARPP and protein phosphatase inhibitor-1),[19] where there is considerable similarity between the primary sequence of these two segments of protein; however, this is the exception rather than the rule.

Phosphorylation site–specific antibodies to phospholamban were produced by immunization of rabbits with phosphorylated-peptide immunogen (residues 9–19 of phospholamban plus C-terminal tyrosine, phosphorylated at either Ser-16 or Thr-17) coupled to a carrier protein, Keyhole limpet hemocyanin.[17] FIGURE 4 displays the initial characterization of the specificity of these antibodies: PS-16, which recognizes Ser-16–phosphorylated forms of PLB; and PT-17, which recognizes Thr-17–phosphorylated forms. The identification of proteins in total heart homogenates (rat heart) phosphorylated *in vitro* by the stimulation of PKA (lanes 1,2) or CaM KII (lanes 3,4) is displayed. PS-16 identifies monomeric and pentameric forms of PLB only in this experiment, and the recognition is entirely dependent on Ser-16 phosphorylation as it is inhibited by the inclusion of Ser-16–phosphorylated peptide (panel D). Similarly, PT-17 identifies Thr-17 forms of PLB (both monomeric and pentameric) specifically, although a minor component of the serum identifies an unrelated protein of 48 kDa.

FIGURE 5 shows a further characterization of the PS-16 antibody, which is able to interact with the monophosphorylated Ser-16 PLB but not the dual-phosphorylated (Ser-16 and Thr-17) PLB. As has already been introduced, the electrophoretic mobility of phosphorylated forms of PLB is progressively reduced as phosphorylation status increases. P_{10} represents the pentamer comprising subunits phosphorylated on Ser-16 and Thr-17 in all cases. Antibody PS-16 is unable to interact with this form of phospholamban, despite its ability to interact with the Ser-16 monophosphorylated

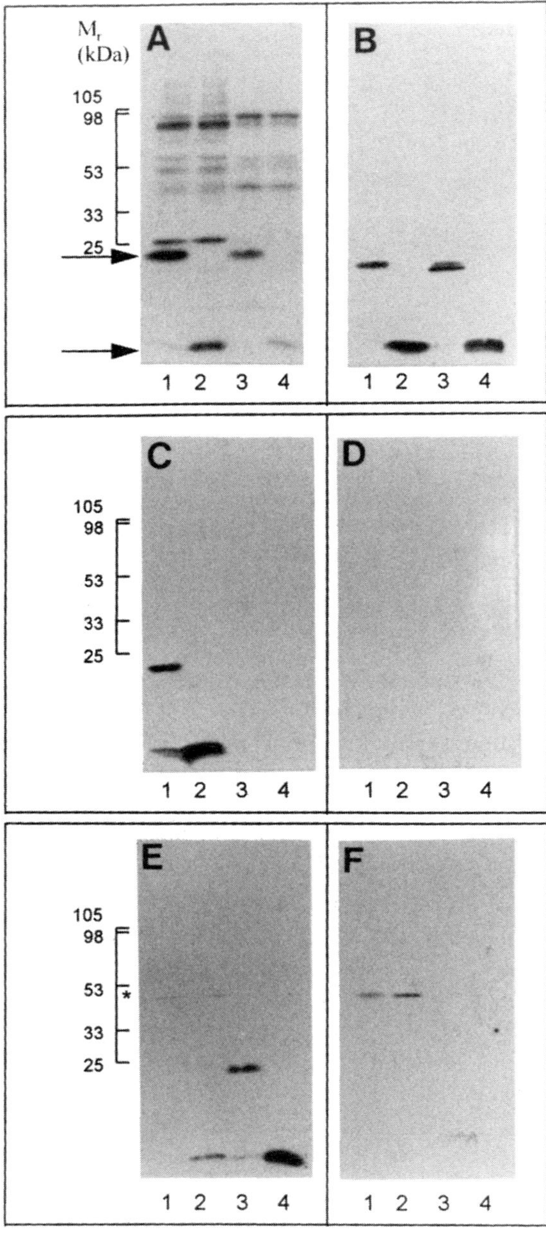

FIGURE 4. Characterization of antibodies to the phosphorylated forms of phospholamban. Rat heart homogenates were phosphorylated *in vitro* by addition of cAMP (*lanes* 1,2) or Ca^{2+}/CaM (*lanes* 3,4) in the presence of γ^{32}P-ATP.[17] Samples in *lanes* 2 and 4 were boiled for 5 min, others were treated at 30 °C for 30 min. Proteins were separated by SDS-PAGE on 5–20% gradient gels and transfered to PVDF membranes. **(A)** Autoradiograph of the blot; **(B)** total phospholamban stain with A1; **(C)** Ser-16 phosphorylated PLB stained with PS-16 (1:10,000); **(D)** PS-16 (1:10,000) + 1 μM Ser-16 phosphopeptide; **(E)** Thr-17 phosphorylated PLB stained with PT-17 (1:5,000); **(F)** PT-17 (1:5,000) + 1 μM Thr-17 phosphopeptide. (Reprinted from Ref. 17 with permission).

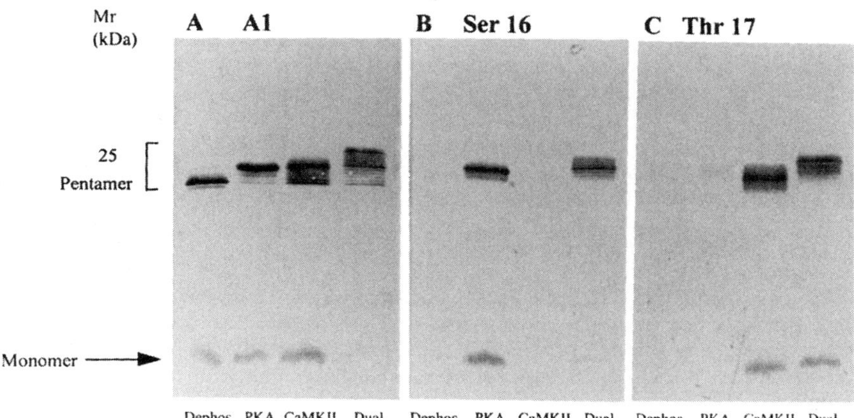

FIGURE 5. PS-16 antibody fails to detect dual phosphorylated PLB. Cardiac SR vesicles proteins were phosphorylated by PK-A, CaM kinase II, or both enzymes as described in Ref. 17. Three µg of dephosphorylated PKA and CaM kinase II, and dual phosphorylated SR samples were separated by SDS-PAGE on 15% acrylamide gels and transferred to PVDF. Identical panels were probed with **(A)** A1 (total PLB), **(B)** PS-16 (Ser-16 phosphorylated PLB), or **(C)** PT-17 (Thr-17 phosphorylated PLB). PS-16 fails to identify the slowest moving species of PLB in the dual phosphorylated sample (P_{10} in FIG. 1).

form of the protein. These observations suggest that Thr-17 must form an important part of the immunorecognition of the PLB target; when this is changed either to phosphothreonine (FIG. 5 and E-G. Krause, Berlin, personal communication) or mutated to Ala (E.G. Kranias, Cincinnati, personal communication), antibody recognition of phosphorylated PLB is lost. A second qualification of the PS-16 antibody has been noted; phospholamban and the 15-kDa plasma membrane protein phospholemman share considerable sequence identity around the phosphorylation site.[20] PS-16 reacts specifically (in a phosphorylation-dependent manner) with a protein of 15 kDa in experiments with intact isolated myocytes (data not shown). This protein is not the phospholamban dimer, as it can not be dissociated upon boiling, and frequently responds to changes in experimental conditions (acidosis, agonist) in a manner unlike that of PLB monomer and pentamer. We suggest that this is most likely the detection of changes in phospholemman phosphorylation, probably of Ser-68 (data not shown).

TIME COURSE OF SER-16 AND THR-17 PHOSPHORYLATION IN ISOLATED VENTRICULAR MYOCYTES

β-Adrenergic stimulation of cardiac muscle has been shown to increase the magnitude of contraction and reduce the time required to complete a cycle of contraction and relaxation.[21] Associated with these changes are increases in the phosphorylation of both Ser-16 and Thr-17 of phospholamban.[15] Ser-16 phosphorylation is the direct result of PKA activation by cAMP, whereas Thr-17 phosphorylation requires activation of calmodulin-dependent kinase II.[22] CaM kinase II activation is a secondary effect of cAMP elevation. The change in Ca^{2+}-handling that results from PKA phosphorylation of targets including phospholamban, the L-type Ca^{2+}-channel, ryanodine receptor, and troponin I is probably responsible for the increase in activity of CaM kinase II. Thus it might be expected that there would be a delay between these two events, the activation of PKA and CaM kinase II. Consistent with this, Wegener *et al.*[15] labeled the ATP pools of guinea pig hearts with ^{32}P and demonstrated that Ser-16 phosphorylation of PLB (PKA mediated) precedes Thr-17 phosphorylation of PLB upon administration of a β-agonist. Using the phosphorylation site–specific antibodies, we have confirmed this result in ferret cardiac myocytes. Ser-16–phosphorylated PLB accumulates rapidly, reaching ~10 pmol/1000 live cells in the first 60 seconds. The abundance of Ser-16–phosphorylated PLB then declines over the subsequent 4 minutes, even in the continued presence of isoprenaline. In contrast, Thr-17–phosphorylated forms of PLB accumulate slowly and progressively, reaching a maximum quantity of ~ 3 pmol/1000 live cells after a 5-minute exposure to isoprenaline (G. A. Drago, J. Colyer, manuscript in preparation). The time delay in Thr-17 phosphorylation compared to Ser-16 phosphorylation is substantial in ferret ventricular myocytes, far greater than was evident in the guinea pig.[15] The temporal separation in the phosphorylation of the two sites might be explained in terms of a two-phase response as outlined above; PKA responds to the rise in cAMP and phosphorylates targets that increase Ca^{2+} in the cytoplasm. This increase in Ca^{2+} stimulates CaM kinase II, which results in Thr-17 phosphorylation of PLB. An alternative explanation for the temporal delay in Thr-17 phosphorylation might be the requirement for a reduced phosphatase activity at the SR in advance of accumulation of Thr-17 phosphorylation of PLB. Mundina-Weilenmann *et al.*[23] noted a β-agonist–independent route to stimulate Thr-17 phosphorylation; this entailed raising extracellular Ca^{2+} (to 3.85 mM) and perfusing the heart with a phosphatase inhibitor, 1 μM okadaic acid. Protein phosphatase–1 is the dominant enzyme with respect to PLB dephosphorylation;[24] thus Mundina-Weilenmann *et al.*[23] concluded that protein phosphatase-1 inhibition was required *in vivo* for significant phosphorylation of Thr-17 to occur. PP-1 inhibition by PKA is well documented (release from protective targeting partner protein, inhibition by inhibitors 1 and 2)[25,26], and thus the temporal separation of Ser-16 and Thr-17 phosphorylation of PLB might be explained by the need to inhibit PP-1 (via PKA actions) prior to accumulation of Thr-17 phosphorylated forms of PLB.

The contribution made by each phosphorylation site to changes in Ca^{2+} handling *in vivo* might be expected (from *in vitro* experimentation)[5] to be proportional to the level of phosphorylation at each site. The independent phosphorylation of Ser-16 or Thr-17 has each been shown to contribute near equally to accelerations in the rate of contraction and the rate of relaxation,[23] and their effects appear to be largely additive. Indeed the amount of Ser-16 phosphorylation and Thr-17 phosphorylation of PLB correlate closely with cAMP concentration, the increase in contraction amplitude, the increase in Ca^{2+} transient amplitude, and the acceleration of Ca^{2+} transient decline (S. Calaghan, E. White and J. Colyer, manuscript in preparation). However, Ser-16 appears to correlate more closely than Thr-17 with three of the four parameters above (t1/2 of Ca^{2+}-transient correlates equally well with both phosphorylation events), and is quantitatively greater, perhaps indicating that Ser-16 phosphorylation plays a more important role in controlling Ca^{2+} handling characteristics in cardiac myocytes than does Thr-17. This is supported by the time dependence of β-stimulation effect and phospholamban phosphorylation. Increases in contraction amplitude and abbreviation of the contractile cycle are observed within the first 60 of β-agonist exposure in ferret myocytes,[27] by which time only Ser-16 phosphorylation of phospholamban has occurred (data not shown).

WHAT PROVOKES PLB PHOSPHORYLATION IN CARDIAC MYOCYTES?

β-Adrenergic stimulation of cardiac myocytes results in the phosphorylation of phospholamban[15] mediated principally via β1-receptor subtype activation.[28] This results in both a positive inotropic response and a positive lusitropic response, with characteristic changes in the shape and kinetics of the Ca^{2+} transient. Changes (increases) in the electrical stimulation rate can also produce changes in the Ca^{2+} transient reminiscent of β-adrenergic stimulation.[29] Is this achieved via phosphorylation of PLB on Thr-17 as postulated by Shouten?[30] Hussain *et al.*[31] confirmed that the abbreviation of the Ca^{2+} transient with increasing electrical stimulation rate was a function of the SR contribution to the Ca^{2+} transient but did not observe an increase in PLB phosphorylation (on Thr-17 or Ser-16). Moreover, they were unable to block the effects of increased stimulation rate on Ca^{2+} handling by application of CaM kinase II inhibitors (KN-62, calmodulin binding domain peptide),[31] which suggests that these changes are independent of CaM kinase II action. As such, phosphorylation of PLB does not represent the molecular mechanism of Ca^{2+} transient adaptation by stimulation rate, and therefore is not the sole means of modulation of Ca^{2+} transient kinetics in cardiac muscle.

Ser-16 phosphorylation is responsive to one final intervention that is independent of β-adrenergic agonists. Depletion of Ca^{2+} from the SR activates processes that result in the phosphorylation of PLB on Ser-16. This would be expected to increase the rate of Ca^{2+} sequestration by the SR and may lead to refilling of the store. We suggest that this is an important control pathway (analogous to store-operated Ca^{2+} entry in non-muscle cells),[32] which can correct the balance between SR and plasma membrane Ca^{2+} transport systems and maintain SR Ca^{2+} load at a level that allows E-C coupling. FIGURE 6 shows an example of the data that have lead to this interpretation. SR Ca^{2+} depletion was prompted by incubation of isolated rat ventricular myocytes with any of three Ca^{2+} pump inhibitors, thapsigargin (TG, 2.5 μM), t-butyl hydroquinone (BHQ, 30 μM), or cyclopiazonic acid (CPA, 50 μM). Each of these interventions reduced the caffeine-dependent Ca^{2+} transient dramatically, consistent with a significant loss of Ca^{2+} from the SR. In response to this depletion of store Ca^{2+} the phosphorylation status of PLB (Ser-16) increased dramatically (FIG. 6). These three Ca^{2+} pump inhibitors are structurally unrelated, but have the common property of depleting the SR of Ca^{2+}, secondary to pump inhibition. This depletion of SR Ca^{2+}, and not the minor increase in $[Ca^{2+}]_i$ that it produces, provides the signal for PLB phosphorylation.

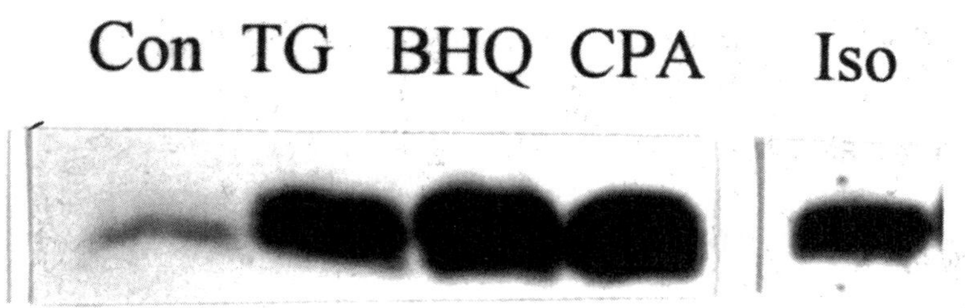

FIGURE 6. Depletion of SR Ca^{2+} stimulates phosphorylation of PLB. Rat ventricular myocytes were treated with 2.5 μM thapsigargin (TG), 30 μM t-butyl hydroquinone (BHQ), or 50 μM cyclopiazonic acid (CPA) for 5 min to deplete the SR of Ca^{2+}. Samples were quenched with SDS-PAGE sample buffer, and total ventricular protein from 10,000 cells was resolved on 15% polyacrylamide SDS-PAGE gels. PS-16 staining of the corresponding immunoblot is presented. (Reprinted with permission from Ref. 33.)

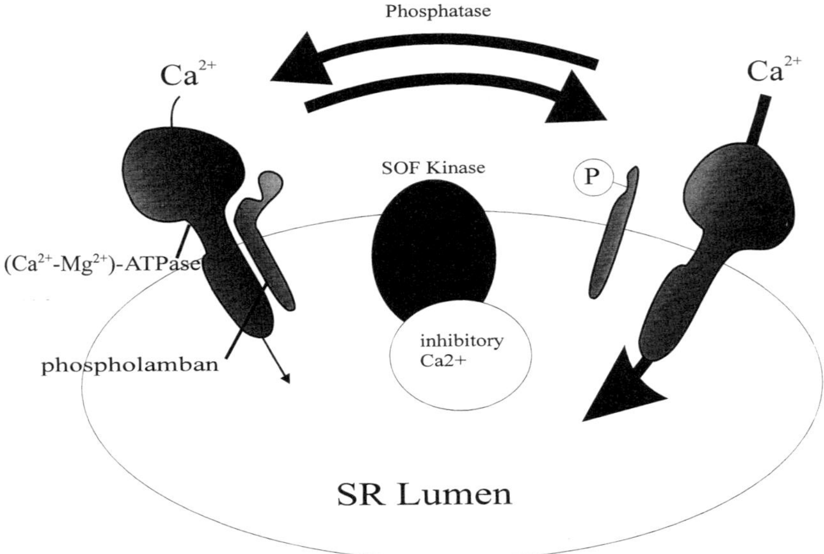

FIGURE 7. A proposed model of signaling generated upon Ca^{2+} store depletion. Sarcoplasmic reticulum is proposed to contain a *s*tate *o*f *f*illing kinase (SOF kinase) that is inhibited through Ca^{2+} binding to a site on a lumen domain of the enzyme. When SR Ca^{2+} falls sufficiently, this mode of inhibition is lost and SOF kinase becomes active and phosphorylates PLB on Ser-16.

The molecular mechanism that signals SR Ca^{2+} load to the cell is under study in my laboratory. A protein kinase responsive to [Ca^{2+}] at suitable concentrations, which phosphorylates Ser-16 of PLB, copurifies with canine cardiac SR vesicles. This enzyme is active at 3 μM Ca^{2+} but is inhibited progressively as the Ca^{2+} rises to 30 and 300 μM. These inhibitory Ca^{2+} concentrations exert their control from the lumenal face of the SR membrane. Thus a summary model of the regulation of PLB phosphorylation by SR Ca^{2+} load is proposed in FIGURE 7. A protein kinase termed SOF kinase (*s*tate *o*f *f*illing) is a component of cardiac sarcoplasmic reticulum. It has access to both the SR lumen and the cytosolic face of the membrane, and is thus perhaps a transmembrane protein. An inhibitory Ca^{2+} binding site of low affinity (K_d ~50 μM) exists in the SR lumenal domain of the protein, whereas the SOF kinase domain is contained within the cytoplasmic domain of the protein. Ca^{2+} binding to SOF kinase is saturated when the store is full, and this inhibits SOF kinase activity. If the Ca^{2+} load of the SR falls, the degree of saturation of this inhibitory Ca^{2+} binding site will also fall, and the inhibition of kinase activity will be incomplete. Phosphorylation of Ser-16 of PLB results from the activity of SOF kinase. This will stimulate SERCA activity and promote refilling of the store (and suppression of SOF kinase activity).

CONCLUSIONS

Phospholamban has been identified as a key component in cardiac muscle Ca^{2+} handling, targeted by β-adrenergic stimuli to increase the speed and magnitude of Ca^{2+}

transients. β-Adrenergic stimulation causes the phosphorylation of PLB on both Ser-16 and Thr-17, both of which produce an identical increase in SERCA2a pump activity. The activation of pump function is in direct proportion to the stoichiometry of phosphorylation, but phosphorylation of both sites on a single molecule of PLB is a redundant move incapable of stimulating pump function above that achieved by phosphorylation of only one residue. In cardiac myocytes, PLB phosphorylation is provoked by β1-adrenergic receptor stimulation, which leads to Ser-16 phosphorylation in advance of Thr-17 phosphorylation. Both phosphorylation events correlate with contractile and Ca^{2+} transient changes *in vivo,* although Ser-16 correlations are generally closer than Thr-17. In terms of the time course of contractile response to β-agonists, the Ser-16 phosphorylation events correlate more closely than Thr-17. Finally, PLB appears to be phosphorylated when the Ca^{2+} load of the SR falls. This represents an important feedback loop capable of promoting Ca^{2+} sequestration by the SR in response to depletion of store Ca^{2+}. A protein kinase that copurifies with the SR vesicles is inhibited by lumenal Ca^{2+}. This kinase becomes active at low $[Ca^{2+}]_{lumen}$ and phosphorylates PLB on Ser-16. We have termed this enzyme SOF kinase, as it is controlled by the *s*tate *of f*illing of cardiac SR.

ACKNOWLEDGMENTS

I would like to thank Drs. Moninder Bhogal, Sarah Calaghan, Guido Drago, Munir Hussain, and Wayne Jackson for their contributions to this work, and Prof. Clive Orchard for his interest and involvement.

REFERENCES

1. Fujii, J., A. Ueno, K. Kitano, S. Tanaka, M. Kadoma & M. Tada. 1987. Complete complementary DNA-derived amino acid sequence of canine cardiac phospholamban. J. Clin. Invest. **79:** 301–304.
2. James, P., M. Inui, M. Tada, M. Chiesi & E. Carafoli. 1989. Nature and site of phospholamban regulation of the Ca^{2+} pump of sarcoplasmic reticulum. Nature **342:** 90–92.
3. Cornea, R. L., L. R. Jones, J. M. Autry & D. D. Thomas. 1997. Mutation and phosphorylation change the oligomeric structure of phospholamban in lipid bilayers. Biochemistry **36:** 2960–2967.
4. Li, C., J. H. Wang & J. Colyer. 1990. Immunological detection of phospholamban phosphorylation states facilitates the description of the mechanism of phosphorylation and dephosphorylation. Biochemistry **29:** 4535–4540.
5. Jackson, W. A. & J. Colyer. 1996. Translation of Ser16 and Thr17 phosphorylation of phospholamban into Ca^{2+}-pump stimulation. Biochem. J. **316:** 201–207.
6. Suzuki, T. & J. H. Wang. 1986. Stimulation of bovine cardiac sarcoplasmic reticulum Ca^{2+} pump and blocking of phospholamban phosphorylation and dephosphorylation by a phospholamban monoclonal antibody. J. Biol. Chem. **261:** 7018–7023.
7. Jackson, W. A. 1996. Regulation of cardiac SR calcium uptake by phosphorylation. Ph.D. thesis, University of Leeds, Leeds, UK.
8. Colyer, J. 1993. Control of the calcium pump of cardiac sarcoplasmic reticulum. A specific role for the pentameric structure of phospholamban? Cardiovasc. Res. **27:** 1766–1771.
9. Toyofuku, T., K. Kurzydlowski, M. Tada & D. H. MacLennan. 1994. Amino acids Lys-Asp-Asp-Lys-Pro-Val^{402} in the Ca^{2+}-ATPase of cardiac sarcoplasmic reticulum are critical for functional association with phospholamban. J. Biol. Chem. **269:** 22929–22932.
10. Sasaki, T., M. Inui, Y. Kimura, T. Kuzuya & M. Tada. 1992. Molecular mechanism of regulation of Ca^{2+} pump ATPase by phospholamban in cardiac sarcoplasmic reticulum—Effects of synthetic phospholamban peptides on Ca^{2+} pump ATPase. J. Biol. Chem. **267:** 1674–1679.

11. Hughes, G., J. M. East & A. G. Lee. 1994. The hydrophilic domain of phospholamban inhibits the Ca^{2+} transport step of the Ca^{2+}-ATPase. Biochem. J. **303:** 511–516.
12. Kimura, Y., K. Kurzydlowski, M. Tada & D. H. MacLennan. 1997. Phospholamban inhibitory function is activated by depolymerization. J. Biol. Chem. **272:** 15061–15064.
13. Kirchberger, M. A., M. Tada & A. M. Katz. 1974. Adenosine 3′:5′-monophosphate–dependent protein kinase–catalyzed phosphorylation reaction and its relationship to calcium transport in cardiac sarcoplamic reticulum. J. Biol. Chem. **249:** 6166–6174.
14. Colyer, J. & J. H. Wang. 1991. Dependence of cardiac sarcoplasmic reticulum calcium pump activity on the phosphorylation status of phospholamban. J. Biol. Chem. **266:** 17486–17493.
15. Wegener, A. D., H. K. B. Simmerman, J. P. Lindemann & L. R. Jones. 1989. Phospholamban phosphorylation in intact ventricles: Phosphorylation of serine 16 and threonine 17 in response to β-adrenergic stimulation. J. Biol. Chem. **264:** 11474–11486.
16. Karczewski, P., S. Bartel & E-G. Krause. 1990. Differential sensitivity to isoprenaline of troponin I and phospholamban phosphorylation in isolated rat hearts. Biochem. J. **266:** 115–122.
17. Drago, G. A. & J. Colyer. 1994. Discrimination between two sites of phosphorylation on adjacent amino acids by phosphorylation site–specific antibodies to phospholamban. J. Biol. Chem. **269:** 25073–25077.
18. Czernik, A. J., J. Mathers & S. M. Mische. 1996. Phosphorylation state–specific antibodies. *In* Neuromethods, Vol 30. Regulatory Protein Modification: Techniques and Protocols. H. C. Hemmings, Ed.: 219–249. Humana Press. Totowa, NJ.
19. Snyder, G. L., J-A. Girault, J. Y. C. Chen, A. J. Czernikl, J. W. Kebabian, J. A. Nathanson & P. Greengard. 1992. Phosphorylation of DARPP-32 and protein phosphatase inhibitor–1 in rat choroid plexus: Regulation by factors other than dopamine. J. Neurosci. **12:** 3071–3083.
20. Palmer, C. J., B. T. Scott & L. R. Jones. 1991. Purification and complete sequence determination of the major plasma membrane substrate for cAMP-dependent protein kinase and protein kinase C in myocardium. J. Biol. Chem. **266:** 11126–11130.
21. Sham, J. S. K., L. R. Jones & M. Morad. 1991. Phospholamban mediates the β-adrenergic–enhanced Ca^{2+}-uptake in mammalian ventricular myocytes. Am. J. Physiol. **261:** H1344–H1349.
22. Simmerman, H. K. B., J. H. Collins, J. L. Theibert, A. D. Wegener & L. R. Jones. 1986. Sequence analysis of phospholamban identification of phosphorylation sites and two major structural domains. J. Biol. Chem. **261:** 13333–13341.
23. Mundina-Weilenmann, C., L. Vittone, M. Ortale, G. Chiappe de Cinglani & A. Mattiazzi. 1996. Immunodetection of phosphorylation sites gives new insights into the mechanisms underlying phospholamban phosphorylation in the intact heart. J. Biol. Chem. **271:** 33561–33567.
24. Steenaart, N. A. E., J. R. Ganim, J. Di Salvo & E. G. Kranias. 1992. The phospholamban phosphatase associated with cardiac sarcoplasmic reticulum is a type 1 enzyme. Arch. Biochem. Biophys. **293:** 17–24.
25. Hubbard, M. J. & P. Cohen. 1993. On target with a new mechanism for the regulation of protein phosphorylation. TIBS **18:** 172–177.
26. Iyer, R. B., S. B. Koritz & M. A. Kirchberger. 1988. A regulation of the level of phosphorylated phospholamban by inhibitor-1 in rat heart preparations in vitro. Mol. Cell. Endocrinol. **55:** 1–6.
27. Bennett, K. L. 1996. The role of phospholamban in the regulation of cardiac contractility. Ph.D. thesis, University of Leeds, Leeds, UK.
28. Xiao, R-P., C. Hohl, R. Altschuld, L. R. Jones, B. Livingston, B. Ziman, B. Tantini & E. G. Lakatta. 1994. β2-Adrenergic receptor-stimulated increase in cAMP in rat heart cells is not coupled to changes in Ca^{2+} dynamics, contractility or phospholamban phosphorylation. J. Biol. Chem. **269:** 19151–19156.
29. Frampton, J. E., S. M. Harrison, M. R. Boyett & C. H. Orchard. 1991. Ca^{2+} and Na+ in rat myocytes showing different force-frequency relationships. Am. J. Physiol. **261:** C739–C750.
30. Schouten, V. J. A. 1990. Interval dependence of force and twitch duration in rat heart ex-

plained by Ca^{2+} pump inactivation in sarcoplasmic reticulum. J. Physiol. (Lond.) **431:** 427–444.

31. HUSSAIN, M., G. A. DRAGO, J. COLYER & C. H. ORCHARD. 1997. Rate-dependent abbreviation of Ca^{2+} transient in rat heart is independent of phospholamban phosphorylation. Am. J. Physiol. **273:** H695–H706.
32. PUTNEY, J. W., JR. 1992. *In* Advances in Second Messenger and Phosphoprotein Research. J. R. Putney, Jr., Ed: 143–151. Raven Press. New York.
33. BHOGAL, M. S. & J. COLYER. 1998. Depletion of Ca^{2+} from the sarcoplasmic reticulum of cardiac muscle prompts the phoshrylation of phospholamban to stimulate store refilling. Proc. Natl. Acad. Sci. USA **95:** 1484–1489.

High-Level Coexpression of the Canine Cardiac Calcium Pump and Phospholamban in Sf21 Insect Cells

JOSEPH M. AUTRY AND LARRY R. JONES[a]

Department of Medicine and Krannert Institute of Cardiology, Indiana University School of Medicine, Indianapolis, Indiana 46202, USA

ABSTRACT: Phospholamban is a pentameric transmembrane phosphoprotein that regulates the activity of the Ca^{2+}-transporting ATPase (SERCA2a) in cardiac sarcoplasmic reticulum. To better understand the structure and function of phospholamban and its mode of regulation of the ATPase, phospholamban and SERCA2a were coexpressed at high levels in Sf21 insect cells using the baculovirus expression system. SERCA2a was expressed as a functionally active Ca^{2+} pump, accounting for ≥ 20% of the total protein in Sf21 cell microsomes. Wild-type phospholamban, as well as phospholamban with different point mutations in the transmembrane region, inhibited both Ca^{2+} transport and ATP hydrolysis by the recombinant Ca^{2+} pump. The inhibition of SERCA2a activity was reversed by an anti–phospholamban monoclonal antibody. The phospholamban molecules studied decreased the apparent Ca^{2+} affinity of the Ca^{2+} pump, but had no effect on enzyme velocity measured at saturating Ca^{2+} concentration. Monomeric phospholamban produced by mutations in the leucine/isoleucine zipper domain decreased the apparent Ca^{2+} affinity the most, giving stronger inhibition of the Ca^{2+} pump than even wild-type phospholamban. Thus, the baculovirus cell expression system is ideally suited for examining functional interactions between phospholamban and SERCA2a. The results obtained suggest that the phospholamban monomer may be the active species inhibiting the Ca^{2+} pump in the cardiac sarcoplasmic reticulum membrane.

In cardiac muscle, the sarcoplasmic reticulum Ca^{2+}-transport ATPase (SERCA2a isoform) is regulated by phospholamban,[1] a small integral membrane phosphoprotein that self-assembles into pentamers in SDS solution[2] and in lipid bilayers.[3] In the dephosphorylated state, phospholamban inhibits the Ca^{2+}-ATPase by decreasing its apparent Ca^{2+} affinity (K_{Ca}).[4,5] Phosphorylation of phospholamban[6,7] or the binding of anti–phospholamban monoclonal antibodies[5,8] to the cytoplasmic phosphorylation domain of phospholamban restores the high Ca^{2+} affinity of the ATPase, increasing Ca^{2+} transport into cardiac sarcoplasmic reticulum at submicromolar Ca^{2+} concentration.

To better understand the molecular mechanism of phospholamban regulation, the baculovirus cell expression system was utilized for investigating phospholamban and Ca^{2+}-ATPase interactions.[9] We observed that phospholamban[10] and SERCA2a[9] were expressed at very high levels in baculovirus-infected *Spodoptera frugiperda* (Sf21) insect cells. Microsomal membranes coexpressing the two proteins exhibited high levels of Ca^{2+} transport and ATP hydrolysis, while cardiac-like coupling[4–8] between phospholamban and SERCA2a was retained.[9] A mutated form of phospholamban producing monomers in SDS[11] and in the lipid bilayer[3]—i.e., L37A-PLB—actually inhibited the ap-

[a] To whom correspondence should be addressed: Krannert Institute of Cardiology, 1111 West 10th Street, Indianapolis, Indiana 46202. Phone: 317-630-6695; fax: 317-630-8595; e-mail: jones@lrdmed.iupui.edu

parent Ca^{2+} affinity of the Ca^{2+} pump more strongly than did wild-type (WT) phospholamban, suggesting that the monomer may be the active component regulating the Ca^{2+} pump in cardiac sarcoplasmic reticulum membranes.[9,12] Here we report on further characterization of the baculovirus system for analyzing phospholamban-SERCA2a regulatory interactions. The effects of additional pentamer-destabilizing mutations in the membrane-spanning domain of phospholamban on SERCA2a activity are described.

HIGH-LEVEL COEXPRESSION OF SERCA2a AND PHOSPHOLAMBAN

We found that the Parr Cell Disruption Bomb was most effective for preparing microsomal membranes in high yield from baculovirus-infected Sf21 insect cells.[9] Forty milligrams of microsomal protein are isolated from 9×10^8 cells in 600 ml suspension culture, which is about one-half the yield of sarcoplasmic reticulum vesicles from one dog heart. Microsomes isolated from Sf21 cells infected with baculovirus encoding SERCA2a (canine isoform) expressed the Ca^{2+} pump at a level approaching that found in native canine cardiac sarcoplasmic reticulum vesicles (FIGS. 1A and 2). Quantitative immunoblotting using the purified canine cardiac Ca^{2+}-ATPase as a standard revealed that the expressed Ca^{2+} pump accounted for 20–25% of the total protein of Sf21 cell microsomes,[9] which is similar to the Ca^{2+} pump content found in canine cardiac sarcoplasmic reticulum vesicles.[13] For comparison, expression of rabbit SERCA1 in COS cells yielded 150 μg of microsomal protein containing 2 μg of Ca^{2+} pump protein.[14] Sf21 microsomes expressing SERCA2a catalyzed active Ca^{2+} transport at a 20-fold higher rate than control microsomes isolated from wild-type baculovirus–infected cells (FIG. 1B). Ca^{2+} activation of Ca^{2+} transport by the recombinant Ca^{2+} pump was found to be half-maximal at approximately 0.1 μM ionized Ca^{2+} concentration, demonstrating that

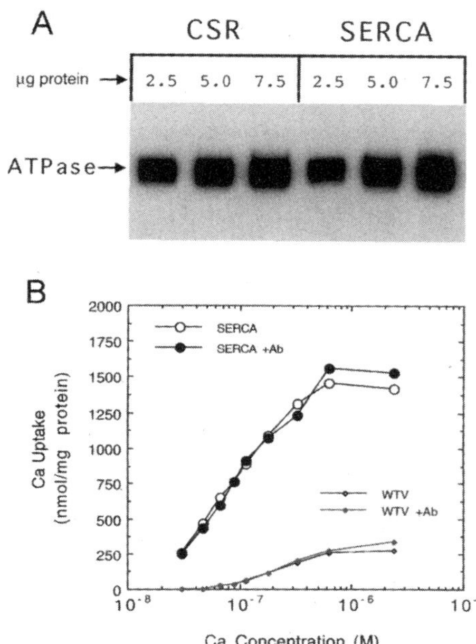

FIGURE 1. High-level expression of canine SERCA2a Ca^{2+} pump. **A:** Sf21 microsomes isolated from SERCA2a baculovirus-infected cells (SERCA) and sarcoplasmic reticulum vesicles isolated from dog heart (CSR) were electrophoresed through 5% polyacrylamide gel and transferred to nitrocellulose for Western blotting. The immunoblot was probed with SERCA2a-specific monoclonal antibody and labeled with ^{125}I-protein A.[9] The amount of membrane protein loaded (μg) is indicated on **top.** ATPase, SERCA2a Ca^{2+} pump. **B:** Ca^{2+} activation of Ca^{2+} transport was measured in Sf21 microsomes from SERCA2a (SERCA) or wild-type (WTV) baculovirus-infected cells. Ca^{2+} uptake at 8 min was determined with *(filled symbols)* or without *(open symbols)* pretreatment by anti–phospholamban monoclonal antibody 2D12.[9]

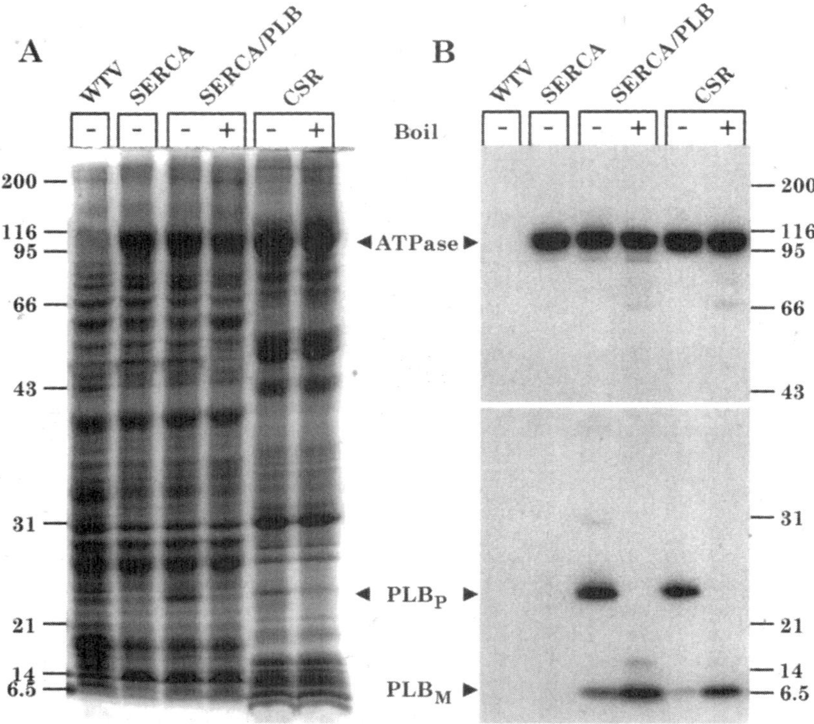

FIGURE 2. SDS-PAGE and immunoblotting of SERCA2a and phospholamban coexpressed in Sf21 microsomes. Sf21 microsomes from wild-type (WTV), SERCA2a (SERCA), and SERCA2a plus phospholamban (SERCA/PLB) baculovirus-infected cells, as well as canine cardiac sarcoplasmic reticulum vesicles (CSR), were subjected to 7.5–15% SDS-PAGE and immunoblotting.[9] Panel **A** shows a Coomassie Blue-stained gel (50 μg of protein/*lane*), and panel **B** shows a corresponding immunoblot (5 μg of protein/*lane*) developed with SERCA2a **(upper)** and phospholamban **(lower)** monoclonal antibodies. ±Boil indicates whether membrane samples were boiled prior to electrophoresis. ATPase, SERCA2a; PLB$_p$, phospholamban pentamer; PLB$_M$, phospholamban monomer.

SERCA2a displays a high Ca^{2+} affinity when expressed in the absence of phospholamban (FIG. 1B and TABLE 1). No endogenous Ca^{2+} pumps in control microsomes were detected by immunoblotting using an antibody specific for SERCA2a (FIG. 2B).

To investigate the role of phospholamban in regulating the cardiac Ca^{2+}-ATPase, we coinfected Sf21 cells with baculoviruses encoding the canine isoforms of both proteins. FIGURE 2 shows that SERCA2a and phospholamban were efficiently coexpressed in Sf21 cell microsomes, in amounts similar to the levels found in canine cardiac sarcoplasmic reticulum vesicles. As a test for functional coupling between the two recombinant proteins, Ca^{2+} transport assays were conducted at low (30 nM) and high (1 μM) ionized Ca^{2+} concentrations in the presence and absence of anti–phospholamban monoclonal antibody 2D12, which blocks the inhibitory interaction between phospholamban and the cardiac Ca^{2+}-ATPase.[5,7,15] At low Ca^{2+} concentration, Ca^{2+} transport by Sf21

TABLE 1. Phospholamban Regulation of SERCA2a Ca^{2+} Affinity in Sf21 Microsomes

Protein Expressed	K_{Ca} Values (nM)			
	Ca^{2+}-ATPase		Ca^{2+} Uptake	
	(–) Ab	(+) Ab	(–) Ab	(+) Ab
SERCA2a	105 ± 10	106 ± 8	95 ± 11	101 ± 10
SERCA2a + WT-PLB	224 ± 44	125 ± 19	168 ± 13	123 ± 6
SERCA2a + L37A-PLB	537 ± 77	185 ± 24	400 ± 30	154 ± 13

NOTE: The ionized Ca^{2+} concentrations giving half-maximal activation of Ca^{2+}-ATPase and Ca^{2+} uptake activities (K_{Ca} values) in Sf21 cell microsomes are reported. Microsomes expressed SERCA2a alone, SERCA2a plus wild-type phospholamban (WT-PLB), or SERCA2a plus monomeric phospholamban (L37A-PLB). Assays were conducted in the presence and absence of anti–phospholamban monoclonal antibody 2D12 (±Ab), as described in the legend to FIG. 1. Results were obtained from three separate microsomal preparations for each condition and are presented as the average ± standard error of the mean.

microsomes containing SERCA2a and phospholamban was stimulated 8-fold by addition of the phospholamban monoclonal antibody (FIG. 3A); at high Ca^{2+} concentration, Ca^{2+} transport by the same microsomes was unaffected by the antibody (FIG. 3B). The same anti–phospholamban monoclonal antibody increased Ca^{2+} uptake by canine cardiac sarcoplasmic reticulum vesicles approximately 10-fold at low Ca^{2+} con-

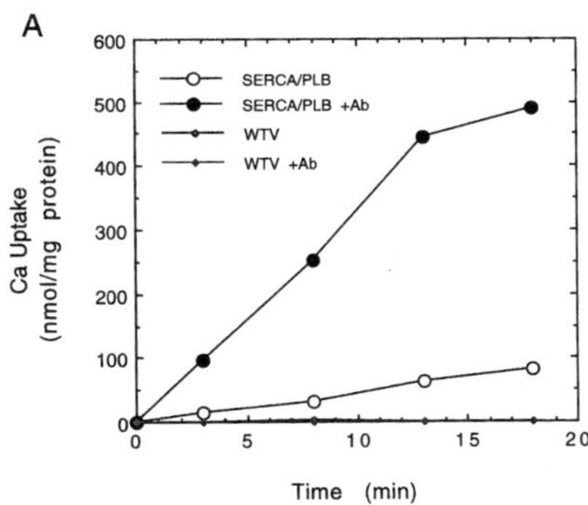

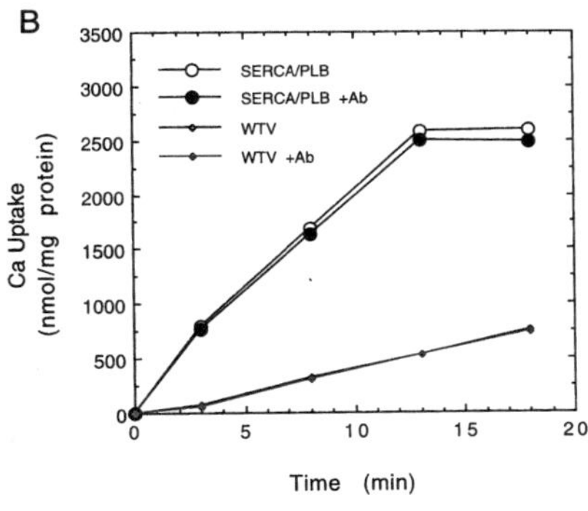

FIGURE 3. Ca^{2+} uptake by Sf21 microsomes coexpressing SERCA2a and phospholamban. Sf21 microsomes coexpressing SERCA2a and phospholamban were assayed for Ca^{2+} uptake at 30 nM ionized Ca^{2+} concentration (panel **A**) and 1 μM ionized Ca^{2+} concentration (panel **B**). Control microsomes (WTV) isolated from wild-type baculovirus–infected cells were also assayed. +Ab *(filled symbols)* denotes microsomes pretreated with phospholamban monoclonal antibody 2D12.

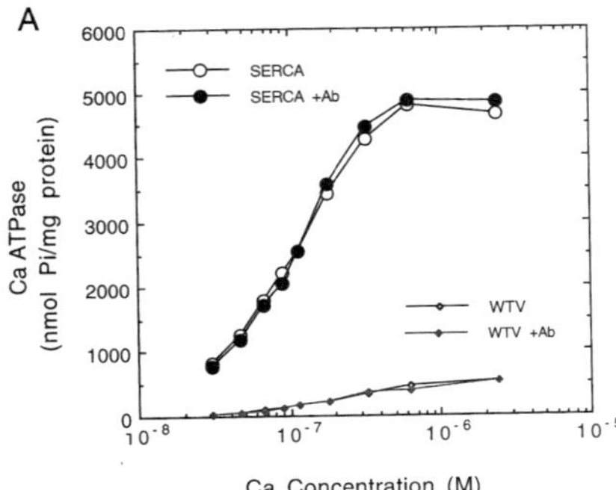

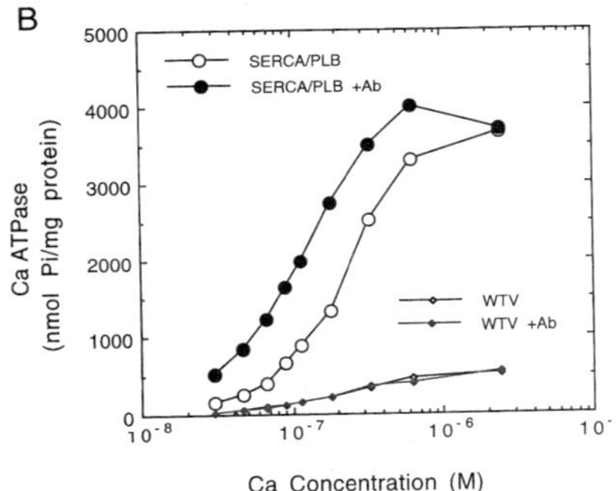

FIGURE 4. Phospholamban regulation of Ca^{2+}-ATPase activity in Sf21 microsomes. Ca^{2+} activation of ATPase activity was measured in Sf21 microsomes from SERCA2a (SERCA)-infected cells (panel **A**) and SERCA2a plus phospholamban (SERCA/PLB)-coinfected cells (panel **B**). Microsomes from wild-type virus (WTV)-infected cells were also assayed. ATPase activities were determined at 8 min of incubation, and basal (Ca^{2+}-independent) ATPase activities have been subtracted from the values reported (see text). *Filled symbols* denote microsomes pretreated with phospholamban monoclonal antibody (+Ab).

centration, but had no effect at saturating Ca^{2+} concentration.[5,10,16] Thus, the functional interaction between the two recombinant proteins expressed in Sf21 cell microsomes is the same as the interaction between phospholamban and SERCA2a in native cardiac sarcoplasmic reticulum vesicles.

Phospholamban regulation of pump function was also investigated by measuring ATP hydrolysis. In membranes containing SERCA2a, the Ca^{2+}-dependent ATPase activity was four times greater than basal (Ca^{2+}-independent) ATPase activity at the lowest ionized Ca^{2+} concentration tested (30 nM), and at least 20 times greater than basal ATPase activity at Ca^{2+} concentrations ($\geq 1\ \mu$M) saturating the high-affinity Ca^{2+} binding sites of SERCA2a.[9] Plots depicting Ca^{2+}-activation of ATP hydrolysis by SERCA2a, expressed in the presence and absence of phospholamban, are shown in FIGURE 4. SERCA2a expressed alone had a high apparent Ca^{2+} affinity (K_{Ca} value = 105 ± 10 nM), which was unaffected by the phospholamban antibody (FIG. 4A and TABLE 1). Coexpression of phospholamban with SERCA2a decreased the apparent Ca^{2+} affinity of the ATPase by a factor of two (K_{Ca} (–Ab) = 224 nM), but this lowering of Ca^{2+} affinity was removed by the anti–phospholamban monoclonal antibody, which shifted the Ca^{2+} activation curve to the left (K_{Ca} (+Ab) = 125 nM) (FIG. 4B and TABLE 1). At the saturating Ca^{2+} concentration of 2.4 μM, the antibody had no effect on ATP hydrolysis (FIG. 4B). Similar results were obtained when Ca^{2+} transport was measured (TABLE 1 and FIG. 3B). Thus, phospholamban acts primarily by decreasing the apparent Ca^{2+} affinity of the pump, whether determined by Ca^{2+} uptake or Ca^{2+}-ATPase assay.

ROLE OF THE PHOSPHOLAMBAN MONOMER IN SERCA2a REGULATION

To investigate the role of the oligomeric structure of phospholamban in ATPase regulation, SERCA2a was coexpressed with several monomeric mutants of phospholamban, in which leucine and isoleucine residues located in the "zipper domain"[11] were individually changed to alanine. Detailed results obtained with one of these mutants, which contains a leucine to alanine substitution at position 37 (L37A-PLB), are presented in FIGURE 5. L37A-PLB has previously been shown to be monomeric in SDS solution[9,11] and in phospholipid bilayers.[3] Coexpression of L37A-PLB monomers with SERCA2a in Sf21 cell microsomes abolished Ca^{2+} transport at low ionized Ca^{2+} concentration (FIG. 5A). Ca^{2+} uptake was dramatically stimulated, however, when the anti–phospholamban monoclonal antibody was added (FIG. 5A). When ATP hydrolysis by the Ca^{2+} pump was measured, L37A-PLB was again observed to be a potent inhibitor of SERCA2a activity, significantly shifting the Ca^{2+} activation curve to the right (FIG. 5B). Therefore, L37A-PLB decreased the apparent Ca^{2+} affinity of SERCA2a ATPase like wild-type phospholamban, but to a much greater extent (fivefold) than did WT-PLB (twofold) (TABLE 1). A similar potent effect of L37A-PLB was noted when Ca^{2+} affinities were monitored by Ca^{2+} transport assay (TABLE 1). These results demonstrate that monomeric phospholamban is actually a stronger inhibitor of Ca^{2+} pump activity than is wild-type phospholamban. However, the basic mechanism of inhibition of SERCA2a by the two species of phospholamban is the same, in that

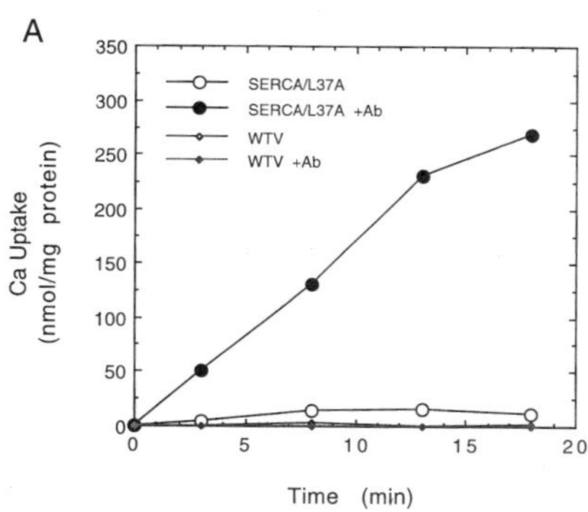

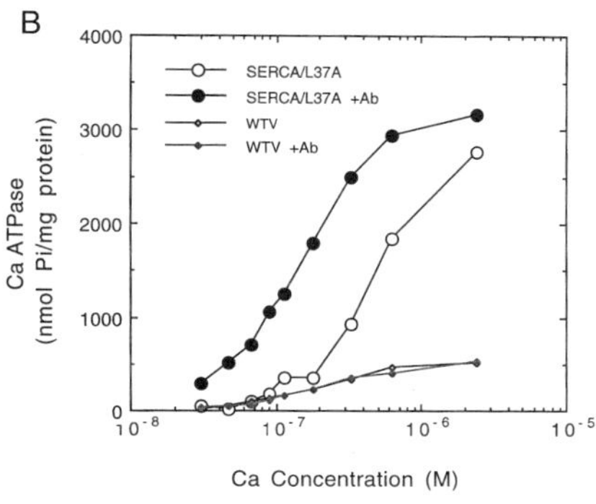

FIGURE 5. Phospholamban monomer effect on Ca^{2+} uptake and Ca^{2+}-ATPase activities. Microsomes were isolated from Sf21 cells infected with SERCA2a- and L37A-PLB–encoding baculoviruses (SERCA/L37A) or with wild-type baculovirus (WTV). Panel **A** shows a time course of Ca^{2+} uptake measured at 30 nM ionized Ca^{2+} concentration, and panel **B** shows the Ca^{2+} dependence of Ca^{2+}-ATPase activity determined at 8 min of incubation, as described in the legend to FIG. 4. Microsomes preincubated with the phospholamban antibody (+Ab) are denoted by *filled symbols.*

the apparent K_{Ca} value is increased with little effect on the V_{max} of the enzyme measured at saturating Ca^{2+} concentration.

Due to the high-level expression of SERCA2a in insect cells, we found that it was possible to measure Ca^{2+} transport and ATPase activity directly in cellular homogenates, obviating the need for isolation of microsomes for reliable detection of activity. Four milligrams of cellular protein are quickly and easily obtained per cell cul-

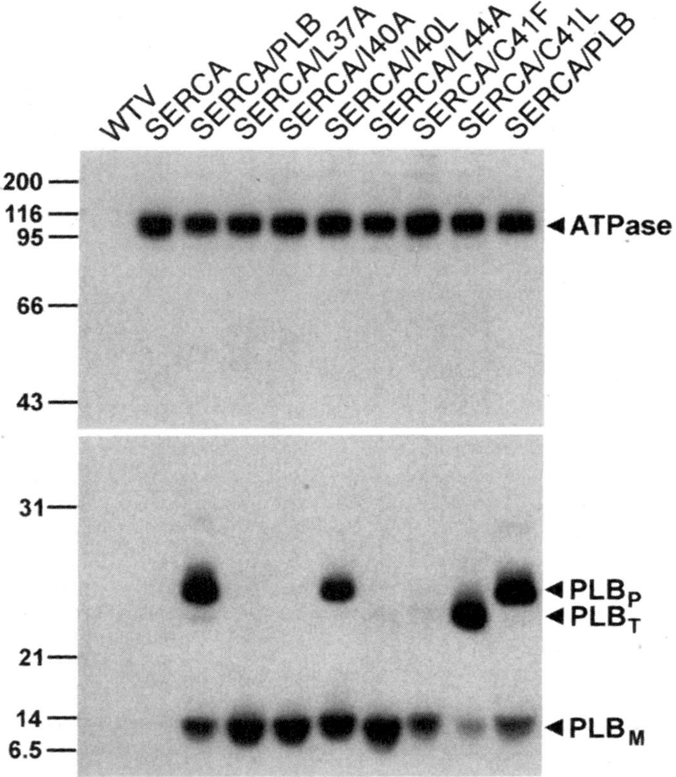

FIGURE 6. Immunoblot showing coexpression of phospholamban mutants with SERCA2a in Sf21 homogenates. Sf21 cells were maintained and infected as described by Autry and Jones,[9] except that 9×10^6 cells were infected in 75-cm^2 dishes. Infected Sf21 cells were harvested by centrifugation and homogenized in 2 ml of medium containing 250 mM sucrose, 30 mM L-histidine (pH 7.4) using a Brinkmann Polytron PT 1200 (Kinematica AG, Luzern, Switzerland). Sf21 cellular homogenates expressing SERCA2a (SERCA), SERCA2a plus wild-type phospholamban (SERCA/PLB), and SERCA2a plus the different phospholamban mutants indicated were subjected to 8% SDS-PAGE and Western blotting as previously described,[9] except that homogenates were solubilized at room temperature in gel loading buffer containing 2.5% SDS for 20 minutes prior to electrophoresis. Control homogenates infected with wild-type baculovirus (WTV) were also run. The immunoblot (10 μg of protein/*lane*) was developed with SERCA2a **(upper)** and phospholamban **(lower)** monoclonal antibodies. Molecular weight standards ($\times 10^{-3}$) are shown on the **left.** ATPase, SERCA2a; PLB_p, phospholamban pentamer; PLB_T, phospholamban tetramer; PLB_M, phospholamban monomer.

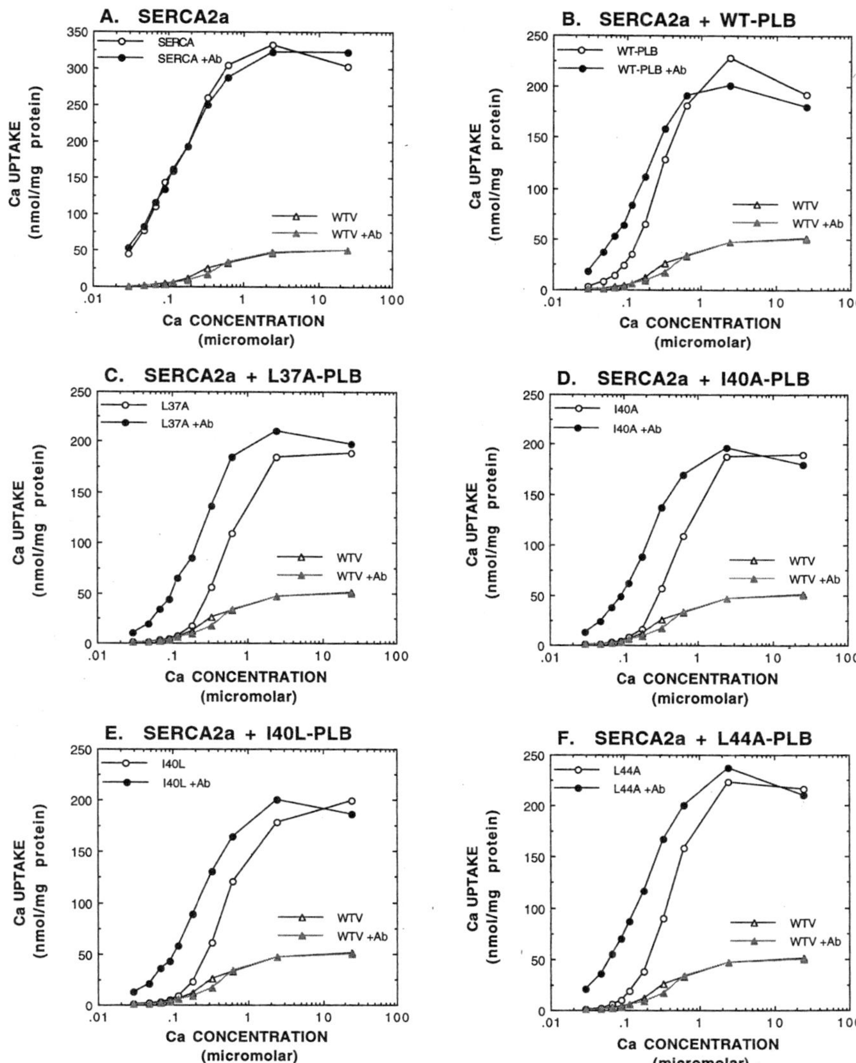

FIGURE 7. Functional coupling of phospholamban monomers to SERCA2a Ca^{2+} pump. A typical experiment measuring Ca^{2+} activation of Ca^{2+} transport by Sf21 cellular homogenates is presented. Homogenates expressing SERCA2a (panel **A**), SERCA2a plus wild-type phospholamban (panel **B**), and SERCA2a plus pentamer–destabilized phospholamban subunits L37A-PLB (panel **C**), I40A-PLB (panel **D**), I40L-PLB (panel **E**), and L44A-PLB (panel **F**) were assayed, along with control homogenates infected with wild-type virus alone (WTV). Ca^{2+} uptake was determined at 8 min as described in Ref. 9, except that 0.5 mM EGTA with 0.050 to 0.525 mM $CaCl_2$ was used to set the desired ionized Ca^{2+} concentrations (0.030 to 25.0 μM Ca^{2+}). Homogenates pretreated with the phospholamban monoclonal antibody (+Ab) are denoted by *filled symbols.*

TABLE 2. Phospholamban Regulation of SERCA2a Ca^{2+} Affinity in Sf21 Homogenates

Protein Expressed	*n*	K_{Ca} Values (nM)	
		(–) Ab	(+) Ab
SERCA2a	6	144 ± 9	137 ± 9
SERCA2a + WT-PLB	6	255 ± 11	138 ± 7
SERCA2a + L37A-PLB	4	450 ± 23	184 ± 21
SERCA2a + I40A-PLB	3	475 ± 25	185 ± 10
SERCA2a + I40L-PLB	3	434 ± 37	195 ± 22
SERCA2a + L44A-PLB	4	422 ± 17	179 ± 3
SERCA2a + C41F-PLB	4	215 ± 22	145 ± 18
SERCA2a + C41L-PLB	4	169 ± 12	135 ± 6

NOTE: The ionized Ca^{2+} concentrations giving half-maximal activation of Ca^{2+} uptake activity (K_{Ca} values) in Sf21 cell homogenates are reported. Homogenates expressed SERCA2a alone, SERCA2a plus wild-type phospholamban (WT-PLB), or SERCA2a plus the different phospholamban mutants indicated. Assays were conducted in the presence and absence of anti–phospholamban monoclonal antibody 2D12 (±Ab), as described in the legend to FIG. 7. Results were obtained from multiple (*n*) homogenate preparations for each condition and are presented as the average ± standard error of the mean.

ture dish (see legend to FIG. 6 for details), which is sufficient material for twenty assays of Ca^{2+} uptake or Ca^{2+}-ATPase activities. FIGURES 6 and 7 and TABLE 2 present immunoblotting and Ca^{2+} uptake results obtained using this homogenate system to analyze the functional effects of several monomer-forming phospholamban mutants coexpressed with SERCA2a. L37A-PLB, which was completely monomeric on SDS-PAGE of homogenates (FIG. 6), decreased the apparent Ca^{2+} affinity of SERCA2a Ca^{2+} pump 2–3-fold more effectively than did wild-type phospholamban (FIG. 7 and TABLE 2), consistent with effects observed with use of microsomal preparations from Sf21 cells (TABLE 1). I40A-PLB and L44A-PLB were also entirely monomeric on SDS-PAGE (FIG. 6), as reported previously by *in vitro* translation assay,[11] and also decreased the apparent Ca^{2+} affinity of SERCA2a as effectively as did L37A-PLB (FIG. 7 and TABLE 2). Although I40L-PLB produces only monomers on SDS-PAGE after being synthesized by *in vitro* translation,[11] a significant amount of pentamer formation was detected when this mutant protein was synthesized by Sf21 cells and subjected to SDS-PAGE (FIG. 6). Surprisingly, I40L-PLB reduced the apparent Ca^{2+} affinity of the Ca^{2+} pump to a degree similar to that produced by the three completely monomeric PLB mutants (FIG. 7 and TABLE 2). C41F-PLB and C41L-PLB produce monomers[17,11] and tetramers,[11] respectively, on SDS-PAGE. C41F-PLB was slightly less effective than WT-PLB in inhibiting SERCA2a (TABLE 2) (see also Toyofuku *et al.*[17]), whereas C41L-PLB did not inhibit the Ca^{2+} pump significantly (TABLE 2). None of the PLB proteins studied (mutated or wild-type) significantly affected SERCA2a activity when Ca^{2+} uptake was measured at saturating ionized Ca^{2+} concentration (≥ 1 μM) (FIG. 7).

DISCUSSION

The baculovirus cell expression system appears to be ideally suited for functional studies examining phospholamban and SERCA2a regulatory interactions. Milligram quantities of highly active SERCA2a are readily obtained in microsomal preparations from Sf21 cells, which is an expression level for Ca^{2+} pumps much higher than that previously reported (for discussion, see REF. 9). Studies on the enzyme kinetics and biophysics of phospholamban-SERCA2a regulatory interactions will be greatly facilitated by use of this high-level expression system.

Successful coexpression of SERCA2a and phospholamban with functional coupling in Sf21 cells has allowed us to test if the phospholamban pentamer is essential for SERCA2a regulation.[9] Results obtained after coexpression of SERCA2a with wild-type phospholamban and several of its pentamer-destabilized mutants indicate that the monomeric species is the most effective inhibitor of Ca^{2+}-transport ATPase activity. Similar results were recently reported by Kimura *et al.*, who coexpressed SERCA2a and phospholamban proteins in HEK-293 cells.[12] Both groups proposed that the phospholamban monomer is an important regulatory component inhibiting the Ca^{2+} pump in cardiac sarcoplasmic reticulum membranes.[9,12]

Although there is good correlation between the monomeric status of phospholamban mutants with the degree of inhibition of the Ca^{2+} pump, certain inconsistencies exist. For instance, I40L-PLB—which contains the similarly sized amino acid leucine at position 40 in the zipper region[11]—was able to partially assemble into pentamers on SDS-PAGE (FIG. 6), yet decreased the apparent Ca^{2+} affinity of the Ca^{2+} pump as potently as the completely monomeric mutants substituted with alanine in the zipper[11] domain (TABLE 2). On the other hand, C41F-PLB, which was mutated in the region directly adjacent to the zipper domain,[11] was totally monomeric (FIG. 6),[11,17] but inhibited SERCA2a no more effectively than did WT-PLB (TABLE 2) (see also Toyofuku *et al.*[17]). Interestingly, the phospholamban tetramer, C41L-PLB (FIG. 6), was unable to give any significant inhibition of the Ca^{2+} pump (TABLE 2).

Thus, circumstantial evidence of the type described above suggests that the phospholamban monomer may be an important regulatory component interacting with the Ca^{2+} pump in the sarcoplasmic reticulum membrane.[9,12] However, it remains to be proved whether the phospholamban pentamer itself is capable of inhibiting SERCA2a, or whether phospholamban monomers dissociating from the pentamer in the membrane[3] are required for enzyme inhibition. Although the active monomer model is an attractive hypothesis to explain the molecular mechanism of phospholamban regulation,[3,9,12,17] further studies with additional mutants, as well as with newly developed biophysical techniques (Cornea *et al.*[3] and Stokes *et al.*[18]), will be required to positively identify the molecular species of native phospholamban that interacts with and inhibits the cardiac Ca^{2+} pump in sarcoplasmic reticulum membranes.

ACKNOWLEDGMENT

We thank Dr. U. Kirchhefer for kindly maintaining high-quality Sf21 cells.

REFERENCES

1. TADA, M., M. A. KIRCHBERGER & A. M. KATZ. 1975. Phosphorylation of a 22,000-dalton component of the cardiac sarcoplasmic reticulum by adenosine 3′:5′-monophosphate–dependent protein kinase. J. Biol. Chem. **250:** 2640–2647.
2. WEGENER, A. D. & L. R. JONES. 1984. Phosphorylation-induced mobility shift in phospholamban in sodium dodecyl sulfate-polyacrylamide gels. J. Biol. Chem. **259:** 1834–1841.
3. CORNEA, R. L., L. R. JONES, J. M. AUTRY & D. D. THOMAS. 1997. Mutation and phosphorylation change the oligomeric structure of phospholamban in lipid bilayers. Biochemistry **36:** 2960–2967.
4. INUI, M., B. K. CHAMBERLAIN, A. SAITO & S. FLEISCHER. 1986. The nature of the modulation of Ca^{2+} transport as studied by reconstitution of cardiac sarcoplasmic reticulum. J. Biol. Chem. **261:** 1794–1800.

5. CANTILINA, T., Y. SAGARA, G. INESI & L. R. JONES. 1993. Comparative studies of cardiac and skeletal sarcoplasmic reticulum ATPases. J. Biol. Chem. **268:** 17018–17025.
6. ODERMATT, A., K. KURZYDLOWSKI & D. H. MACLENNAN. 1996. The V_{max} of the Ca^{2+}-ATPase of cardiac sarcoplasmic reticulum (SERCA2a) is not altered by Ca^{2+}-calmodulin–dependent phosphorylation or by interaction with phospholamban. J. Biol. Chem. **271:** 14206–14213.
7. REDDY, L. G., L. R. JONES, R. C. PACE & D. L. STOKES. 1996. Purified, reconstituted cardiac Ca^{2+}-ATPase is regulated by phospholamban but not by direct phosphorylation with Ca^{2+}/calmodulin–dependent protein kinase. J. Biol. Chem. **271:** 14964–14970.
8. MORRIS, G. L., H.-C. CHENG, J. COLYER & J. H. WANG. 1991. Phospholamban regulation of cardiac sarcoplasmic reticulum (Ca^{2+}-Mg^{2+})–ATPase. J. Biol. Chem. **266:** 11270–11275.
9. AUTRY, J. M. & L. R. JONES. 1997. Functional coexpression of the canine cardiac Ca^{2+} pump and phospholamban in *Spodoptera frugiperda* (Sf21) cells reveals new insights on ATPase regulation. J. Biol. Chem. **272:** 15872–15880.
10. REDDY, L. G., L. R. JONES, S. E. CALA, J. J. O'BRIAN, S. A. TATULIAN & D. L. STOKES. 1995. Functional reconstitution of recombinant phospholamban with rabbit skeletal Ca^{2+}-ATPase. J. Biol. Chem. **270:** 9390–9397.
11. SIMMERMAN, H. K. B., Y. M. KOBAYASHI, J. M. AUTRY & L. R. JONES. 1996. A leucine zipper stabilizes the pentameric membrane domain of phospholamban and forms a coiled-coil pore structure. J. Biol. Chem. **271:** 5941–5946.
12. KIMURA, Y., K. KURZYDLOWSKI, M. TADA & D. H. MACLENNAN. 1997. Phospholamban inhibitory function is activated by depolymerization. J. Biol. Chem. **272:** 15061–15064.
13. JONES, L. R., S. H. PHAN & H. R. BESCH, JR. 1978. Gel electrophoretic and density gradient analysis of the K^+,Ca^{2+}-ATPase and the Na^+,K^+-ATPase activities of cardiac membrane vesicles. Biochim. Biophys. Acta **514:** 294–309.
14. CLARKE, D. M., K. MARUYAMA, T. W. LOO, E. LEBERER, G. INESI & D. H. MACLENNAN. 1989. Functional consequences of glutamate, aspartate, glutamine, and asparagine mutations in the stalk sector of the Ca^{2+}-ATPase of sarcoplasmic reticulum. J. Biol. Chem. **264:** 11246–11251.
15. SHAM, J. S. K., L. R. JONES & M. MORAD. 1991. Phospholamban mediates the β-adrenergic–enhanced Ca^{2+} uptake in mammalian ventricular myocytes. Am. J. Physiol. **261:** H1344–H1349.
16. BRIGGS, F. N., K. F. LEE, A. W. WECHSLER & L. R. JONES. 1992. Phospholamban expressed in slow-twitch and chronically stimulated fast-twitch muscles minimally affects calcium affinity of sarcoplasmic reticulum Ca^{2+}-ATPase. J. Biol. Chem. **267:** 26056–26061.
17. TOYOFUKU, T., K. KURZYDLOWSKI, M. TADA & D. H. MACLENNAN. 1994. Amino acids Glu^2 to Ile^{18} in the cytoplasmic domain of phospholamban are essential for functional association with the Ca^{2+}-ATPase of sarcoplasmic reticulum. J. Biol. Chem. **269:** 3088–3094.
18. YOUNG, H. S., L. G. REDDY, L. R. JONES & D. L. STOKES. 1998. Co-reconstitution and co-crystallization of phospholamban and Ca^{2+}-ATPase. Ann. N.Y. Acad. Sci. This volume.

Co-reconstitution and Co-crystallization of Phospholamban and Ca^{2+}-ATPase[a]

HOWARD S. YOUNG,[b] LAXMA G. REDDY,[c] LARRY R. JONES,[d] AND DAVID L. STOKES[b]

[b]*Skirball Institute of Biomolecular Medicine, New York University Medical Center, 540 First Avenue, New York, New York 10012, USA*

[c]*Department of Biochemistry, University of Minnesota, 435 Delaware Street SE, Minneapolis, Minnesota 55455, USA*

[d]*Krannert Institute of Cardiology, Indiana University Medical School, 1111 West 10th Street, Indianapolis, Indiana 46202, USA*

ABSTRACT: Significant advances have recently been made in understanding the regulation of Ca^{2+}-ATPase by phospholamban and in modeling their structures. However, these insights would be furthered by determining the 3-D structure of both proteins within the membrane, thus revealing the structural basis for their interaction. To this end, we have developed methods for reconstituting purified Ca^{2+}-ATPase with recombinant phospholamban. After reconstitution at high lipid-to-protein ratios, we have verified their functional association by measuring calcium transport and ATPase activity. Furthermore, we have grown co-crystals after reconstitution at low lipid-to-protein ratios. The structure of Ca^{2+}-ATPase has recently been solved by cryoelectron microscopy at 8-Å resolution, thus revealing transmembrane α-helices. Using a variety of constraints, we have associated these helices with the predicted transmembrane sequences to produce a detailed model for the packing of transmembrane helices. Structure determination of the co-crystals is currently underway, which we hope will eventually reveal the interaction of phospholamban with Ca^{2+}-ATPase at a similar level of detail.

In recent years, many different approaches have been taken to address the structure of phospholamban (PLB). These include saturation mutagenesis, Fourier transform infrared spectroscopy, and NMR.[1] As a result, an attractive model has evolved, in which the monomeric form of PLB binds to and regulates Ca^{2+}-ATPase, whereas the pentameric form consists of a five-stranded, coiled coil that serves as an inactive pool of PLB. This model is supported by spectroscopic studies of membrane-bound PLB that provide evidence for a dynamic equilibrium between various oligomeric states.[2] Furthermore, recent mutagenesis studies have established a strong correlation between the oligomeric state of PLB in SDS gels and its ability to regulate Ca^{2+}-ATPase.[3,4] The sites of interaction between PLB and Ca^{2+}-ATPase have been addressed by cross-linking[5] and also by site-directed mutagenesis of both Ca^{2+}-ATPase[6] and PLB.[7,8] In some cases, it was concluded that a sequence in Ca^{2+}-ATPase near its phosphorylation site governed the interaction;[6,9] yet in other cases, the full regulatory capacity has been attributed to the transmembrane domain of PLB.[7] Indeed, disparate results have been obtained in a variety of other attempts to determine the distinct roles of the transmembrane and cytoplasmic domains of PLB,[10–15] but it seems reasonable that both domains contribute to the binding and regulation. As yet, there is little in-

[a] This work has been partially supported by NIH Grants HL48807 (to D.L.S.) and HL06308 (to L.R.J.), and by NIH postdoctoral fellowship GM18281 (to H.S.Y.).

formation about the structural details of this interaction, and we have therefore undertaken to solve the crystal structure of PLB and Ca^{2+}-ATPase by cryoelectron microscopy. Thus, we hope ultimately to reveal the elements of secondary structure involved in this interaction and conformational changes in Ca^{2+}-ATPase that reflect the regulation.

To accomplish this goal, the first, and often most daunting, step is to produce crystals of the proteins in question. Unlike X-ray crystallographers, who must solubilize membrane proteins in detergent before attempting to grow large, isotropic crystals, we require relatively small crystals that are confined within a single membrane, which are called two-dimensional crystals because the unit cell does not repeat in the direction normal to the bilayer. Given that skeletal Ca^{2+}-ATPase forms tubular crystals within the membrane of native sarcoplasmic reticulum (SR),[16] our first crystallization trials employed cardiac SR, in which cardiac Ca^{2+}-ATPase (SERCA2a) and PLB are present and functionally coupled. However, the greater heterogeneity of this preparation, in terms both of protein composition and of the distribution of microsomes from various membrane sources (e.g., SR, plasma membrane, mitochondrial membranes), appeared to prevent any sort of crystallization. We therefore decided to co-reconstitute Ca^{2+}-ATPase and PLB into proteoliposomes and thereafter to attempt co-crystallization.

In order to maximize our chances for crystallization, we characterized the functionality of the proteins throughout the steps of purification and reconstitution.[14,17] In the case of Ca^{2+}-ATPase, this consisted of measuring both ATPase activity and calcium transport; a successful reconstitution should not only preserve high activities, but should also maintain good coupling between ATP hydrolysis and calcium transport. In the case of PLB, regulation of both ATPase activity and calcium transport was documented. Given the strong consensus for PLB lowering the calcium affinity of Ca^{2+}-ATPase without affecting activity at saturating calcium concentrations (V_{max}),[4,18–20] we generally screened our preparations with ATPase and calcium transport assays at high (pCa 5.4) and at low (pCa 6.8) calcium concentrations: suppression of activity at low calcium concentration reflects the shift in calcium affinity, whereas the higher, saturating calcium concentration serves as a control for other effects such as vesicle leakiness. The reversibility of the regulation was usually checked with a monoclonal antibody to PLB, which has been shown to mimic the effect of phosphorylation;[21] we explicitly verified this effect both with cyclic AMP–dependent protein kinase and with calcium/calmodulin–dependent protein kinase (TABLE 1 and FIG. 1). The fact that our preparations demonstrated this wide range of specific effects on Ca^{2+}-ATPase activity strongly suggests that the functional association between Ca^{2+}-ATPase and PLB was preserved after reconstitution.

Our desire to measure calcium transport placed restrictions on the lipid-to-protein ratio that we could use during reconstitution. Specifically, this assay requires that vesicles have a large internal volume to prevent a buildup of calcium during the time required for this assay.[22] For this reason, initial reconstitution trials were conducted at a high lipid-to-protein ratio (40–80:1 by weight), to limit the number of Ca^{2+}-ATPase molecules in any given vesicle. Furthermore, high concentrations of oxalate (50–100 mM) were trapped inside these vesicles to keep the internal calcium low by precipitation of calcium oxalate. Both Triton X-100 and $C_{12}E_8$ detergents effectively preserved Ca^{2+}-ATPase activity after solubilization, but removal of these detergents by dialysis was problematic, given their extremely low critical micellar concentration. We therefore used BioBeads SM2 to remove these nonionic detergents,[23] which allowed us to control the rate of reconstitution by adjusting the rate of BioBead addition (30 min–4 h in our work). We used detergent-solubilized, purified protein as starting material for reconstitution, and, in most cases, skeletal Ca^{2+}-ATPase was co-reconstituted with recombinant PLB. This skeletal Ca^{2+}-ATPase was purified by Reactive red affinity chromatog-

TABLE 1. Functional Characterization of Ca^{2+}-ATPase and PLB Co-reconstitution

	Calcium Transport µmoles/mg/min						ATPase Activity µmoles/mg/min					
	pCa 6.8[a]			pCa 5.4			pCa 6.8			pCa 5.4		
		ab/k[b]	Ctrl		ab/k	Ctrl		ab/k	Ctrl		ab/k	Ctrl
Wild-type PLB[c]												
SERCA1 + ab	0.13	0.25	0.27	4.73	4.87	4.87	0.46	0.83	0.70	2.50	2.65	2.54
SERCA2 + ab	0.40	0.70	0.71	2.44	2.75	2.81	0.44	0.79	0.78	1.64	1.83	1.70
SERCA2 + PKA	0.22	0.34	0.34	2.77	2.87	2.79	—	—	—	—	—	—
SERCA2a + CamK	0.30	0.48	0.43	2.52	2.67	2.61	—	—	—	—	—	—
SERCA1[d]												
PLB 26–52	0.06	—	0.14	2.39	—	3.70	0.54	—	0.48	3.63	—	3.98
PLB 1–31	0.21	—	0.17	4.18	—	4.10	0.39	—	0.38	2.77	—	2.71
PLB L37A[e]	0.36	1.02	0.92	3.93	4.28	4.02	0.04	0.26	0.21	3.00	3.34	3.79
PLB WT[f]	—	—	—	—	—	—	0.12	0.20	0.50	5.73	6.17	5.66
PLB L37A[f]	—	—	—	—	—	—	0.01	0.13	0.30	3.49	2.86	3.31

[a] Effects at low calcium concentration (pCa 6.8) reflect a shift in the calcium affinity, whereas effects at high calcium concentration reflect a change in V_{max}. Data derived predominantly from References 14 and 17.

[b] In some experiments, a PLB monoclonal antibody (ab) was used, and in other experiments a protein kinase was used to disrupt the interaction between PLB and Ca^{2+}-ATPase.

[c] In this group of experiments, wild-type PLB was reconstituted with either skeletal muscle Ca^{2+}-ATPase (SERCA1) or cardiac muscle Ca^{2+}-ATPase (SERCA2a). The effects of PLB were tested either with the monoclonal antibody (ab), with cAMP-dependent protein kinase (PKA), or calcium/calmodulin-dependent protein kinase (CamK).

[d] In this group of experiments, SERCA1 was reconstituted with several variants of PLB, consisting of the membrane domain (PLB 26–52), the cytoplasmic domain (PLB 1–31), or the single-site mutant L37A.

[e] These results are unpublished work of L. G. Reddy, L. R. Jones & D. D. Thomas.

[f] These experiments were done at very low lipid-to-protein ratios (1:2), which prevent the measurement of calcium transport.

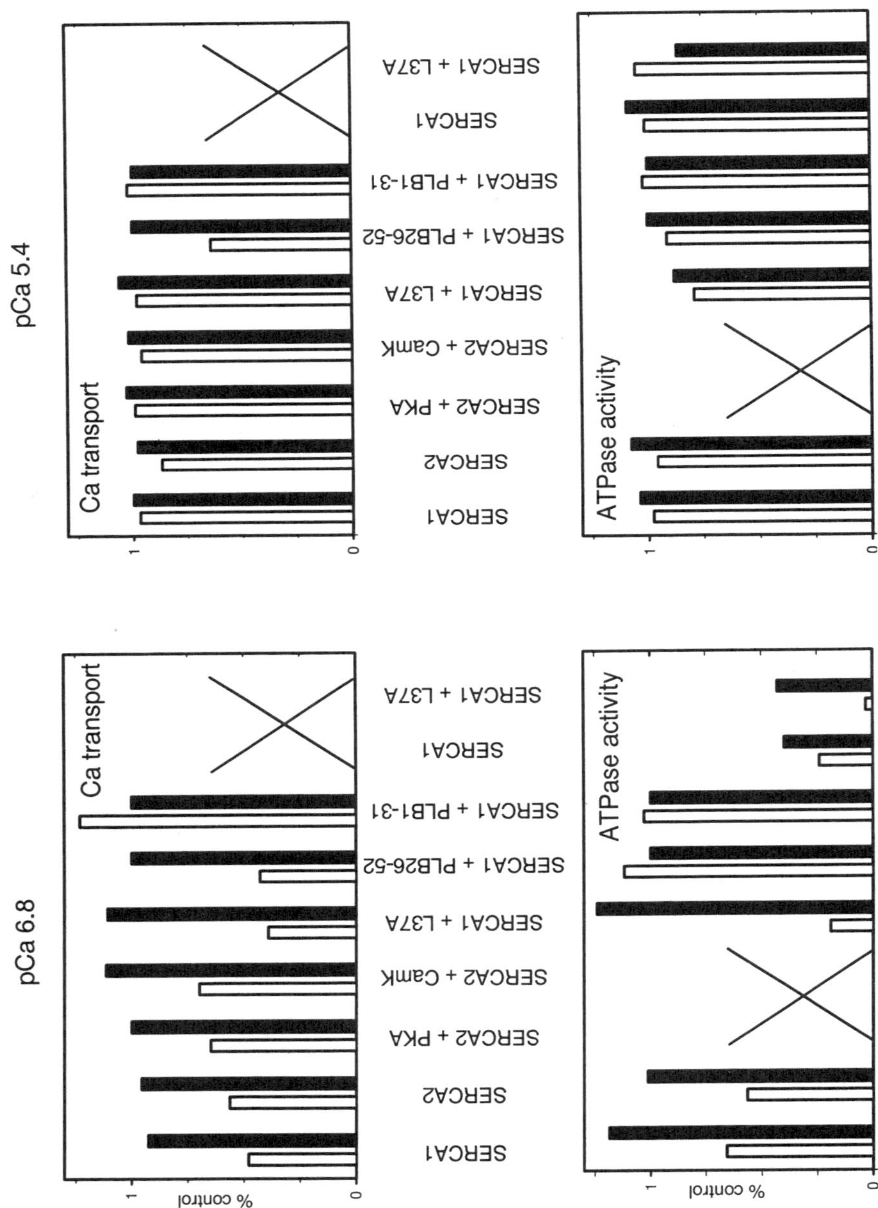
pCa 6.8
pCa 5.4
Ca transport
ATPase activity
% control
0
1
SERCA1
SERCA2
SERCA2 + PKA
SERCA2 + CamK
SERCA1 + L37A
SERCA1 + PLB26-52
SERCA1 + PLB1-31
SERCA1
SERCA1 + L37A

FIGURE 1. Quantitation of PLB regulation of Ca^{2+}-ATPase in reconstituted proteoliposomes. This data has been taken from TABLE 1[14,17] and normalized relative to the control activity in each group. The white and black *bars* of each pair correspond to activities of reconstituted preparations assayed in the absence and presence of the monoclonal PLB antibody, respectively (except in the case of PKA and CamK, which used cAMP-dependent protein kinase and calcium/calmodulin-dependent protein kinase, respectively, instead of the antibody). The **top two plots** represent calcium uptake measured by filtration and scintillation counting of ^{45}Ca, whereas the **bottom two plots** represent ATPase activities measured by determination of free phosphate using malachite green. The **plots on the left** correspond to minimal calcium concentrations (pCa 6.8) where the effect of antibody (or phosphorylation) should be maximal. The **plots on the right** are at saturating calcium concentrations (pCa 5.4) where there should be no effect given that PLB shifts the apparent calcium affinity of Ca^{2+}-ATPase without affecting V_{max}. Except where indicated, reconstitutions included wild-type PLB, and stimulation was accomplished with the antibody. Except for the two conditions on the **far right of each plot,** reconstitutions were done with high lipid-to-protein ratios (40–80:1 by weight); the **two conditions on the far right of each plot** were done at very low ratios (1:2), and used for crystallization. Thus, most reconstitutions provided the expected inhibition at low calcium concentrations that was reversed either by antibody or by phosphorylation. This reversal was not complete at low lipid-to-protein ratios, possibly due to steric hindrance caused by high packing densities or by increased vesicle aggregation. L37A was generally more effective than wild-type PLB, especially at low lipid-to-protein ratios. Finally, the isolated cytoplasmic (PLB_{1-31}) and transmembrane (PLB_{26-52}) domains of PLB were ineffective at regulation: PLB_{1-31} had no effect at all, whereas PLB_{26-52} affected only calcium transport, but did so at both low and high calcium concentrations.

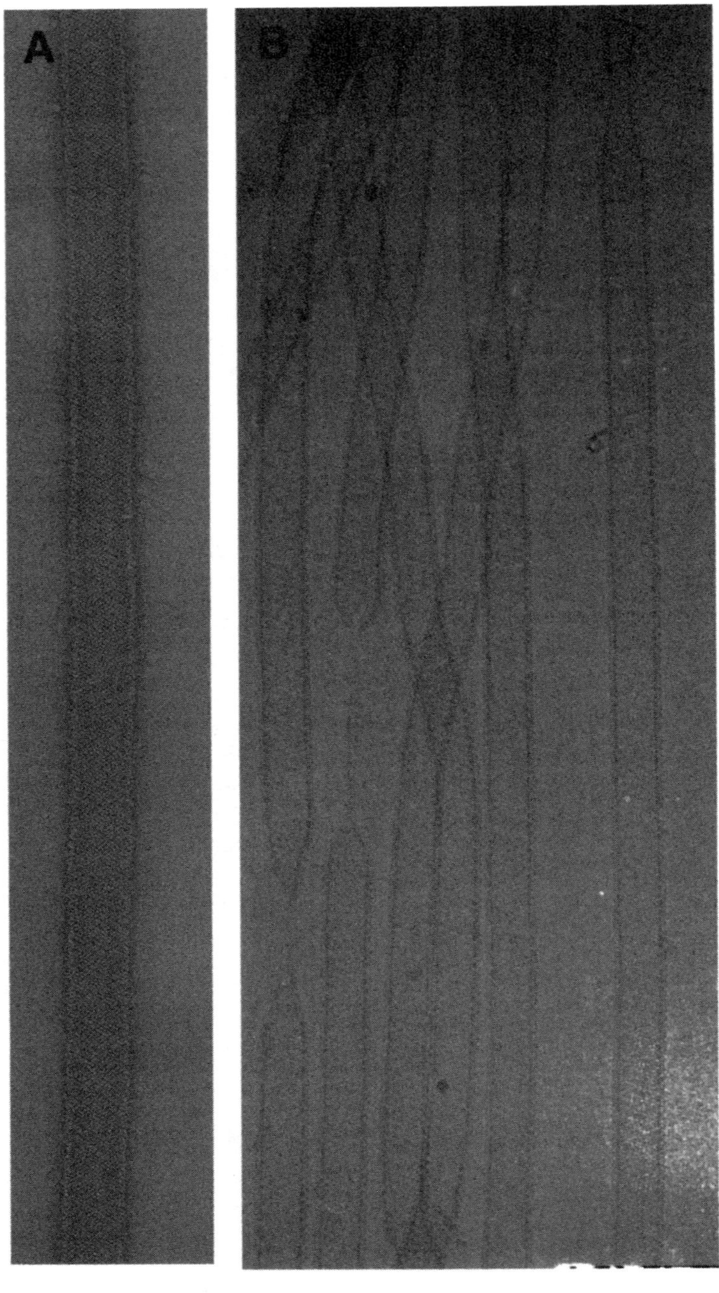
A
B

raphy in $C_{12}E_8$, which produced a highly active (10 μmoles/mg/min at 25 °C) and partially delipidated (~25 moles lipid/mole protein) enzyme. PLB was purified in octylglucoside by monoclonal antibody affinity chromatography after overexpression in a culture of Sf9 cells infected by baculovirus carrying the gene for PLB.[14] We also devised a method for affinity purification of cardiac Ca^{2+}-ATPase with Affi blue for use in some of the reconstitutions.[17] This isoform proved to be inherently more labile, and significant modifications were necessary to preserve its activity. Due to this increased lability, to the much smaller quantities of cardiac SR obtained in routine preparations, and to the reported similarity in the regulation of skeletal Ca^{2+}-ATPase by PLB,[18] we used the skeletal isoform for the ensuing co-crystallization work.

During initial studies we found that PLB was not efficiently incorporated into lipid vesicles by simply using BioBeads to remove the octylglucoside. However, good incorporation was observed when PLB was dried down with lipids into a thin film and resuspended in aqueous buffer in the presence of a small amount of trifluoroethanol. The resulting proteoliposomes were then fully solubilized with either $C_{12}E_8$, Triton X-100 or octylglucoside and added to $C_{12}E_8$-solubilized Ca^{2+}-ATPase. Reconstitution was accomplished by adding BioBeads in the ratio of 20:1 (hydrated beads by weight) for $C_{12}E_8$ or 40:1 for Triton X-100. Detergent removal was virtually complete after 30 min if all the BioBeads were added at once, thus constituting what we considered to be a fast reconstitution. (Keep in mind, however, that other studies employing dilution or detergent adsorption to hydrophobic columns undoubtedly resulted in much faster reconstitutions.) Alternatively, BioBeads were added incrementally over a 4-hour period at room temperature, providing a much slower reconstitution (though not as slow as dialysis would be, especially for detergents with such low critical micellar concentrations). It was previously determined that such slow detergent removal produced a heterogeneous population of proteoliposomes, which comprised a lipid-rich fraction and a protein-rich fraction.[23] For functional assays, we wanted a homogeneous distribution of proteins in relatively large proteoliposomes and, indeed, we found rapid removal of Triton-X100 to be most satisfactory. In particular, ATPase activities were consistently higher after purification and reconstitution than in SR. Perhaps more significant were the excellent rates of calcium transport, which produced coupling ratios of Ca^{2+}:ATP close to the theoretical limit of 2:1 at pCa 5.4 (TABLE 1 and FIG. 1).

For assessing the association between Ca^{2+}-ATPase and PLB, either skeletal or cardiac Ca^{2+}-ATPase was reconstituted with a variety of PLB constructs (TABLE 1). Using wild-type PLB at physiologically relevant stoichiometries (~ 3:1 molar ratio of PLB to Ca^{2+}-ATPase), we obtained equivalent levels of regulation with either skeletal or cardiac Ca^{2+}-ATPase. A monoclonal antibody to PLB (2D12) was used to reverse fully the inhibitory effect of PLB,[21] and we explicitly showed that phosphorylation by either cAMP-dependent protein kinase or calcium/calmodulin–dependent protein kinase was equally effective at this reversal (TABLE 1 and FIG. 1). Also, we found that neither the

←

FIGURE 2. Tubular crystals from co-reconstituted Ca^{2+}-ATPase and PLB. These crystals were grown in our standard, decavanadate-containing crystallization solutions and exhibited the same crystal lattice as tubes grown within the native membrane of skeletal SR. The diameter of the thinnest tubes (650 Å) tends to be somewhat larger than for SR (600 Å). Panel **A** shows a negatively stained, flattened tube in which one can see the "dimer ribbons" of molecules running at ~ 30° relative to the diameter (i.e., relative to a horizontal line across the tube). Panel **B** shows frozen-hydrated tubes, which have reversed contrast (protein is white in **A** and black in **B**). In this case, tubes are suspended in vitreous ice over a hole in the carbon support and therefore retain their cylindrical shape. Various constrictions are observed in the tubes, which are probably caused by turbulence in the solution when the excess solution is removed by blotting immediately prior to rapid freezing.

transmembrane domain nor the cytoplasmic domain of PLB inhibited Ca^{2+}-ATPase, even when added in excess. In line with recent mutagenesis results, the single-site PLB mutant L37A was found to be more effective in inhibition than wild-type PLB,[3,4] supporting the hypothesis that the PLB monomer—which is produced by this particular mutation—is the species responsible for regulation of Ca^{2+}-ATPase and that the pentamer is an inactive storage form of PLB in the membrane.

Our next goal was to produce preparations suitable for crystallization trials, and this required reconstitutions at much lower lipid-to-protein ratios (<1:1) in order to facilitate protein-protein interactions.[24] Although measurement of calcium uptake is impossible at such high protein densities, measurement of ATPase activity indicated that Ca^{2+}-ATPase was still highly active and interacting with PLB (TABLE 1 and FIG. 1). The inhibition produced by L37A was particularly high, suggesting that the high protein density in SR is necessary to promote the interaction between PLB and Ca^{2+}-ATPase. The monoclonal antibody was rather ineffective in reversing this inhibition, possibly due to steric hindrance caused either by the high protein density or vesicle aggregation.

We found that reconstitution of Ca^{2+}-ATPase alone was strongly affected by the detergent used and the rate of its removal. Fast (complete after 15–30 min) removal of Triton X-100 resulted in a homogeneous population of vesicles, whereas slow (3–4 h) removal of $C_{12}E_8$ resulted in two distinct populations of vesicles. These two populations could be distinguished in electron micrographs and could be separated by sucrose gradient centrifugation. Analysis of the protein and lipid composition of the two populations revealed that the low-density, lightly staining vesicles were virtually pure lipid, whereas the denser, darkly staining vesicles were densely packed with protein (lipid-to-protein ratio of ~1:2). Furthermore, quantitation of fluorescein isothiocyanate labeling indicated that virtually all the Ca^{2+}-ATPase molecules were facing the same direction in these vesicles, making this an attractive preparation for crystallization. Indeed, arrays readily formed on the surface of these vesicles after incubation in our standard, decavanadate-containing solutions. However, the small size of vesicles (0.1 μm) limited the extent of arrays, and we therefore subjected them to cycles of freeze-thaw with the intention of inducing fusion. Rather than fusion, however, this procedure tended to cause aggregation of vesicles. Nevertheless, tubular crystals grew out of the vesicle aggregates after incubation in crystallization solutions. The frequency of these crystals was influenced by the lipid composition, and we specifically found that inclusion of lipids that destabilize bilayers (phosphatidyl ethanolamine and phosphatidic acid) was helpful in producing tubes. We postulated that these aggregates represent an ill-defined phase from which protein and lipid can be recruited by the elongating tubular crystal. The crystal lattice in the tubes is the same as that in tubes grown directly from SR,[25] thus confirming the functionality of the protein and its one-sided orientation after reconstitution.

Inclusion of PLB in these reconstitutions actually promoted the formation of tubular crystals, which could be due to one or more of the following effects: (a) the marked increase in vesicle aggregation, (b) the stabilization of the E_2 conformation of Ca^{2+}-ATPase by PLB, or (c) an effect of PLB on the physical properties of the aggregates or of the bilayer. Both wild-type PLB and L37A have been used in these co-crystallizations, and both produce tubular crystals (FIGS. 2 and 3). The molar stoichiometry of PLB to Ca^{2+}-ATPase in the vesicles used for crystallization was determined by SDS-PAGE and densitometry, which included known amounts of PLB and Ca^{2+}-ATPase to construct a standard curve. After initially including an 8-fold excess of PLB, we found the crystallization vesicles to contain a 4–6-mole excess of PLB, presumably due to inefficiencies in reconstitution of PLB or to a more homogeneous distribution of PLB in the two populations of vesicles. Given the evidence for a dynamic exchange of PLB between monomers and pentamers,[2] we felt that this range of molar ratios was physiologically

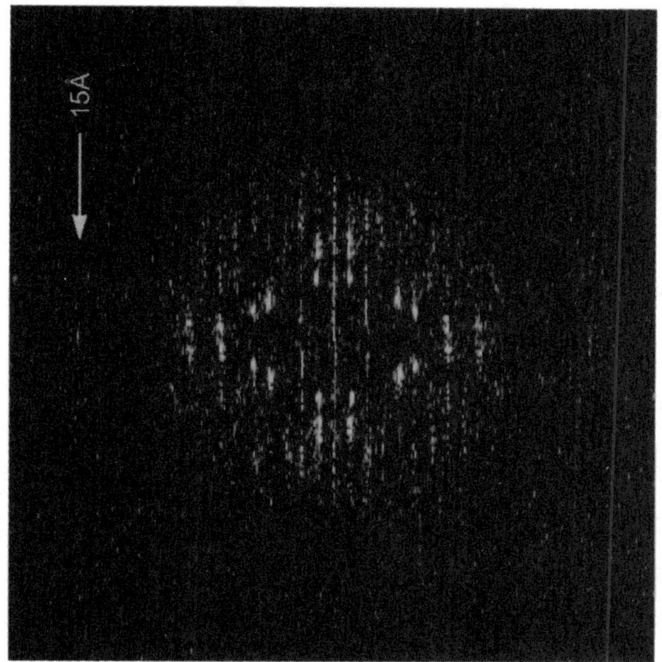

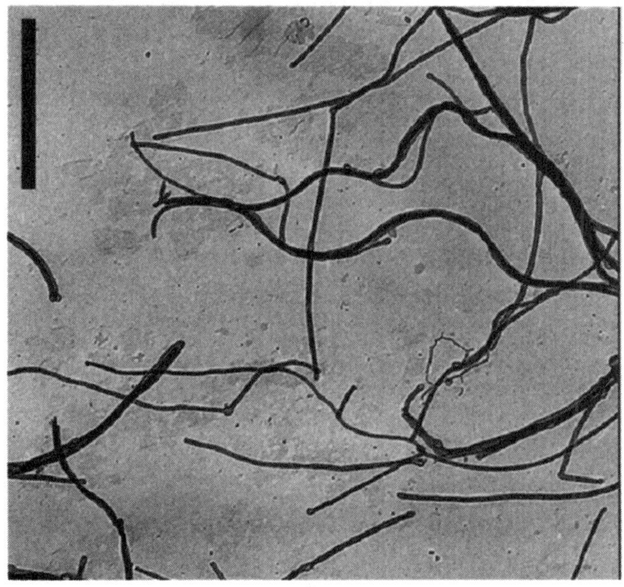

FIGURE 3. Tubular crystals from co-reconstituted Ca^{2+}-ATPase and PLB. On the **left** is a low-magnification image of negatively stained tubes showing the preponderance of tubular crystals (*scale bar* represents 5 μm). The frequency of these tubes is very much increased when PLB is included in the reconstitution, suggesting an effect of PLB either in stabilizing the relevant conformation of Ca^{2+}-ATPase or in altering the properties of the bilayer. On the **right** is a computed Fourier transform from a digitized image showing layer lines characteristic of helical symmetry. These layer lines frequently extend to 15-Å resolution, and five such images have so far been included in a 3-D reconstruction of the Ca^{2+}-ATPase-PLB complex.

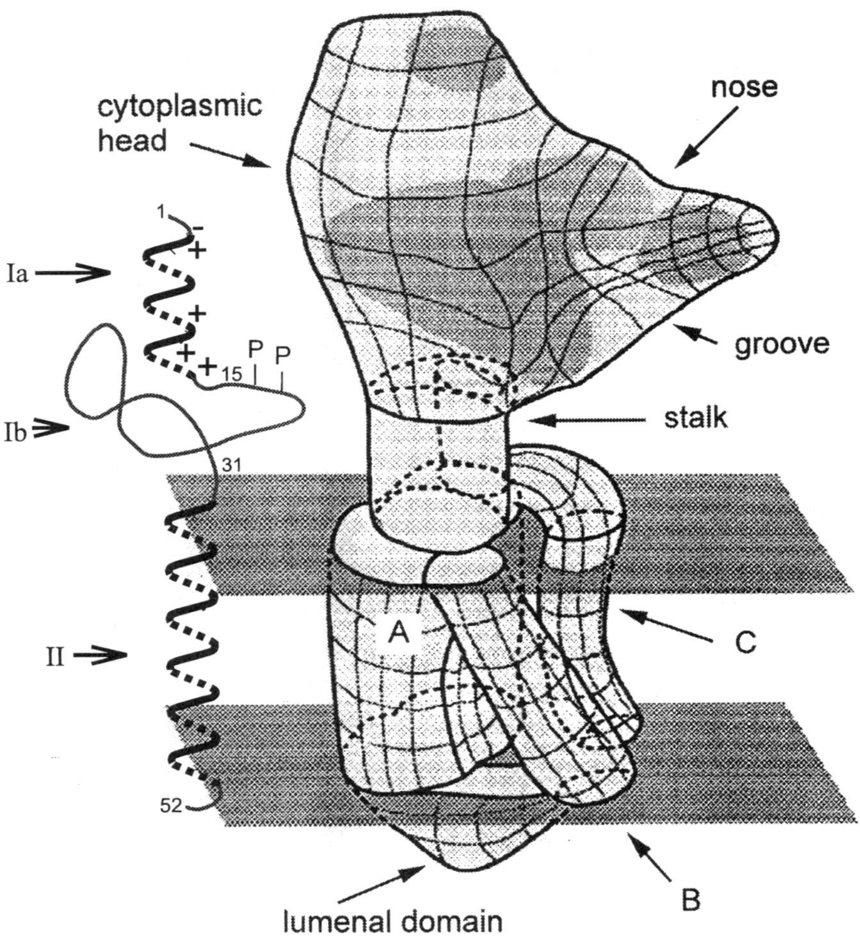

FIGURE 4. Cartoons of the structures for Ca^{2+}-ATPase and PLB. Ca^{2+}-ATPase is shown on the **right;** the shape is based on 3-D reconstructions from native SR crystals.[25, 28] A large cytoplasmic head and beak is connected to the membrane by a narrow stalk. The transmembrane domain is divided into three parts, labeled A, B, and C. The lumenal domain is relatively small, comprising only ~15% of the molecular mass. The PLB monomer is ~5% of the mass of Ca^{2+}-ATPase and is shown schematically on the **left.** PLB is composed of a cytoplasmic domain of 31 residues (subdivided into domains Ia and Ib) and a transmembrane domain of 21 residues (domain II).

appropriate. After crystallization, the presence of tubes was determined after negative staining (FIG. 3a), and specimens were prepared for electron microscopy by rapid freezing in a thin meniscus of crystallization buffer. This is a widespread and popular method for preserving molecular structure, and we were therefore surprised to observe disordering of tubes apparently induced solely by this freezing. Several factors seem to contribute to this disordering, including an excess of PLB in the vesicles used for reconstitution. This is perhaps an indication that the monomeric form of PLB is interacting with Ca^{2+}-ATPase and the excess PLB is serving to destabilize the bilayers. The relative stability of tubular crystals formed from reconstituted Ca^{2+}-ATPase alone suggest that the particular choice of lipids or presence of residual detergent is not responsible for the disorder. In the case of the PLB mutant, L37A, this instability occurs at lower PLB-to-Ca^{2+}-ATPase ratios (>2:1), though tubular crystals have been successfully formed at a 1:1 ratio, which seems physiologically appropriate given the monomeric state of this mutant and its increased affinity for Ca^{2+}-ATPase.[3,4]

Computer processing of electron micrographs of frozen-hydrated tubes indicates that the co-crystals have the same packing as crystals containing Ca^{2+}-ATPase alone, either reconstituted[24] or in SR membranes.[25–27] The tubular shape of crystals suggests the presence of helical symmetry. Indeed, rows of molecules are built from dimers that self-associate into ribbons and that spiral around the tube at an angle of ~25–30° relative to its radial axis (FIG. 2a). The diameter of the tubes is innately variable, and we always choose the thinnest tubes for imaging to provide some constraint on the range of helical symmetries; a wider tube accommodates a larger number of dimers in one turn of the fundamental helix, thus changing the helical symmetry. Averaging of tubes is required to increase the signal-to-noise ratio along the layer lines that compose the Fourier transform (FIG. 3b); a variety of defocus values are necessary to fill in the zeros in this Fourier transform, the positions of which depend on the precise value of defocus used to record the image. Traditionally, this averaging has been done in Fourier space (i.e., simply averaging data from like layer lines), and a single 3-D map has been calculated from this averaged Fourier data. However, new techniques have recently been developed to average these 3-D maps in real space, thus relaxing the requirement for tubes with precisely the same helical symmetry. Such a strategy has been used for maps at 8-Å resolution from SR[28] and may prove invaluable for our work with these co-crystals. The tubular co-crystals are wider (650 Å) than those from SR containing Ca^{2+}-ATPase alone (550–600 Å) and have a correspondingly larger number of molecules in the fundamental helix (28 vs. 22–25 for SR tubes). Even when the crystal lattice is preserved, tubes often have bubbles or constrictions along their length and are generally more curved than their counterparts from SR (FIG. 2b). As a result, the Fourier data is so far not as good, and our preliminary 3-D map (average of 5 tubes) to ~14 Å is considerably noisier than previous maps from SR.[25, 28] Nevertheless, the overall shape of the molecule is the same: a large cytoplasmic head and nose connected to the membrane by a narrow stalk, a small lumenal domain, and a transmembrane domain that can be divided into three main parts (FIG. 4). PLB is expected to contribute predominantly to the transmembrane region and perhaps also to the stalk, but unfortunately the transmembrane densities in the map always have lower contrast and are therefore more subject to noisy data. It is therefore difficult to say anything definitive at this time about the presence of PLB or its effects on Ca^{2+}-ATPase structure. However, there is some evidence of extra transmembrane density next to the A transmembrane domain (FIG. 4) and also evidence for conformational changes in both membrane and stalk domains. However, such conclusions will have to await further image processing to improve the reliability of the current map. A concomitant increase in resolution may also be necessary to reveal the oligomeric state of PLB in the membrane, and comparative studies with the PLB mutant L37A should help resolve the respective roles of the various oligomeric states that have been observed by SDS-PAGE.

REFERENCES

1. STOKES, D. L. 1997. Keeping calcium in its place: Ca^{2+}-ATPase and phospholamban. Curr. Opin. Struct. Biol. **7:** 550–556.

2. CORNEA, R. L., L. R. JONES, J. M. AUTRY & D. D. THOMAS. 1997. Mutation and phosphorylation change the oligomeric structure of phospholamban in lipid bilayers. Biophys. J. **36:** 2960–2967.
3. KIMURA, Y., K. KURZYDLOWSKI, M. TADA & D. H. MACLENNAN. 1997. Phospholamban inhibitory function is enhanced by depolymerization. J. Biol. Chem. **272:** 15061–15064.
4. AUTRY, J. M. & L. R. JONES. 1997. Functional co-expression of the canine cardiac Ca^{2+} pump and phospholamban in *Spodoptera frugiperda* (Sf21) cells reveals new insights on ATPase regulation. J. Biol. Chem. **272:** 15872–15880.
5. JAMES, P., M. INUI, M. TADA, M. CHIESI & E. CARAFOLI. 1989. Nature and site of phospholamban regulation of the Ca^{2+} pump of sarcoplasmic reticulum. Nature **342:** 90–92.
6. TOYOFUKU, T., K. KURZYDLOWSKI, M. TADA & D. H. MACLENNAN. 1994. Amino acids Lys-Asp-Asp-Lys-Pro-Val^{402} in the Ca^{2+}-ATPase of cardiac sarcoplasmic reticulum are critical for functional association with phospholamban. J. Biol. Chem. **269:** 22929–22932.
7. KIMURA, Y., K. KURZYDLOWSKI, M. TADA & D. H. MACLENNAN. 1996. Phospholamban regulates the Ca^{2+}-ATPase through intramembrane interactions. J. Biol. Chem. **271:** 21726–21731.
8. TOYOFUKU, T., K. KURZYDLOWSKI, M. TADA & D. H. MACLENNAN. 1994. Amino acids Glu^2 to Ile^{18} in the cytoplasmic domain of phospholamban are essential for functional association with the Ca^{2+}-ATPase of sarcoplasmic reticulum that affect functional association with phospholamban. J. Biol. Chem. **268:** 2809–2815.
9. TOYOFUKU, T., K. KURZYDLOWSKI, M. TADA & D. H. MACLENNAN. 1993. Identification of regions in the Ca^{2+}-ATPase of sarcoplasmic reticulum that affect functional association with phospholamban. J. Biol. Chem. **268:** 2809–2815.
10. HUGHES, G., A. P. STARLING, R. P. SHARMA, J. M. EAST & A. G. LEE. 1996. An investigation of the mechanism of inhibition of the Ca^{2+}-ATPase by phospholamban. Biochem. J. **318:** 973–979.
11. SASAKI, T., M. INUI, Y. KIMURA, T. KUZUYU & M. TADA. 1992. Molecular mechanism of regulation of Ca^{2+} pump ATPase by phospholamban in cardiac sarcoplasmic reticulum. J. Biol. Chem. **267:** 1674–1679.
12. KIM, H. W., N. A. E. STEENAART, D. G. FERGUSON & E. G. KRANIAS. 1990. Functional reconstitution of the cardiac sarcoplasmic reticulum Ca^{2+}-ATPase with phospholamban in phospholipic vesicles. J. Biol. Chem. **265:** 1702–1709.
13. JONES, L. R. & L. J. FIELD. 1993. Residues 2–25 of phospholamban are insufficient to inhibit the Ca^{2+} transport ATPase of cardiac sarcoplasmic reticulum. J. Biol. Chem. **268:** 11486–11488.
14. REDDY, L. G., L. R. JONES, S. E. CALA, J. J. O'BRIAN, S. A. TATULIAN & D. L. STOKES. 1995. Functional reconstitution of recombinant phospholamban with rabbit skeletal Ca-ATPase. J. Biol. Chem. **270:** 9390–9397.
15. VORHERR, T., M. CHIESI, R. SCHWALLER & E. CARAFOLI. 1992. Regulation of the calcium ion pump of sarcoplasmic reticulum: Reversible inhibition by phospholamban and by the calmodulin binding domain of the plasma membrane ion pump. Biochemistry **31:** 371–376.
16. DUX, L. & A. MARTONOSI. 1983. Two-dimensional arrays of proteins in sarcoplasmic reticulum and purified Ca^{2+}-ATPase vesicles treated with vanadate. J. Biol. Chem. **258:** 2599–2603.
17. REDDY, L. G., L. R. JONES, R. C. PACE & D. L. STOKES. 1996. Purified, reconstituted cardiac Ca^{2+}-ATPase is regulated by phospholamban but not by direct phosphorylation with Ca^{2+}/calmodulin-dependent protein kinase. J. Biol. Chem. **271:** 14964–14970.
18. CANTILINA, T., Y. SAGARA, G. INESI & L. R. JONES. 1993. Comparative studies of cardiac and skeletal sarcoplasmic reticulum ATPases: Effect of phospholamban antibody on enzyme activation. J. Biol. Chem. **268:** 17018–17025.
19. KIMURA, Y., M. INUI, M. KADOMA, Y. KIJIMA, T. SASAKI & M. TADA. 1991. Effects of monoclonal antibody against phospholamban on calcium pump ATPase of cardiac sarcoplasmic reticulum. J. Mol. Cell. Cardiol. **23:** 1223–1230.
20. FUJII, J., K. MARUYAMA, M. TADA & D. H. MACLENNAN. 1990. Co-expression of slow-twitch/cardiac muscle Ca^{2+}-ATPase (SERCA2) and phospholamban. FEBS Lett. **273:** 232–234.

21. BRIGGS, F. N., K. F. LEE, A. W. WECHSLER & L. R. JONES. 1992. Phosopholamban expressed in slow-twitch and chronically stimulated fast-twitch muscles minimally affects calcium affinity of sarcoplasmic reticulum Ca-ATPase. J. Biol. Chem. **267:** 26056–26061.
22. LEVY, D., M. SEIGNEURET, A. BLUZAT & J.-L. RIGAUD. 1990. Evidence for proton countertransport by the sarcoplasmic reticulum Ca^{2+}-ATPase during calcium transport in reconstituted proteoliposomes with low ionic permeability. J. Biol. Chem. **265:** 19524–19534.
23. LEVY, D., A. GULIK, A. BLUZAT & J.-L. RIGAUD. 1992. Reconstitution of the sarcoplasmic reticulum Ca^{++}-ATPase: Mechanisms of membrane protein insertion into liposomes during reconstitution procedures involving detergents. Biochim. Biophys. Acta **1107:** 283–298.
24. YOUNG, H. S., J.-L. RIGAUD, J.-J. LACAPERE, L. G. REDDY & D. L. STOKES. 1997. How to make tubular crystals by reconstitutioin of detergent-solubilized Ca^{2+}-ATPase. Biophys. J. **72:** 2545–2558.
25. TOYOSHIMA, C., H. SASABE & D. L. STOKES. 1993. Three-dimensional cryo-electron microscopy of the calcium ion pump in the sarcoplasmic reticulum membrane. Nature **362:** 469–471.
26. TAYLOR, K. A., L. DUX & A. MARTONOSI. 1986. Three-dimensional reconstruction of negatively stained crystals of the Ca^{++}-ATPase from muscle sarcoplasmic reticulum. J. Mol. Biol. **187:** 417–427.
27. CASTELLANI, L., P. M. HARDWICKE & P. VIBERT. 1985. Dimer ribbons in the three-dimensional structure of sarcoplasmic reticulum. J. Mol. Biol. **185:** 579–594.
28. ZHANG, P., C. TOYOSHIMA, K. YONEKURA, N. M. GREEN & D. L. STOKES. 1988. Structure of the calcium pump from sarcoplasmic reticulum at 8Å resolution. Nature **392:** 835–839.

Molecular Regulation of Phospholamban Function and Gene Expression[a]

MICHIHIKO TADA,[b] MASANORI YABUKI, AND TOSHIHIKO TOYOFUKU

Department of Medicine and Pathophysiology, Osaka University Medical School, Yamada-oka 2-2, Suita, Osaka 565, Japan

ABSTRACT: Ca-ATPase regulates intracellular Ca levels by pumping Ca into sarcoplasmic reticulum. Phospholamban (PLN) functions as an inhibitory cofactor for cardiac Ca-ATPase (SERCA2). To define the molecular mode of interaction between two proteins, interaction sites have been identified. Studies using photoactivated cross-linker and chimeric Ca-ATPase between SERCA2 and nonmuscle Ca-ATPase (SERCA3) indicated that potential binding residues are located just downstream of the active ATPase site (Asp351) of SERCA2. Site-directed mutagenesis study of this region showed that six residues, Lys-Asp-Asp-Lys-Pro-Val402, of SERCA2 are functionally important for the interaction. Further, mutagenesis study of PLN showed that the cytoplasmic region of PLN contains a potential binding site with SERCA2. The unique expression of PLN in cardiac cells has been analyzed by the transcriptional level of its gene using luciferase activity and Gel shift assays. CCAAT-box in the 5′-upstream region was found to be essential for its expression by associating with Y-box binding transcriptional factors.

An increasing body of knowledge has indicated that phosphoester phosphorylation of key proteins, catalyzed by protein kinases, assumes pivotal roles in signal transduction in mammalian cells including cardiomyocytes. Phospholamban was first found as an intrinsic protein factor in cardiac muscle sarcoplasmic reticulum (SR) to serve as a substrate for cAMP-dependent protein kinase (PKA)[1,2] and subsequently for calmodulin-dependent protein kinase.[3] These findings were accompanied by a series of documentations that Ca-ATPase in cardiac SR, forming a functional unit with phospholamban, is controlled by phosphorylation and dephosphorylation of phospholamban.[4–6] Phospholamban was also found to be expressed in slow-twitch skeletal and smooth muscle SR, along with Ca-ATPase.[7] Also indicated was the possibility that the dephospho-form of phospholamban functions as an inhibitory cofactor of Ca-ATPase, with its phosphorylation serving to suppress the inhibition, thus augmenting the Ca-ATPase activity.[5,8,9] Since intracellular Ca transients, primarily modulated by Ca channels and pumps in SR and plasma membranes, determine the mode of contractility of the myofibrillar apparatus, the phospholamban function is recognized as an interfacial key to cross the two intracellular messengers, Ca and cAMP, with each other at the membrane of SR. Thus, under β-adrenergic stimulation of cardiomyocytes, cAMP-catalyzed phosphorylation of phospholamban markedly augments SR Ca pump activity, thus resulting in the inotropic and chronotropic effects of the myocardium.

[a] This work was supported by grants to M.T. from the International Human Frontier Science Program Organization and Grants-in-Aid for Scientific Research from the Ministry of Education, Science and Culture of Japan.

[b] Address for correspondence: Michihiko Tada, M.D., Ph.D., Department of Medicine and Pathophysiology, Osaka University Medical School, Yamada-oka 2-2, Suita, Osaka 565, Japan. e-mail: mtada@mr-path.med.osaka-u.ac.jp

TABLE 1. Expression and Chromosomal Localization of Sarco- and Endoplasmic Reticulum Ca-ATPases and Phospholamban

	Gene	Tissue					Chromosome
		Fast	Slow	Cardiac	Smooth	Nonmuscle	
Ca^{2+}-ATPase	SERCA1	$+^{a,b}$	−	−	−	−	16
	SERCA2	−	$+^{a}$	$+^{a}$	$+^{b}$	$+^{b}$	12
	SERCA3	−	+	+	+	+	17
Phospholamban		−	+	+	+	−	6

[a,b] Expression of alternatively spliced forms.

This article reviews several features of utmost importance in the phospholamban-Ca-ATPase system, leading to the hypothesis that a protein-protein interaction between these SR proteins mediates cAMP-dependent modulation of Ca signaling in cardiac muscle cells. We also show our attempts at describing the mechanism by which the phospholamban gene is regulated—a mechanism that is potentially responsible for this gene's unique and specified expression in cardiac muscle as well as in slow-twitch skeletal and smooth muscles.

EXPRESSION OF Ca-ATPase AND PHOSPHOLAMBAN GENES

Cardiac and skeletal muscles show a high degree of homology in the expression of key functional proteins, involved in excitation-contraction coupling. In cardiac muscle SR, the isoforms expressed are typically different from those expressed in skeletal muscle. There are at least three kinds of Ca-ATPase genes expressed in sarco- and endoplasmic reticulum (SER)[10] (TABLE 1). While SERCA1 is expressed in fast-twitch skeletal muscle, SERCA2 is expressed in cardiac and slow-twitch skeletal muscle, smooth muscle, and nonmuscle tissues. SERCA3 is expressed in a broad variety of muscle and nonmuscle tissues. SERCA1 and SERCA2 genes are located on human chromosomes 16 and 12, respectively. Phospholamban gene, located on human chromosome 6, is expressed in cardiac, slow-twitch skeletal, and smooth muscles, but not in nonmuscle cells including brain, liver, and kidney. Thus, phospholamban gene is coexpressed with Ca pump ATPase in SR of cardiac, slow-twitch skeletal and smooth muscles, which are the products of SERCA2 genes.

SR Ca-ATPase ACTIVITY IS REGULATED BY PHOSPHOLAMBAN PHOSPHORYLATION

Phospholamban was shown to directly alter the key elementary steps of Ca ATPase when presteady steps were analyzed by enzyme kinetic studies. The Ca transport cycle of Ca-ATPase exhibits a complex series of intermediate reaction steps that involve the sequential formation and degradation of phosphorylated intermediates (EP).[4,11] During the transport cycle, the ATPase enzyme undergoes distinct conformational changes. The enzyme exists in two different conformational states, E_1 and E_2, which exhibit different affinities for Ca.[12] The E_1 form has a high affinity for Ca, and the E_2 form has a low affinity. The phosphorylated intermediate EP is also shown to exhibit two comparable forms, E_1P and E_2P. Ca-ATPase thus translocates Ca according to the reaction sequence shown in Equation 1[5]:

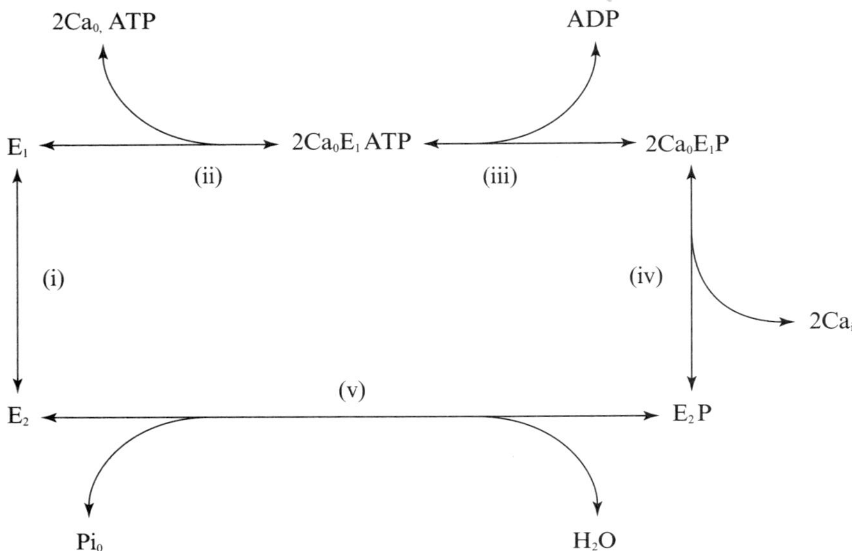

where i and o refer to the intraluminal and cytoplasmic sides of SR membrane, respectively. In this reaction, conversions of E_2 to E_1 and E_1P to E_2P [steps (i) and (iv)] are the rate-limiting steps.[5]

Phosphorylation of phospholamban enhances ATPase activity and Ca uptake activity by increasing the Ca affinity of Ca-ATPase.[1,13] This activation of the ATPase reaction is due to the acceleration of the turnover of the enzyme reaction.[14] Pre–steady state kinetic studies revealed that the two rate-limiting steps, step (i) and (iv), are accelerated by phospholamban phosphorylation.[12,15] Since these correspond to the conformational transition steps of the ATPase enzyme, phospholamban exerts its action by regulating the cation-induced conformational change of the ATPase molecule.

MOLECULAR STRUCTURE OF PHOSPHOLAMBAN

Phospholamban was first found to exist as an oligomer in the presence of a strong detergent such as sodium dodecyl sulfate (SDS) and becomes a 6-kDa monomer in a temperature-dependent manner[3] and by phosphorylation. The result of a low-angle laser light-scattering technique,[16] together with the pattern of temperature-dependent and phosphorylation-dependent mobility shift,[17] indicated that phospholamban is a pentamer composed of five identical monomers.

Purification of canine phospholamban[18,19] and its amino acid[20,21] and cDNA sequencing[22] revealed its molecular structure. The phospholamban monomer deduced from the amino acid sequence is 52 amino acids long, which corresponds to the calculated molecular weight of 6080 Da.[21,22] Since phospholamban is encoded by only one gene, which is located on human chromosome 6,[23] the oligomer should be composed of five identical monomers (homopentamer). FIGURE 1 shows the secondary structural model of phospholamban, deduced from the amino acid sequence analyses. This peptide is distinctly amphipathic, in that the NH2-terminal half (Met1 to Asn 30,

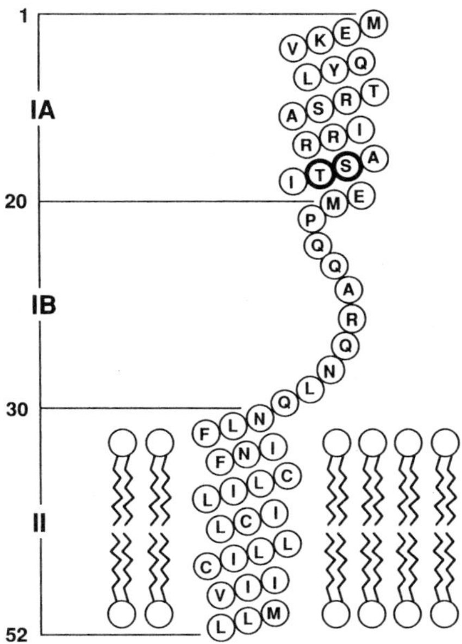

FIGURE 1. Secondary structure of canine phospholamban monomer. The two a helices, domain IA and domain II, are connected by domain IB, which forms a random structure. Domain I is exposed at the cytoplasmic surface, whereas domain II is anchored in the SR membrane. The circled residues S and T represent Ser16 and Thr17, which are phosphorylated by cAMP-dependent and Ca/-calmodulin-dependent protein kinase, respectively.

named domain I) is hydrophilic and exposed at the cytoplasmic surface, whereas the COOH-terminal half (Leu 31 to Leu 52, named domain II) is extremely hydrophobic and embedded within the SR membrane.[24] The circular dichroism analysis indicated that this molecule is rich in alpha helices; two helices (domain IA and II) are connected by the less structured domain IB.[25,26]

Domain I contains specific phosphorylation sites; Ser16 and Thr17 are the sites for phosphorylation, catalyzed by cAMP-dependent protein and Ca/calmodulin-dependent protein kinases.[20,27] Two Arg residues, Arg13 and 14, adjacent to the two phosphorylatable residues, were proved to be essential for phosphorylation,[27] in accord with the consensus sequence for protein kinase substrate. Domain II contains the key amino acids for oligomeric organization. By site-directed mutagenesis,[27] replacement of one or more of Cys 36, 41, and 46 reduced the stability of phospholamban oligomer. However, these Cys residues in the neighboring monomers could not form disulfide bonds for oligomer formation, because these Cys residues existed as free SH groups.[20] Instead, formation of hydrogen bonds between neighboring Cys residues is likely responsible for pentamer structure formation. The size, hydrophobicity, and polarity of the side chains of Cys residues probably match the microenvironment, allowing the hydrophobic residues in neighboring helices to create optimal stabilizing forces in the SR membrane.

PROTEIN-PROTEIN INTERACTION BETWEEN Ca-ATPase AND PHOSPHOLAMBAN MOLECULES

It is important to note that phospholamban phosphorylation enhances two rate-limiting steps in the reaction sequence of ATP hydrolysis, because these are the steps at which a significant conformational change of the Ca-ATPase occurs with the great alteration of Ca affinity of enzyme in the E_1-E_2 model. Chemical and molecular biological evidence supports the hypothesis that phospholamban exerts its action on Ca-ATPase through a direct protein-protein interaction.

Phospholamban-Interacting Site of Ca-ATPase

Studies using a cross-linking agent demonstrated a direct interaction between Ca-ATPase and phospholamban.[28] The Lys residue of purified phospholamban (Lys3) was conjugated with Denny-Jaffe cross-linking reagent. Light activation of conjugated phospholamban incubated with purified Ca-ATPase from cardiac muscle resulted in the formation of a complex only when phospholamban was in the unphosphorylated state and the Ca-ATPase was in the Ca-free state (E_2 conformation). The domain of the ATPase that interacts with phospholamban was identified by sequencing the photo affinity-labeled peptide. This peptide, whose two Lys residues (Lys 397 and Lys 400) were labeled, was found to originate from a region that is just six amino acids on the COOH-terminal side of the phosphorylation domain (FIGURE 2). The amino acid sequence in the phosphorylation site among three SERCA isoforms and cation-transporting ATPases shares a high degree of homology, whereas the putative phospholamban-binding domain is present only in SR type ATPase, especially SERCA1 and 2, but not SERCA3. A synthetic peptide covering this sequence was able to compete for phospholamban with cardiac Ca-ATPase.[29]

The functional significance of this sequence for phospholamban interaction was confirmed by the *in vitro* coexpression system of two proteins in COS-1 cells.[30,31] When SERCA1 or 2 was coexpressed with phospholamban, pCa curves were shifted toward higher Ca^{2+} concentrations, compared with those without phospholamban, indicating that phospholamban suppresses the ATPase activity. When SERCA3 was coexpressed with phospholamban, no effect on the pCa curve was seen, in agreement with the amino acid sequence data, in which SERCA3 is devoid of a phospholamban-interacting region.[30] A series of chimeric Ca-ATPase between SERCA2 and SERCA3 were constructed and used in a coexpression system so as to identify the region functionally important for phospholamban interaction.[30] By analyzing the effects of coexpressed phospholamban on Ca dependency for chimeric Ca-ATPases, the region between amino

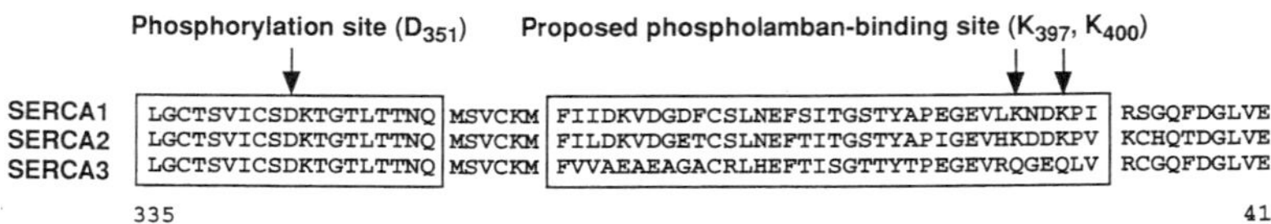

FIGURE 2. Comparison of amino acid sequence around phospholamban-binding region in SERCA isoforms. Phospholamban was conjugated with ^{125}I-labeled Denny-Jaffe reagent. Light activation of conjugated phospholamban incubated with purified ATPase resulted in the formation of a complex. The phospholamban-ATPase complex was cleaved at azo linkage sodium dithionite. This cleavage left the ^{125}I-label attached to the domain that interacts with phospholamban. The ATPase was then digested with CNBr and fractionated using reverse-phase HPLC followed by ion exchange column chromatography. The ^{125}I-labeled peptides were sequenced. The lysine at position 397 and 400 are bound with the cross-linking reagent, and the aspartic acid at position 351 is the phosphorylation site.

acids 365 and 412 of SERCA2 covering the putative phospholamban-binding domain, as described above, was revealed to be important for protein-protein interaction. When a series of mutations were made in SERCA2 between amino acids 365 and 412 and the mutants were coexpressed with phospholamban, only mutation of amino acids Lys 397 to Val 402 affected phospholamban association with the Ca-ATPase.[31]

The finding that the phospholamban-binding domain exists in close proximity to the active phosphorylation site of Ca-ATPase (Asp 351) suggests that binding of phospholamban to this site could exert significant effects on steps involving phosphorylation of Ca-ATPase. Together with kinetic studies, it is plausible that phospholamban may shift the E_1/E_2 equilibrium of SERCA in favor of the E_2 conformation through modifying the constraints on its molecule.

Ca-ATPase–Interacting Site of Phospholamban

Anti-phospholamban monoclonal antibody A1, the epitope of which was identified as a region involving Arg9, enhanced the Ca uptake of cardiac SR vesicles.[32–34] The antibody activated the Ca uptake and ATPase activity by increasing the affinity for Ca. Phospholamban coexpressed with SERCA2 in COS-1 cells diminished the affinity of the ATPase for Ca.[31]

Mutant phospholamban with replacement of amino acid residues in domain I showed that not only positively and negatively charged side chain but also hydrophobic side chain of amino acid residues in domain IA of phospholamban are involved in this interaction,[31] which are summarized in TABLE 2. On the basis of the predicted structural model of domain IA (FIG. 1), charged amino acid residues are clustered on

TABLE 2. Effects of Mutated Amino Acid Residues in Domain I of Phospholamban on the Ca Dependency for SERCA2

Phospholamban Coexpression	SERCA2 Activity (K_m)	Charge Changes
Without	6.73 ± 0.03	
With mutation		
None	6.42 ± 0.04*	0
(A) Relationship to charge		
E2A	6.70 ± 0.03	+1
K3E	6.70 ± 0.04	−2
R9E	6.69 ± 0.04	−2
R13E	6.75 ± 0.03	−2
R14E	6.74 ± 0.02	−2
S16-P	6.70 ± 0.05	−2
(B) Relationship to hydropathy		
V4A	6.62 ± 0.04	
L7A	6.64 ± 0.05	
I12A	6.63 ± 0.05	
I18A	6.67 ± 0.04	

NOTE: The K_m values represent the concentration of Ca that supported half-maximal Ca uptake by SERCA2, coexpressed with wild-type and mutant phospholambans. These values are presented in relation to changes in charge or hydrophobicity of the cytoplasmic region of phospholamban. The asterisk indicates that the K_m values for SERCA2 expressed alone and coexpressed with wild-type phospholamban are statistically significant ($p < 0.01$).

TABLE 3. Effects of Phospholamban Peptides on Reconstituted Cardiac SR Ca-ATPase Activity[36]

Peptides	Molar Ratio	n	V_{max} (nmol/mg/min)	K_{Ca} (μM)
Control		4	653.0 ± 28.3	0.49 ± 0.02
+ PLN 1-31	[330]	4	420.2 ± 12.4[a]	0.51 ± 0.05
Control		3	634.5 ± 112.4	0.52 ± 0.02
+ PLN 28-47	[100]	3	657.7 ± 43.5	1.33 ± 0.30[a]
Control		4	627.8 ± 63.6	0.51 ± 0.04
+ PLN 8-47	[100]	3	625.3 ± 51.8	1.18 ± 0.20[a]
+ PLN 8-47-P	[100]	3	669.0 ± 68.4	0.72 ± 0.09

NOTE: Purified canine cardiac Ca-ATPase in leaky vesicles of phospholipid was preincubated with synthetic partial phospholamban peptide corresponding to the NH2-terminal hydrophilic domain (PLN 1-31) or was incorporated into liposomes with synthetic phospholamban peptides containing the COOH-terminal hydrophobic sequence (PLN 28–47, PLN 8–47) by the freeze-thaw sonication method before ATPase assay. For phosphorylation of PLN 8–47, liposomes containing the peptides were first phosphorylated by cAMP-dependent protein kinase. The phosphorylated vesicles were then collected by ultracentrifugation. A molar ratio between the peptides and ATPase is indicated in brackets. V_{max} and K_{ca} were determined from Ca-dependent profiles of ATPase activity using the double reciprocal plot of Lineweaver and Burk. Data are mean ± SD. [a]$p < 0.05$ vs. control by unpaired t-test.

one side of an α-helical wheel, while hydrophobic residues are on the other side. Thus, if the cytoplasmic domain IA formed an amphipathic α-helix, it could fit compactly into a complementary pocket in its interaction with SERCA2, thereby accounting for the hydrophobic and electrostatic contributions to the interaction between two proteins. Together with the evidence that the phospholamban-interacting site exists in the unique sequence near the phosphorylation site (Asp351) of Ca-ATPase, the cytoplasmic part of phospholamban would play an important role in the functional interaction with SERCA2.

An experiment brought about by the reconstitution of synthesized phospholamban peptides and the purified Ca-ATPase addressed the new aspects of a protein-protein interaction between two proteins, as summarized in TABLE 3.[35,36] The peptide corresponding to 25 amino acid residues from the NH2-terminus (Met 1 to Arg 25) inhibited Ca uptake, and this inhibition was diminished by phosphorylation of the peptide. The synthetic peptide corresponding to domain I of phospholamban (Met 1 to Asn 31) inhibits purified cardiac SR Ca-ATPase activity in a dose-dependent manner, and this inhibition is diminished by phosphorylation of the peptide.[36] However, the affinity of ATPase activity for Ca was not changed by these maneuvers, suggesting that this peptide affected only V_{max} of Ca-ATPase activity. On the other hand, peptides containing domain II, the intramembrane portion of phospholamban, decreased the Ca affinity of ATPase; and phosphorylation of the peptide relieved this inhibitory effect. This novel mechanism by transmembrane interaction between phospholamban and Ca-ATPase has been recently proved by studies using site-directed mutagenesis.[37,38] These results indicate that, in terms of phospholamban-mediated regulation of Ca-ATPase, not only the cytoplasmic domain but also the intramembrane portion of phospholamban are required. As the peptides devoid of NH2-terminal 7 residues had no effect on the V_{max}, the residues responsible for the V_{max} effect could reside in the NH2-terminal portion. The COOH-terminal intramembrane domain could contribute to the effects on Ca affinity.

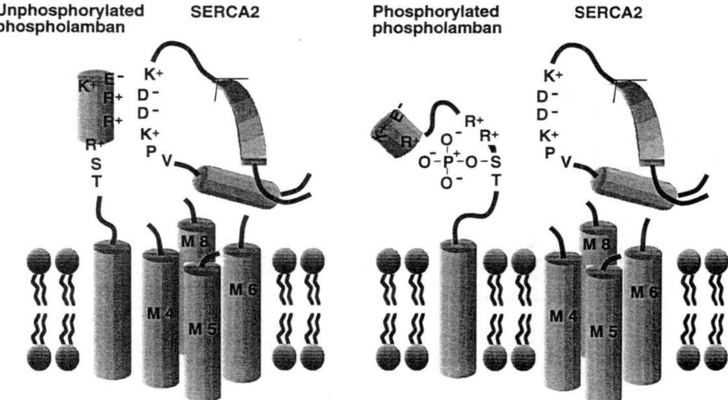

FIGURE 3. Diagrammatic representation of the interaction between phospholamban and Ca-ATPase. The interaction between phospholamban and the Ca-ATPase is proposed to take place in the cytoplasmic and transmembrane parts of two proteins. Unphosphorylated phospholamban suppresses the Ca-ATPase activity by associating charged amino residues in domain IA with the six serial amino acid residues Lys-Asp-Asp-Lys-Pro-Val402 in the cytoplasmic region of the Ca-ATPase, in which the association of transmembrane parts is stable. Phosphorylation of Ser16 in the domain IA of phospholamban induces its conformational change, resulting in the dissociation from the Ca-ATPase in the cytoplasmic and transmembrane parts.

Molecular Mode of Protein-Protein Interaction

Taking kinetic and chemical properties into consideration, we propose the possible mode of interactions between cytoplasmic domains of phospholamban and Ca-ATPase (FIG. 3). When phospholamban is in the unphosphorylated state, the sequence Lys-Asp-Asp-Lys-Pro-Val in the phospholamban-binding domain of Ca-ATPase, rich in charged residues, may contribute to the interaction with charged residues of phospholamban. Such an electrostatic milieu may be perturbed when the phosphate is incorporated into Ser and/or Thr residues of phospholamban, thus resulting in the dissociation of the interaction sites. Domain II of phospholamban may not be a mere anchor, but plays an important role in the interaction between the two proteins in addition to domain I.

CHARACTERIZATION OF 5′ UPSTREAM REGION OF THE PHOSPHOLAMBAN GENE

Regulation of phospholamban gene expression plays a key role in its unique tissue distribution and responses to the physiological condition. In order to analyze the transcriptional regulation of phospholamban gene, rabbit phospholamban gene was cloned. Phospholamban gene is composed of two exons and 5′ upstream regulatory region, containing muscle-specific elements and hormone responsive elements, especially thyroid hormone. The transcriptional levels of phospholamban gene were analyzed by measuring the luciferase activities of the chimeric constructs, in which successively 5′-truncated segments of this gene were introduced into the luciferase reporter gene. Dele-

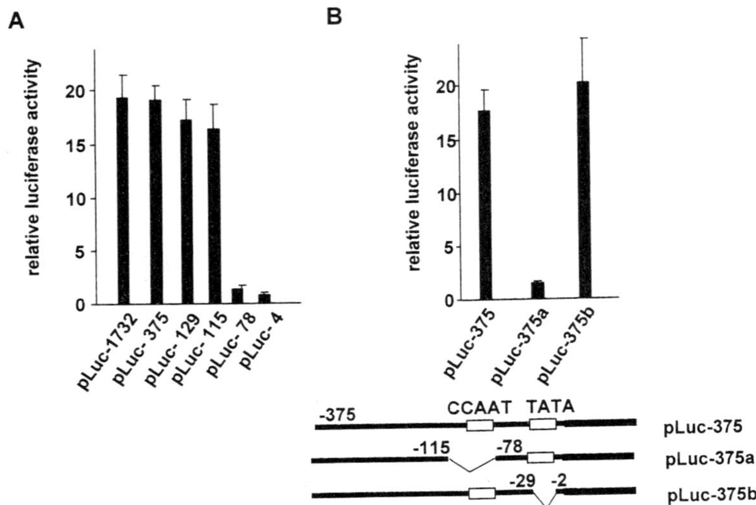

FIGURE 4. Luciferase activities of phospholamban-luciferase fusion constructs transfected into cardiac myocytes. **(A)** Deletion constructs containing different lengths of the 5′-upstream region of the phospholamban gene were transfected into rat neonatal cardiac myocytes. Luciferase activities are calculated as percentages of the *renilla* luciferase activity of pRL-CMV in each experiment. **(B)** Internal deletion constructs of the 5′-upstream region of the phospholamban gene were transfected into rat neonatal cardiac myocytes. The position numbers are counted from the transcription start site. The luciferase construct ligated with the fragment −375/+84 was designated as pLuc-375. The internal deleted constructs, pLuc-375a, pLuc-375b, and pLuc-375c, were generated by PCR-directed mutagenesis using the fragment −375/+84 of the phospholamban gene.

tion from −115 to −78 base pair (bp) from the transcriptional start site led to the 90% loss of luciferase activity of phospholamban gene in cultured rat cardiac myocytes (FIG. 4-A). Internal deletion construct lacking nucleotide from −115 to −78 bp of phospholamban gene lost 90% of its activity, while the construct lacking TATA-box of phospholamban gene did not change its activities compared with the wild-type construct (FIG. 4-B). Nucleotide sequence analysis showed that the region from −115 to −78 bp contains the NF-Y/CP1 binding motif. The NF-Y/CP1 binding motif contains inverted CCAAT core sequence and has been shown to positively regulate a number of eukaryotic promoters. Although transcriptional factors for this motif are ubiquitously expressed in the adult tissues, there is increasing evidence that they also play a role in the maintenance of tissue-specific expression[39,40] (FIG. 5).

Gel shift assay using this nucleotide sequence with nuclear proteins extracted from cardiac myocytes showed that this nucleotide sequence was able to bind to the protein of nuclear extract (FIG. 6-A). Several transcriptional factors have been reported to specifically bind to the NF-Y/CP1 binding motif: EFI_A/YB-1, NF-YA, and NF-YB.[39,40] In order to determine whether the NF-Y/CP1 binding proteins participate in the binding of the transcriptional factor to the NF-Y/CP1 binding motif of phospholamban gene, we used antibodies against NFYA, NFYB, and EFI_A/YB-1. Antibodies against NFYA, NFYB, but not EFI_A/YB-1 effectively removed the binding of nuclear extract to the NF-Y/CP1 binding motif in gel shift assay (FIG. 6-B). These results indicated that

A **Promoter Region of Phospholamban Gene**

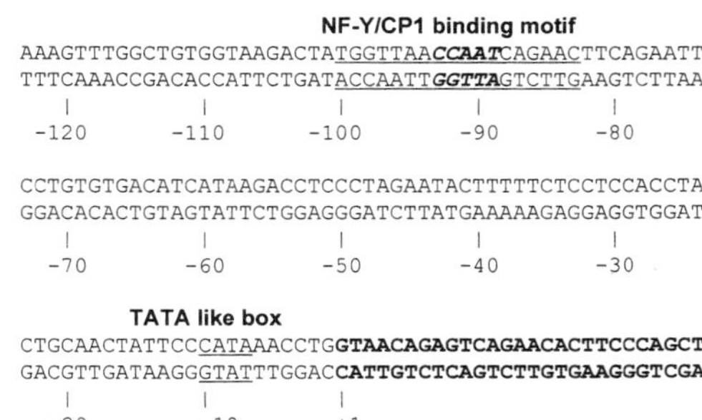

B **Sequence Comparison of NF-Y/CP1 Binding Motif in PLN Gene with Other Homologue**

Binding sites	Binding proteins	Promoters
TGGTTAA*CCAAT*CAGAAC		PLN
CTTTTAA*CCAAT*CAGAAT	NF-Y	MHC II E a *
GCGCCAG*CCAAT*GAGCGC	CP-1	α-Globin
GTCTCCA*CCAAT*GGGAGG	CBF	α2(I)collagen *
ACTTCCA*CCAAT*CGGCAT	EF1	RSV LTR *
CCCATGA*CCACT*TTTGGC	EF1/YB1	MLC2v *

FIGURE 5. Nucleotide sequences of the 5′ upstream region of phospholamban gene covering nucleotide sequence from –115 to –78 base pairs. **(A)** The 5′ upstream region of phospholamban gene contains NFY/CP1 binding site from –100 to –83 bp. **(B)** Sequence comparisons of NF-Y/CP1 binding motif in phospholamban gene with other homologues. All sites contain the CCAAT core sequence and similar flanking sequences. *Asterisks* indicate the antisense sequences of promoters. Abbreviations: MHC II-Eα, major histocompatibility complex class II-Eα; RSV-LTR, Rous sarcoma virus long terminal repeat; MLC-2v, myosin light-chain 2v.

a major component of the NF-Y/CP1 binding activity in cardiac myocytes consists of a complex of these factors. We therefore concluded that the NF-Y/CP1 binding motif of the phospholamban gene is essential for its expression by associating with the NF-Y/CP1 binding transcriptional factors.

PHYSIOLOGICAL AND PATHOPHYSIOLOGICAL SIGNIFICANCE OF SR Ca-ATPase–PHOSPHOLAMBAN SYSTEM

The increase of cAMP and resultant activation of PKA caused by β-adrenergic stimulation alter a number of intracellular events in cardiac muscle. FIGURE 7 represents the effects of protein phosphorylation, catalyzed by PKA, on Ca signaling processes in SR and sarcolemmal membranes. Increased Ca channel activity sarcolemmal membrane due to PKA-phosphorylation of Ca channel increases the amount of Ca available for the acceleration and enhancement of muscle contractility directly and by activating the Ca-induced Ca release mechanism in SR. Increased Ca uptake through the Ca-ATPase–phospholamban system by PKA accelerates the rate of muscle relaxation. Eventual increases in Ca storage in SR can be added to the amount of

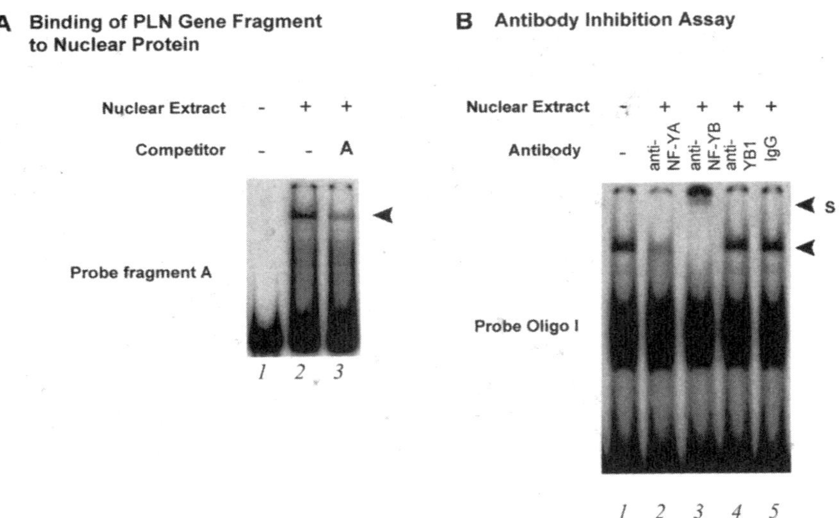

FIGURE 6. Gel shift assays of the fragment of phospholamban gene in the presence of nuclear protein extracts from rat cardiac myocytes. **(A)** End-labeled fragment A covering from –131 to +81 bp was incubated with nuclear extract in the absence or presence of unlabeled competing fragment A. *Lane 1,* control without added nuclear extract; *lane 2,* with nuclear extract; *lane 3,* with 100-fold molar excess of unlabeled competing fragment A in the presence of nuclear extract. **(B)** End-labeled oligonucleotide covering from –102 to –76 bp was incubated with nuclear extract in the presence or absence of specific antibody and subjected to gel shift assay. *Lane 1,* with nuclear extract without antibody; *lane 2,* with nuclear extract and anti–NF-YA antibody; *lane 3,* with nuclear extract and anti–NF-YB antibody; *lane 4,* with nuclear extract and anti–EFI_A/YB-1 antibody; *lane 5,* with nuclear extract and rabbit IgG. The nuclear protein–oligonucleotide complex is indicated by *arrowheads;* supershifted band is indicated by *arrowhead* plus S.

Ca available for subsequent contraction through the Ca-induced Ca release mechanism in SR, resulting in the augmentation of muscle contraction. Recent studies on transgenic mice lacking phospholamban as a result of gene targeting have given us more insights into our understanding of the role of phospholamban in mediating the contractile response of the heart to β-adrenergic agonists.[41,42]

There is evidence for long-term alterations of Ca-ATPase activity under different pathophysiological conditions[43,44] in addition to the short-term alteration. Cardiac hypertrophy and heart failure, which are induced by thyroid hormone, pressure overload, and volume overload, have been investigated extensively. With hyperthyroidism, the rate of Ca uptake in the heart by SR was significantly increased, but the Ca storage capacity and the steady state level of Ca were unaltered.[43] Under these conditions, phospholamban mRNA levels were reduced, while Ca-ATPase mRNA levels were not reduced in hyperthyroidism.[44,45] In isolated cultured cardiac myocytes, the exposure to thyroid hormone resulted in the marked reduction of phospholamban mRNA, while Ca-ATPase mRNA was found to be increased significantly.[46] Thus, increase in Ca uptake in hyperthyroidism can be explained by the change in stoichiometry of these proteins. Although the stoichiometry of these proteins in cardiac SR remains unclear, one of the adaptive mechanisms of the Ca signaling process in response to specific condi-

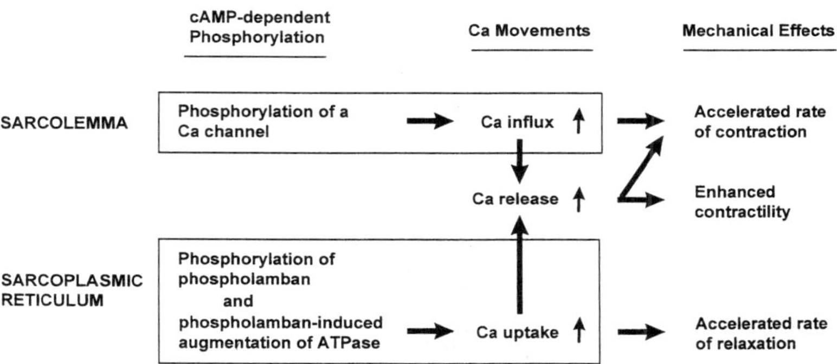

FIGURE 7. Role of membrane phosphorylation in calcium fluxes across sarcolemma and sarcoplasmic reticulum in cardiac muscle.

tions in cardiac muscle would be achieved by changes of the molar ratio of Ca signaling proteins.

REFERENCES

1. Tada, M., M. A. Kirchberger, D. I. Repke & A. M. Katz. 1974. The stimulation of calcium transport in cardiac sarcoplasmic reticulum by adenosine 3′:5′-monophosphate–dependent protein kinase. J. Biol. Chem. **249**(19): 6174–6180.
2. Tada, M., M. A. Kirchberger & A. M. Katz. 1975. Phosphorylation of a 22,000-dalton component of the cardiac sarcoplasmic reticulum by adenosine 3′:5′-monophosphate–dependent protein kinase. J. Biol. Chem. **250**(7): 2640–2647.
3. Le Peuch, C. J., J. Haiech & J. G. Demaille. 1979. Concerted regulation of cardiac sarcoplasmic reticulum calcium transport by cyclic adenosine monophosphate dependent and calcium-calmodulin–dependent phosphorylations. Biochemistry **18**(23): 5150–5157.
4. Tada, M., T. Yamamoto & Y. Tonomura. 1978. Molecular mechanism of active calcium transport by sarcoplasmic reticulum. Physiol. Rev. **58**(1): 1–79.
5. Tada, M. & A. M. Katz. 1982. Phosphorylation of the sarcoplasmic reticulum and sarcolemma. Annu. Rev. Physiol. **44:** 401–423.
6. Tada, M., M. Kadoma, M. Inui & J. Fujii. 1988. Regulation of Ca2+-pump from cardiac sarcoplasmic reticulum. Methods Enzymol. **157:** 107–154.
7. Fujii, J., J. Lytton, M. Tada & D. H. MacLennan. 1988. Rabbit cardiac and slow-twitch muscle express the same phospholamban gene. FEBS Lett. **227**(1): 51–55.
8. Tada, M. 1992. Molecular structure and function of phospholamban in regulating the calcium pump from sarcoplasmic reticulum. Ann. N. Y. Acad. Sci. **671:** 92–103.
9. Toyofuku, T., K. Kurzydlowski, M. Tada & D. H. MacLennan. 1994. Amino acids Lys-Asp-Asp-Lys-Pro-Val402 in the Ca(2+)-ATPase of cardiac sarcoplasmic reticulum are critical for functional association with phospholamban. J. Biol. Chem. **269**(37): 22929–22932.
10. Burk, S. E., J. Lytton, D. H. MacLennan & G. E. Shull. 1989. cDna cloning, functional expression, and mRna tissue distribution of a third organellar Ca2+ pump. J. Biol. Chem. **264**(31): 18561–18568.
11. de Meis, L. & A. Vianna. 1979. Energy interconversion by the Ca^{2+}-dependent ATPase of the sarcoplasmic reticulum. Annu. Rev. Biochem. **48:** 275–292.
12. Tada, M., M. Yamada, M. Kadoma, M. Inui & F. Ohmori. 1982. Calcium transport by cardiac sarcoplasmic reticulum and phosphorylation of phospholamban. Mol. Cell. Biochem. **46**(2): 73–95.

13. Kirchberger, M. A., M. Tada & A. M. Katz. 1974. Adenosine 3′:5′-monophosphate–dependent protein kinase–catalyzed phosphorylation reaction and its relationship to calcium transport in cardiac sarcoplasmic reticulum. J. Biol. Chem. **249**(19): 6166–6173.
14. Tada, M., F. Ohmori, M. Yamada & H. Abe. 1979. Mechanism of the stimulation of Ca2+-dependent ATPase of cardiac sarcoplasmic reticulum by adenosine 3′:5′-monophosphate–dependent protein kinase. Role of the 22,000-dalton protein. J. Biol. Chem. **254**(2): 319–326.
15. Tada, M., M. Yamada, F. Ohmori, T. Kuzuya, M. Inui & H. Abe. 1980. Transient state kinetic studies of Ca2+-dependent ATPase and calcium transport by cardiac sarcoplasmic reticulum. Effect of cyclic AMP-dependent protein kinase–catalyzed phosphorylation of phospholamban. J. Biol. Chem. **255**(5): 1985–1992.
16. Watanabe, Y., Y. Kijima, M. Kadoma, M. Tada & T. Takagi. 1991. Molecular weight determination of phospholamban oligomer in the presence of sodium dodecyl sulfate: Application of low-angle laser light scattering photometry. J. Biochem. Tokyo **110**(1): 40–45.
17. Wegener, A. D., H. K. Simmerman, J. Liepnieks & L. R. Jones. 1986. Proteolytic cleavage of phospholamban purified from canine cardiac sarcoplasmic reticulum vesicles. Generation of a low resolution model of phospholamban structure. J. Biol. Chem. **261**(11): 5154–5159.
18. Inui, M., M. Kadoma & M. Tada. 1985. Purification and characterization of phospholamban from canine cardiac sarcoplasmic reticulum. J. Biol. Chem. **260**(6): 3708–3715.
19. Jones, L. R., H. K. Simmerman, W. W. Wilson, F. R. Gurd & A. D. Wegener. 1985. Purification and characterization of phospholamban from canine cardiac sarcoplasmic reticulum. J. Biol. Chem. **260**(12): 7721–7730.
20. Simmerman, H. K., J. H. Collins, J. L. Theibert, A. D. Wegener & L. R. Jones. 1986. Sequence analysis of phospholamban. Identification of phosphorylation sites and two major structural domains. J. Biol. Chem. **261**(28): 13333–13341.
21. Fujii, J., M. Kadoma, M. Tada, H. Toda & F. Sakiyama. 1986. Characterization of structural unit of phospholamban by amino acid sequencing and electrophoretic analysis. Biochem. Biophys. Res. Commun. **138**(3): 1044–1050.
22. Fujii, J., A. Ueno, K. Kitano, S. Tanaka, M. Kadoma & M. Tada. 1987. Complete complementary DNA-derived amino acid sequence of canine cardiac phospholamban. J. Clin. Invest. **79**(1): 301–304.
23. Fujii, J., A. Zarain Herzberg, H. F. Willard, M. Tada & D. H. MacLennan. 1991. Structure of the rabbit phospholamban gene, cloning of the human cDNA, and assignment of the gene to human chromosome 6. J. Biol. Chem. **266**(18): 11669–11675.
24. Tada, M. & M. Kadoma. 1989. Regulation of the Ca2+ pump ATPase by cAMP-dependent phosphorylation of phospholamban. Bioessays **10**(5): 157–163.
25. Simmerman, H. K., D. E. Lovelace & L. R. Jones. 1989. Secondary structure of detergent-solubilized phospholamban, a phosphorylatable, oligomeric protein of cardiac sarcoplasmic reticulum. Biochim. Biophys. Acta **997**(3): 322–329.
26. Girardet, J. L. & Y. Dupont. 1992. Ellipticity changes of the sarcoplasmic reticulum Ca(2+)-ATPase induced by cation binding and phosphorylation. FEBS Lett. **296**(1): 103–106.
27. Fujii, J., K. Maruyama, M. Tada & D. H. MacLennan. 1989. Expression and site-specific mutagenesis of phospholamban. Studies of residues involved in phosphorylation and pentamer formation. J. Biol. Chem. **264**(22): 12950–12955.
28. James, P., M. Inui, M. Tada, M. Chiesi & E. Carafoli. 1989. Nature and site of phospholamban regulation of the Ca2+ pump of sarcoplasmic reticulum. Nature **342** (6245): 90–92.
29. Vorherr, T., M. Chiesi, R. Schwaller & E. Carafoli. 1992. Regulation of the calcium ion pump of sarcoplasmic reticulum: Reversible inhibition by phospholamban and by the calmodulin binding domain of the plasma membrane calcium ion pump. Biochemistry **31**(2): 371–376.
30. Toyofuku, T., K. Kurzydlowski, M. Tada & D. H. MacLennan. 1993. Identification of regions in the Ca(2+)-ATPase of sarcoplasmic reticulum that affect functional association with phospholamban. J. Biol. Chem. **268**(4): 2809–2815.
31. Toyofuku, T., K. Kurzydlowski, M. Tada & D. H. MacLennan. 1994. Amino acids

Glu2 to Ile18 in the cytoplasmic domain of phospholamban are essential for functional association with the Ca(2+)-ATPase of sarcoplasmic reticulum. J. Biol. Chem. **269**(4): 3088–3094.

32. SUZUKI, T. & J. H. WANG. 1986. Stimulation of bovine cardiac sarcoplasmic reticulum Ca2+ pump and blocking of phospholamban phosphorylation and dephosphorylation by a phospholamban monoclonal antibody. J. Biol. Chem. **261**(15): 7018–7023.
33. MORRIS, G. L., H. C. CHENG, J. COLYER & J. H. WANG. 1991. Phospholamban regulation of cardiac sarcoplasmic reticulum (Ca(2+)–Mg2+)-ATPase. Mechanism of regulation and site of monoclonal antibody interaction. J. Biol. Chem. **266**(17): 11270–11275.
34. KIMURA, Y., M. INUI, M. KADOMA, Y. KIJIMA, T. SASAKI & M. TADA. 1991. Effects of monoclonal antibody against phospholamban on calcium pump ATPase of cardiac sarcoplasmic reticulum. J. Mol. Cell Cardiol. **23**(11): 1223–1230.
35. KIM, H. W., N. A. STEENAART, D. G. FERGUSON & E. G. KRANIAS. 1990. Functional reconstitution of the cardiac sarcoplasmic reticulum Ca2(+)-ATPase with phospholamban in phospholipid vesicles. J. Biol. Chem. **265**(3): 1702–1709.
36. SASAKI, T., M. INUI, Y. KIMURA, T. KUZUYA & M. TADA. 1992. Molecular mechanism of regulation of Ca2+ pump ATPase by phospholamban in cardiac sarcoplasmic reticulum. Effects of synthetic phospholamban peptides on Ca2+ pump ATPase. J. Biol. Chem. **267**(3): 1674–1679.
37. KIMURA, Y., K. KURZYDLOWSKI, M. TADA & D. H. MACLENNAN. 1996. Phospholamban regulates the Ca2+-ATPase through intramembrane interactions. J. Biol. Chem. **271**(36): 21726–21731.
38. KIMURA, Y., K. KURZYDLOWSKI, M. TADA & D. H. MACLENNAN. 1997. Phospholamban inhibitory function is activated by depolymerization. J. Biol. Chem. **272**(24): 15061–15064.
39. WOLFFE, A. P. 1994. Structural and functional properties of the evolutionarily ancient Y-box family of nucleic acid binding proteins. Bioessays **16**(4): 245–251.
40. ZOU, Y. & K. R. CHIEN. 1995. EFIA/YB-1 is a component of cardiac HF-1A binding activity and positively regulates transcription of the myosin light-chain 2v gene. Mol. Cell. Biol. **15**(6): 2972–2982.
41. HOIT, B. D., S. F. KHOURY, E. G. KRANIAS, N. BALL & R. A. WALSH. 1995. In vivo echocardiographic detection of enhanced left ventricular function in gene-targeted mice with phospholamban deficiency. Circ. Res. **77**(3): 632–637.
42. LUO, W., B. M. WOLSKA, I. L. GRUPP, J. M. HARRER, K. HAGHIGHI, D. G. FERGUSON, J. P. SLACK, G. GRUPP, T. DOETSCHMAN, R. J. SOLARO & E. G. KRANIAS. 1996. Phospholamban gene dosage effects in the mammalian heart. Circ. Res. **78**(5): 839–847.
43. SUKO, J. 1973. The calcium pump of cardiac sarcoplasmic reticulum. Functional alterations at different levels of thyroid state in rabbits. J. Physiol. Lond. **228**(3): 563–582.
44. NAGAI, R., A. ZARAIN HERZBERG, C. J. BRANDL, J. FUJII, M. TADA, D. H. MACLENNAN, N. R. ALPERT & M. PERIASAMY. 1989. Regulation of myocardial Ca2+-ATPase and phospholamban mRNA expression in response to pressure overload and thyroid hormone. Proc. Natl. Acad. Sci. USA **86**(8): 2966–2970.
45. ARAI, M., K. OTSU, D. H. MACLENNAN & M. PERIASAMY. 1992. Regulation of sarcoplasmic reticulum gene expression during cardiac and skeletal muscle development. Am. J. Physiol. **262**(3 Pt. 1): C614–620.
46. KIMURA, Y., K. OTSU, K. NISHIDA, T. KUZUYA & M. TADA. 1994. Thyroid hormone enhances Ca2+ pumping activity of the cardiac sarcoplasmic reticulum by increasing Ca2+ ATPase and decreasing phospholamban expression. J. Mol. Cell. Cardiol. **26**(9): 1145–1154.

Potential for Pharmacology of Ryanodine Receptor/Calcium Release Channels[a]

LE XU, ASHUTOSH TRIPATHY, DANIEL A. PASEK, AND GERHARD MEISSNER[b]

Department of Biochemistry and Biophysics, University of North Carolina, Chapel Hill, North Carolina 27599-7260, USA

ABSTRACT: Calcium release channels, known also as ryanodine receptors (RyRs), play an important role in Ca^{2+} signaling in muscle and nonmuscle cells by releasing Ca^{2+} from intracellular stores. Mammalian tissues express three different RyR isoforms comprising four 560-kDa (RyR polypeptide) and four 12-kDa (FK506 binding protein) subunits. The large protein complexes conduct monovalent and divalent cations and are capable of multiple interactions with other molecules. The latter include small diffusible endogenous effector molecules including Ca^{2+}, Mg^{2+}, adenine nucleotides, sufhydryl modifying reagents (glutathione, NO, and NO adducts) and lipid intermediates, and proteins such as protein kinases and phosphatases, calmodulin, immunophilins (FK506 binding proteins), and in skeletal muscle the dihydropyridine receptor. Because of their role in regulating intracellular Ca^{2+} levels and their multiple ligand interactions, RyRs constitute an important, potentially rich pharmacological target for controlling cellular functions. Exogenous effectors found to affect RyR function include ryanoids, toxins, xanthines, anthraquinones, phenol derivatives, adenosine and purinergic agonists and antagonists, NO donors, oxidizing reagents, dantrolene, local anesthetics, and polycationic reagents.

In striated muscle, an action potential triggers the rapid intracellular release of Ca^{2+} by a mechanism commonly referred to as excitation-contraction (E-C) coupling. The two major membrane structures involved in E-C coupling are a transverse (T-) tubule membrane system of invaginations through which muscle contraction is triggered, and an intracellular Ca^{2+} storing and Ca^{2+} releasing membrane system, the sarcoplasmic reticulum (SR), which contains an ATP-dependent Ca^{2+} pump and a Ca^{2+} release channel. The release channels typically span the narrow gap where the SR and the T-tubule are within ~15 nm of each other (for review see Refs. 1–4). The SR Ca^{2+} release channels are also known as feet or junctional processes, and as ryanodine receptors (RyR) because they bind the plant alkaloid ryanodine with high affinity and specificity. They may, at least in skeletal muscle, be directly linked to another Ca^{2+} channel (L-type) in the T-tubule membrane, also known as the dihydropyridine receptor (DHPR). However, the relative number of RyRs and DHPRs varies, ranging from about 10 RyRs per DHPR in cardiac muscle to a 1:1 stoichiometry in fast-twitch mammalian skeletal muscle. Also, in some species and tissues such as avian heart or mammalian atrium, many SR Ca^{2+} release channels are located in the interior cytoplasm far away from L-type Ca^{2+} channels.[5,6] Accordingly, not all RyRs may be linked or closely apposed to DHPRs in striated muscle.

[a] Support from United States Public Health Service grants AR18687 and HL27430 is gratefully acknowledged.

[b] Corresponding author. Phone: 919-966-5021; fax: 919-966-2852; e-mail: gmeissne.biochem @mhs.unc.edu

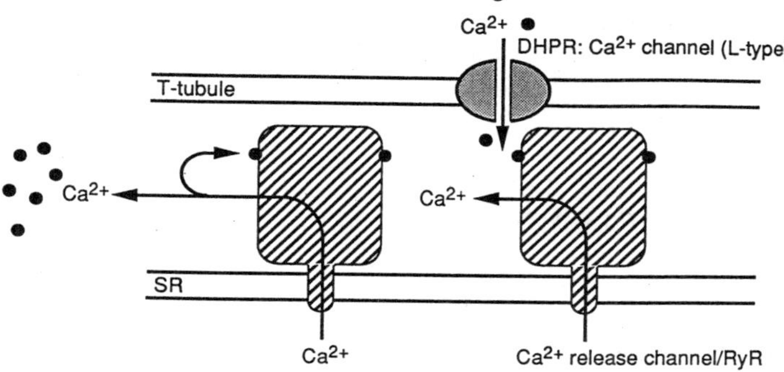

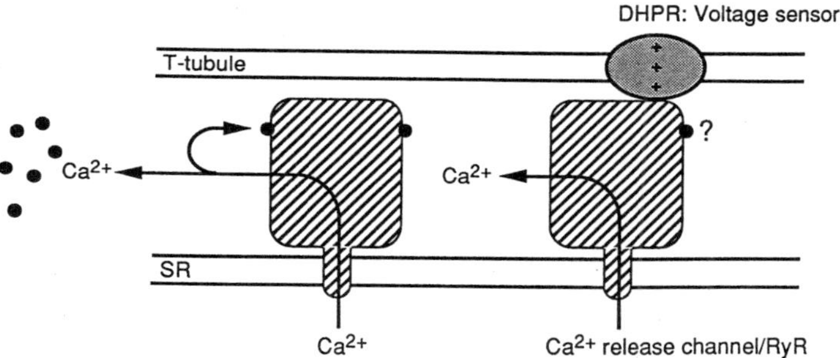

FIGURE 1. Models of excitation-contraction coupling.

Different excitation-contraction coupling mechanisms exist in skeletal and cardiac muscles (for review see Refs. 7–9). In cardiac muscle, L-type Ca^{2+} channels located in the surface membrane and T-tubule mediate the influx of Ca^{2+} during an action potential by functioning as voltage-dependent Ca^{2+} channels. The resulting rise in intracellular Ca^{2+} concentration triggers the massive release of Ca^{2+} by opening closely apposed SR Ca^{2+} release channels (FIG. 1). This process is known as calcium-induced Ca^{2+} release (CICR). Ca^{2+} passing through the release channels can regulate channel activity by having access to cytosolic Ca^{2+} activation and inactivation sites. Intracellular Ca^{2+} transients have been suggested to arise as the sum of localized Ca^{2+} release events called Ca^{2+} sparks. The opening of a single T-tubule Ca^{2+} channel is apparently sufficient to evoke a Ca^{2+} spark by activating a "functional Ca^{2+} release unit," which may consist of one or more RyRs.[10]

In vertebrate skeletal muscle, a different mechanism of E-C coupling, referred to as the mechanical coupling mechanism, has been formulated. Morphological, biophysical, and pharmacological evidence as well as molecular expression studies have suggested a direct interaction between SR Ca^{2+} release channels and T-tubule DHPRs.[1,2,4,8,9] The latter function in skeletal muscle E-C coupling as voltage sensors rather than Ca^{2+}

channels (FIG. 1). A more recent view is that Ca^{2+} ions initially released by DHPR-linked Ca^{2+} release channels open channels that are not linked to DHPRs. Accordingly, E-C coupling in vertebrate skeletal muscle appears to be regulated by a dual mechanism involving both DHPR-dependent and Ca^{2+}-dependent mechanisms. Other proteins have been suggested to have an important role in the coupling of the DHPR and RyR in skeletal muscle.[1–4]

MAMMALIAN TISSUES EXPRESS THREE RyRs

Mammalian tissues express three structurally and functionally related M_r~560,000 RyR polypeptides that are encoded by three different genes. The primary structure of the skeletal muscle RyR (RyR1), cardiac muscle (RyR2), and brain (RyR3) RyRs has been determined by cDNA cloning and sequencing.[1–4] The skeletal and cardiac isoforms are also expressed in brain and other tissues at low levels. In turn, the brain RyR is expressed as a minor component in skeletal and cardiac muscles—however, apparently without being essential for striated muscle function.[11] The RyRs have been isolated as 30 S protein complexes comprised of four large M_r ~560,000 subunits[4] and (in the case of RyR1 and RyR2) four small (FK506 binding protein, M_r ~12,000) subunits.[12] They all share a high-affinity binding site for [^{3}H]ryanodine and a high-conductance pathway for Ca^{2+} and monovalent cations, but display differences in their *in vitro* regulation by Ca^{2+} and other endogenous effector molecules (TABLE 1).

Analysis of the hydropathy of the predicted amino acid sequence has provided some

TABLE 1. Properties of Mammalian RyR/Ca^{2+} Release Channel Complexes

	RyR1[a] (Skeletal Muscle)	RyR2[a] (Cardiac Muscle)	RyR3[b] (Brain)
Sedimentation coefficient	30 S	30 S	30 S
Subunit composition: RyR polypeptide and FKBP	4 + 4	4 + 4	4 + ?
Amino acid residues/RyR polypeptide	~5035	~4970	~4870
Single-channel conductance			
In 50 mM Ca^{2+}	~145 pS	~145 pS	~110 pS
In 250 mM K^+	~775 pS	~775 pS	~775 pS
Endogenous effectors			
Activation by µM Ca^{2+}	Yes	Yes	Yes
Regulation by DHPR/voltage-sensor	Yes	No	No
Activation by adenine nucleotides	Yes	Yes	Yes
Inhibition by mM Ca^{2+} and Mg^{2+}	Yes	Yes	Yes
Regulation by MgATP	Yes	Yes	
Regulation by monovalent ions	Yes	Yes	Yes
Activation/inhibition by calmodulin	Yes/Yes	No/Yes	Yes/Yes
Regulation by protein phosphorylation	Yes	Yes	
Activation by acylcarnitines	Yes	Yes	
Regulation by sulfhydryl reacting/NO-generating compounds	Yes	Yes	

[a] Refs. 1–4.
[b] Refs. 13, 14.

valuable clues regarding the disposition of the M_r ~560,000 polypeptides in the SR membrane.[1–4] Two major structural regions have been deduced: (i) a carboxy-terminal pore region, which exhibits a high extent of similarity in amino acid sequence and is made up of at least 4 transmembrane segments (16 or more per tetrameric RyR); and (ii) a large more variable extramembrane region, which corresponds to the cytoplasmic foot structure. Primary sequence predictions also suggest the presence of several phosphorylation sites and sites for binding of cytoplasmic Ca^{2+}, ATP, and calmodulin. One phosphorylation site, several calmodulin binding sites, and Ca^{2+}-sensitive channel domains (for the skeletal RyR only) have been experimentally confirmed.

REGULATION BY ENDOGENOUS EFFECTORS

The *in vitro* function of RyR ion channels has been primarily studied by three complementary techniques: (i) measurement of macroscopic Ca^{2+} fluxes to and from SR vesicles, (ii) recording of microscopic monovalent ion and Ca^{2+} currents through single channels incorporated into planar lipid bilayers using SR vesicles and purified RyRs, and (iii) measurement of [^{3}H]ryanodine binding. These studies have shown that the RyRs are cation-selective channels capable of multiple interactions with other molecules (TABLE 1).

The RyRs display an unusually large ion conductance for monovalent cations (~775 pS with 250 mM K^+ as the current carrier, FIG. 2) and divalent cations (~145 pS with 50 mM Ca^{2+}).[4] They are ligand-gated channels with Ca^{2+} ions being important, if not the principal, activators and regulators of the channels. In the absence of other effectors, the skeletal muscle and cardiac RyRs are activated by µM cytosolic Ca^{2+} and inhibited by mM cytosolic Ca^{2+}, as determined in single channel measurements (FIG. 2). Typically, cardiac muscle Ca^{2+} release channels are activated to a greater extent than skeletal channels when Ca^{2+} is the sole activating ligand, and require higher concentrations of Ca^{2+} for inhibition than skeletal RyRs. Biomodal Ca^{2+} dependence of channel activity on Ca^{2+} suggests the presence of high-affinity (activating) and low-affinity (inhibitory) Ca^{2+} binding sites that are accessible from the cytosolic side and have been presumed to be located on the large cytosolic foot region of RyRs. In addition, SR lumenal Ca^{2+} flowing through the open skeletal and cardiac muscle RyRs may regulate channel activity by having access to the cytosolic Ca^{2+} activation and Ca^{2+} inactivation sites[16,17] (for a different view see Ref. 18). Other possible Ca^{2+}-dependent mechanisms are RyR adaptation[19] (but see also Refs. 20, 21) and regulation by SR lumenal (calsequestrin) and cytosolic (calmodulin) Ca^{2+} binding proteins.[3,4]

RyRs are activated by adenine nucleotides and inhibited by Mg^{2+}. Among adenine nucleotides, cyclic ADP-ribose has been reported to be the most effective,[22] although a physiological role of this compound in cardiac muscle has been questioned.[23] Other adenine nucleotides (ATP, ADP, AMP) activate the skeletal muscle Ca^{2+} release channel in the absence of Ca^{2+} (and Mg^{2+}) but are less effective in activating the cardiac isoform at low [Ca^{2+}]. In the absence of Mg^{2+}, µM Ca^{2+} and mM ATP nearly fully activate both channel forms. The presence of Mg^{2+} and ATP results in formation of a MgATP complex, which is an important allosteric modulator of RyRs.[4]

Contracting muscle produces both reactive nitrogen and oxygen intermediates. In favor of a functional role of these compounds, redox-active compounds have been shown to modulate E-C coupling and antioxidant enzymes to inhibit force production.[24] Both L-type Ca^{2+} channels[25] and Ca^{2+} release channels[3,26] contain sulfhydryls whose oxidation modulates function. The cardiac channel is S-nitrosylated endogenously, and S-nitrosylation by exogenous NO-generating molecules of up to 12

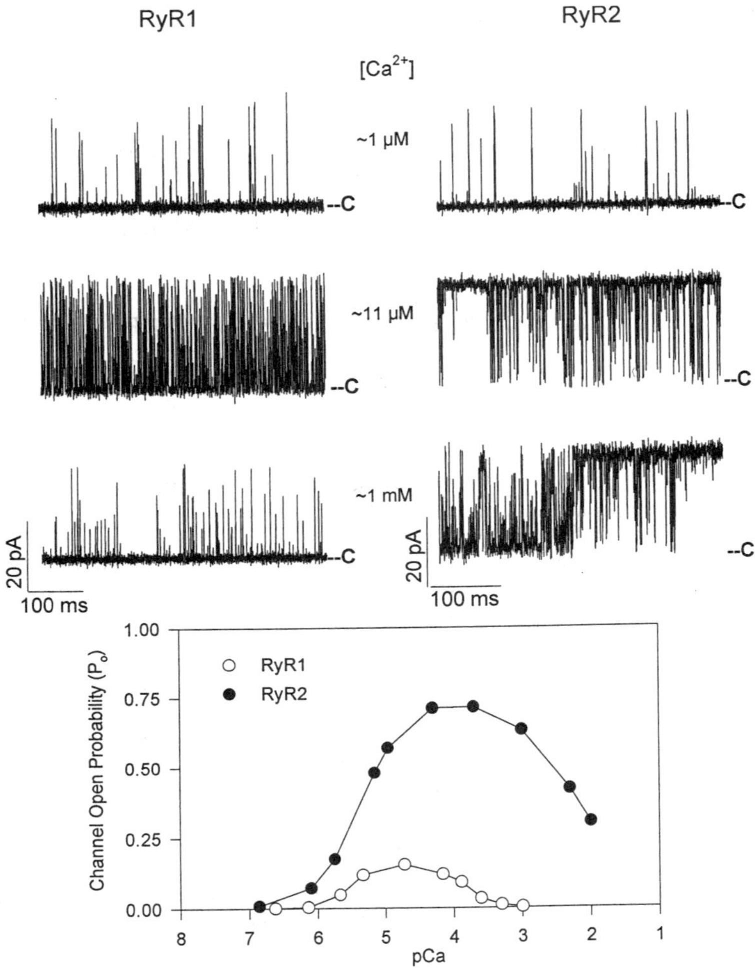

FIGURE 2. Ca^{2+}-dependence of single purified skeletal muscle (RyR1) and cardiac muscle (RyR2) Ca^{2+} release channels. In the **upper two panels,** single-channel currents were recorded as described[15] at +40 mV (RyR1) and +35 mV (RyR2) in symmetrical 250 mM KCl, 20 mM KPipes, pH 7.35 media containing the indicated concentrations of free cytosolic Ca^{2+}. Lumenal free [Ca^{2+}] was ≤10 μM. *Bars on the right* (--) represent the closed (C) channels. The **lower panel** shows channel open probability (P_o) as a function of cytosolic free [Ca^{2+}].

sites/RyR led to cardiac channel activation.[27] Other diffusible transmitter molecules that must be considered to regulate cardiac RyR activity include lipid metabolites such as acylcarnitines and sphingosine[4] and polyamines such as spermine.[28] Moreover, a complex regulation of RyR activities by endogenous and exogenous kinases has been described.[1–4]

REGULATION BY EXOGENOUS EFFECTORS

Because of their multiple ligand interactions, RyRs constitute an abundant target for controlling cellular functions. A large number of exogenous effectors have been found to affect RyR function including ryanoids, toxins, xanthines, NO donors, local anesthetics, and polycationic reagents (TABLE 2). These drugs are currently extensively used for studying structure-activity relationships of RyRs. However, their use as potential therapeutic agents for controlling intracellular Ca^{2+} release from SR has been limited so far due to a lack of target specificity; ryanoids, some toxins, and dantrolene (a muscle relaxant used in the prevention and treatment of malignant hyperthermia[3]) appear to be the exception.

Below we will discuss studies in which we have used skeletal muscle and cardiac muscle SR membrane and purified RyR preparations to determine the functional interaction of RyRs with pharmacological agents. We will focus on a few selected drugs and describe the ways in which these drugs modify the conductance and gating behavior of single channels incorporated into planar lipid bilayers as well as affect the Ca^{2+}-dependence of [^{3}H]ryanodine binding. High-affinity [^{3}H]ryanodine binding is a very convenient way of assessing the functional interaction of RyRs with endogenous and exogenous effectors because as a general rule conditions that open RyR ion channels,

TABLE 2. Pharmacological Modulators of Mammalian RyR/Ca^{2+} Release Channels and Their Potential Target Sites

Pharmacological Modulator[a]	Action	Target Site
DHPR antagonists	Inhibition of RyR	Dihydropyridine receptor
Ryanoids,[b] ryanotoxin	Modification of conductance	?
Xanthines[b]	Activation	Modulators of Ca^{2+} activation sites
Antraquinones		
Doxorubicin	Activation/inhibition	?
Phenol derivatives		
4-Chloro-m-cresol[b]	Activation	?
Adenosine/purinergic agonists/antagonists[b]	Activation	ATP binding site(s)
Suramin[b]	Activation	?
Digitalis glycosides[b]	Activation (cardiac ?)	?
Calmodulin antagonists	?	Calmodulin regulatory sites
Modulators of FKBP	Activation (skeletal)	FK506 binding protein
Modulators of kinases/phosphatases	Activation/Inhibition	Phosphorylation sites
Modulators of lipid metabolism	?	?
Modulators of nitric oxide synthase, NO-generating compounds	Activation/inhibition	?
Local anesthetics		
Tetracaine[b]	Inhibition	?
Dantrolene	Inhibition	?
Polycationic reagents		
Ruthenium red[b]	Inhibition	Ca^{2+} site(s)/channel pore

[a] Ref. 3.
[b] See also FIGS. 5–11 and text.

such as the presence of μM Ca^{2+} or mM ATP, increase the affinity of [^{3}H]ryanodine binding.[3,4,29] Since the action of the drugs is in general dependent on the ionic composition of the assay media, we determined the latter activities under conditions relevant physiologically. Specifically, we took into account that Ca^{2+}-dependent RyR activity is affected by [MgATP], free [Mg^{2+}], ionic composition, and redox state.[3,15,26,30,31] Total cellular [ATP] and free [Mg^{2+}] range from 5–10 mM[32,33] and from 0.7–1.0 mM,[34] respectively. K^+ concentration is ~150 mM.[35] Cl^- activate the skeletal and cardiac RyRs,[30,31] but Cl^- concentration in muscle cells is quite low (~5–20 mM).[35] As discussed above, ryanodine receptors contain sulfhydryl groups that are important to their function.[3] These may be in a reduced state *in vivo* because cells maintain a reducing environment by containing thiol-reducing compounds, the most abundant being glutathione.[36] Accordingly, to better simulate the *in vivo* action of the drugs, we chose to determine the Ca^{2+}-dependence of [^{3}H]ryanodine binding in FIGURES 3 and 6–10 in 125 mM Kglutamate, 5 mM KCl media in the presence of 5 mM MgAMPPCP (~0.7 mM free Mg^{2+} at ~1 μM Ca^{2+}) and 5 mM glutathione. FIGURE 3 shows the effects of 5 mM MgAMPPCP (AMPPCP is a nonhydrolyzable ATP analog) and 5 mM glutathione on the Ca^{2+} activation profiles of the skeletal and cardiac RyRs. Addition of 5 mM MgAMPPCP increased the levels of [^{3}H]ryanodine binding and rendered the channels less sensitive to inhibition by mM Ca^{2+}. Greater than 0.5 mM free Ca^{2+} concentrations were not tested in the presence of AMPPCP because of difficulties in keeping Ca^{2+} in solution. FIGURE 3 further shows

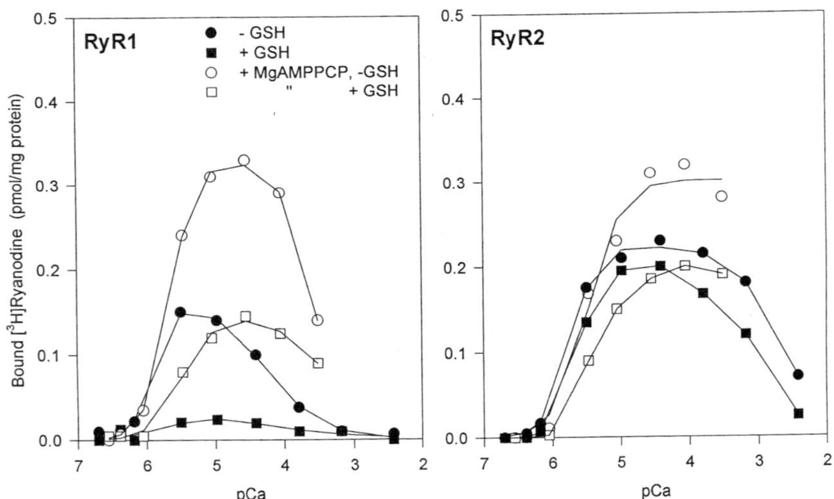

FIGURE 3. Effects of MgAMPPCP and glutathione on Ca^{2+}-dependence of [^{3}H]ryanodine binding to skeletal (RyR1) and cardiac (RyR2) ryanodine receptors. Specific [^{3}H]ryanodine binding to skeletal muscle and cardiac muscle SR membranes was determined at ~24 °C as described[31] in the absence and presence of 5 mM MgAMPPCP and/or 5 mM glutathione in 0.125 M Kglutamate, 5 mM KCl, pH 7 medium containing 2 nM [^{3}H]ryanodine, and the indicated concentrations of free Ca^{2+}. Continuous lines were obtained assuming that the receptors possess cooperatively interacting high-affinity Ca^{2+} activation and low-affinity Ca^{2+}-inactivation sites (scheme 1 and equation 1 of Ref. 31). Note: In this and the following figures, B_{max} values of high-affinity [^{3}H]ryanodine binding ranged from 12–18 and 3–4 pmol/mg protein for skeletal and cardiac muscle SR vesicles, respectively.

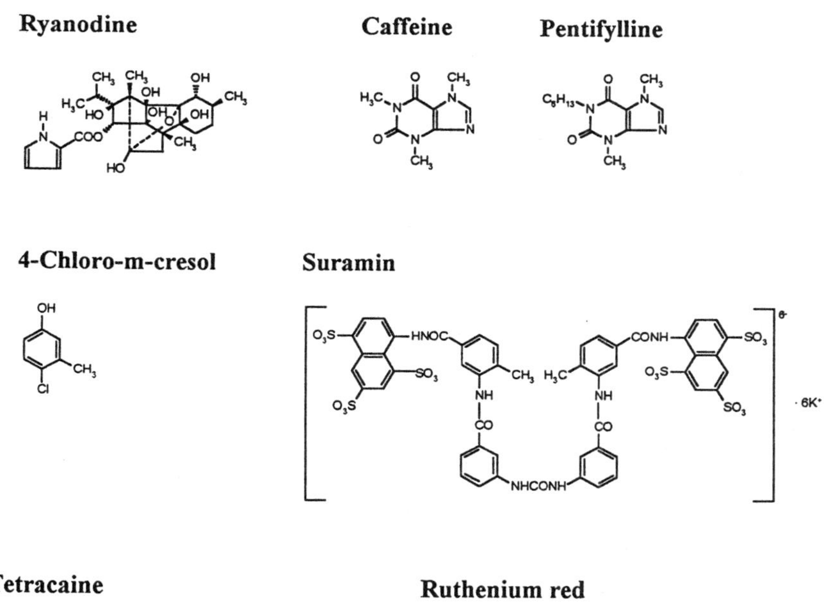

FIGURE 4. Chemical structures of exogenous effectors of RyRs.

that the addition of 5 mM glutathione reduced the levels of [^{3}H]ryanodine binding to a greater extent for the skeletal than cardiac RyR. The Ca^{2+}-dependence of [^{3}H]ryanodine binding was not greatly affected by glutathione in the 0.125 M Kglutamate, 5 mM KCl media containing and lacking 5 mM MgAMPPCP.

The action of the following drugs (for structures see FIG. 4) is described below: (i) ryanodine, a highly specific plant alkaloid that locks RyR ion channels into a subconductance state at nanomolar concentrations, whereas it fully closes them at micromolar concentrations; (ii) caffeine and pentifylline, two xanthines that lower the threshold of Ca^{2+} activation of RyRs; (iii) 4-chloro-m-cresol and suramin, two unrelated potent activators of RyRs; (iv) tetracaine, a local anesthetic that inhibits RyRs by an allosteric mechanism; and (v) ruthenium red, a potent inhibitor of RyRs. In addition, we shall briefly comment on the action of adenosine agonists and digitalis glycosides, which have been reported to activate the cardiac but not skeletal RyR.

Ryanodine

Ryanodine is a neutral plant alkaloid that is isolated from the stems of the South American shrub, *Ryania speciosa* (FIG. 4).[29] The pharmacological effects of ryanodine were initially recognized in muscles, where depending on muscle activity and type, it can either cause contracture or a decline in contractile force. Single-channel measurements

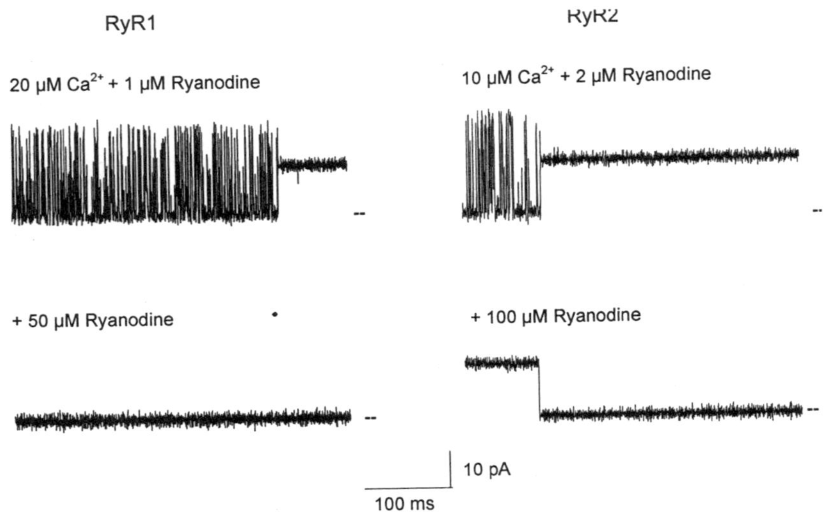

FIGURE 5. Effect of ryanodine on single purified skeletal **(left panel)** and cardiac **(right panel)** RyRs reconstituted into a planar lipid bilayer. Channels were recorded in symmetrical 250 mM KCl medium containing the indicated concentrations of free cytosolic Ca^{2+}. Shown is the appearance of a sudden subconductance state with a conductance about half of that of the unmodified channel and channel open probability (P_o) of ~1, several minutes after the addition of 1–2 μM ryanodine to the cytosolic (cis) chamber of the bilayer apparatus. The **lower trace** shows the transition from the subconductance state to a fully closed state within ~1 min after the addition of 50–100 μM ryanodine. *Bars on right* (- -) represent closed states of the channel.

have provided more direct insights into the action of ryanodine by showing that ryanodine modifies both the conductance and gating behavior of the skeletal and cardiac RyRs. In FIGURE 5, single K^+-conducting, Ca^{2+}-activated skeletal (left panel) and cardiac (right panel) Ca^{2+} release channels are shown. Similarly to what has previously been shown,[4] both channels entered into a long-lasting subconductance state following the addition of 1–2 μM ryanodine to the cytosolic side of the bilayer chamber. The subsequent addition of 50–100 μM ryanodine led to full closing of both channels. A characteristic property of both the subconductance and fully closed channel states is their insensitivity to regulation by other ligands such as Ca^{2+}, ATP, or Mg^{2+}, which otherwise greatly affect the gating behavior of the channels.[4] [^{3}H]Ryanodine binding studies have suggested that binding to a high-affinity site locks the skeletal muscle channel into the open subconductance state and binding of one or more ryanodine to low-affinity sites closes the channel[37] (for a different view see Ref. 38). In this regard it should be noted that, in order to reduce the times required to observe the otherwise very slow interactions of ryanodine with the channel, ryanodine concentrations of FIGURE 5 were in excess to those required to occupy the high- and low-affinity sites.

Ryanodine has had a major impact on the study of the mechanism of excitation-contraction coupling. The tritiated compound (commercially available with a specific activity of >50 Ci/mmol, Dupont NEN, Boston, MA) binds with high affinity and specificity to the Ca^{2+} release channels, giving these their alternate name. Because the drug dissociates slowly from the membrane-bound or detergent-solubilized receptors, [^{3}H]ryanodine binding has been found to be an ideal probe in the isolation of RyRs from a variety of tissues and species.[4] Ryanodine is also extensively used in demonstrating the presence of intracellular RyRs as well as assessing the role of intracellular Ca^{2+} stores in controlling cytosolic Ca^{2+} concentrations. Action of ryanodine is use dependent; and, as pointed out above, the affinity of [^{3}H]ryanodine binding is increased by channel activators such as μM Ca^{2+}.[3,4,29]

Because of their high selectivity, ryanoids have the potential to serve as therapeutic agents in controlling intracellular Ca^{2+} concentrations. However, naturally occurring ryanoids in general essentially irreversibly activate RyRs and therefore are too potent modulators of SR Ca^{2+} release to be suitable as therapeutic agents. Efforts are currently underway to synthesize ryanoids that modify the activity of RyRs in a more manageable manner.[29]

Xanthines

Methylxanthines (dimethyl-, theophylline, and theobromine; trimethyl-, caffeine) are common components of the diet for most people. Methylxanthines evoke the release of Ca^{2+} from intracellular membrane compartments by rendering RyRs more sensitive to activation by Ca^{2+};[30,31] however, their specificity is less than that of the ryanoids.[39] [^{3}H]Ryanodine binding measurements with skeletal muscle SR membranes at a high salt (1 M KCl) and low Ca^{2+} (<1 nM) concentration indicated that pentifylline (1-hexyl-3,7-dimethylxanthine) was the most effective of 30 xanthines tested.[40] Single-channel data of FIGURE 6 confirm that pentifylline is more effective than caffeine in activating the submaximally Ca^{2+}-activated skeletal Ca^{2+} release channel as well as cardiac Ca^{2+} release channel. The two bottom panels of FIGURE 6 compare the effects of 5 mM caffeine and 1 mM pentifylline on the Ca^{2+}-dependence of [^{3}H]ryanodine binding to cardiac SR membranes in the 0.125 M Kglutamate, 5 mM glutathione medium in the absence and presence of 5 mM MgAMPPCP. In the presence of 5 mM MgAMPPCP, 5 mM caffeine and 1 mM pentifylline were equally effective in rendering the cardiac muscle RyR more sensitive to Ca^{2+} activation by shifting the Ca^{2+} activation curve to the left and increasing the maximum level of [^{3}H]ryanodine binding. In the absence of MgAMPPCP, both xanthines also rendered the cardiac RyR more sensitive to activation by Ca^{2+}. However, whereas 5 mM caffeine raised the maximum level of [^{3}H]ryanodine twofold, curiously no increases above the control level were obtained for pentifylline. These results raise the interesting possibility that allosteric effectors such as MgAMPPCP affect the interaction between the xanthine and Ca^{2+} regulatory sites of cardiac RyR.

Like ryanodine, caffeine is extensively used to assess the role of sarco-/endoplasmic reticulum in controlling cellular Ca^{2+} concentrations. The use of caffeine offers several advantages in that it rapidly and reversibly causes sarco-/endoplasmic reticulum Ca^{2+} release. Two major limitations of caffeine are that relatively high concentrations are needed for activation and that the specificity is not as absolute as that of ryanodine. Further studies are needed to better understand the ways in which xanthines activate RyRs so that analogs can be synthesized that interact specifically and with high potency with RyRs.

4-Chloro-m-cresol

4-Chloro-m-cresol is a potent activator of RyR in skeletal muscle, where it is used as a diagnostic agent to distinguish between normal and malignant hyperthermia–susceptible muscles.[41] 4-Chloro-m-cresol increased [^{3}H]ryanodine binding to the skeletal RyR in a Ca^{2+}-dependent manner, and in single-channel measurements activated the

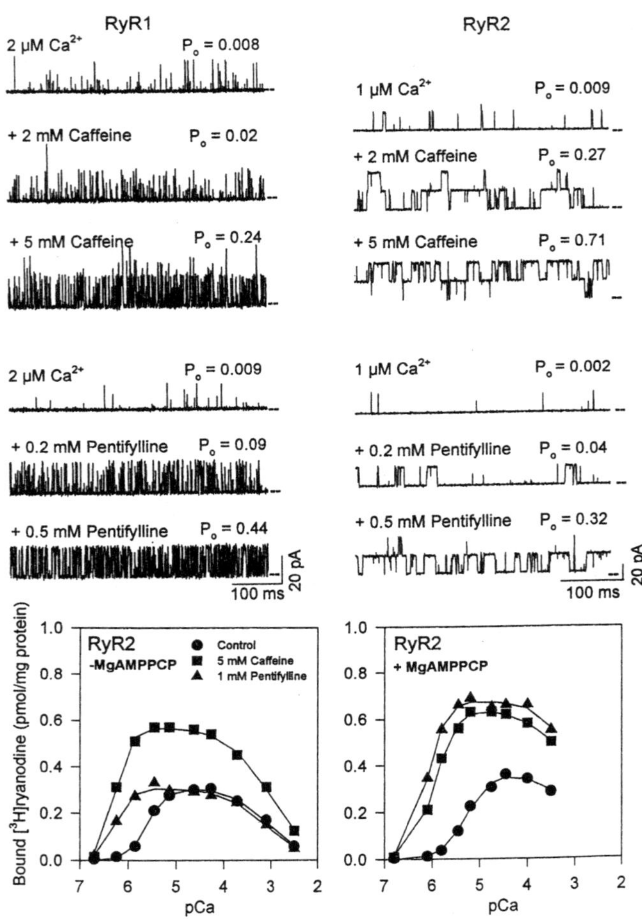

FIGURE 6. Effects of caffeine and pentifylline on skeletal **(left panels)** and cardiac **(right panels)** RyR/Ca^{2+} release channels. Two purified skeletal and cardiac muscle channels were recorded as in FIG. 2 in the presence of indicated cytosolic free [Ca^{2+}] and indicated concentrations of caffeine **(top panels)** and pentifylline **(middle panels).** Specific [^{3}H]ryanodine binding to cardiac SR membranes was determined as in FIG. 3 in the presence of 5 mM glutathione, and presence and absence of 5 mM MgAMPCP in media containing the indicated concentrations of free Ca^{2+}, caffeine, and pentifylline **(bottom panels).**

skeletal RyR to a greater extent when applied to the lumenal instead of the cytosolic side, suggesting binding sites different from those for Ca^{2+} and adenine nucleotides.[41] FIGURE 7 shows that 4-Chloro-m-cresol also activates the cardiac RyR when added to either side of the bilayer, but also shows that in the case of the cardiac RyR 4-chloro-m-cresol was most effective when added to the cytosolic side of the bilayer. 4-Chloro-m-cresol increased [^{3}H]ryanodine binding to the skeletal and cardiac RyRs in the pres-

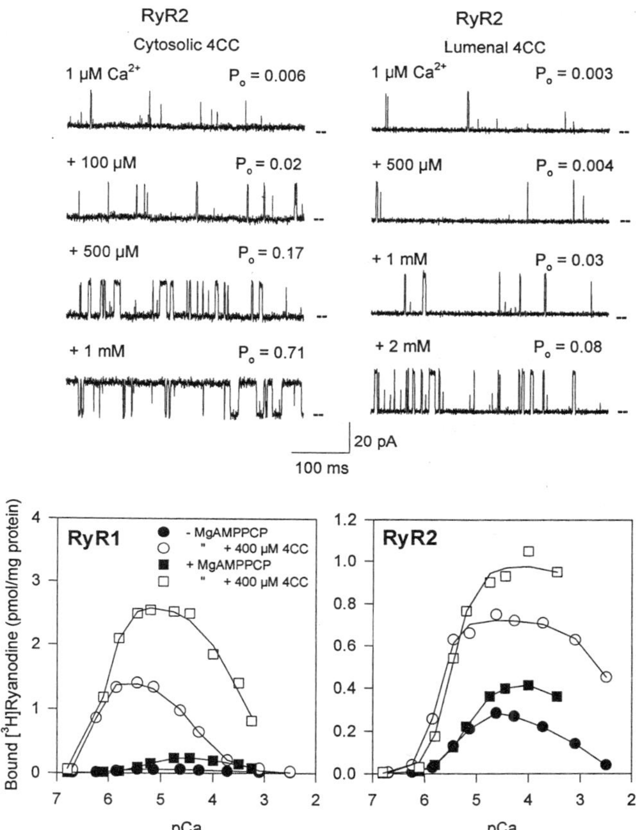

FIGURE 7. Effects of 4-chloro-m-cresol on skeletal (RyR1) and cardiac (RyR2) Ca^{2+} release channels. Single purified cardiac muscle channels were recorded as in FIG. 2 in the presence of 1 µM cytosolic and <0.1 µM lumenal Ca^{2+}, respectively, and indicated concentrations of cytosolic **(top left panel)** and lumenal **(top right panel)** 4-chloro-m-cresol (4CC). Specific [^{3}H]ryanodine binding to skeletal **(bottom left panel)** and cardiac **(bottom right panel)** SR membranes was determined as in FIG. 3 in the presence of 5 mM glutathione, and presence and absence of 5 mM MgAMPCP in media containing the indicated concentrations of free Ca^{2+} and 4-chloro-m-cresol.

ence and absence of MgAMPPCP ($EC_{50} \approx$ 100–200 µM at 7 µM free Ca^{2+}, unpublished studies) without significantly changing the Ca^{2+}-activation profiles (FIG. 7). Taken together, these results indicate that 4-chloro-m-cresol activates both channel forms by a similar mechanism that involves binding to sites different from those for Ca^{2+} and ATP.

Suramin

Suramin is an antiparasitic and antitumor agent and is known to inhibit ATP-dependent enzyme[42] and P2-purinoceptor activities.[43] Suramin activated the skele-

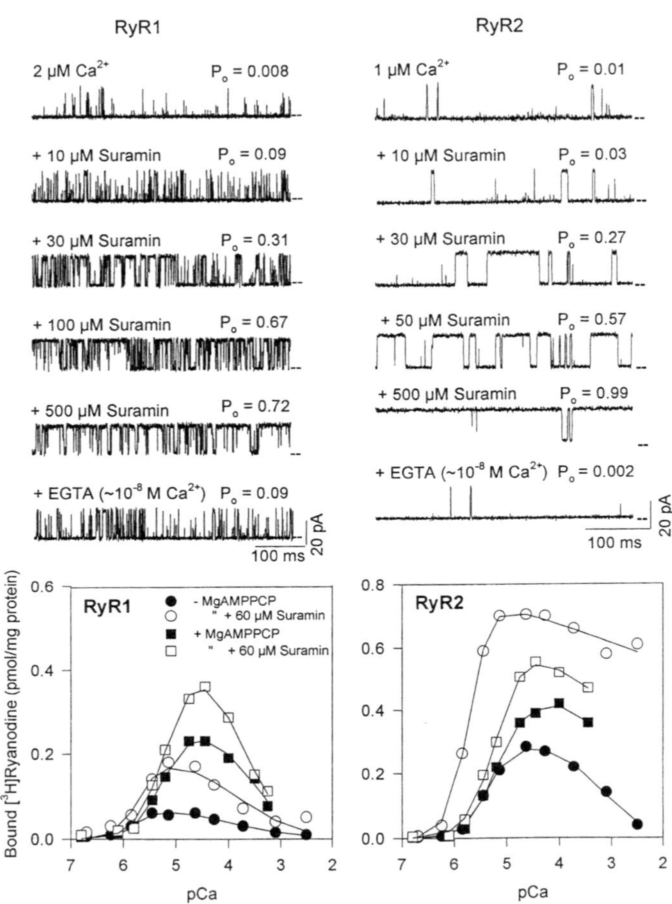

FIGURE 8. Effects of suramin on single-channel activities of and [^{3}H]ryanodine binding to skeletal (RyR1) and cardiac (RyR2) Ca^{2+} release channels. Single purified skeletal **(top left panel)** and cardiac **(top right panel)** Ca^{2+} release channels were recorded as in FIG. 2 in the presence of indicated concentrations of free cytosolic Ca^{2+} and cytosolic suramin. Specific [^{3}H]ryanodine binding to skeletal **(bottom left panel)** and cardiac **(bottom right panel)** SR membranes was determined as in FIG. 3 in the presence of 5 mM glutathione, and presence and absence of 5 mM MgAMPCP in media containing the indicated concentrations of free Ca^{2+} and suramin.

tal[42,44,45] and cardiac[45] RyRs in a Ca^{2+}-independent manner with[45] or without[44] changing single-channel conductance by apparently binding to a site different from that for adenine nucleotides[44,45] (for a different view see Ref. 42). FIGURE 8 shows that 500 μM cytosolic suramin almost fully activates the submaximally Ca^{2+}-activated skeletal and cardiac RyRs without a significant change in single-channel conductance. Decrease in cytosolic [Ca^{2+}] <0.1 μM resulted in a major reduction of channel activities, which suggested that the action of suramin is influenced by cytosolic Ca^{2+}. Lumenal suramin was without effect. [^{3}H]ryanodine binding studies confirmed that suramin activates the skeletal and cardiac RyRs in a Ca^{2+}-dependent manner (FIG. 8). Activation was observed in the presence and absence of MgAMPPCP, supporting the view of binding of suramin to a site different from that of ATP.

Adenosine Receptor Agonists

We tested the effects of the following four potent adenosine receptor agonists[43]: N-p-aminophenethyladenosine (APNEA), N^6-cyclohexyladenosine (CHA), N-ethylcarboxamidoadenosine (NECA), and CGS-21680. In the absence of MgAMPPCP at a free [Ca^{2+}] of 25 μM and agonist concentration of 10 μM, CGS-21680 was the most effective in stimulating [^{3}H]ryanodine binding to cardiac RyR (unpublished studies). CGS-21680 apparently activated the RyR by binding to the receptor's ATP binding site(s) because it had no noticeable effect on [^{3}H]ryanodine binding in the presence of 5 mM MgAMPPCP. These results suggest that because of a high cellular MgATP concentration, adenosine receptor agonists may have only a very limited capability of releasing Ca^{2+} from intracellular ryanodine-sensitive stores.

Digitalis Glycosides

Digitalis glycosides (digoxin, digitoxin) have been reported to activate the cardiac but not skeletal muscle RyR at therapeutic (1–10 nM) concentrations.[46] We observed only a modest (<2-fold) activation of single cardiac Ca^{2+} release channel by 1–10 nM digitoxin. Similarly, digitoxin and digoxin only minimally (<1.5-fold) stimulated [^{3}H]ryanodine binding at concentrations of 10–100 nM.

Tetracaine

Tetracaine is a local anesthetic known to inhibit Ca^{2+} release from SR.[3] FIGURE 9 shows that, as previously observed for the skeletal muscle RyR,[47] channel open probability of cardiac RyR was lowered by the addition of tetracaine to either the cytosolic or lumenal side of the bilayer. Tetracaine inhibited the cardiac RyR by inducing long channel closings and was most effective when added to the cytosolic side of the bilayer. The two lower panels of FIGURE 9 compare the effects of tetracaine on the Ca^{2+}-dependence of [^{3}H]ryanodine binding to skeletal and cardiac SR membranes in 0.125 M Kglutamate, 5 mM glutathione medium in the absence and presence of 5 mM MgAMPPCP. In the absence of MgAMPPCP at 25 μM free Ca^{2+}, tetracaine inhibited [^{3}H]ryanodine binding to the two RyRs with a similar IC_{50} of ~50 μM (unpublished studies). The addition of MgAMPPCP affected the two RyRs differently. Under this condition, a more than 5-fold higher tetracaine concentration was required for the half-maximum inhibition of [^{3}H]ryanodine binding to the cardiac RyR ($IC_{50} \approx 450$ μM vs. 75 μM for skeletal RyR, unpublished studies).

Ruthenium Red

Ruthenium red is a polycationic reagent that is effective in inhibiting SR Ca^{2+} release channels at nanomolar concentrations.[3] Single-channel recordings of FIGURE 10 (left

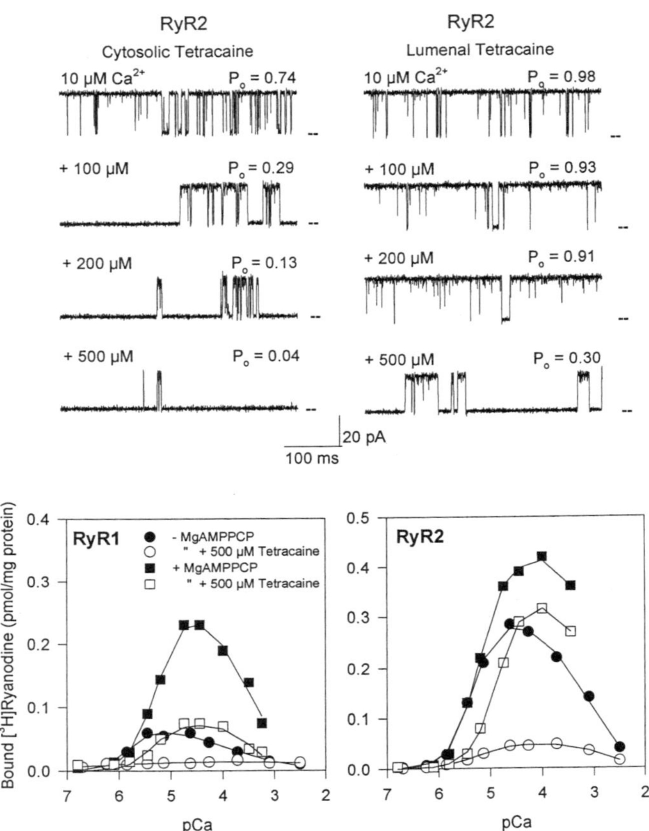

FIGURE 9. Effects of tetracaine on skeletal and cardiac RyR/Ca^{2+} release channels. Single purified cardiac muscle channels were recorded as in FIG. 2 in the presence of 10 μM cytosolic and <0.1 μM lumenal Ca^{2+}, respectively, and indicated concentrations of cytosolic **(top left panel)** and lumenal **(top right panel)** tetracaine. Specific [^{3}H]ryanodine binding to skeletal **(bottom left panel)** and cardiac **(bottom right panel)** SR membranes was determined as in FIG. 3 in the presence of 5 mM glutathione, and presence and absence of 5 mM MgAMPCP in media containing the indicated concentrations of free Ca^{2+} and tetracaine.

panel) show that ruthenium red inhibits the Ca^{2+}-activated cardiac RyR by inducing long channel closings without changing single-channel conductance. The channel was half-maximally inhibited at a ruthenium red concentration of ~20 nM. The right panel of FIGURE 10 shows that appreciably higher ruthenium red concentrations were required to half-maximally inhibit [^{3}H]ryanodine binding to cardiac SR membranes (IC_{50} ~0.3 μM and > 1 μM in absence and presence of 5 mM MgAMPPCP, respectively). The reasons for the different IC_{50} values are unclear. One possible reason is that different assay media were used. Also, despite extensive use, the mechanism(s) by which ruthenium red inhibits RyRs is (are) not well understood. Ruthenium red blocked single

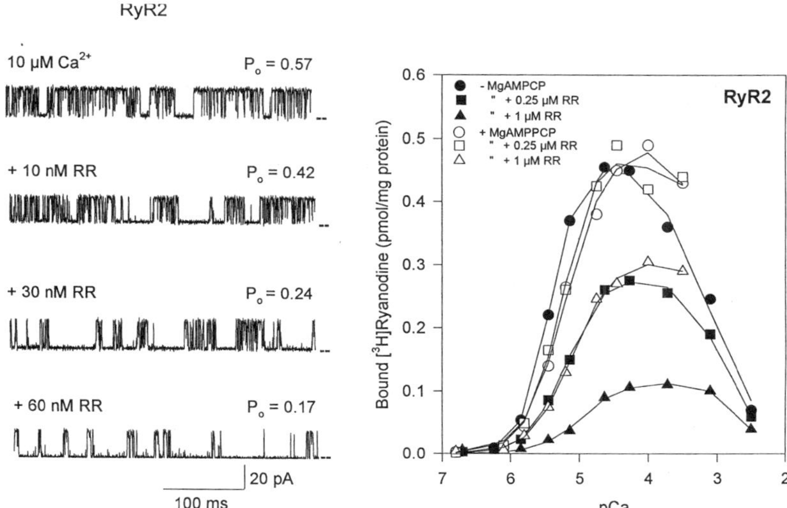

FIGURE 10. Effects of ruthenium red on single-channel activities and [^{3}H]ryanodine binding to cardiac Ca^{2+} release channels. Single purified cardiac muscle channels were recorded as in FIG. 2 in the presence of 10 µM cytosolic and <0.1 µM lumenal Ca^{2+}, respectively, and indicated concentrations of cytosolic ruthenium red **(left panel).** Specific [^{3}H]ryanodine binding to cardiac muscle SR membranes was determined as in FIG. 3 in the presence of 5 mM glutathione, and presence and absence of 5 mM MgAMPPCP in media containing the indicated concentrations of free Ca^{2+} and ruthenium red **(right panel).**

ryanodine-modified skeletal channels by binding to multiple sites located in the conductance pore of the channel.[48] In overlay studies with skeletal RyR fusion peptides, ruthenium red bound to several Ca^{2+} binding peptides.[49] In our preliminary experiments, a similar inhibition was observed at positive and negative holding potentials, which suggests that ruthenium red inhibited channel activity by binding to sites (Ca^{2+} binding sites?) outside the electric field.

CONCLUDING REMARKS

In conclusion, RyR/Ca^{2+} release channels constitute a potentially rich target for controlling cellular functions. A large number of pharmacological agents affect RyR function including ryanoids, toxins, xanthines, adenosines, NO donors, local anesthetics, and polycationic reagents. Few, if any, of these have been determined to be specific for RyR1 vs. RyR2. However, the potential of these drugs to serve as molecular targets for studying structure-activity relationships of RyRs is beginning to be realized. In turn, it is hoped that this information will help in the development of low-molecular-weight, membrane-permeable, nontoxic agents that display high affinity and target specificity and therefore have the potential to serve as therapeutic agents for controlling intracellular Ca^{2+} release from SR.

REFERENCES

1. Franzini-Armstrong, C. & F. Protasi. 1997. Ryanodine receptors of striated muscles: A complex channel capable of multiple interactions. Physiol. Rev. **77:** 699–729.
2. Sutko, J. L. & J. A. Airey. 1996. Ryanodine receptor Ca^{2+} release channels: Does diversity in form equal diversity in function? Physiol. Rev. **76:** 1027–1071.
3. Zucchi, R. & S. Ronca-Testoni. 1997. The sarcoplasmic reticulum Ca^{2+} channel/ryanodine receptor: Modulation by endogenous effectors, drugs and disease states. Pharmacol. Rev. **49:** 1–51.
4. Meissner, G. 1994. Ryanodine receptor/Ca^{2+} release channels and their regulation by endogenous effectors. Annu. Rev. Physiol. **56:** 485–508.
5. Junker, J., J. R. Sommer, M. Sar & G. Meissner. 1994. Extended junctional sarcoplasmic reticulum of avian cardiac muscle contains functional ryanodine receptors. J. Biol. Chem. **269:** 1627–1634.
6. Carl, S. L., K. Felix, A. H. Caswell, N. R. Brandt, W. J. Ball, Jr., P. L. Vaghy, G. Meissner & D. G. Ferguson. 1995. Immunolocalization of sarcolemmal dihydropyridine receptor and sarcoplasmic reticular triadin and ryanodine receptor in rabbit ventricle and atrium. J. Cell Biol. **129:** 673–682.
7. Wier, W. G. 1990. Cytoplasmic Ca^{2+} in mammalian ventricle: Dynamic control by cellular processes. Annu. Rev. Physiol. **52:** 467–485.
8. Rios, E. & G. Pizarro. 1991. Voltage sensor of excitation-contraction coupling in skeletal muscle. Physiol. Rev. **71:** 849–908.
9. Schneider, M. F. 1994. Control of calcium release in functioning skeletal muscle fibers. Annu. Rev. Physiol. **56:** 463–484.
10. Santana, L. F., H. Cheng, A. M. Gomez, M. B. Cannell & W. J. Lederer. 1996. Relation between the sarcolemmal Ca^{2+} current and Ca^{2+} sparks and local control theories for cardiac excitation-contraction coupling. Circ. Res. **78:** 166–171.
11. Takeshima, H., T. Ikemoto, M. Nishi, N. Nishiyama, M. Shimuta, Y. Sugitani, J. Kuno, I. Saito, H. Saito, M. Endo, M. Iino & T. Noda. 1996. Generation and characterization of mutant mice lacking ryanodine receptor type 3. J. Biol. Chem. **271:** 19649–19652.
12. Timerman, A. P., H. Onoue, H. B. Xin, S. Barg, J. Copello, G. Wiederrecht & S. Fleischer. 1996. Selective binding of FKBP12.6 by the cardiac ryanodine receptor. J. Biol. Chem. **271:** 20385–20391.
13. Murayama, T. & Y. Ogawa. 1997. Characterization of type 3 ryanodine receptor (RyR3) of sarcoplasmic reticulum from rabbit skeletal muscles. J. Biol. Chem. **272:** 24030–24037.
14. Chen, S. R. W., X. Li, K. Ebisawa & L. Zhang. 1997. Functional characterization of the recombinant type 3 Ca^{2+} release channel (ryanodine receptor) expressed in HEK293 cells. J. Biol. Chem. **272:** 24234–24246.
15. Xu, L., G. Mann & G. Meissner. 1996. Regulation of cardiac Ca^{2+} release channel (ryanodine receptor) by Ca^{2+}, H^+, Mg^{2+}, and adenine nucleotides under normal and simulated ischemic conditions. Circ. Res. **79:** 1100–1109.
16. Tripathy, A. & G. Meissner. 1996. Sarcoplasmic reticulum lumenal Ca^{2+} has access to cytosolic activation and inactivation sites of skeletal muscle Ca^{2+} release channel. Biophys. J. **70:** 2600–2615.
17. Xu, L. & G. Meissner. 1997. Regulation of cardiac calcium release channel (ryanodine receptor) by lumenal Ca^{2+}. Biophys. J. **72:** A375.
18. Sitsapesan, R. & A. J. Williams. 1994. Regulation of the gating of the sheep cardiac sarcoplasmic reticulum Ca^{2+} release channel by luminal Ca^{2+}. J. Membrane Biol. **137:** 215–226.
19. Gyorke, S. & M. Fill. 1993. Ryanodine receptor adaptation: Control mechanism of Ca^{2+}-induced Ca^{2+} release in heart. Science **260:** 807–809.
20. Sitsapesan, R., R. A. P. Montgomery & A. J. Williams. 1995. New insights into the gating mechanisms of cardiac ryanodine receptors revealed by rapid changes in ligand concentration. Circ. Res. **77:** 765–772.
21. Schiefer, A., G. Meissner & G. Isenberg. 1995. Ca^{2+} activation and Ca^{2+} inactivation of canine reconstituted cardiac sarcoplasmic reticulum Ca^{2+}-release channels. J. Physiol. **489:** 337–348.

22. SITSAPESAN, R., S. J. MCGARRY & A. J. WILLIAMS. 1994. Cyclic ADP-ribose competes with ATP for the adenine nucleotide binding site on the cardiac ryanodine receptor Ca^{2+}-release channel. Circ. Res. **75:** 596–600.
23. GUO, X., M. A. LAFLAMME & P. L. BECKER. 1996. Cyclic ADP-ribose does not regulate sarcoplasmic reticulum Ca^{2+} release in intact cardiac myocytes. Circ. Res. **79:** 147–151.
24. KOBZIK, L., M. B. REID, D. S. BREDT & J. S. STAMLER. 1994. Nitric oxide in skeletal muscle. Nature **372:** 546–548.
25. CAMPBELL, D. L., J. S. STAMLER & H. C. STRAUSS. 1996. Redox modulation of L-type calcium channels in ferret ventricular myocytes. J. Gen. Physiol. **108:** 277–293.
26. ZABLE, A. C., T. G. FAVERO & J. J. ABRAMSON. 1996. Glutathione modulates ryanodine receptor from skeletal muscle sarcoplasmic reticulum. Evidence for redox regulation of the Ca^{2+} release mechanism. J. Biol. Chem. **272:** 7069–7077.
27. XU, L. J., P. EU, G. MEISSNER & J. S. STAMLER. 1998. Activation of the cardiac calcium release channel (ryanodine receptor) by poly-S-nitrosylation. Science **279:** 234–237.
28. UEHARA, A., M. FILL, P. VELEZ, M. YASUKOCHI & I. IMANAGA. 1996. Rectification of rabbit cardiac ryanodine receptor current by endogenous polyamines. Biophys. J. **71:** 769–777.
29. SUTKO, J. L., J. A. AIREY, W. WELCH & L. RUEST. 1997. The pharmacology of ryanodine and related compounds. Pharmacol. Rev. **49:** 53–98.
30. MEISSNER, G., E. RIOS, A. TRIPATHY & D. A. PASEK. 1997. Regulation of skeletal muscle Ca^{2+} release channel (ryanodine receptor) by Ca^{2+} and monovalent cations and anions. J. Biol. Chem. **272:** 1628–1638.
31. LIU, W., D. A. PASEK & G. MEISSNER. 1998. Modulation of Ca^{2+}-gated cardiac muscle Ca^{2+} release channel/ryanodine receptor by mono- and divalent cations. Am. J. Physiol. **274:** C120–C128.
32. HOHL, C. M., A. A. GARLEB & R. A. ALTSCHULD. 1992. Effects of simulated ischemia and reperfusion on the sarcoplasmic reticulum of digitonin-lysed cardiomyocytes. Circ. Res. **70:** 716–723.
33. KORETSUNE, Y., M. C. CORRETTI, H. KUSUOKA & E. MARBAN. 1991. Mechanism of early ischemic contractile failure: Inexcitability, metabolic accumulation, or vascular collapse? Circ. Res. **68:** 255–262.
34. MURPHY, E., C. STEENBERGEN, L. A. LEVY, B. RAJU & R. E. LONDON. 1989. Cytosolic free magnesium levels in ischemic rat heart. J. Biol. Chem. **264:** 5622–5627.
35. VON ZGLINICKI, T. & M. BIMMLER. 1987. The intracellular distribution of ions and water in rat liver and heart muscle. J. Microscopy **146:** 77–85.
36. DENEKE, S. M. & B. L. FANBURG. 1989. Regulation of cellular glutathione. Am. J. Physiol. **257:** L163–L173.
37. LAI, F. A., M. MISRA, L. XU, H. A. SMITH & G. MEISSNER. 1989. The ryanodine receptor-Ca^{2+} release channel complex of skeletal muscle sarcoplasmic reticulum. Evidence for a cooperatively coupled, negatively charged homotetramer. J. Biol. Chem. **264:** 16776–16785.
38. BUCK, E., I. ZIMANYI, J. J. ABRAMSON & I. N. PESSAH. 1992. Ryanodine stabilizes multiple conformational states of the skeletal muscle calcium release channel. J. Biol. Chem. **267:** 23560–23567.
39. SAWYNOK, J & T. L. YAKSH. 1993. Caffeine as an analgesic adjuvant: A review of pharmacology and mechanisms of action. Pharmacol. Rev. **45:** 43–85.
40. LIU, W. & G. MEISSNER. 1997. Structure-activity relationship of xanthines and skeletal muscle ryanodine receptor/Ca^{2+} release channel. Pharmacology **54:** 135–143.
41. HERRMANN-FRANK, A., M. RICHTER, S. SARKOZI, U. MOHR & F. LEHMANN-HORN. 1996. 4-Chloro-m-cresol, a potent and specific activator of the skeletal muscle ryanodine receptor. Biochim. Biophys. Acta **1289:** 31–40.
42. EMMICK, J. T., S. KWON, K. R. BIDASEE, K. T. BESCH & H. R. BESCH, JR. 1994. Dual effect of suramin on calcium fluxes across sarcoplasmic reticulum vesicle membranes. J. Pharm. Exp. Ther. **269:** 717–724.
43. KEBABIAN, J. W. & J. L. NEUMEYER. 1994. The RBI Handbook of Receptor Classification. Research Biochemicals International. Natick, MA.
44. HOHENEGGER, M., M. MATYASH, K. POUSSU, A. HERRMANN-FRANK, S. SARKOZI, F. LEHMANN-HORN & M. FREISSMUTH. 1996. Activation of the skeletal muscle ryanodine receptor by suramin and suramin analogs. Mol. Pharmacol. **50:** 1443–1453.

45. SITSAPESAN, R. & A. J. WILLIAMS. 1996. Modification of the conductance and gating properties of ryanodine receptors by suramin. J. Membr. Biol. **153:** 93–103.
46. MCGARRY, S. J. & A. J. WILLIAMS. 1993. Digoxin activates sarcoplasmic reticulum Ca^{2+}-release channels: A possible role in cardiac inotropy. Br. J. Pharmacol. **108:** 1043–1050.
47. XU, L., R. JONES & G. MEISSNER. 1993. Effects of local anesthetics on single channel behavior of skeletal muscle calcium release channel. J. Gen. Physiol. **101:** 207–233.
48. MA, J. 1993. Block by ruthenium red of the ryanodine-activated calcium release channel of skeletal muscle. J. Gen. Physiol. **102:** 1031–1056.
49. CHEN, S. R. W., L. ZHANG & D. H. MACLENNAN. 1992. Characterization of a Ca^{2+} binding and regulatory site in the Ca^{2+} release channel (ryanodine receptor) of rabbit skeletal muscle sarcoplasmic reticulum. J. Biol. Chem. **267:** 23318–23326.

FKBP12 Modulates Gating of the Ryanodine Receptor/Calcium Release Channel[a]

KAROL ONDRIAS,[b] STEVEN O. MARX,[c] MARTA GABURJAKOVA,[b] AND ANDREW R. MARKS[c,d]

[b]*Institute of Molecular Physiology and Genetics, Slovak Academy of Sciences, Vlarska 5, 83334 Bratislava, Slovak Republic*
[c]*Molecular Cardiology Program, Department of Medicine, Columbia University College of Physicians and Surgeons, New York, New York 10032, USA*

ABSTRACT: Excitation-contraction (EC) coupling in muscle requires the activation of intracellular calcium release channels (CRC). Four type 1 ryanodine receptor (RyR1) molecules form each tetrameric CRC. Each RyR1 contains a binding site for the FK506 binding protein (FKBP12), a *cis-trans* peptidyl-prolyl isomerase that is required for coordinated gating of the four RyR1 subunits comprising the channel.[1,2] When FKBP12 is bound to RyR1, it stabilizes the four subunits that form each CRC. We propose that binding of one FKBP12 to each RyR1 lowers the energy of twisted-amide peptidyl-prolyl bonds and stabilizes RyR1 in a conformation that permits coordinated gating of the four RyR1 subunits.

In skeletal muscle the ryanodine receptor (RyR1)/calcium release channel (CRC) on the sarcoplasmic reticulum (SR) is required for muscle contraction.[3] Activation of RyR1 is thought to be triggered by a direct protein-protein interaction with a cytoplasmic loop of the voltage-dependent calcium channel (VDCC) on the transverse tubule.[4] The FK506 binding protein (FKBP12) is one of a family of *cis-trans* peptidyl-prolyl isomerases referred to as immunophilins because they bind the immunosuppressant drugs FK506 and rapamycin.[5] In skeletal muscle FKBP12 binds with high affinity to RyR1 and stabilizes the channel structure.[1,2] When FKBP12 is not bound to RyR1, the channel no longer opens to its full conductance (~120 pS with Ca^{2+} as the current carrier), but rather behaves as though each of the four subunits were an independently gated channel.[2] This gating behavior results in a binomial distribution of subconductance states with amplitudes of 1/4, 1/2, and 3/4 of the full conductance of the channel.[2]

Coexpression of recombinant RyR1 with FKBP12 in insect cells (Sf9) eliminates subconductance states resulting in channels that open to the full conductance of 120 pS.[2] Expression of RyR1 without FKBP12 or addition of FK506 or rapamycin (to compete FKBP12 off of RyR1) causes subconductance states to reappear.[2]

[a] This work was supported by the Richard and Lynne Kaiser Family Foundation and by grants to A.R.M. from the National Institutes of Health (NS29814 and HL56180), the American Heart Association, and the Muscular Dystrophy Association. A.R.M. is a Bristol-Meyers Squibb Established Investigator of the American Heart Association. S.O.M. is a Clinician-Scientist Awardee of the American Heart Association.

[d]Address for correspondence: Andrew R. Marks, M.D., Director, Molecular Cardiology P&S 9-401, Columbia University College of Physicians and Surgeons, 630 West 168th Street, Box 65, New York, New York 10032. Phone: 212-305-0270; fax: 212-305-3690; e-mail: arm42@columbia.edu

RyR1 channels on the SR membrane are densely packed square structures that appear to be in contact with their neighbors at each of four corners.[6,7] The biophysical properties of RyR1 have been examined using channels fused to planar lipid bilayers under conditions such that a single channel is active at any given time. RyR1 contains an FKBP12 binding site that includes the tetrapeptide Ser-Leu-Pro-Leu. The twisted amide in the leucyl-prolyl bond is a high-affinity substrate for FKBP12.[9] However, since FKBP12 remains bound to RyR1 even during extensive purification,[1] it is unlikely that this leucyl-prolyl bond undergoes isomerization from *cis* to *trans* in the intact RyR1 channel, as this would result in a lowering of the affinity of the substrate/binding site for FKBP12.[8] Therefore, we propose a model for the mechanism underlying the regulatory effects of FKBP12 on RyR1 (see FIG. 1). Our model is based on the concept that the FKBP12 binding site of RyR1 includes a leucyl-prolyl bond that is constrained in a twisted amide conformation. The substructures of FK506 and rapamycin mimic the twisted amide conformation of peptidyl-prolyl bonds and have high affinity for FKBP12.[9] The twisted amide conformation is a high-energy structure and is inherently unstable, but binding of FKBP12 lowers the energy by about ~6 kcal/mol and stabilizes the channel structure.[9,10] However, we propose that the *cis-trans* isomerization of the leucyl-prolyl bond in RyR1 does not occur (due to spacial constraints imposed by the structure of the channel protein). Thus, FKBP12 remains tightly bound to RyR1, lowering the energy of the channel complex by 24 kcal/mol when all four FKBP12 binding sites are occupied, and the stabilized channel structure gates as a single channel comprised of four RyR1 molecules.

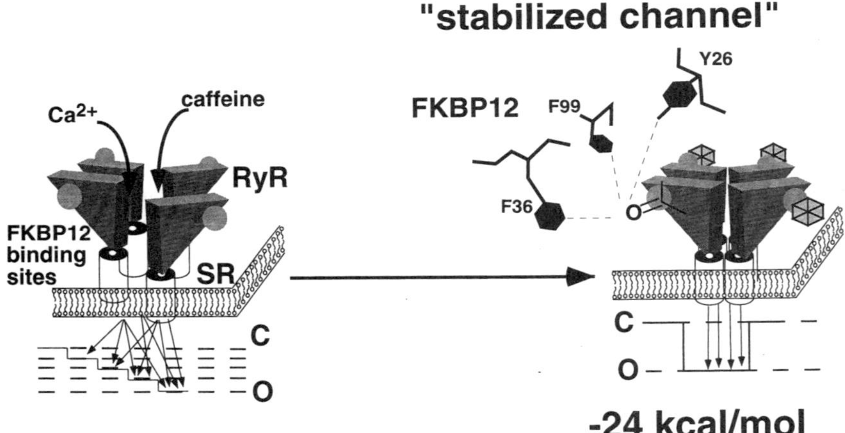

FIGURE 1. Model for FKBP12 interaction with the RyR1. RyR1s represented as a tetrameric structure with four pores through the SR membrane. This unproved model is based on data suggesting that the subconductance states observed in the recombinant channel in the absence of FKBP12 are distributed in a binomial fashion and are multiples of 1/4 of the full channel conductance.[2] Each RyR has one FKBP12 binding site. Binding of FKBP12 to RyR1 could lower the energy of each of the peptidyl-prolyl bonds in the binding site by 6 kcal/mol by stabilizing twisted-amide structures, resulting in a net lowering of energy for the channel complex of 24 kcal/mol. Highly conserved aromatic residues in FKBP12 are known to be clustered around the C8 carbonyl of the rapamycin and FK506 substructures and could interact with carbonyl in the twisted-amide conformation of the leucyl-prolyl bond in the FKBP12 binding site on RyR1.

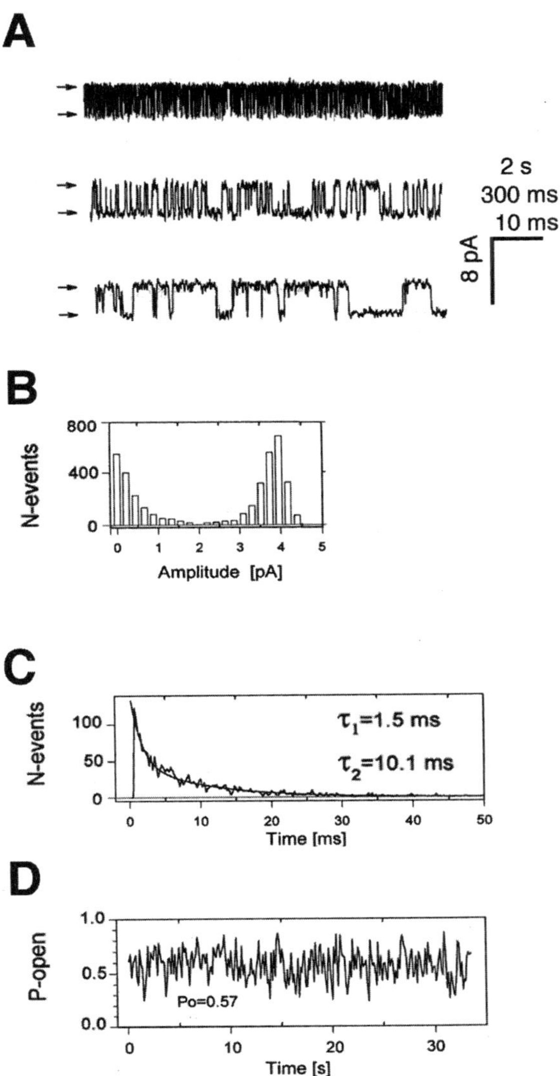

FIGURE 2. RyR1 coexpressed with FKBP12. **(A)** Tracings show the activity of a single recombinant RyR1 channel in the bilayer. **(B)** Current amplitude histogram for a single RyR1 channel. **(C)** Mean open times for a single RyR1. **(D)** The open probability for a single RyR1 channel. In these experiments recombinant RyR1 was expressed in insect cells (Sf9), purified on a sucrose gradient, and reconstituted into liposomes; and these RyR1-containing liposomes were fused to planar lipid bilayers. The conditions for single-channel recordings were: (1) *trans* chamber 53 mM $Ca(OH)_2$; (2) *cis* chamber 0.5 mM $CaCl_2$, 1 mM $MgCl_2$, pH 7.35. The channels were activated with 5 mM caffeine. Recordings were at 0 mV; channel openings are in the upward direction. The *arrows* at left of the tracings in **A** indicate the 0- and 4-pA current levels.

METHODS

Expression and Purification of RyR1

Full-length RyR1 cDNA was expressed in Sf9 cells as previously described.[2] Recombinant and rabbit skeletal muscle RyR1 were purified by sucrose density centrifugation essentially as described elsewhere.[11]

Single-Channel Recordings Using Planar Lipid Bilayers

RyR1 protein was reconstituted into unilamellar vesicles, which were then fused to black lipid membranes using a chamber similar to that described previously.[2,12] Black lipid membranes[12] were formed across a hole (diameter 0.05–0.3 μm) separating *cis* and *trans* chambers. *Cis* and *trans* chambers were filled with the following solutions to measure the Ca^{2+} current through the RyR1 channel: *cis* solution, 250 mM Hepes, 125 mM Tris, 0.05–0.1 mM $CaCl_2$, pH 7.35; *trans* solution, 53 mM $Ca(OH)_2$, 250 mM Hepes, pH 7.35. The *trans* chamber was connected to the head-stage input of an Axon 200 amplifier (Axon Instruments) by a Ag/AgCl electrode and agar/KCl bridges. The *cis* chamber was held at ground with a similar electrode. Single-channel currents were continuously monitored and recorded with a digital audio tape (DAT) and with a chart recorder. Recordings were filtered through a low-pass Bessel (Frequency Devices, Haverhill, MA) at 2 kHz and digitized at 0.5 kHz. Single-channel properties were evaluated using the PClamp 6 program. Analysis of single-channel behavior was performed as previously described.[2]

RESULTS

Multiple studies have reported the single-channel properties of RyR1 examined in planar lipid bilayers.[2,11,13–19] In the present study the charge carrier was 53 mM Ca^{2+}, which reproducibly results in single RyR1 channel openings with amplitudes of ~4 pA (0 mV potential across the bilayer membrane) yielding a conductance of ~120 pS. This is the same conductance reported for the recombinant RyR1[2,16] and for the native RyR1 isolated from skeletal muscle.[15,20] Recombinant RyR1 was coexpressed with FKBP12 in insect (Sf9) cells, purified, incorporated into lipid vesicles, and fused to planar lipid bilayers resulting in stable channels opening to the full single-channel conductance of 4 pA (FIG. 2A, B). The mean open times (fit with two exponentials) of τ_1 = 1.5 ms and τ_2 = 10.1 ms (FIG. 2C) and the open probability P_o = 57% (FIG. 2D) were typical for RyR1 (activated with 5 mM caffeine).

We have previously reported that coexpression of RyR1 with FKBP12 or addition of FKBP12 to an RyR1 channel in the bilayer stabilized the channel, resulting in openings to the full conductance for a single channel.[2] As shown in FIGURE 3, approximately 30 minutes after addition of FKBP12 to a bilayer containing recombinant RyR1, a single channel exhibiting multiple subconductance states converted to a stable single channel with full conductance (current amplitude = 4 pA).

FIGURE 4 shows the effects of addition of rapamycin (10 nM) to the *cis* (cytosolic) side of the bilayer containing a recombinant RyR1 channel coexpressed with FKBP12 (FIG. 4A). Approximately 10 minutes after the addition of rapamycin, which competes FKBP12 off of RyR1, the subunits of the channel were destabilized and the channel exhibited multiple subconductance states (FIG. 4B).

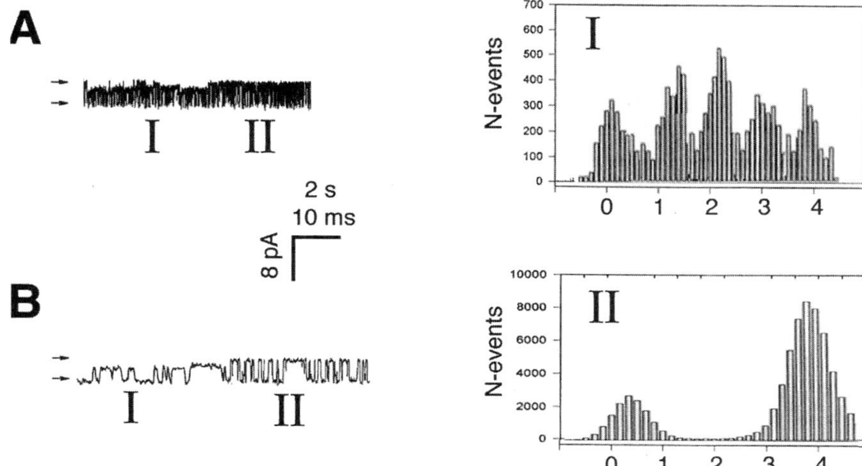

FIGURE 3. Addition of FKBP12 to recombinant RyR1 channels alters gating. **(A)** Compressed time scale showing the transition from a single channel with multiple subconductance states (labeled "I") to a single channel with full openings (labeled "II"). **(B)** Expanded time scale showing the transition from single channel with subconductance states to a single channel with full openings. Amplitude histograms on the **right** correspond to regions labeled "I" and "II." Recordings were at 0 mV; channel openings are in the upward direction. The *arrows* at left of the tracings in **A** and **B** indicate the 0- and 4-pA current levels.

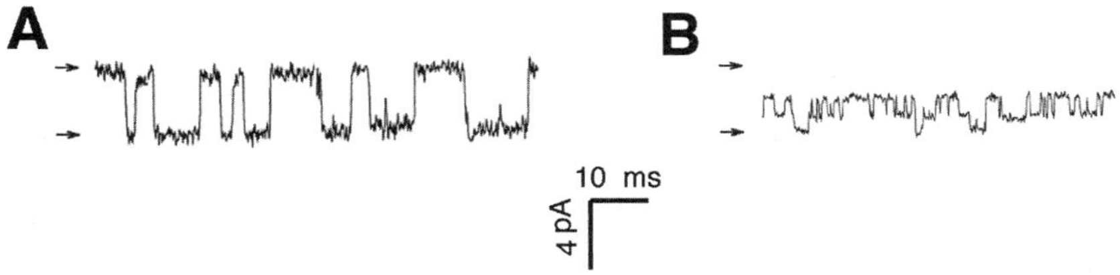

FIGURE 4. Removal of FKBP12 destabilizes recombinant RyR1 channels. **(A)** A recombinant RyR1 channel exhibiting full conductance openings. **(B)** The same channel following addition of rapamycin to remove FKBP12 from RyR1shows subconductance states in the destabilized channel following rapamycin. Recordings were at 0 mV; channel openings are in the upward direction. The *arrows* at left of the tracings in **A** and **B** indicate the 0- and 4-pA current levels.

Similar effects were observed (FIG. 5) when rapamycin was added to native channels isolated from rabbit skeletal muscle (FKBP12 remains tightly bound to RyR1 during purification).

DISCUSSION

The present study demonstrates the role of FKBP12 in the gating of RyR1 channels in planar lipid bilayers, which may represent an important feature of E-C coupling *in*

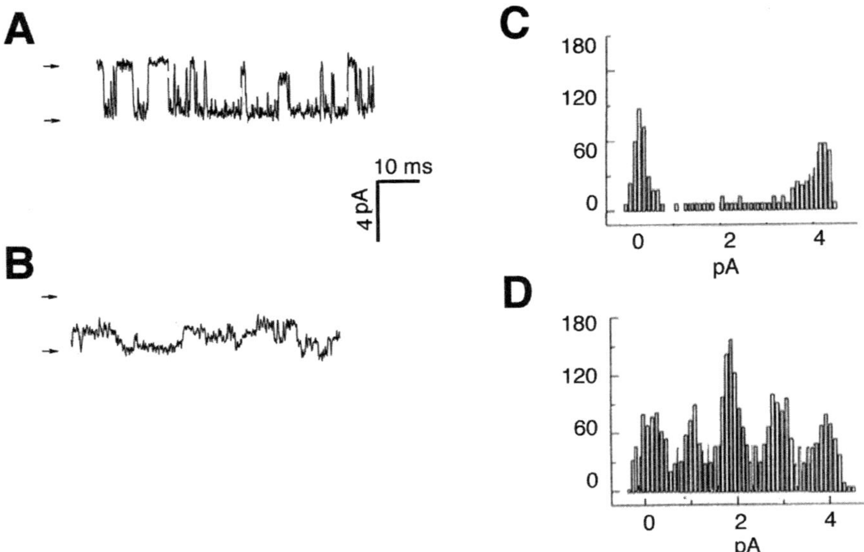

FIGURE 5. Rapamycin destabilizes RyR1 channels purified from skeletal muscle. **(A)** RyR1 channel from rabbit skeletal muscle exhibiting full conductance openings. **(B)** The same channel following addition of rapamycin (10 nM). Amplitude histograms showing **(C)** currents of ~4 pA for full conductance stabilized channels and **(D)** multiple subconductance states for the channel following addition of rapamycin. Recordings were at 0 mV; channel openings are in the upward direction. The *arrows* at left of the tracings in **A** and **B** indicate the 0- 4-pA current levels.

vivo. We have observed similar findings using cardiac RyR2,[14] suggesting that gating may be a common feature of the role of FKBP12 in regulating RyR of striated muscles. Indeed, a recent report of an FKBP12 null mouse showed that there was subconductance in both RyR1 from skeletal muscle and in RyR2 from cardiac muscle.[21]

Both rapamycin and FK506 inhibit the stabilizing effect of FKBP12 on RyR1 at nanomolar concentrations.[2] FK506 and rapamycin share a substructure that mimics the twisted amide transition state of a peptidyl-prolyl bond.[9] FKBP12 binds with nanomolar affinity to RyR1 and has a slow off-rate,[22] suggesting that the leucyl-prolyl bond in the RyR1 binding site for FKBP12 may be constrained in a transition-state conformation that is similar to the twisted amide structure.[9] If the leucyl-prolyl bond were not constrained in a twisted amide conformation, *cis-trans* isomerization of the bond would occur and FKBP12 would not remain bound to RyR1, as the affinity for either the *cis* or *trans* conformation of the leucyl-prolyl bond is lower than that for the transition state.[9]

Both FK506 and rapamycin alter the contractile properties of intact skeletal muscle[2] and of cardiac myocytes.[23] Despite these observations, complaints of defects in muscle function are not frequent among patients taking FK506 or rapamycin as immunosuppressants. This is likely due to the fact that the immunosuppressant effects of both drugs are gain-of-function phenomena and require low intracellular concentrations, whereas the effects on striated muscles are stoichiometric. If, indeed, FKBP12 plays an important role in E-C coupling, gene targeting resulting in an FKBP12-

deficient mouse would be expected to result in a defect in skeletal muscle function, although this defect could be subtle, such as a mild skeletal muscle weakness. Although there were no gross defects in skeletal muscle function in the FKBP12 null mouse, further studies using muscle from this mutant mouse should prove informative in this regard.[21]

ACKNOWLEDGMENT

The authors thank Daniel and Sarah Marks for help in the preparation of this manuscript.

REFERENCES

1. JAYARAMAN, T. *et al.* 1992. FK506 binding protein associated with the calcium release channel (ryanodine receptor). J. Biol. Chem. **267:** 9474–9477.
2. BRILLANTES, A.-M. B. *et al.* 1994. Stabilization of calcium release channel (ryanodine receptor) function by FK-506 binding protein. Cell **77:** 513–523.
3. TAKESHIMA, H. *et al.* 1994. Excitation-contraction uncoupling and muscular degeneration in mice lacking functional skeletal muscle ryanodine-receptor gene. Nature **369:** 556–559.
4. TANABE, T. *et al.* 1990. Regions of the skeletal muscle dihydropyridine receptor critical for excitation-contraction coupling. Nature **346:** 567–569.
5. MARKS, A. R. 1996. Cellular functions of immunophillins. Physiol. Rev. **76:** 631–649.
6. FRANZINI-ARMSTRONG, C. & G. NUNZI. 1983. Junctional feet and membrane particles in the triad of a fast twitch muscle fiber. J. Muscle Res. Cell. Motil. **4:** 233–252.
7. SAITO, A. *et al.* 1988. Ultrastructure of the calcium release channel of sarcoplasmic reticulum. J. Cell. Biol. **107:** 211–219.
8. VAN DUYNE, G. D. *et al.* 1993. Atomic structures of the human immunophilin FKBP-12 complexes with FK506 and rapamycin. J. Mol. Bio. **229:** 105–124.
9. ALBERS, M. W., C. T. WALSH & S. L. SCHREIBER. 1990. Substrate specificity of the human rotamase FKBP: A view of FK506 and rapamycin as leucine-(twisted amide)-proline mimics. J. Org. Chem. **55:** 4984–4986.
10. ROSEN, M. K. *et al.* 1990. Inhibition of FKBP rotamase activity by immunosuppressant FK506: Twisted amide surrogate. Science **248:** 863–866.
11. LINDSAY, A. & A. WILLIAMS. 1991. Functional characterization of the ryanodine receptor from sheep cardiac muscle sarcoplasmic reticulum. Biochem. Biophys. Acta **1064:** 89–102.
12. MILLER, C. 1986. Ion Channel Reconstitution. Plenum. New York.
13. CORONADO, R. *et al.* 1992. Planar bilayer recording of ryanodine receptors of sarcoplasmic reticulum. Methods Enzymol. **207:** 699–707.
14. KAFTAN, E., A. R. MARKS & B. E. EHRLICH. 1996. Effects of rapamycin on ryanodine receptor/calcium release channels from skeletal and cardiac muscle. Circ. Res. **78:** 990–997.
15. LAI, F. A. *et al.* 1988. Purification and reconstitution of the calcium release channel from skeletal muscle. Nature **331:** 315–319.
16. ONDRIAS, K. *et al.* 1996. Single channel properties and calcium conductance of the cloned expressed ryanodine receptor/calcium release channel. *In* Organellar Ion Channels and Transporters: **51:** 29–45. Society of General Physiologists. Woods Hole, MA.
17. TINKER, A., A. R. G. LINDSAY & A. J. WILLIAMS. 1992. A model for ionic conduction in the ryanodine receptor channel of sheep cardiac muscle sarcoplasmic reticulum. J. Gen. Phys. **100:** 495–517.
18. TINKER, A. & A. J. WILLIAMS. 1992. Divalent cation conduction in the ryanodine receptor channel of sheep cardiac muscle sarcoplasmic reticulum. J. Gen. Physiol. **100:** 479–493.
19. WILLIAMS, A. 1992. Ion conduction and discrimination in the sarcoplasmic reticulum ryanodine receptor/calcium-release channel. J. Muscle Res. & Cell Motil. **13:** 7–26.
20. SMITH, J. S., R. CORONADO & G. MEISSNER. 1986. Single channel measurements of the calcium release channel from skeletal muscle sarcoplasmic reticulum. J. Gen. Physiol. **88:** 573–588.

21. SHOU, W. *et al.* 1998. Cardiac defects and altered ryanodine function in mice lacking FKBP12. Nature **391:** 489–492.
22. TIMERMAN, A. P. *et al.* 1995. Characterization of an exchange reaction between soluble FKBP-12 and the FKBP-ryanodine receptor complex. Modulation by FKBP mutants deficient in peptidyl-prolyl isomerase activity. J. Biol. Chem. **270:** 2451–2459.
23. MCCALL, E. *et al.* 1996. Effects of FK-506 on contraction and Ca2+ transients in rat cardiac myocytes. Circ. Res. **79:** 1110–1121.

Factors That Control Sarcoplasmic Reticulum Calcium Release in Intact Ventricular Myocytes[a]

DONALD M. BERS,[b] LI LI, HIROSHI SATOH,[c] AND EILEEN McCALL[d]

Department of Physiology, Loyola University Chicago, Stritch School of Medicine, Maywood, Illinois 60514, USA

ABSTRACT: Much has been discovered studying sarcoplasmic reticulum (SR) Ca release channels in SR vesicles and lipid bilayers. We have focused on how SR Ca release is regulated in intact mammalian ventricular myocytes, using fluorescent Ca indicators, voltage clamp, and confocal microscopy. Three major factors appear to contribute to the probability of spontaneous localized SR Ca release events (or Ca "sparks") in resting myocytes: (1) cytosolic [Ca], (2) SR Ca content, and (3) time after previous activity (i.e., recovery from adapted or inactivated state). These same three factors function during excitation-contraction (E-C) coupling and can explain rest potentiation of twitches, increased fractional SR Ca release at higher SR Ca loads, and Ca overload. Since SR Ca release is sensitive to both I_{Ca} and SR Ca load, we have controlled (and measured) these parameters. At constant SR Ca load and I_{Ca} in intact cells we have found that SR Ca release is increased by Ca-calmodulin–dependent protein kinase (CaMKII) and FK506 (which may interfere with the interaction between the Ca release channel and the FK binding protein) and is reduced by the Ca channel agonist Bay K 8644, CaMKII inhibitors, and during ventricular hypertrophy. Thus the regulation of the SR Ca release channel in the intact cell is an important factor in cellular cardiac function.

Electrophysiological studies of the cardiac ryanodine receptor (RyR) incorporated into lipid bilayers and Ca flux studies in isolated sarcoplasmic reticulum (SR) vesicles have been extremely valuable.[1–3] Indeed, the ability to incorporate the cardiac RyR into lipid bilayers and record current carried by single RyR channels has provided unique insights into the properties of these channels, including their conductance, open time, open probability, and factors that alter channel gating properties.[1–11] These studies in the well-controlled bilayer chamber environment have provided detailed evaluations of the regulation of RyR channel gating by Ca, ATP, Mg, caffeine, ryanodine, phosphorylation, and other factors. These types of studies have been essential in the continuing development of our comprehensive understanding of cardiac excitation-contraction (E-C) coupling.[1,8,10]

[a] This work was supported by grants from the United States Public Health Service (HL-30077, HL-44583, and HL-52478).

[b] Address for correspondence: Donald M. Bers, Ph.D., Department of Physiology, Loyola University Chicago, Stritch School of Medicine, 2160 South First Avenue, Maywood, Illinois 60153. Phone: 708-216-1018; fax: 708-216-6308; e-mail: dbers@luc.edu

[c] Current address: Department of Internal Medicine III, Hamamatsu University School of Medicine, 3600 Handa-cho, Hamamatsu 431-31, Japan.

[d] Current address: Lily Research Laboratories, Cardiovascular Research, Lily Corporate Center, Indianapolis, Indiana 46285.

In addition to these studies of the RyR in relative isolation, it is equally important to evaluate how the SR Ca release channel behaves in intact cells in its normal physiological environment. The importance of this is underscored by the many factors and associated proteins that are able to modulate RyR gating and the fact that the unitary flux is so large that even small gating changes could greatly alter physiological function of the SR Ca release channel during the cellular Ca transient and contraction in the heart. The work we will discuss here focuses on factors that alter or regulate SR Ca release channel function in the intact mammalian ventricular myocyte. This work complements and extends work in more isolated systems, but has the inherent disadvantage that the complex cellular environment makes it harder to maintain control of all of the potentially relevant factors. On the other hand, the importance of this kind of data makes these kind of studies crucial. We have generally used fluorescent Ca indicators to measure intracellular [Ca] ($[Ca]_i$), often in combination with whole-cell voltage clamp to allow control of membrane potential (E_m) while allowing measurement of transmembrane currents (e.g., Ca current, I_{Ca}, and Na/Ca exchange current, $I_{Na/Ca}$). Many of these voltage clamp studies are also done with the perforated patch variation, which prevents the dialysis of cellular proteins by the patch pipette. These studies help build a more comprehensive understanding of cardiac E-C coupling and the regulation of SR Ca release in the native physiological environment.

We describe three major intrinsic factors that contribute to the probability of spontaneous localized SR Ca release events (or Ca "sparks") in resting myocytes: (1) cytosolic [Ca], (2) SR Ca content, and (3) time after previous activity (i.e., recovery from adapted or inactivated state). These same three factors function during E-C coupling and can explain rest potentiation of twitches, increased fractional SR Ca release at higher SR Ca loads, and Ca overload. Since SR Ca release is sensitive to both I_{Ca} and SR Ca load, we have controlled (and measured) these parameters. At constant SR Ca load and I_{Ca} in intact cells we have found that SR Ca release is increased by CaMKII and the immunosupressant drug FK506 (which may interfere with the interaction between the Ca release channel and endogenous FK-506 binding proteins) and is reduced by the Ca channel agonist Bay K 8644, CaMKII inhibitors, and during ventricular hypertrophy and heart failure. Thus, understanding the regulation of the SR Ca release channel in the intact cellular environment is a critical part in the comprehensive understanding of cellular cardiac function.

GENERAL METHODS

The experiments described here were performed with ventricular myocytes isolated from either rat, rabbit, or ferret hearts using standard methods. A superfusion chamber was mounted on the stage of an inverted microscope equipped for epifluorescence measurement of $[Ca]_i$ using the indicator indo-1, cell shortening using a video edge detector, ionic currents using whole-cell voltage clamp and incorporating a rapid solution switching device. Some experiments were also done using laser scanning confocal fluorescence microscopy (LSCFM). The details of the experimental methods are described more completely in the individual papers from which the figures below and the data discussed were obtained.[12–14] The normal conditions for these experiments were usually a default rate of stimulation (0.5 Hz), at 23 °C, and a modified normal Tyrode's solution (NT) containing (in mM): 140 NaCl, 6 KCl, 1 $MgCl_2$, 2 $CaCl_2$ (1 in rat experiments), 10 glucose, and 5 HEPES at pH 7.40.

Ca SPARKS AS FUNDAMENTAL EVENTS IN SR Ca RELEASE

Basic Properties of Ca Sparks

Ca sparks were first described as local spontaneous SR Ca release events in ventricular myocytes by Cheng *et al.*[15] using confocal microscopy. These localized Ca transients or Ca sparks are due to SR Ca release via RyR channels and represent release through either a single channel or, more likely, via a small cluster of RyR release channels working as a single functional unit.[16,17] Ca sparks can also be activated by Ca entry via L-type Ca current (I_{Ca}).[18,19] Indeed, the global Ca transient during the normal twitch is also made up of a very large number of Ca sparks occurring throughout the cell almost simultaneously.[20] Although individual Ca sparks are generally not distinguishable during the normal twitch, this is because the Ca sparks are synchronized by the action potential and L-type Ca current, and thus overlapping in both time and space. The decline of local $[Ca]_i$ during the Ca spark is largely due to Ca diffusing away from the site of release, but SR Ca reuptake also contributes significantly to $[Ca]_i$ decline.[21] Thus the rate of SR Ca pumping can effect the spatial and temporal spread of Ca sparks and may thereby influence their ability to activate neighboring regions.

An example of spontaneous Ca sparks in a resting ventricular myocyte is shown in FIGURE 1. FIGURE 1A shows a two-dimensional LSCFM image of a myocyte that happened to catch two separate Ca sparks (indicated by arrows). To increase temporal resolution it has been customary to use the line scan mode of the confocal microscope. In this cell we scanned the whole length of the cell every 4 ms along a line avoiding nuclei. FIGURE 1B shows part of a line scan image with a single prominent Ca spark. In this case distance along the cell length is shown in the vertical dimension and time along the horizontal dimension. FIGURE 1C shows the local $[Ca]_i$ in the narrow region of the cell where the Ca spark occurs (indicated by the bar in FIGURE 1B). The surface plot in FIGURE 1D shows the time and spatial dependence of local $[Ca]_i$ during this single Ca spark.

During rest there must be a finite rate of Ca leak from the SR. In the steady state this resting Ca leak may be compensated by Ca reuptake by the SR Ca-ATPase, such that the SR Ca content does not change. In some cell types this is the normal observation (e.g., rat ventricular myocytes), while in other cells the rate of resting Ca leak exceeds the rate of reuptake such that a net loss of Ca occurs during rest (e.g., in rabbit or guinea-pig ventricular myocytes).[1,22] The reasons for the different effects of rest on SR in different mammalian species will be discussed more explicitly below.

The finite SR Ca leak rate could, in principle, result from several pathways. However, it seems likely that much, if not all of this resting leak is through occasional openings of SR Ca release channels and Ca sparks. Bassani and Bers[23] measured the rate of unidirectional Ca leak from the SR in intact rat and rabbit ventricular myocytes as 0.3 μmol/l cytosol using global Ca measurements. Cheng *et al.*[15] estimated the Ca flux associated with a spark as $\sim 2 \times 10^{-19}$ mol, consistent with a single RyR current of 4 pA for 10 ms (40 fC). To explain a resting SR Ca leak rate of 0.3 μmol/l cytosol would require about 50 Ca sparks/s in the cell (or $\sim 2 \bullet \text{pL}^{-1} \bullet \text{s}^{-1}$). The 40-fC Ca spark flux used by Cheng *et al.*[15] may be at the upper limit of single RyR channel current under physiological conditions, where a single RyR channel flux of 6 fC (2 pA × 3 ms)[9] may be more realistic. This would be consistent with 6–7 RyR release channels contributing to the Ca flux at a single Ca spark.

It seems clear that the normal Ca transient during the twitch in ventricular myocytes is composed of a temporal and spatial summation of many Ca sparks, which are synchronized by the action potential and activation of Ca influx via Ca channels.[18,19] To attain the peak SR Ca release flux estimated by Wier *et al.*[24] (3 mM/s) would require si-

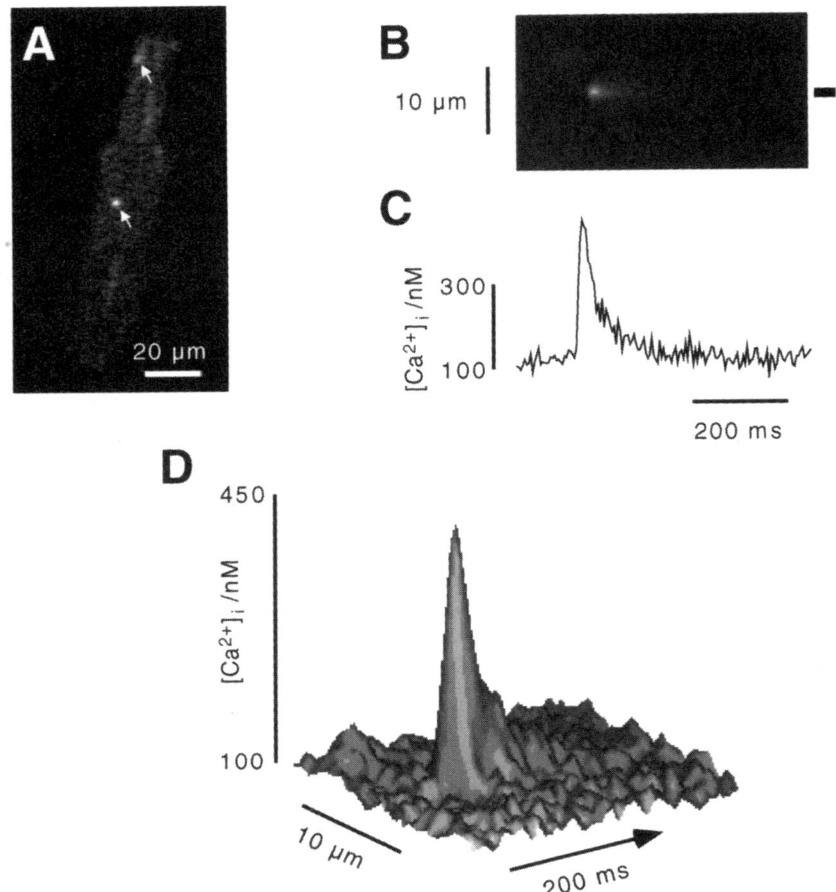

FIGURE 1. Typical Ca sparks in an isolated mouse ventricular myocyte. **A.** Two-dimensional laser scanning confocal fluorescence image of a single myocyte loaded with the Ca-sensitive indicator fluo-3, exhibiting two Ca sparks *(arrows)*. **B.** Line scan image along the long axis of a mouse ventricular myocyte (only part of the scanned cell length is shown). Scans were repeated every 4 ms and stacked from left to right. Distance along the cell is in the vertical direction. **C.** Line graph of $[Ca]_i$ measured at the spot indicated by the *bar* in B for the same line scan image (~1 µm). **D.** 3-D surface plot of $[Ca]_i$ during a Ca spark, indicating the temporal and spatial spread of Ca. (Original figure prepared by Dr. Jörg Hüser.)

multaneous activation of about 9,000 Ca sparks per 30-pL cell (within a few ms). If a Ca spark were due to a single RyR, this would require only 0.5% of the ~1.7 million RyR in a 30-pL rat ventricular myocyte.[25] Even if 6–7 RyR are required to produce the 40 fC of Ca flux above, this would still require only 3.4% of the total number of cellular RyRs. Furthermore, a total SR Ca release flux of 60 µmol/l cytosol[13] would also require only ~9,000 Ca sparks (based on 40 fC/spark) or 3–4% of the cellular RyR (based on 6 fC/RyR). Thus twitch activation requires only a small percentage of available release channels to function at any given twitch.

This low percentage of RyR required for activation is particularly interesting in the light of estimates of the fraction of L-type Ca channels required to produce the measured cellular Ca current (also only in the range of 3%).[26] Santana *et al.*[27] also inferred that the opening of a single L-type Ca channel can trigger a Ca spark and that the spark probability depends on the square of the local [Ca] in the space between the sarcolemmal Ca channel and the RyR. Thus spark frequency and SR Ca release clearly depend critically on the local cytosolic [Ca], and this is a cornerstone of Ca-induced Ca release as the E-C coupling mechanism in cardiac muscle.

SR Ca Load and Recovery Time Affect Spontaneous Resting Ca Spark Frequency

In addition to the local $[Ca]_i$, there are other factors that can alter Ca spark probability in resting ventricular myocytes. FIGURE 2 shows some results from Satoh *et al.*,[14] who studied the frequency of Ca sparks in both rabbit and rat ventricular myocytes. In rabbit ventricular myocytes there is a gradual decrease in Ca spark frequency after the last steady state stimulated twitch, whereas in the rat just the opposite is the case. The decrease in Ca spark frequency in rabbit is paralleled by a gradual decline in the amplitude of the post-rest twitch global Ca transients. This process is classically referred to as rest decay. This Ca transient decline was also paralleled by a gradual decline in SR Ca content assessed by caffeine-induced Ca_i transients. This resting loss in SR Ca can be completely prevented by switching to a Na-free, Ca-free solution during the rest period; and this changes the decline in Ca spark frequency in rabbit to a gradual increase that closely resembles that seen in the control rat. Thus it appears that the decline in Ca spark frequency during rest in rabbit can be attributed to a time-dependent decrease in SR Ca content. When the SR Ca load is changed in other ways (e.g., changing stimulation frequency or extracellular [Ca]) the Ca spark frequency parallels this, even when there is no change in the diastolic $[Ca]_i$ or time since the last stimulation. Clearly intra-SR Ca can modulate Ca spark frequency. This is also consistent with single-channel recordings where luminal Ca appears to increase open probability under a number of experimental conditions.[28,29]

Rat ventricular myocytes in FIGURE 2 under control conditions (and rabbit cells rested in 0Na, 0Ca) exhibit an increase in the Ca spark frequency during the first 10–20 seconds of rest. This frequency appears to reach a maximal value, and this is associated with a rest potentiation of the post-rest twitch Ca transient. This occurs without any change in SR Ca content during the rest as assessed by caffeine-induced Ca transients. It can also be seen without any increase in resting $[Ca]_i$. In fact, we demonstrated that the 7-nM rise in global diastolic $[Ca]_i$ in this circumstance in rat cells was caused by the increasing Ca spark frequency (rather than the rise in $[Ca]_i$ causing the increase in Ca spark frequency). Thus there is a clear time-dependent recovery after the last activation for the microscopic SR Ca release units to become available for Ca sparks with the control probability (and this requires several seconds to become complete). A somewhat faster component of Ca spark restitution has also been reported ($t_{1/2}$ ~0.5 s),[30] and these two phases of restitution may well coexist.

From the foregoing we conclude that the probability of an SR Ca release event depends on at least three key factors: (1) local $[Ca]_i$ as in Ca-induced Ca release, (2) intra-SR Ca load, perhaps attributable to a luminal effect of Ca, and (3) recovery of the SR Ca release channel from inactivation or adaptation.[8,11] However, the interaction of these factors is probably complex. One situation where this was brought to light by Satoh *et al.*[14] is when cellular Ca load approaches the overloaded state. In this case the

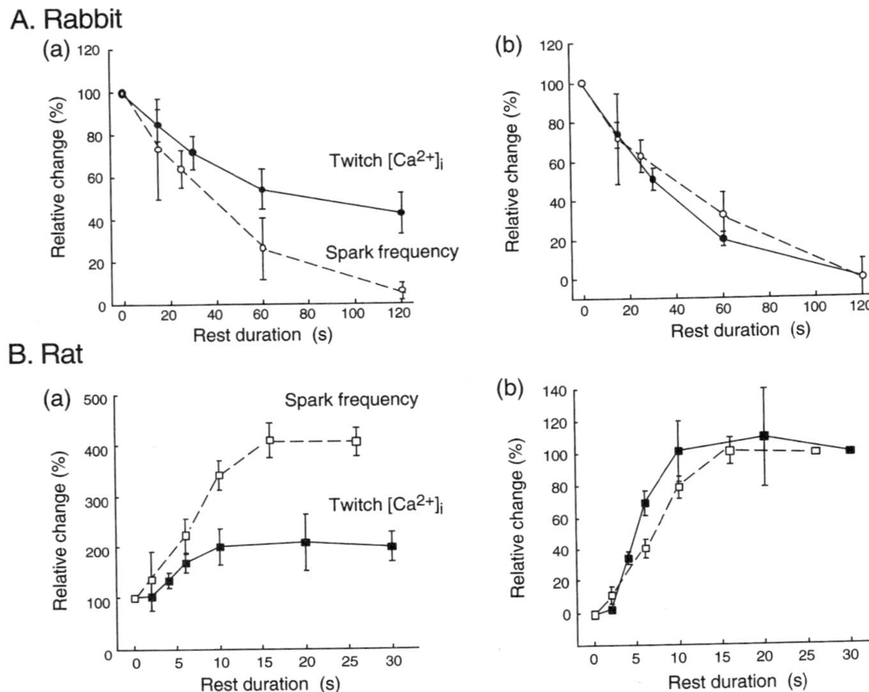

FIGURE 2. Frequency of Ca sparks in **(A)** rabbit and **(B)** rat ventricular myocytes during rest, after 1-Hz stimulation. The Ca spark frequency was normalized to the number of sparks observed during the first 2 s of rest in rabbit and rat *(solid symbols and lines)*. These initial values were ~90 and 40 sparks•pL^{-1}•s^{-1} for rabbit and rat, respectively, but by 15 s of rest this difference was reversed. The amplitude of the first post-rest global twitch Ca transient was normalized to the 1-Hz steady state twitch Ca transient *(broken lines)*. In **(b)** the data from **(a)** were further normalized to minimum and maximum values to allow more clear kinetic comparision between post-rest twitch $[Ca]_i$-transients and spark frequency. (Reprinted from Satoh *et al.*[14] with permission.)

relatively spark-free period after the twitch (attributed to the recovery of SR Ca release channels) was abolished.

REST POTENTIATION AND REST DECAY IN INTACT MYOCYTES

To extend the results from FIGURE 2 to a more macroscopic level we will discuss functional parallels observed in whole-cell Ca transients during twitches (FIG. 3). Rabbit and guinea-pig ventricular myocytes typically exhibit rest decay of twitches that is paralleled by decline in SR Ca content where caffeine-induced contractures and Ca transients were used to assess SR Ca content.[22,31,32] This can be seen in the two control (NT) curves in FIGURE 3A (where twitch refers to post-rest twitch amplitude and Caff reflects the SR Ca content). When the myocytes are incubated in 0Na, 0Ca solution during the rest, the gradual decline in SR Ca content is prevented, and rabbit exhibits

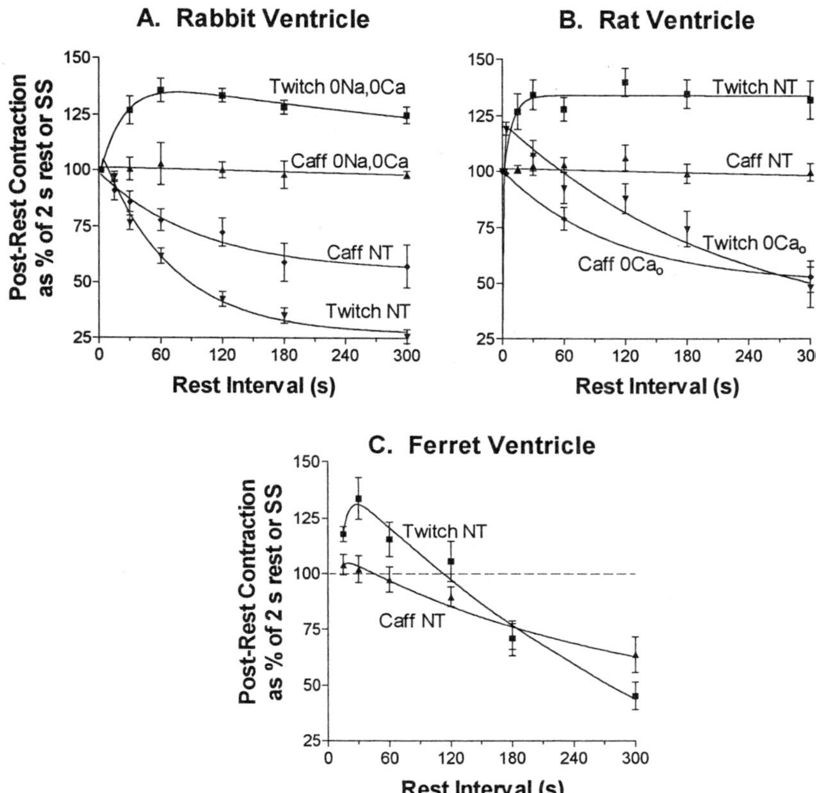

FIGURE 3. Amplitude of post-rest contractions in rabbit, rat, and ferret ventricular myocytes. Both post-rest twitches and caffeine-induced contractures (Caff) were measured either in a modified normal Tyrode's solution (NT), when Na/Ca exchange was blocked during the rest (0Na,0Ca), or after predepletion of $[Na]_i$ and rest in Ca-free 140 mM Na solution (0Ca$_o$). Caff data are indicative of SR Ca load. Data were fit with the expression $A \bullet \exp(-t/\tau_{RD})(1-\exp(-t/\tau_{RP})) + B$, where τ_{RP} is the time constant for recovery of E-C coupling, τ_{RD} is the time constant of rest decay of SR Ca content, B is a residual baseline, and A is a proportionality constant. (Data is from Bers *et al.*[31] and Bassani & Bers[32] and has been combined and reanalyzed.)

rest potentiation of twitches very much like that shown for the rat ventricular myocytes in NT in FIGURE 3B. Rat ventricular myocytes can be caused to exhibit rest decay as in the control rabbit, but this requires manipulation of the [Na] and/or [Ca] gradients.[32] When rat myocytes are depleted of intracellular Na and then exposed to a Ca-free, 140-mM Na solution during rest (to enhance the ability of Na/Ca exchange to extrude Ca from the cells), rat ventricular myocytes exhibit rest decay of twitches and SR Ca content (0Ca$_o$ in FIG. 3B).

Ferret ventricular myocytes exhibit intermediate responses (FIG. 3C). Under control conditions (NT) there is a monotonic decline in SR Ca content, but rest potentiation is seen at shorter rest intervals (up to 2 min) and rest decay at longer rests. It is now clear that most of the early rest potentiation in ferret is due to the recovery of E-C coupling from refractoriness, because there is no increase in SR Ca, action potential, or Ca current.[31] This behavior resembles that in the control rat and in the rabbit when SR Ca depletion is prevented by 0Na,0Ca. At longer rests in ferret, the SR Ca content is declining, and this may limit the twitch amplitude at longer times. Indeed, the curve fit for the ferret twitch data in FIGURE 3C reflects a simple model where twitch amplitude is proportional to the product of two exponentials, one the slow decline of SR Ca available ($\tau \sim 250$ s), the other an exponentially recovering fraction of SR Ca release (reflecting the faster recovery of E-C coupling, $\tau \sim 6$ s). Thus, these two aspects have opposite effects, with recovery of E-C coupling dominant at short times and the SR Ca content at long times in ferret. In contrast, control rabbit is dominated by rest decay and control rat by rest potentiation. It may be useful to consider where some other common experimental species fit in this comparison.[1,31] Guinea-pig ventricle behaves much like rabbit in this regard, being dominated by rest decay. Mouse ventricle shows mainly rest potentiation like the rat, while feline, canine, and human ventricle seem to be most like ferret, exhibiting a combination of rest potentiation and rest decay.

It is also worth clarifying why rabbit and ferret SR lose Ca during rest and why 0Na, 0Ca solution prevents resting loss (or gain) of SR Ca. Na/Ca exchange is the main cellular competitor with the SR Ca-ATPase.[1] Thus as Ca leaks from the SR, its fate is to be transported either back into the SR by the Ca-ATPase or out of the cell by Na/Ca exchange. In 0Na, 0Ca solution the Na/Ca exchange is completely blocked, so virtually all of the Ca leaked by the SR is resequestered and there is no loss in content with time (as in FIG. 3A). When the Na/Ca exchange is functional, the SR may be slowly depleted and the rate will depend on how well the Na/Ca exchange competes with the SR Ca pump. In rabbit ventricle the Na/Ca exchanger is relatively potent in this regard, whereas in rat a weaker Na/Ca exchanger coupled with a stronger SR Ca-ATPase[13] makes the Na/Ca exchange less effective. In addition Shattock and Bers[33] reported higher resting $[Na]_i$ in rat ventricle, which would even further limit the ability of this system to extrude Ca during rest.

E-C COUPLING: I_{Ca}, SR Ca LOAD, AND FRACTIONAL SR Ca RELEASE

Fabiato[34] showed that for a given SR Ca content the amount of Ca released is graded as a function of the amount of triggering Ca. This classic and still incompletely understood graded behavior of Ca-induced Ca-release is illustrated in FIGURE 4. As test pulse voltage is varied, the amplitude of contraction (and underlying Ca transient) parallels the amplitude of the Ca current (I_{Ca}). FIGURE 4B shows another way to look at the same type of data. In this case contraction amplitude is plotted directly as a function of I_{Ca}, where each point on the loop is from a different test potential (E_m). It is important to note that each test pulse is preceded by a series of at least five conditioning pulses to ensure that the SR Ca content is the same for each test pulse. When the SR Ca load was decreased by reducing the intensity of the conditioning train, there was a smaller contraction for a given I_{Ca}. Thus there is lower SR Ca release at lower load. There is also little hysteresis in these loops, which suggests that there is little intrinsic E_m-dependence of SR Ca release, in agreement with other results.[35,36] Indeed, what hysteresis there is is such that the same I_{Ca} at negative voltages is slightly more efficacious in producing SR Ca release. This is consistent with results of Wier *et al.*[24] and may be due to larger single-channel currents at negative E_m, making them more likely to trigger Ca release from local RyRs. It should also be noted that these experiments were done under conditions of very low $[Na]_i$ so that Ca entry via Na/Ca exchange was prevented. With high $[Na]_i$ larger contractions and Ca transients can be observed for a given I_{Ca} at positive E_m. Indeed, several studies have suggested that Ca entry via Na/Ca

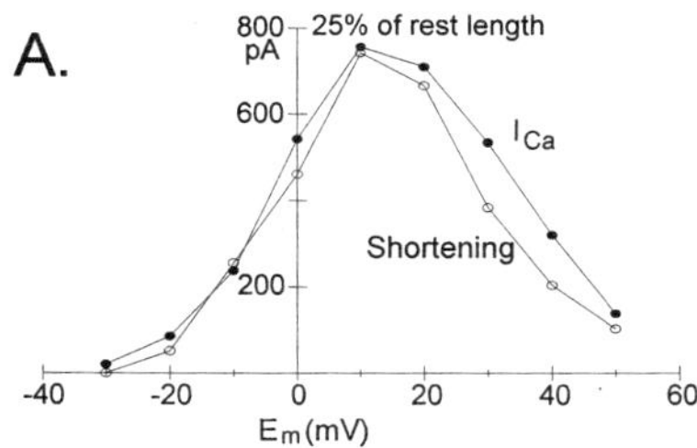

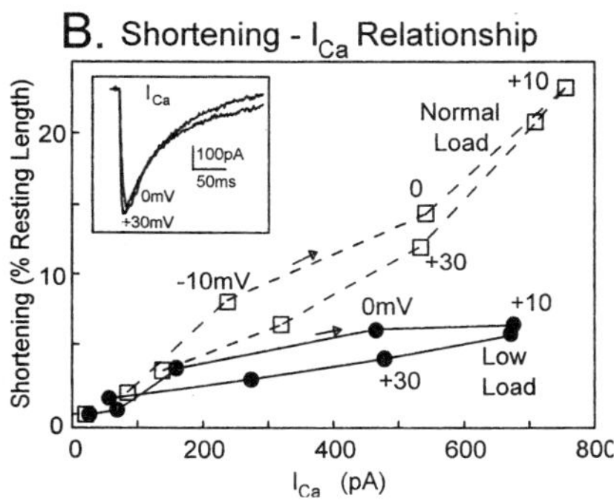

FIGURE 4. Ca-induced Ca release in E-C coupling in a ferret ventricular myocyte. **A.** Bell-shaped I_{Ca}- and contraction-voltage relationships. A set of five conditioning pulses (from –70 mV to 0 mV) preceded the test pulses to different potentials (E_m). Contraction and I_{Ca} were recorded simultaneously. **B.** Contraction amplitude is plotted as a function of I_{Ca} for normal load as in **A** and for a low SR Ca load (after a weaker train of conditioning pulses). The **inset** shows raw current traces from the normal curve at –30 and 0 mV. (Reprinted from Bassani *et al.*[41] with permission.)

exchange can contribute to the trigger for SR Ca release under certain conditions.[37–39] Precisely how much this contributes to the physiological triggering of SR Ca release remains to be elucidated.

Although these types of studies have been very powerful, they have not provided quantitative information about exactly what fraction of SR Ca is released at a twitch and how this is modified by changes in either triggering I_{Ca} or by the level of SR Ca load. Bassani *et al.*[40,41] developed an experimental strategy to examine these issues, using Ca transients in intact ferret ventricular myocytes evoked by action potentials and application of caffeine. FIGURE 5 shows their results. In FIGURE 5A the SR Ca load was kept constant and the fractional SR Ca release was measured at different levels of Ca current trigger (in this case by changing $[Ca]_o$). As when I_{Ca} was changed by altering test potential, increasing trigger I_{Ca} produced parallel increases in the fraction of SR Ca released. This is expected according to Ca-induced Ca release, but this data provides an indication of what fraction of SR Ca gets released under normal conditions (~35% in ferret) and over what dynamic range it is modulated (from 10 to 60%) as the I_{Ca} trigger is varied by changing $[Ca]_o$ over a 16-fold range.

The converse experiment is illustrated in FIGURE 5B, where SR Ca load was varied with a constant I_{Ca} trigger. The normal SR Ca load at 0.5-Hz stimulation was 91 µmol/l cytosol, and 35% was released at the normal twitch. When cells were paced at 0.8 Hz and at high $[Ca]_o$ (8 mM), the SR Ca load reached a maximum of 95 µmol/l cytosol. This maximal point was when the cells were on the verge of Ca overload (i.e., just below the frequency where large spontaneous SR Ca release and waves occurred). It was somewhat surprising that the twitch Ca transients were so much larger with only a 4% increase in SR Ca load. Indeed, the amount of SR Ca released was almost doubled (from 32 to 56 µmol/l cytosol), but most of this increase was due to an increase in fractional SR Ca release (from 35 to 59%) rather than the amount available for release. It is possible that the SR Ca load is limited by the thermodynamic capacity of the SR

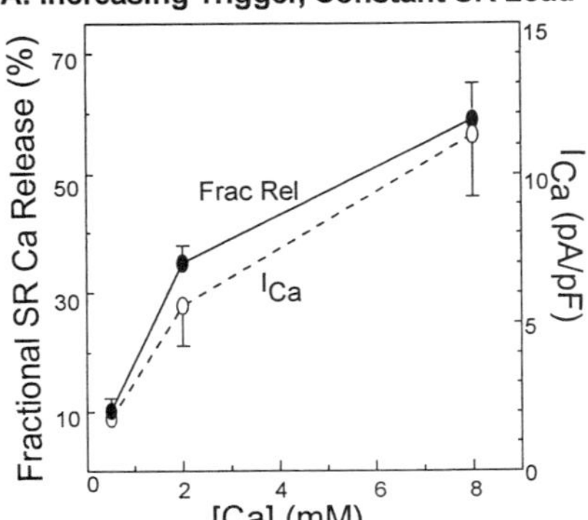

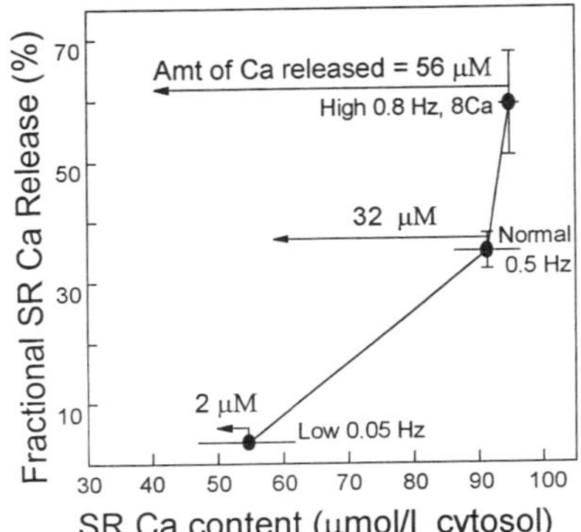

FIGURE 5. Modulation of fractional SR Ca release by varying I_{Ca} trigger and SR Ca load during the twitch in ferret ventricular myocytes. **A.** Cells were loaded to a constant level (by stimulation at 0.5 Hz), and $[Ca]_o$ was changed just prior to the test contraction where the fraction of SR Ca release is measured. Thus, increasing trigger (at constant SR Ca load) increases fractional release. Parallel voltage clamp experiments were done to evaluate how I_{Ca} changes over this range of $[Ca]_o$. **B.** Using a constant trigger (with 2 mM $[Ca]_o$) the SR of cells were Ca loaded to different levels by varying frequency (as indicated) and also increasing $[Ca]_o$ at the highest load. SR Ca content was measured by translating the peak and resting $[Ca]_i$ during caffeine-induced contractures to total cytosolic [Ca], using measured values for cytosolic Ca buffering.[83] (Reprinted from Bassani *et al.*[41] with permission.)

Ca-ATPase to generate a free *trans* SR [Ca] gradient.[42] It is also possible that under our normal conditions the intra-SR Ca buffers such as calsequestrin become saturated so that there is little increase in SR Ca content with more aggressive stimulation, for a given increase in intra-SR free [Ca] ($[Ca]_{SR}$). This possible rise in $[Ca]_{SR}$ may in turn exert some effect to increase RyR gating and thereby fractional release. Whether luminal Ca exerts this effect directly on the RyR or via some less direct means cannot be assessed in these whole-cell measurements, but luminal Ca has been reported to increase RyR open probability in single channels.[28,29] In the skeletal muscle RyR the effect of luminal Ca to increase open probability has been attributed to Ca coming out through the channel acting at a cytoplasmic site,[43] but this may not be the case in the cardiac channel.[29]

Luminal Ca may thus be an important integral control of SR Ca release. Furthermore, what is usually referred to as spontaneous SR Ca release associated with cellular Ca overload, may really be release triggered by intra-SR Ca. Furthermore, The increase in fractional SR Ca release works synergistically with increases in Ca load and may even be the more important factor at relatively high SR Ca loads.

The effects of reduction of SR Ca load are also of interest (FIG. 5B). When SR Ca load is decreased by greatly reducing the frequency of stimulation, the fractional SR Ca release is dramatically reduced. In FIGURE 5B reduction of SR load by only 40% almost abolished SR Ca release. That is, only 4% of the SR Ca load was released (2 µmol/l cytosol), and this amount is much less than even the amount of Ca that enters the cell via I_{Ca} (5–12 µmol/l cytosol).[44] Thus at low levels of SR Ca load, the SR nearly stops participating in E-C coupling even though there is still a large pool of Ca available for release (55 µmol/l cytosol).

From the foregoing sections it is clear that at both microscopic and whole-cell levels, the SR Ca release by the RyR in its normal cellular environment is regulated by $[Ca]_i$, $[Ca]_{SR}$, and recovery time from a previous activation. In addition, it is well known that the RyR can be modulated by many other endogenous as well as exogenous moieties. In the following sections effects of several specific modulators on SR Ca release in the intact ventricular myocyte will be discussed.

CaMKII INCREASES FRACTIONAL SR Ca RELEASE

Endogenous effector systems may be important in the regulation of E-C coupling. Ca-calmodulin–dependent protein kinase (CaMKII) is a ubiquitous Ca-dependent second messenger system that has been implicated in the control of processes from gene transcription to active cellular memory. The cardiac RyR has also been identified as a specific target for CaMKII phosphorylation,[45] and several reports have examined the effects of exogenous CaMKII on the RyR in bilayers and SR vesicles.[45,46] However, these results have not provided a clear understanding of how this modulation works in the intact cell. Indeed, the cyclical nature of the cardiac Ca transient and its physiological modulation by heart rate and hormones make it particularly important to evaluate effects of CaMKII on SR Ca release in the intact cell.

Li *et al.*[47] evaluated the effects of endogenous CaMKII on E-C coupling in intact ventricular myocytes. These studies were performed using the perforated patch variation of whole-cell voltage clamp. This allows measurement of currents without dialyzing cell proteins or small regulatory molecules out of the cell. Thus the physiological environment is especially well preserved. Since we know that SR Ca load and I_{Ca} can strongly affect the amount of SR Ca release, I_{Ca} and SR Ca load must be measured and controlled in these cellular experiments. This way the influence of other agents on the E-C coupling process can be appropriately evaluated. Thus, if we can make the SR Ca load the same and the I_{Ca} trigger the same, we can examine how agents (such as the CaMKII inhibitor KN-93) alter the relationship between trigger Ca and SR Ca release. FIGURE 6 shows voltage clamp experiments from Li *et al.*[47] and indicates how the SR Ca load at the end of a train of conditioning voltage clamp pulses was matched in the absence and presence of the CaMKII inhibitor KN-93. After a series of five conditioning voltage clamp pulses were given, 10 mM caffeine was rapidly applied, causing release of the SR Ca content. The maintained caffeine exposure prevented reaccumulation of Ca by the SR. The peak of the caffeine-induced contracture and Ca transient give two estimates of SR Ca content (see FIG. 6, left). In addition, during the caffeine application almost all of the SR Ca is extruded by Na/Ca exchange,[12,13,48] which produces an inward current ($I_{Na/CaX}$). This $I_{Na/CaX}$ can be integrated to provide an additional measure of the SR Ca content.[49,50] Because KN-93 slightly decreases I_{Ca}, a somewhat more aggressive series of conditioning pulses was often required to obtain matching SR Ca loads with KN-93 vs. control. The bar graph in FIGURE 6C indicates that the SR Ca load achieved with KN-93 was the same as in control.

Having established an unchanged SR Ca load, Li *et al.*[47] could assess the relationship between trigger I_{Ca} and SR Ca release. In FIGURE 7A it can be seen that for a given I_{Ca} (and SR Ca load), the contraction produced with CaMKII blocked was much smaller. The mean twitch contractions and Ca transients in the presence of KN-93 were 39 ± 4% and 49 ± 6% of control (for matched SR Ca load and I_{Ca}). This effect was consistent throughout the E_m range studied. Furthermore, the depressant effect on E-C coupling was partially reversible and could not be mimicked by KN-92, an analog of KN-93 that does not inhibit CaMKII. Moreover, if weaker conditioning trains were used, then KN-93 had little or no effect. This is consistent with CaMKII normally

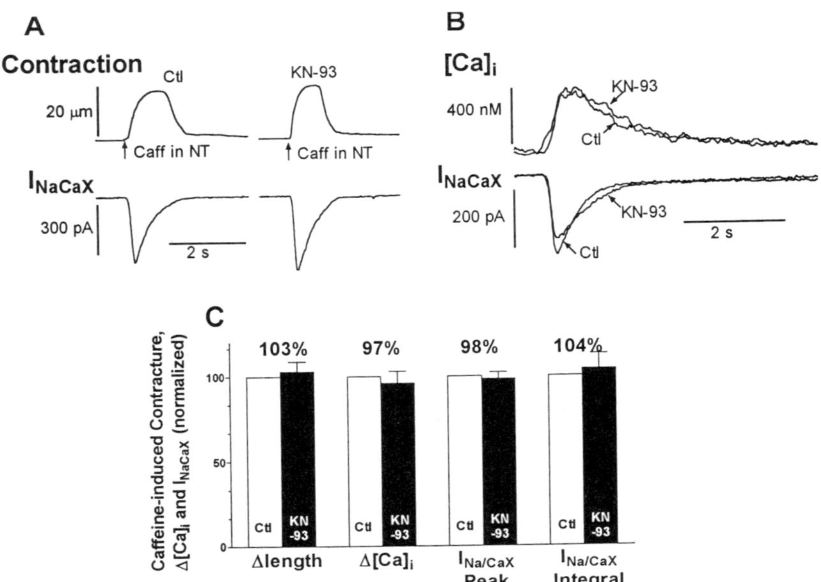

FIGURE 6. Testing the matching of SR Ca load in the study of CaMKII effects on E-C coupling. After a train of conditioning pulses, caffeine was applied to release SR Ca (**A** and **B**). The amplitude of the resulting contraction, Ca transient, and Na/Ca exchange current ($I_{Na/CaX}$) and the integral of Ca extruded by $I_{Na/CaX}$ are all quantitative indices of the SR Ca content. The bar graph **(C)** shows pooled results for these measures in the absence and presence of KN-93. (Modified from Li *et al.*[47] with permission.)

being activated by the Ca transients during the conditioning pulses. Complementary studies by duBell *et al.*[51] showed that dialysis of voltage clamped ventricular myocytes (using ruptured patch) with exogenous phosphatases also inhibited E-C coupling (although the specific protein kinase pathway involved was not delineated). These results suggest that endogenous CaMKII–dependent phosphorylation of the RyR may be a physiologically important regulator of SR Ca release in intact cells. This same general protocol we devised for studying the effects of CaMKII on E-C coupling above has also been used to study several other modulators in the intact cellular environment.

OTHER FACTORS THAT ALTER E-C COUPLING

E-C Coupling is Altered by FK-506

Immunophillin FK binding proteins (FKBPs) are peptide isomerases and also bind to and copurify with the RyR.[52–54] These FKBPs are the targets for the immunosuppresant drugs FK-506 and rapamycin, and these agents can cause dissociation of FKBP from the RyR.[52] FK-506, rapamycin, or direct removal of FKBP from the RyR has been reported to alter RyR channel gating in bilayer studies,[55–58] although Barg *et al.*[59] found that removal of FKBP modulated gating of only the skeletal and not the cardiac RyR. For the cardiac RyR Kaftan *et al.*[58] found that removal of FKBP destabilizes

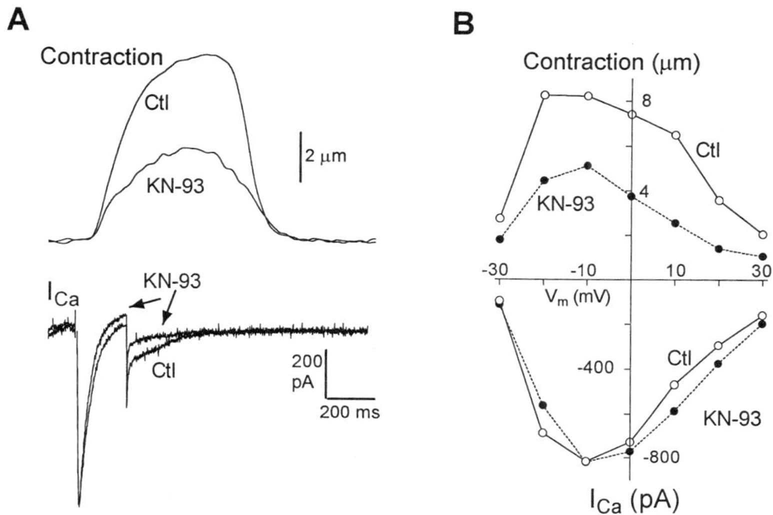

FIGURE 7. The CaMKII inhibitor KN-93 depresses E-C coupling at constant SR Ca load with simultaneous recording of I_{Ca} and cell contraction. **A.** For the same SR Ca load and I_{Ca} the contraction is much smaller in the presence of the CaMKII inhibitor KN-93. The larger tail current in control is due to larger inward $I_{Na/CaX}$ (secondary to the larger Ca transient). **B.** Complete E_m-dependence for an experiment as in **A** where I_{Ca} was not much depressed by KN-93. (Modified from Li *et al.*[47] with permission.)

the gating of the channel such that there is an overall increase in open probability with the appearance of subconductance states. Indeed, when exogenous recombinant FKBP was added to recombinant RyR in bilayers, the channel gating properties with FKBP were restored.

Whole-cell studies have been undertaken to better understand how FKBP may alter SR Ca release in the intact cell.[60–62] McCall *et al.*[60] found that FK-506 increased twitch Ca transients, even when the SR Ca content was unchanged (FIG. 8). They also found that there was no effect on I_{Ca}, suggesting that FK-506 enhanced E-C coupling. On the average FK-506 also increased resting Ca spark frequency by a factor of four and increased steady state SR Ca content. Thus the six cells in FIGURE 8 were a selected subset that happened not to show a net change in SR Ca content. This was convenient for the sake of comparing twitch Ca transients at constant SR Ca load, but normally the SR Ca load was also increased.[60] Given the higher Ca spark rate and greater SR Ca release during twitches, one might have expected lower SR Ca load. However, FK-506 also depressed Na/Ca exchange, and it is possible that the inhibition of the Na/Ca exchange allows more Ca to remain in the cell and SR (explaining the enhanced SR Ca load). Xiao *et al.*[61] found similar results with higher concentrations of FK-506 (50 μM) with respect to Ca transients, I_{Ca} and sparks, but they found that the Ca sparks were longer in duration and that there was also a population of lower-amplitude events. These Ca spark results corresponded to some RyR bilayer findings[58] and was also consistent with their observation of a slowing of RyR adaptation in bilayers. At lower FK-506 concentration (5–10 μM) McCall *et al.*[60] did not find measurable changes in either Ca spark amplitude or duration. In addition to its effects on the SR Ca release process,

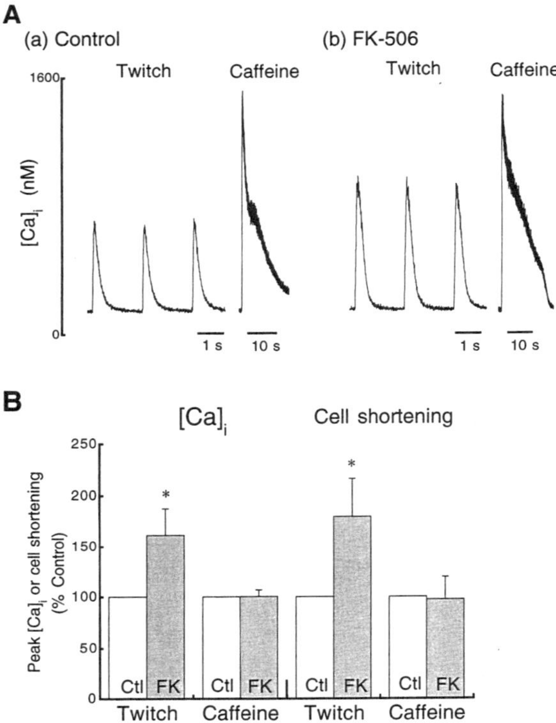

FIGURE 8. Effects of FK-506 on Ca transients and contractions during twitches and caffeine-induced contractures in rat ventricular myocytes. **A.** FK-506 (5 μM) increased twitch Ca transients (measured with fluo-3) even when SR Ca content was not altered (based on caffeine-induced Ca transients). **B.** Pooled data from a subset of six cells that did not show the more typical increase in SR Ca content with FK-506 (allowing simpler conclusions). The observation that neither caffeine-induced Ca transients nor contractures were modified also suggests no change in myofilament Ca sensitivity with FK-506. (Reprinted from McCall *et al.*[60] with permission.)

duBell *et al.*[62] showed that 25 μM FK-506 inhibits outward K currents in ventricular myocytes, causing prolongation of the action potential duration. This action potential duration effect may also contribute to the positive inotropic action of FK-506 reported in the other studies. Endogenous FKBP may have a stabilizing effect on the RyR in intact cells. This may limit SR Ca release during twitches and also limit spontaneous SR Ca release, which can be arrhythmogenic.

Bay K 8644 Alters SR Ca Release at Rest and During E-C Coupling

Bay K 8644 is a well-known L-type Ca channel agonist that prolongs the openings of single Ca channel and thereby substantially increases I_{Ca}.[63] Hryshko *et al.*[64,65] first reported that Bay K 8644 also greatly accelerated the rest decay of twitches in canine ventricle. McCall *et al.*[66] followed up these observations using ferret ventricle and found that this accelerated rest decay was due to rapid depletion of SR Ca during rest. They also demonstrated that Bay K 8644 increased ryanodine binding in intact myocytes, but this effect was abolished by cellular disruption. Finally, they demonstrated that the Bay K 8644–induced acceleration of resting SR Ca loss was still present in the complete absence of extracellular Ca and when Na/Ca exchange was prevented. This proved that resting Ca influx was not involved in triggering the loss of SR Ca. Satoh *et al.*[67] also showed that Bay K 8644 dramatically increased the frequency of Ca sparks in ferret ventricular myocytes (even in Ca-free solution) and that this effect could be inhibited by nifedipine. This increased SR Ca leak then explained the faster resting SR Ca loss. These studies led to the working hypothesis depicted in FIGURE 9. This cartoon illustrates that there may be a relatively direct, Ca influx–independent pathway whereby Bay K 8644 binds to the dihydropyridine receptor (DHPR) and propagates some conformational change to the resting cardiac RyR to increase its open probability.[66] This intriguing hypothesis probably merits further study. It may also be worth noting that given the stoichiometry of RyR to DHPR in ferret ventricular myocytes (10:1)[25] this sort of direct effect could involve a maximum of only 10% of the RyRs in the cell. Additionally, even if there is such a relatively direct physical link,[68] this does not necessarily imply that it is the same link as in skeletal muscle, where this sort of link is thought to mediate E_m-dependent SR Ca release during E-C coupling.[69,70]

McCall and Bers[71] extended these studies with Bay K 8644 to do the type of E-C coupling experiments described above for CaMKII (in FIG. 7). FIGURE 10 shows the somewhat surprising result that Bay K 8644 depressed E-C coupling. That is, for a given I_{Ca} and SR Ca content, the contraction was smaller after exposure to 100 nM Bay K 8644 (note that manipulation of E_m or $[Ca]_o$ was used to achieve comparable I_{Ca} and SR Ca load with Bay K 8644). One explanation for this depression of E-C coupling is that once Bay K 8644 binds to the DHPR (which increases diastolic RyR

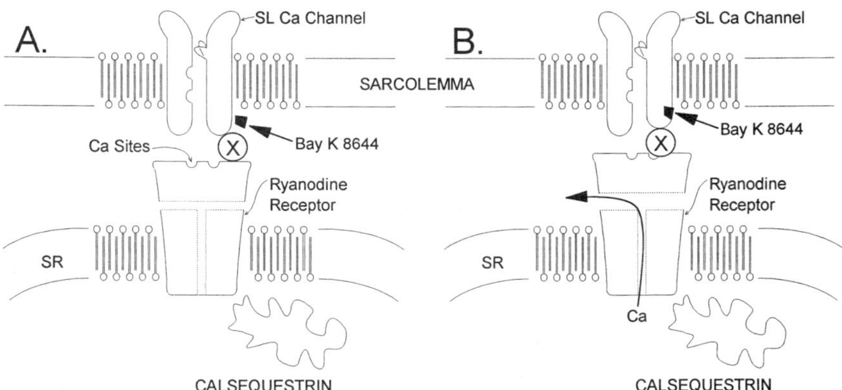

FIGURE 9. Simplified schematic diagram of how Bay K 8644 might cause increased RyR gating via an effect on the dihydropyridine receptor. Bay K 8644 may bind to the dihydropyridine receptor on the L-type Ca channel, and this may alter RyR state by a relatively direct (Ca influx independent) coupling, perhaps through an intermediate protein (X).

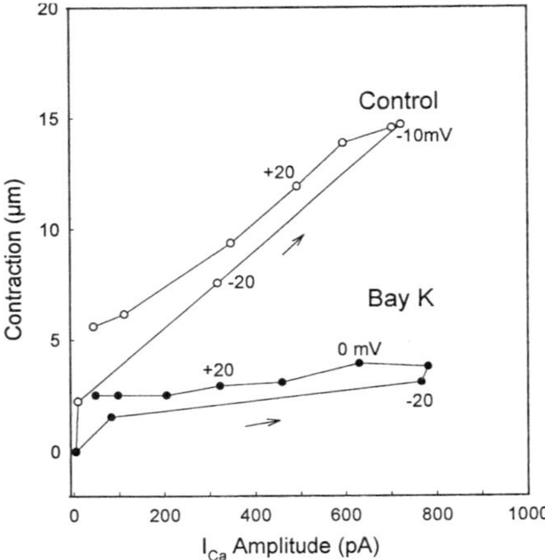

FIGURE 10. Bay K 8644 depresses the efficacy of I_{Ca} to activate SR Ca release in ferret ventricular myocytes. Conditioned current-voltage relationships were assessed in the absence and presence of 100 nM Bay K 8644 (as in FIGS. 4 and 7). The SR Ca content was verified to be the same for both conditions using caffeine-induced contractures. Lower $[Ca]_o$ or manipulation of E_m was used to obtain comparable load and I_{Ca} in the presence of Bay K 8644 compared to control. (Reprinted from McCall & Bers[71] with permission).

openings indirectly), the RyR becomes less sensitive to activating Ca coming from the sarcolemmal Ca channel (cartooned in FIG. 9 as linker X partially blocking a possible Ca activating site). While this may be an interesting untested possibility, there is another, simpler explanation that does not require this scheme. Since Bay K 8644 increases some of the single-channel open times dramatically from 0.5–1 ms to 10–20 ms,[63] fewer individual sarcolemmal Ca channels are expected to have opened for a given peak I_{Ca} (because more of them will remain open). If the first 0.5–1 ms of channel opening is sufficient for activation of the neighboring RyR, then longer opening of individual sarcolemmal Ca channels is essentially wasted in terms of activation of SR Ca release. Thus, Bay K 8644 may cause a given whole-cell I_{Ca} to be less efficacious simply because of the way it alters single-channel gating of the L-type Ca channel.

Cardiac Hypertrophy and Heart Failure Alter E-C Coupling

Cardiac pathophysiological research has also benefited from the types of studies described above. The SR has been increasingly implicated in the progression of cellular dysfunction in hypertrophy and heart failure.[72] Indeed, down-regulation of the SR Ca-ATPase has been reported in several experimental animal models of hypertrophy[73–75] and also in the failing human heart.[76–78] Consequently much work has focused on the SR Ca-ATPase and its possible involvement in slowed relaxation and $[Ca]_i$ decline and reduced SR Ca loading. On the other hand, Brilliantes *et al.*[79] reported a decrease in RyR mRNA expression in human heart failure. With SR Ca-ATPase it may be reasonable to expect that the Ca transport dysfunction may be roughly in proportion to the number of pumps expressed. For the RyR, relatively subtle changes in channel gating could have profound effects on cellular Ca regulation (diastolic and systolic). Thus, functional effect of RyR regulation could be out of proportion with expression of the protein. Unfortunately, there has not been extensive study with the type of controlled experiments described here in ventricular myocytes isolated from failing and nonfailing human ventricle.

On the other hand, two recent studies have used these strategies in the study of ventricular myocytes isolated from hypertrophic and failing rat ventricles.[80,81] Gómez *et al.*[80] studied hypertensive salt-sensitive Dahl rats (Dahl-SS) with ventricular hypertrophy and also a line of spontaneously hypertensive rats that develop congestive heart failure (SH-HF). The hypertrophic myocytes isolated from Dahl-SS hearts had normal spontaneous Ca sparks, I_{Ca} density, RyR number, RyR single-channel properties, and SR Ca content. However, a given I_{Ca} produced a smaller number of Ca sparks as well as reduced global Ca transients compared to controls. They inferred that this reflected a depression of E-C coupling in the hypertrophied myocytes (as with KN-93 in FIG. 7), and myocytes from the SH-HF showed the same effect. In the Dahl-SS rats the depression of E-C coupling could be overcome by activation with β-adrenergic agonists, but this was not the case with the SH-HF rats. They speculated that there might be some kind of spatial defect in hypertrophy and failure (a larger gap between RyR and DHPR), such that a given I_{Ca} influx could not activate the nearby RyRs as well as in control. There is no structural evidence for this speculative hypothesis, but functionally any effect that reduces the apparent sensitivity of SR Ca release to a given I_{Ca} trigger would fit the data (and the geometric idea is intriguing). Stimulation of I_{Ca} by isoproterenol could then have allowed E-C coupling to be restored (although there was no control for intrinsic effects of cyclic AMP–dependent protein kinase on E-C coupling).

In studies of a more moderate model of chronic pressure overload hypertrophy in the rat (induced by coarctation of the abdominal aorta for 16 weeks), McCall *et al.*[81] and Delbridge *et al.*[82] also found normal I_{Ca} density, numbers, and affinity of RyR and SR Ca content in these significantly hypertrophied left ventricular myocytes. At normal $[Ca]_o$ there was also no depression of E-C coupling (in experiments like those in FIG. 7). However, when $[Ca]_o$ was reduced to 0.5 mM, there was a substantial depression of E-C coupling in hypertrophic myocytes vs. those from sham-operated animals (even though SR Ca loads were still comparable between the groups). This is entirely consistent with the results of Gómez *et al.*[80] with more severe hypertrophy and heart failure. With the less severe hypertrophy the defect may be more subtle and the normal I_{Ca} trigger may be just strong enough to mask the developing pathophysiology. Indeed, this could mark the state prior to overt heart failure.

Thus, defects in the regulation of SR Ca release must be considered in pathophysiological alterations in cardiac function. These sorts of controlled studies are really just beginning. Even in the case of reduced SR Ca-ATPase expression and SR Ca accumulation, this bears consideration. This is especially the case because any reduction in optimal steady state SR Ca loading will not only reduce the amount of Ca available for release, but also the fraction of SR Ca released (e.g., as shown in FIG. 5B).

SUMMARY

This paper emphasizes the importance of studying the behavior of SR Ca release and the RyR in the normal cellular environment. Complementary electrophysiological and Ca measurements in intact single cells with studies of more isolated and inherently controllable systems (such as SR vesicles and RyR in bilayers) will continue to be valuable in building a more integrated and comprehensive understanding of how SR Ca release is regulated in physiological and pathophysiological contexts. The studies described here have shown that the RyR is sensitive to $[Ca]_i$, $[Ca]_{SR}$, and time after the last activation, where increasing any of these can increase SR Ca release. Endogenous CaMKII and FK-506 also appear to increase the efficacy of E-C coupling, while Bay K 8644 and cardiac hypertrophy or failure may lead to a decrease in the efficacy of a given I_{Ca} trigger to release SR Ca, even with the same SR Ca load.

ACKNOWLEDGMENTS

The authors acknowledge the talented contributions of Drs. Rosana Bassani, José Bassani, Lothar Blatter, Kenneth S. Ginsburg, and Weilong Yuan. Dr. Jörg Hüser prepared FIGURE 1 from his experiments. We thank Ms. Christina Hovance and Mr. Steven Scaglione for careful work in isolating cardiac myocytes.

REFERENCES

1. BERS, D. M. 1991. Excitation-Contraction Coupling and Cardiac Contractile Force. Kluwer Academic Press. Dordrecht, Netherlands.
2. MEISSNER, G & J. S. HENDERSON. 1987. Rapid calcium release from cardiac sarcoplasmic reticulum vesicles is dependent on Ca^{2+} and is modulated by Mg^{2+}, adenine nucleotide, and calmodulin. J. Biol. Chem. **262:** 3065–3073.
3. CORONADO, R., J. MORISETTE, M. SUKHAREVA, & D. M. VAUGHAN. 1994. Structure and function of the ryanodine receptors. Am. J. Physiol. **266:** C1485–C1504.
4. MEISSNER, G. 1986 Ryanodine activation and inhibition of the Ca^{2+} release channel of sarcoplasmic reticulum. J. Biol. Chem. **261:** 6300–6306.
5. ROUSSEAU, E. & G. MEISSNER. 1989. Single cardiac sarcoplasmic reticulum Ca^{2+}-release channel: Activation by caffeine. Am. J. Physiol. **256:** H328–H333.
6. ROUSSEAU, E., J. S. SMITH, J. S. HENDERSON & G. MEISSNER. 1986. Single channel and $^{45}Ca^{2+}$ flux measurements of the cardiac sarcoplasmic reticulum calcium channel. Biophys. J. **50:** 1009–1014.
7. ROUSSEAU, E., J. S. SMITH & G. MEISSNER. 1987. Ryanodine modifies conductance and gating behavior of single Ca^{2+} release channel. Am. J. Physiol. **253:** C364–C368.
8. GYÖRKE, S. & M. FILL. 1993. Ryanodine receptor adaptation: Control mechanism of Ca^{2+}-induced Ca^{2+} release in heart. Science **260:** 807–809.
9. TINKER, A., LINDSAY, A. R. G. & A. J. WILLIAMS. 1993. Cation conductance in the calcium release channel of the cardiac sarcoplasmic reticulum under physiological and pathophysiological conditions. Cardiovasc. Res. **27:** 1820–1825.
10. VALDIVIA, H. H., J. H. KAPLAN, G. C. R. ELLIS-DAVIES & W. J. LEDERER. 1995. Rapid adaptation of cardiac ryanodine receptors: Modulation by Mg^{2+} and phosphorylation. Science **267:** 1997–1999.
11. SCHIEFER, A., G. MEISSNER & G. ISENBERG. 1995. Ca^{2+} activation and Ca^{2+} inactivation of cardiac sarcoplasmic reticulum Ca^{2+}-release channels. J. Physiol. **489:** 337–348.
12. BASSANI, R. A., J. W. M. BASSANI & D. M. BERS. 1992. Mitochondrial and sarcolemmal Ca transport can reduce $[Ca]_i$ during caffeine contractures in rabbit cardiac myocytes. J. Physiol. **453:** 591–608.
13. BASSANI, J. W. M., R. A. BASSANI & D. M. BERS. 1994. Relaxation in rabbit and rat cardiac cells: Species-dependent differences in cellular mechanisms. J. Physiol. **476:** 279–293.
14. SATOH, H., L. A. BLATTER & D. M. BERS. 1997. Effects of $[Ca]_i$, Ca^{2+} load and rest on Ca^{2+} spark frequency in ventricular myocytes. Am. J. Physiol. **272:** H657–668.
15. CHENG, H., W. J. LEDERER & M. B. CANNELL. 1993. Calcium sparks: Elementary events underlying excitation-contraction coupling in heart muscle. Science **262:** 740–744.
16. TSUGORKA, A., E. RIOS & L. A. BLATTER 1995. Imaging elementary events of calcium release in skeletal muscle cells. Science **269:** 1723–1726.
17. PARKER, I., W. J. ZANG & W. G. WIER. 1996. Ca^{2+} sparks involving multiple Ca^{2+} release sites along Z-lines in rat heart cells. J. Physiol. **497:** 31–38.
18. CANNELL, M. B., H. CHENG & W. J. LEDERER. 1995. The control of calcium release in heart muscle. Science **268:** 1045–1049.
19. LÓPEZ-LÓPEZ, J. R., P. S. SHACKLOCK, C. W. BALKE & W. G. WIER. 1995. Local calcium transients triggered by single L-type calcium channel currents in cardiac cells. Science **268:** 1042–1045.
20. CANNELL, M. B., H. CHENG & W. J. LEDERER. 1994. Spatial non-uniformities in $[Ca^{2+}]$i during excitation-contraction coupling in cardiac myocytes. Biophys. J., **67:** 1942–1956.
21. GÓMEZ, A. M., H. CHENG, W. J. LEDERER & D. M. BERS. 1996. Ca diffusion and SR trans-

port both contribute to the $[Ca]_i$ decline during Ca sparks in rat ventricular myocytes. J. Physiol. **496:** 575–581.
22. BERS, D. M. 1989. SR Ca loading in cardiac muscle preparations based on rapid cooling contractures. Am. J. Physiol. **256:** C109–C120.
23. BASSANI, R. A. & D. M. BERS. 1995. Rate of diastolic Ca release from the sarcoplasmic reticulum of intact rabbit and rat ventricular myocytes. Biophys. J. **68:** 2015–2022.
24. WIER, W. G., T. M. EGAN, J. R. LÓPEZ-LÓPEZ & C. W. BALKE. 1994. Local control of excitation-contraction coupling in rat heart cells. J. Physiol., **474:** 463–471.
25. BERS, D. M. & V. M. STIFFEL. 1993. The ratio of ryanodine: Dihydropyridine receptors in cardiac and skeletal muscle and implications for E-C coupling. Am. J. Physiol., **264:** C1587–C1593.
26. LEW, W. Y. W., L. V. HRYSHKO & D. M. BERS. 1991. Dihydropyridine receptors are primarily functional L-type Ca channels in rabbit ventricular myocytes. Circ. Res. **69:** 1139–1145.
27. SANTANA, L. F., H. CHENG, A. M. GÓMEZ, M. B. CANNELL & W. J. LEDERER. 1996. Relation between the sarcolemmal Ca^{2+} current and Ca^{2+} sparks and local control theories for cardiac excitation-contraction coupling. Circ. Res.; **78:** 166–171.
28. R. SITSAPESAN & A. J. WILLIAMS. 1994. Regulation of the gating of the sheep cardiac sarcoplasmic reticulum Ca^{2+}-release channel by luminal Ca^{2+}. J. Membr. Biol. **137:** 215–226.
29. LUKYANENKO, V., I. GYÖRKE & S. GYÖRKE. 1996. Regulation of calcium release by calcium inside the sarcoplasmic reticulum in ventricular myocytes. Pflügers Arch. **432:** 1047–1054.
30. CHENG, H. M. R. LEDERER, W. J. LEDERER & M. B. CANNELL. 1996. Calcium sparks and $[Ca^{2+}]_i$ waves in cardiac myocytes. Am. J. Physiol. **270:** C148–C159.
31. BERS, D. M., R. A. BASSANI, J. W. M. BASSANI, S. BAUDET & L. V. HRYSHKO. 1993. Paradoxical twitch potentiation after rest in cardiac muscle: Increased fractional release of SR calcium. J. Mol. Cell. Cardiol. **25:** 1047–1057.
32. R. A. BASSANI & D. M. BERS. 1994. Na-Ca exchange is required for rest-decay but not for rest-potentiation of twitches in rabbit and rat ventricular myocytes. J. Mol. Cell. Cardiol. **26:** 1335–1347.
33. SHATTOCK, M. J. & D. M. BERS. 1989. Rat vs. rabbit ventricle: Ca flux and intracellular Na assessed by ion-selective microelectrodes. Am. J. Physiol. **256:** C813–C822.
34. A. FABIATO. 1985. Time and calcium dependence of activation and inactivation of calcium-induced release of calcium from the sarcoplasmic reticulum of a skinned canine cardiac Purkinje cell. J. Gen. Physiol. **85:** 247–290.
35. NIGGLI, E. & W. J. LEDERER. 1990. Voltage-independent calcium release in heart muscle. Science **250:** 565–568.
36. NÄBAUER, M., G. CALLEWART, L. CLEEMANN & M. MORAD. 1989. Regulation of calcium release is gated by calcium current, not gating charge, in cardiac myocytes. Science **244:** 800–803.
37. BERS, D. M, D. M. CHRISTENSEN & T. X. NGUYEN. 1988. Can Ca entry via Na-Ca exchange directly activate cardiac muscle contraction? J. Mol. Cell. Cardiol. **20:** 405–414.
38. LEBLANC, N. & J. R. HUME. 1990. Sodium current-induced release of calcium from cardiac sarcoplasmic reticulum. Science **248:** 372–376.
39. LEVI, A. J., K. W. SPITZER, O. KOHMOTO & J. H. B. BRIDGE. 1994. Depolarization-induced Ca entry via Na-Ca exchange triggers SR release in guinea pig cardiac myocytes. Am. J. Physiol. **266:** H1422–H1433.
40. BASSANI, J. W. M., R. A. BASSANI & D. M. BERS. 1993. Twitch-dependent SR Ca accumulation and release in rabbit ventricular myocytes. Am. J. Physiol. **265:** C533–C540.
41. BASSANI, J. W. M., W. YUAN & D. M. BERS. 1995. Fractional SR Ca release is altered by trigger Ca and SR Ca content in cardiac myocytes. Am. J. Physiol. **268:** C1313–C1319.
42. SHANNON, T. R. & D. M. BERS. 1997. Assessment of intra-SR free [Ca] and buffering in rat heart. Biophys. J. **73:** 1524–1531.
43. A. TRIPATHY & G. MEISSNER. 1996. Sarcoplasmic reticulum lumenal Ca^{2+} has access to cytosolic activation and inactivation sites of skeletal muscle Ca^{2+} release channel. Biophys. J. **70:** 2600–2615.
44. YUAN, W., K. S. GINSBURG & D. M. BERS. 1996. Comparison of sarcolemmal Ca channel current in rabbit and rat ventricular myocytes. J. Physiol. **493:** 733–746.
45. WITCHER, D. R., R. J. KOVACS, H. SCHULMAN, D. C. CEFALI & L. R. JONES. 1991. Unique

phosphorylation site on the cardiac ryanodine receptor regulates calcium channel activity. J. Biol. Chem. **266:** 11144–11152.

46. HAIN, J., H. ONOUE, M. MAYRLEITNER, S. FLEISCHER & H. SCHINDLER. 1995. Phosphorylation modulates the function of the calcium release channel of sarcoplasmic reticulum from cardiac muscle. J. Biol. Chem. **270:** 2074–2081.
47. LI, L., H. SATOH, K. S. GINSBURG & D. M. BERS. 1997. The effects of CaMKII on cardiac excitation-contraction coupling in ferret ventricular myocytes. J. Physiol. **501:** 17–32.
48. NEGRETTI, N., S. C. O'NEILL & D. A. EISNER. 1993. The relative contributions of different intracellular and sarcolemmal systems to relaxation in rat ventricular myocytes. Cardiovasc. Res. **27:** 1826–1830.
49. VARRO, A., N. NEGRETTI, S. B. HESTER & D. A. EISNER. 1993. An estimate of the calcium content of the sarcoplasmic reticulum in rat ventricular myocytes. Pflügers Arch. **423:** 158–160.
50. DELBRIDGE, L. M. D., J. W. M. BASSANI & D. M. BERS. 1996. Steady-state twitch Ca fluxes and cytosolic Ca buffering in rabbit ventricular myocytes. Am. J. Physiol. **39:** C192–C199.
51. DUBELL, W. H., W. J. LEDERER & T. B. ROGERS. 1996. Dynamic modulation of cardiac excitation-contraction coupling by protein phosphatases in rat ventricular myocytes. J. Physiol. **493:** 793–800.
52. JAYARAMAN, T., A. M. BRILLANTES, A. P. TIMERMAN, A. P. FLEISCHER, H. ERDJUMENT-BROMAGE, P. TEMPST & A. R. MARKS. 1992. FK506 binding protein associated with the calcium release channel (ryanodine receptor). J. Biol. Chem. **267:** 9474–9477.
53. TIMERMAN, A. P., E. OGUNBUNMI, E. FREUND, G. WIEDERRECHT, A. MARKS & S. FLEISCHER. 1993. The calcium release channel of sarcoplasmic reticulum is modulated by FK-506 binding protein. J. Biol. Chem. **268:** 22992–22999.
54. TIMERMAN, A. P., T. JAYARAMAN, G. WIEDERRECHT, H. ONOUE, A. R. MARKS & S. FLEISCHER. 1994. The ryanodine receptor from canine heart sarcoplasmic reticulum is associated with a novel FK-506 binding protein. Biochem. Biophys. Res. Commun. **198:** 701–706.
55. BRILLANTES, A. B., K. ONDRIAS, A. SCOTT, E. KOBRINSKY, E. ONDRIASOVA, M. C. MOSCHELLA, T. JAYARAMAN, M. LANDERS, B. E. EHRLICH & A. R. MARKS. 1994. Stabilization of calcium release channel (ryanodine receptor) function by FK-506 binding protein. Cell **77:** 513–523.
56. AHERN, G. P., P. R. JUNANKAR, & A. F. DULHUNTY. 1994. Single channel activity of the ryanodine receptor calcium release channel is modulated by FK-506. FEBS Letts. **352:** 369–374.
57. CHEN, S. R. W., L. CHANG & D. H. MACLENNAN. 1994. Assymetrical blockade of the Ca release channel (ryanodine receptor) by 12-KDa FK-506 binding protein. Proc. Natl. Acad. Sci. USA; **91:** 11953–11957.
58. KAFTAN, E., A. R. MARKS & B. E. EHRLICH. 1996. Effects of rapamycin on ryanodine receptor/calcium release. Circ. Res. **78:** 990–997.
59. BARG, S., J. A. COPELLO & S. FLEISCHER. 1997. Different interactions of cardiac and skeletal muscle ryanodine receptors with FK-506 binding protein isoforms. Am. J. Physiol. **272:** C1726–C1733.
60. MCCALL, E., L. LI, H. SATOH, L. A. BLATTER & D. M. BERS. 1996. Effects of FK-506 on contraction and Ca transients in cardiac myocytes. Circ. Res. **79:** 1108–1119.
61. XIAO, R. P., H. H. VALDIVIA, K. BOGDANOV, C. VALDIVIA, E. G. LAKATTA & H. CHENG. 1997. The immunophilin FK506-binding protein modulates Ca^{2+} release channel closure in rat heart. J. Physiol. **500:** 343–354.
62. W. H. DUBELL, P. A. WRIGHT, W. J. LEDERER & T. B. ROGERS. 1997. Effects of the immunosupressant FK506 on excitation-contraction coupling and outward K^+ currents in rat ventricular myocytes. J. Physiol. **501:** 509–516.
63. HESS, P., J. B. LANSMAN & R. W. TSIEN. 1984. Different modes of Ca channel gating behavior favored by dihydropyridine Ca agonists and antagonists. Nature **311:** 538–544.
64. HRYSHKO, L. V., R. BOUCHARD, T. CHAU & D. BOSE. 1989. Inhibition of rest potentiation in canine ventricular muscle by BAY K 8644: Comparison with caffeine. Am. J. Physiol. **257:** H399–H406.

65. HRYSHKO, L. V., T. KOBAYASHI & D. BOSE. 1989. Possible inhibition of canine ventricular sarcoplasmic reticulum by BAY K 8644. Am. J. Physiol. **257:** H407–H414.
66. MCCALL, E., L. V. HRYSHKO, V. M. STIFFEL, D. M. CHRISTENSEN & D. M. BERS. 1996. Functional linkage between the cardiac dihydropyridine and ryanodine receptor: Acceleration of rest decay by Bay K 8644. J Mol. Cell. Cardiol. **28:** 79–93.
67. SATOH, H., D. M. BERS, & L. M. BLATTER. 1996. Modulation of spatial and temporal characteristics of calcium sparks: Effects of BayK 8644, caffeine and ryanodine. Biophys. J. **70:** 274.
68. SLAVIK, K. J., J-P WANG, B. AGHDASI, J-Z. ZHANG, F. MANDEL, N. MALOUF & S. L. HAMILTON. 1997. A carboxy-terminal peptide of the α_1-subunit of the dihydropyridine receptor inhibits Ca^{2+} release channels. Am. J. Physiol. **272:** C1475–C1481.
69. RÍOS, E. & G. PIZARRÓ. 1988. Voltage sensors and calcium channels of excitation-contraction coupling. News Physiol. Sci. **3:** 223–227.
70. TANABE, T., K. G. BEAM, B. A. ADAMS, T. NIIDOME & S. NUMA. 1990. Regions of the skeletal muscle dihydropyridine receptor critical for excitation-contraction coupling. Nature **356:** 567–569.
71. MCCALL, E. & D. M. BERS. 1996. Bay K 8644 depresses excitation-contraction coupling in cardiac muscle. Am. J. Physiol. **270:** C878–C884.
72. ARAI, M., H. MATSUI & M. PERIASAMY. 1994. Sarcoplasmic reticulum gene expression in cardiac hypertrophy and heart failure. Circ. Res. **74:** 555–564.
73. DE LA BASTIE, D., D. LEVITSKY, L. RAPPAPORT, J-J. MERCADIER, F. MAROTTE, C. WISNEWSKY, V. BROVKOVICH, K. SCHWARTZ & A-M. LOMPRE. 1990. Function of the sarcoplasmic reticulum and expression of its Ca^{2+}-ATPase gene in pressure overload-induced cardiac hypertrophy in the rat. Circ. Res. **66:** 554–564.
74. FELDMAN, A. M., E. O. WEINBERG, P. E. RAY & B. H. LORELL. 1993. Selective changes in cardiac gene expression during compensated hypertrophy and the transition to cardiac decompensation in rats with chronic aortic banding. Circ. Res. **73:** 184–192.
75. QI, M., T. R. SHANNON, D. E. EULER, D. M. BERS & A. M. SAMAREL. 1997. Downregulation of sarcoplasmic reticulum Ca^{2+}-ATPase during the progression of pressure overload left ventricular hypertrophy. Am. J. Physiol. **272:** H2416–H2424.
76. MERCADIER, J. J., A. M. LOMPRE, P. DUC, K. R. BOEHLER, J. B. FRAYSSE, C. WISNEWSKI, P. D. ALLEN, M. KOMAJDA & K. SCHWARTZ. 1990. Altered sarcoplasmic reticulum Ca^{2+}-ATPase gene expression in the human ventricle during end-stage heart failure. J. Clin. Invest. **85:** 305–309.
77. TAKAHASHI, T., P. D. ALLEN & S. IZUMO. 1992. Expression of A-, B-, and C-type natriuretic peptide genes in failing and developing human ventricles: Correlation with expression of the Ca^{2+}-ATPase gene. Circ. Res. **71:** 9–17.
78. HASENFUSS, G., H. REINECKE, R. STUDER, M. MEYER, B. PIESKE, J. HOLTZ, C. HOLUBARSCH, H. POSIVAL, H. JUST, & H. DREXLER. 1994. Relation between myocardial function and expression of sarcoplasmic reticulum Ca^{2+} ATPase in failing and nonfailing human myocardium. Circ. Res. **75:** 434–442.
79. BRILLANTES, A. M., P. ALLEN, T. TAKAHASHI, S. IZUMO & A. R. MARKS. 1992. Differences in cardiac calcium release channel (ryanodine receptor) expression in myocardium from patients with end-stage heart failure caused by ischemic versus dilated cardiomyopathy. Circ. Res. **71:** 18–26.
80. GÓMEZ, A. M., H. H. VALDIVIA, H. CHENG, M. R. LEDERER, L. F. SANTANA, M. B. CANNELL, S. A. MCCUNE, R. A. ALTSCHULD & W. J. LEDERER. 1997. Defective excitation-contraction coupling in experimental hypertrophy and heart failure. Science **276:** 800–805.
81. MCCALL, E., K. S. GINSBURG, R. A. BASSANI, J. W. M. BASSANI, T. R. SHANNON & D. M. BERS. 1998. Effects of cardiac hypertrophy in the rat on cellular Ca fluxes and excitation-contraction coupling. Am. J. Physiol. **274:** H1348–H1360.
82. DELBRIDGE, L. M. D., H. SATOH, W. YUAN, J. W. M. BASSANI, M. QI, K. S. GINSBURG, A. M. SAMAREL & D. M. BERS. 1997. Cardiac myocyte volume, Ca^{2+} fluxes and sarcoplasmic reticulum loading in pressure overload hypertrophy. Am. J. Physiol. **272:** H2425–H2435.
83. HOVE-MADSEN, L. & D. M. BERS. 1993. Passive Ca buffering and SR Ca uptake in permeabilized rabbit ventricular myocytes. Am. J. Physiol. **264:** C677–C686.

Models for the Transmembrane Region of the Phospholamban Pentamer: Which Is Correct?[a]

PAUL D. ADAMS,[b] ALBERT S. LEE,[b] AXEL T. BRÜNGER,[b,c] AND DONALD M. ENGELMAN[b,d]

[b]*Department of Molecular Biophysics and Biochemistry, Yale University, New Haven, Connecticut 06520, USA*

[c]*The Howard Hughes Medical Institute, Yale University, New Haven, Connecticut 06520, USA*

ABSTRACT: Phospholamban is a 52–amino acid protein that assembles into a pentamer in the membranes of the sarcoplasmic reticulum. Pentamer formation is driven in large part by interactions of the transmembrane regions of the protein, which are thought to be arranged as interacting α-helices. The structural properties of phospholamban have been studied by mutagenesis and optical spectroscopy, resulting in a large database. In this discussion, we present advances in computational modeling, which identifies two probable structures for the transmembrane pentamer. A new approach to mutagenesis is described, which should lead to a clear distinction between the two possible models.

Phospholamban is thought to have a role in the regulation of the calcium ATPase activity in the sarcoplasmic reticulum via an inhibitory association that can be reversed by phosphorylation. The phosphorylation of phospholamban is initiated by β-adrenergic stimulation, identifying phospholamban as an important component in the stimulation of cardiac activity by β-agonists. The protein was discovered in 1974[1,2] and has been the subject of numerous functional studies. Its role in regulation of the sarcoplasmic calcium pumps has led to a high level of interest in studying its properties.

The protein is a 52–amino acid transmembrane protein that assembles into pentamers that are observed to be stable under conditions of sodium dodecyl sulphate polyacrylamide gel electrophoresis (SDS-PAGE).[3] It has been shown that interactions of the transmembrane helices alone are sufficient to drive pentamer formation, giving rise to interest in the way that this part of the structure is organized.

In the following, we present a succinct summary of the foundations of work on phospholamban structure, followed by a discussion of recent modeling efforts and a description of a new approach using mutagenesis that we expect, in combination with the modeling, to lead to a unique choice of structural model.

[a] This work was supported by grants from the National Institutes of Health, PO1395461, National Science Foundation, DMB8805587, funds from Boehringer Ingelheim Inc., and the National Foundation for Cancer Research to D.M.E.; and by a grant from the National Science Foundation, ACS 93-181159 to A.T.B. The coordinates of the second phospholamban model found in this study will be deposited in the Brookhaven Protein Data Bank.

[d] Corresponding author. Phone: 203-432-6143; fax: 203-432-6946.

BASICS OF PHOSPHOLAMBAN STRUCTURE

A summary of information in this area is available in a review.[4] Sequence analysis of the polypeptide reveals two distinct regions. The cytoplasmic portion corresponds approximately to the amino terminal half of the protein, and contains the serine and threonine residues phosphorylated by regulatory kinases.[5] The carboxy-terminal half of the polypeptide is predominantly hydrophobic and is believed to traverse the bilayer as an alpha helix.[6] The complete cDNA sequence is available for a number of species (see Ref. 4), including the human sequence.[7]

As has been mentioned above, phospholamban tends to appear as a pentamer on SDS-PAGE. The most populated forms of phospholamban are those of monomer and pentamer,[8] and boiling reduces the apparent size of the protein reversibly.[3] Most convincingly, patterns of phosphorylation at S16 and T17 are revealed in electrophoretic patterns compatible with pentamer formation.[5]

Various techniques have been used to establish the secondary structure of the transmembrane region, most notably circular dichorism,[6] and Fourier transform infrared spectroscopy.[6,9] The results of these studies suggest that the transmembrane domain forms an alpha helical structure approximately perpendicular to the plane of the lipid bilayer in which they are embedded. Mutagenesis studies originally undertaken by MacLennan and colleagues[10] were aimed at understanding the structural roles of different amino acids in the membrane region. Subsequent work using chimeric constructs expressed in *E. coli* explored a wider range of sequence alterations.[11] Assays were run using SDS-PAGE to determine influences of substitutions on pentamer formation, resulting in the data shown in FIGURE 1. These results were subsequently confirmed by work using alanine and phenalanine substitutions throughout the transmembrane sequence.[12] A comparison of the results of these studies is shown in FIGURE 2. Clearly, there is a repeating pattern of disruption when substitutions are made along the length of the polypeptide suggesting interacting surfaces of helices. To explain these mutagenesis results, molecular modeling studies were undertaken.

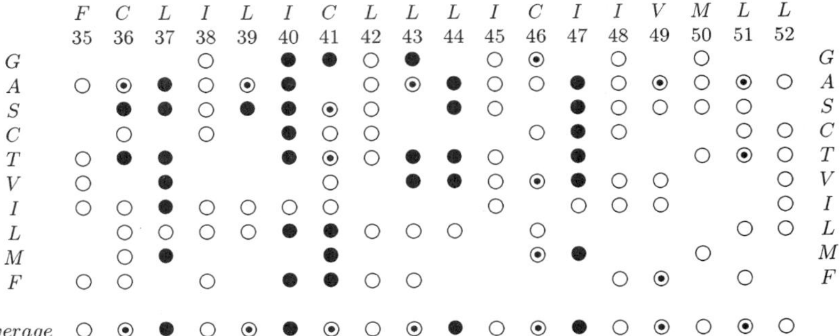

FIGURE 1. Effect of conservative substitutions on the oligomeric state of the chimeric phospholamban protein. Oligomerization properties of point mutants of the phospholamban transmembrane domain were determined by SDS-PAGE/Western blot analysis. Sensitive residues are denoted by *filled circles,* insensitive residues by *open circles,* and semisensitive residues by *half-filled circles.*

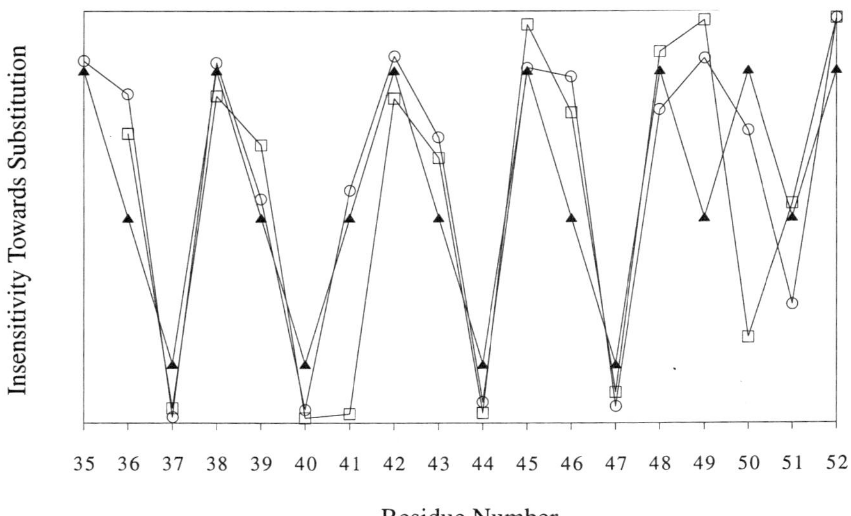

FIGURE 2. Insensitivity of amino acids in the transmembrane domain of phospholamban toward substitution, when assayed for pentamerization in two different mutagenesis studies. *Solid triangles* present the results of Engelman and coworkers[11]; *open circles* are the result of alanine substitutions, and *open squares* phenylalanine substitutions, both from the work of Jones and coworkers.[12]

MOLECULAR MODELING

By employing a global conformational search coupled with molecular dynamics simulations, a set of favored structures was obtained.[13] Two conceptual approaches were used: one method employed an extensive exploration of the interaction of two monomers, subsequently testing whether favored monomer-monomer interactions could be propagated into pentamers. The other method was based on an exploration of a set of symmetric rotations of helices arranged in a pentamer. Both right- and left-handed initial crossing angles were explored in both cases, and in each case a set of possible structures was obtained.[13] A single model was initially suggested on the basis of these explorations. Subsequently, improvements to the modeling procedures have been implemented, resulting in the identification of a second possible structure, indistinguishable from the originally proposed structure on energetic grounds, and similar in the extent to which it appears compatible with the mutagenesis data. This result is described in the following section.

IMPROVED MODELING STUDIES

We have revisited the modeling of the phospholamban pentamer with improved global searching strategies. This extended global searching method was also successfully applied to the transmembrane region of glycophorin.[14] In addition to the improvements described in Reference,[14] the revised modeling of phospholamban utilized three major extensions to the method. The energy calculations carried out during the molecular dynamics and conjugate gradient minimization protocols used the united atom OPLS force field.[15] This provided a more accurate representation of the forces between the atoms in the five helices, resulting in more accurate structures at the end of the global searching procedure. In addition, the molecular dynamics simulations were carried out in torsion angle space—i.e., bond lengths and bond angles remained fixed

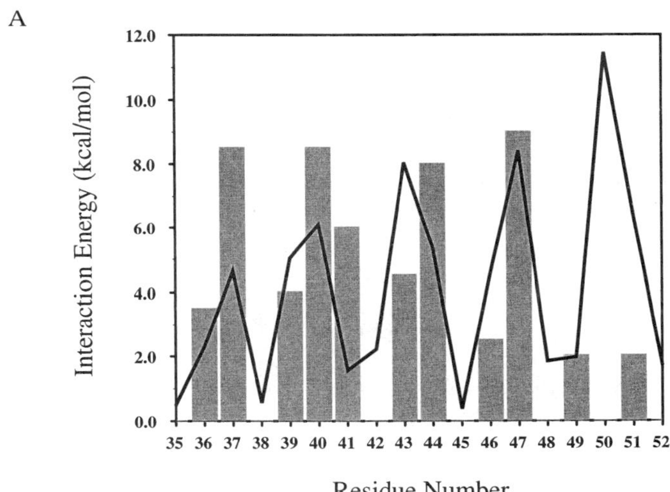

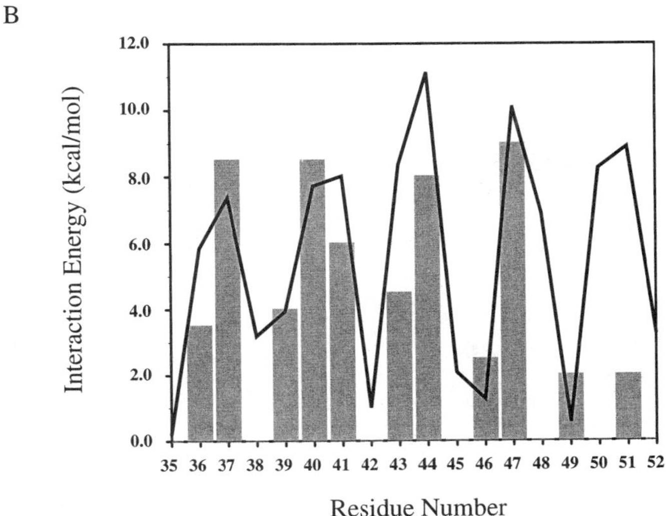

FIGURE 3. Average interaction energy per residue *(solid line)* compared to the sensitivity of each residue to mutation *(vertical bars)*. **(A)** The original phospholamban model.[13] **(B)** The new model found in this modeling study.

during the calculations.[16] The use of this reduced representation of the molecule restricted searching to chemically reasonable conformations. Finally, side chain conformations started from energetically favorable rotamer states. This served to improve the starting structures prior to global searching.

The existing global computational searching method[14] and the improvements outlined above were combined in our recent modeling of the phospholamban pentamer. The search was limited to a symmetric pentamer, with the rotation angle about the long axis of each helix varied from 0° to 360° in 20° steps. To further increase sampling, four trials were carried out from the same starting position, using different initial random velocities in each case. Calculations were performed for both left-handed and right-handed crossing angles between the five helices. The search generated a total of 144 structures, which were compared on the basis of their root mean square coordinate deviation (RMSD) from one another. These deviations were used to group the structures into clusters. This generated 9 clusters that satisfied the selection criteria of at least 10 structures in a cluster with a maximum RMSD of 1.5 Å. The coordinates of all the structures in a cluster were then used to generate a single average structure.[13,14]

The nine models produced as a result of this computational searching were then compared to the experimental mutagenesis data.[13] Only two models showed any correlation to the experimental mutagenesis data, and both have left-handed crossing angles. The model that had been identified by previous global searching methods was present (FIGURE 3A), with a pentamer bundle crossing angle of 12°. However, in contrast to the previous work, an additional model was present with a similarly good match to the experimental data (FIGURE 3B). This new model possesses a very similar pentamer bundle crossing angle of 14°. Analysis of the two models shows that the difference between them is a rotation of approximately 50° around the long axis of the 5 alpha-helices. This results in residues that were previously in the interface between neighboring helices (FIGURE 4A) now being positioned at the center of the pentamer bundle (FIGURE 4B). This packing arrangement is very similar to the "leucine-zipper" struc-

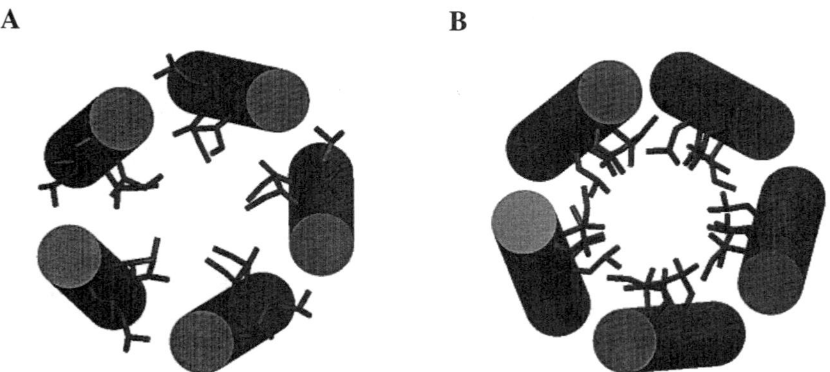

FIGURE 4. Structures of the two models found by the global searching method that are consistant with the mutagenesis data. Both models are viewed along the fivefold bundle axis, with helices shown as *cylinders*. Residues that show extreme sensitivity to mutation (L37, I40, L44, I47) are shown. **(A)** The original phospholamban model.[13] **(B)** The additional model found in this modeling study. The main difference between these models is a rotation of approximately 50° around the long axis of each helix.

ture postulated by Jones and coworkers on the basis of experimental mutagenesis and helical-wheel diagrams.[12]

The two models generated by the global computational search were extensively compared with the experimental mutagenesis data. However, no clear criteria for favoring one structure over the other can be found. As a result of the close packing of the five helices in the pentamer and the large contact area between neighboring helices, both models show a similar trend in interaction energy between residues (FIGURE 3). However, there are significant differences for residues 38, 41, 44, and 48. These differences are a result of the anticlockwise rotation of the helices by 50°, when looking from amino to carboxy terminus, going from the previously predicted to the newly predicted model.

Thus, it is seen that two structures exist that cannot be easily distinguished on the basis of existing mutagenesis data or energy calculations. In the following, a method is proposed and tested to distinguish between these alternatives. It is felt that this general approach may be useful for a number of membrane structural studies in the future.

DESIGN AND TESTING OF COMPLEMENTARY MUTATIONS

The extensive mutagenesis performed on the transmembrane domain residues of phospholamban established the existence of a high degree of sequence specificity in oligomerization.[11] Even seemingly conservative substitutions (e.g., Leu37⇒Ile, Ile40⇒Leu, Ile47⇒Val) disrupted pentamerization of the *Staphylococcal nuclease*/phospholamban chimeric protein used in the study. The transmembrane domain of phospholamban is composed of predominantly aliphatic residues, and the energy of association is thought to be driven by van der Waals interactions, which are maximized by the precise packing of complementary helix faces. It is this necessity for tight packing of side chains along the helix-helix interfaces that forms the basis of designing complementary mutations.

A mutation is complementary if it is able to compensate for the disruptive effects of an initial mutation, thus reestablishing pentamerization. Complementarity is possible only if the two mutated residues are proximal in space and form tight packing interactions. If the fit is too tight, steric collisions force the helices apart, thus weakening or abolishing favorable helix interactions. If the fit is loose, favorable van der Waals energy is reduced, weakening the interaction between the helices. Since the two models differ in the identity of the residues defining helix-helix interfaces, two positions that interact in one model, but not in the other, can be used to design complementary mutants. A complementary mutation would thus support one model and disprove the other, resolving any ambiguity.

Based on the first phospholamban model of Adams *et al.* (FIGURE 5a), a Leu39⇒Val (FIGURE 5b) mutation was predicted to complement the disruptive Cys41⇒Met (FIGURE 5c) mutation as seen in FIGURE 5d. The steric clash introduced by the bulky Met group at position 41, indicated by the overlap of van der Waals surfaces, was predicted to be alleviated by reducing the size of the side chain at position 39 from Leu to Val. This prediction was tested by creating the double mutant and measuring oligomer formation under SDS-PAGE by Western blotting. Preliminary evidence indicates that pentamerization is reestablished for the double mutant.

At the time of this prediction, only the first model was available.[13] The two mutations, when modeled in the second phospholamban structure described in this paper (FIGURE 5e), also demonstrated complementarity (FIGURE 5h). The experimental result is therefore consistent with the two models predicted. The ambiguity of which model is correct thus remains. However, the Leu39⇒Val/Cys41⇒Met double mutant demonstrates the feasibility of designing model-based complementary mutations. With this new approach

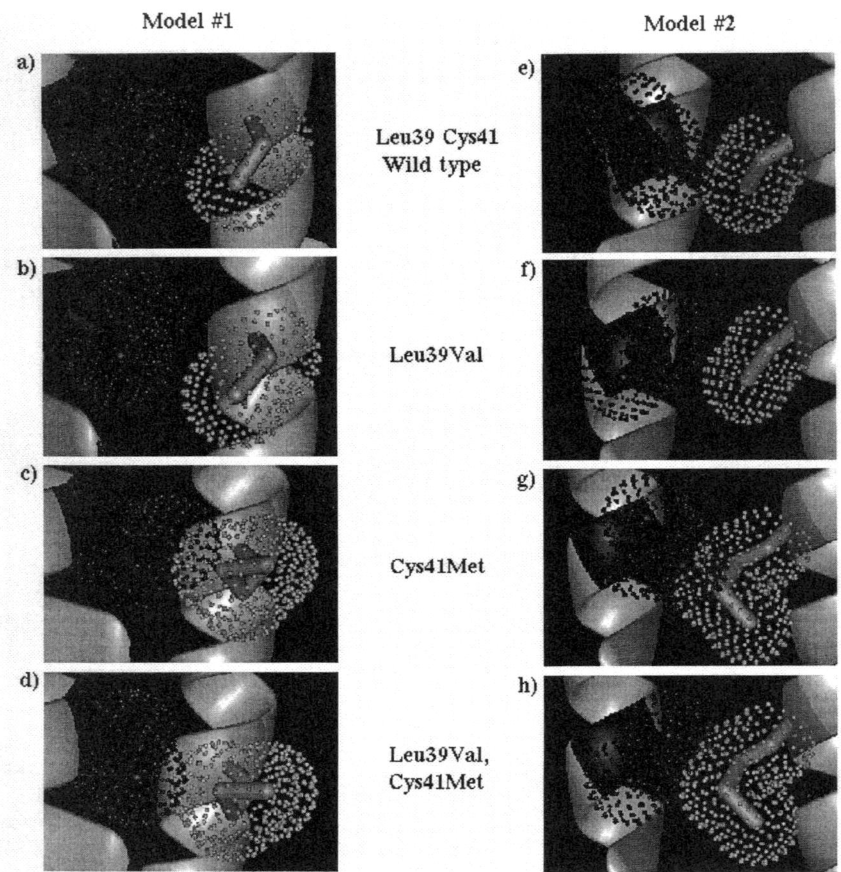

FIGURE 5. Complementary mutation design. Van der Waals representations of residues 39 and 41 in the two phospholamban models: **(a)** the model of Adams *et al.*; **(e)** the new model described in this study. For each model the effects of single and double mutations are shown: Leu39⇒Val **(b** and **f)**, Cys41⇒Met **(c** and **g)**, and Leu39⇒Val/Cys41⇒Met **(d** and **h)**. Dark grey van der Waals surfaces and bonds correspond to residue 39, while light grey corresponds to residue 41. All hydrogens and residues other than 39 and 41 are omitted. Only one 39/41 interaction out of the five present in the pentamer is illustrated.

to mutagenesis, the two models can be tested by looking at other pairs of residues. By choosing residues that interact in only one model, a clear distinction will be possible.

CONCLUSIONS

Improvements to the modeling procedures have given rise to increased ambiguity, but better definition. There are now two models that appear plausible on computational grounds, one of which is that originally proposed,[13] and the other is similar to the model suggested by Jones[12] on the basis of helical wheel diagrams and mutagenesis. It is not possible to distinguish between these two models on the basis of current information. Thus, we have developed an approach using model-derived complementary mutation studies to arrive at a firm conclusion. The initial test of these methods, while not resulting in a decision concerning which model is correct, suggests that the approach is feasible and may be generally useful.

REFERENCES

1. KATZ, A. M., M. TADA, & M. A. KIRCHBERGER. 1975. Control of calcium transport in the myocardium by the cyclic AMP-protein kinase system. Adv. Cyclic Nucleotide Res. **5:** 453–472.
2. KIRCHBERGER, M. A. & T. ANTONETZ. 1982. Phospholamban: Dissociation of the 22,000 molecular weight protein of cardiac sarcoplasmic reticulum into 11,000 and 5,500 molecular weight forms. Biochem. Biophys. Res. Commun. **105**(1): 152–156.
3. LAMERS, J. M. & J. T. STINIS. 1982. Phosphorylation of low-molecular-weight proteins in preparations of rat heart sarcolemma and sarcoplasmic reticulum. Adv. Myocardiol. **3:** 289–297.
4. ARKIN, I. T., P. D. ADAMS, A. T. BRUNGER, S. O. SMITH & D. M. ENGELMAN. 1997. Structural perspectives of phospholamban, a helical transmembrane pentamer. Annu. Rev. Biophys. Biomol. Struct. **26:** 157–179.
5. SIMMERMAN, H. K., J. H. COLLINS, J. L. THEIBERT, A. D. WEGENER & L. R. JONES. 1986. Sequence analysis of phospholamban. Identification of phosphorylation sites and two major structural domains. J. Biol. Chem. **261**(28): 13333–13341.
6. ARKIN, I. T., M. ROTHMAN, C. F. LUDLAM, S. AIMOTO, D. M. ENGELMAN *et al.* 1995. Structural model of the phospholamban ion channel complex in phospholipid membranes. J. Mol. Biol. **248**(4): 824–834.
7. FUJII, J., A. ZARAIN-HERZBERG, H. F. WILLARD, M. TADA & D. H. MACLENNAN. 1991. Structure of the rabbit phospholamban gene, cloning of the human cDNA, and assignment of the gene to human chromosome 6. J. Biol. Chem. **266**(18): 11669–11675.
8. WEGENER, A. D., H. K. SIMMERMAN, J. P. LINDEMANN & L. R. JONES. 1989. Phospholamban phosphorylation in intact ventricles. Phosphorylation of serine 16 and threonine 17 in response to beta-adrenergic stimulation. J. Biol. Chem. **264**(19): 11468–11474.
9. TATULIAN, S. A., L. R. JONES, L. G. REDDY, D. L. STOKES & L. K. TAMM. 1995. Secondary structure and orientation of phospholamban reconstitute in supported bilayers from polarized attenuated total reflection FTIR spectroscopy. Biochemistry **34**(13): 4448–4456.
10. FUJII, J., K. MARUYAMA, M. TADA & D. H. MACLENNAN. 1989. Expression and site-specific mutagenesis of phospholamban. Studies of residues involved in phosphorylation and pentamer formation. J. Biol. Chem. **264**(22): 12950–12955.
11. ARKIN, I. T., P. D. ADAMS, K. R. MACKENZIE, M. A. LEMMON, A. T. BRÜNGER & D. M. ENGELMAN. 1994. Structural organization of the pentameric transmembrane α-helices of phospholamban, a cardiac ion channel. EMBO J. **13:** 4757–4764.
12. SIMMERMAN, H. K., Y. M. KOBAYASHI, J. M. AUTRY & L. R. JONES. 1996. A leucine zipper stabilizes the pentameric membrane domain of phospholamban and forms a coiled-coil pore structure. J. Biol. Chem. **271**(10): 5941–5946.
13. ADAMS, P. D., I. T. ARKIN, D. M. ENGELMAN & A. T. BRÜNGER. 1995. Computational searching and mutagenesis suggest a structure for the pentameric transmembrane domain of phospholamban. Nat. Struc. Biol. **2**(2): 154–162.
14. ADAMS, P. D., D. M. ENGELMAN & A. T. BRÜNGER. 1997. An improved prediction for the structure of the dimeric transmembrane domain of glycophorin A obtained through global searching. Proteins **26:** 257–261.
15. JORGENSEN, W. L. & J. TIRADO RIVES. 1988. The OPLS potential functions for proteins energy minimizations for crystals of cyclic peptides and crambin. J. Am. Chem. Soc. **110**(6): 1657–1666.
16. RICE, L. M. & A. T. BRÜNGER. 1994. Torsion angle dynamics: Reduced variable conformational sampling enhances crystallographic structure refinement. Proteins **19:** 277–290.

Direct Spectroscopic Detection of Molecular Dynamics and Interactions of the Calcium Pump and Phospholamban[a]

DAVID D. THOMAS,[b] LAXMA G. REDDY, CHRISTINE B. KARIM, MING LI, RAZVAN CORNEA, JOSEPH M. AUTRY,[c] LARRY R. JONES,[c] AND JOHN STAMM

Department of Biochemistry, University of Minnesota Medical School, Minneapolis, Minnesota 55455, USA

[c]*Krannert Institute of Cardiology, Indiana University School of Medicine, Indianapolis, Indiana 46202, USA*

ABSTRACT: In order to test molecular models of cardiac calcium transport regulation, we have used spectroscopy to probe the structures, dynamics, and interactions of the Ca pump (Ca-ATPase) and phospholamban (PLB) in cardiac sarcoplasmic reticulum (SR) and in reconstituted membranes. Electron paramagnetic resonance (EPR) and phosphorescence of probes bound to the Ca pump show that the activity of the pump is quite sensitive to its oligomeric interactions. In cardiac SR, PLB aggregates and inhibits the pump, and both effects are reversed by PLB phosphorylation. Previous analyses of PLB's oligomeric state were only in detergent solutions, so we used EPR and fluorescence to determine the oligomeric structure of PLB in its native state in lipid bilayers. Wild-type PLB is primarily oligomeric in the membrane, while the mutant L37A-PLB is monomeric. For both proteins, phosphorylation shifts the dynamic monomer-oligomer equilibrium toward oligomers, and induces a similar structural change, as indicated by tyrosine fluorescence; yet L37A-PLB is more effective than wild-type PLB in inhibiting and aggregating the pump. Fluorescence energy transfer shows that the Ca pump increases the fraction of monomeric PLB, indicating that the pump preferentially binds monomeric PLB. These results support a *reciprocal aggregation model for Ca pump regulation,* in which the Ca pump is aggregated and inhibited by association with PLB monomers, and phosphorylation of PLB reverses these effects while decreasing the concentration of PLB monomers. To investigate the structure of the PLB pentamer in more detail, we measured the reactivities of cysteine residues in the transmembrane domain of PLB, and recorded EPR spectra of spin labels attached to these sites. These results support an atomic structural model, based on molecular dynamics simulations and mutagenesis studies, in which the PLB pentamer is stabilized by a leucine-isoleucine zipper within the transmembrane domain.

Active calcium transport into the sarcoplasmic reticulum of cardiac muscle is catalyzed by the Ca pump (Ca-ATPase, SERCA2a) and regulated by phospholamban (PLB), a 52-amino-acid protein that inhibits the pump at submicromolar [Ca^{2+}] until PLB is phosphorylated under beta-adrenergic stimulation (reviewed in Ref. 1). This is a complex regulatory mechanism in which dynamic protein-protein interactions are proposed to play crucial roles. For example, it has been proposed, on the basis of SDS-PAGE, that PLB is a pentameric complex in the membrane,[2] that phosphorylation results in the dissociation of an inhibitory complex between PLB and the pump,[3] and that

[a] This work was supported by grants from the National Institutes of Health to D.D.T. (GM27906) and L.R.J. (HL06308 and HL49428). L.G.R. and C.B.K. were supported by grants from the American Heart Association.

[b] Phone: 612-625-0957; fax: 612-624-0632; e-mail: ddt@ddt.biochem.umn.edu

PLB regulates the oligomeric state of the pump.[4] In order to test and refine these hypotheses, we have used spectroscopic probes to detect directly the molecular dynamics and oligomeric interactions of these two proteins in native and reconstituted membranes. This work was facilitated not only by the development of spectroscopic probe technology, but also by methods for functional co-reconstitution of PLB and the Ca pump,[5,6] and by molecular genetic techniques that made possible the expression and purification of PLB and its mutants in mg quantities[5,7] and the functional coexpression of PLB with the Ca-ATPase.[8,9]

OLIGOMERIC INTERACTIONS OF THE CA PUMP

Our early work on protein and lipid dynamics in skeletal SR established principles that proved essential in understanding the more complex mechanism of regulation of calcium pumping in the heart. It had been shown that optimal activity of the skeletal muscle Ca pump appears to require a fluid lipid environment, but it was not clear how lipid affects the structure and dynamics of the pump. Therefore, we measured the rotational dynamics of the Ca pump on the microsecond time scale, using saturation transfer electron paramagnetic resonance (EPR)[10] and time-resolved phosphorescence anisotropy (TPA),[11] and we found that the Ca-sensitive ATPase activity of the pump correlated much better with rotational mobility of the pump protein than with other physical parameters, such as lipid fluidity. In particular, it was found that the Ca-ATPase could be strongly inhibited and aggregated by the addition of melittin, a cationic amphipathic peptide, without any significant change in lipid fluidity.[12,13] Similar effects of Ca-ATPase inhibition and aggregation were observed with lidocaine, a cationic amphipathic local anesthetic, whereas general anesthetics tended to disaggregate and activate the pump.[14,15] This inhibition, as in the case of other agents that aggregate the Ca-ATPase, was found to be correlated with stabilization of the E2 (low–Ca affinity) form of the Ca pump.[16]

EFFECT OF PHOSPHOLAMBAN ON OLIGOMERIC INTERACTIONS OF THE Ca PUMP

We used TPA to show that, at low [Ca^{2+}], the Ca pump is less mobile (more aggregated) in cardiac SR than in skeletal SR, and that phosphorylation of PLB in cardiac SR decreases pump aggregation as it relieves the PLB-induced inhibition of the Ca-ATPase, suggesting that the regulation of Ca pump aggregation plays an important role in the function of PLB in the heart[4] (FIG. 1). We proposed that in the absence of phosphorylation, the cationic phospholamban pentamer binds to the anionic Ca pump and induces pump aggregation, resulting in inhibition (FIG. 1, top), but upon phosphorylation the cationic charge on PLB is greatly reduced, decreasing affinity for the pump and relieving inhibition (FIG. 1, bottom). In order to verify this mechanism in a more controlled system, we co-reconstituted PLB with the Ca pump in lipid bilayers (FIG. 2, bottom) and found that PLB inhibits the SERCA1 (skeletal) as well as the SERCA2 (cardiac) isoform of the pump, that this inhibition is reversed by either phosphorylation or PLB antibody[5,6] (FIG. 3, bottom), and that PLB aggregates the pump, as indicated by TPA (Reddy and Thomas, unpublished).

OLIGOMERIC INTERACTIONS OF PHOSPHOLAMBAN

PLB was proposed to be a stable pentamer, based on mobility in SDS-PAGE,[2] so we set out to determine the oligomeric state of PLB in a lipid bilayer. EPR spectra of spin-

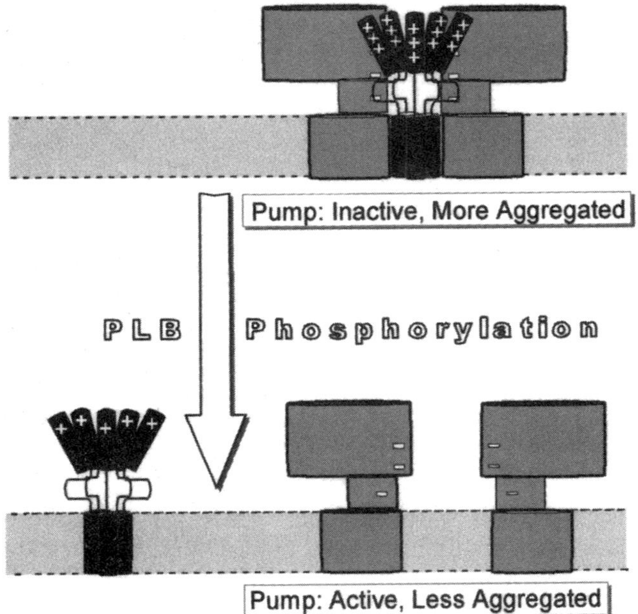

FIGURE 1. Model for the regulation of the Ca pump *(gray)* by the phospholamban pentamer *(black),* based on phosphorescence anisotropy data showing that PLB phosphorylation disaggregates and activates the Ca pump.[4]

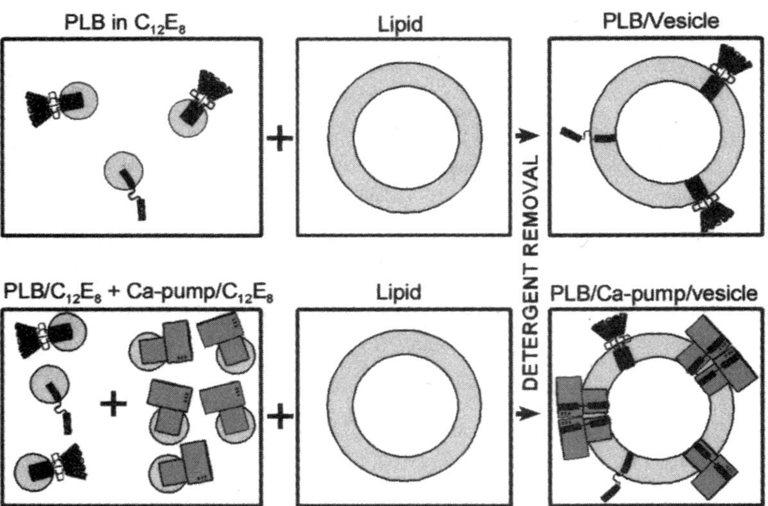

FIGURE 2. Reconstitution of PLB in lipid vesicles without **(top)** and with **(bottom)** the Ca pump. The proteins are dissolved in the detergent $C_{12}E_8$ **(left),** lipid vesicles are added, and detergent is removed, producing vesicles with proteins inserted **(right).**[5]

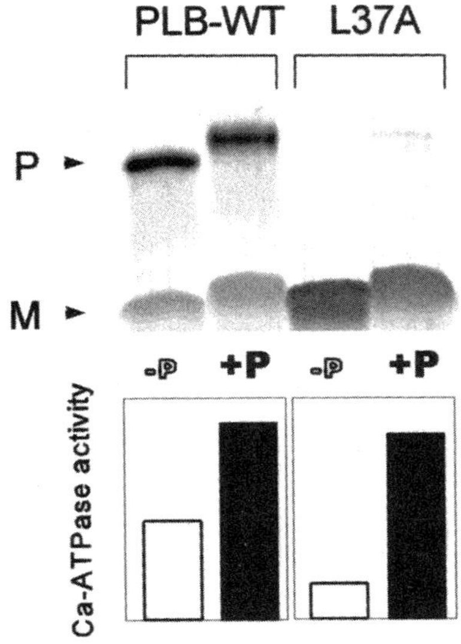

FIGURE 3. Oligomeric state on SDS-PAGE **(top)** and regulation of Ca-ATPase activity in reconstituted membranes **(bottom)** for WT-PLB **(left)** and mutant L37A-PLB **(right),** in the absence (–P) and presence (+P, equivalent to PLB phosphorylation) of PLB antibody.

labeled phospholipids can be used to count the number of boundary lipids in contact with the protein surface, and thus to measure the perimeter of the protein, which is quite sensitive to its oligomeric state (FIG. 4). We combined PLB with a mixture containing detergent, phospholipid, and phospholipid spin label (14-PCSL), then removed detergent, resulting in reconstituted PLB in lipid vesicles (FIG. 2, top). We found that the

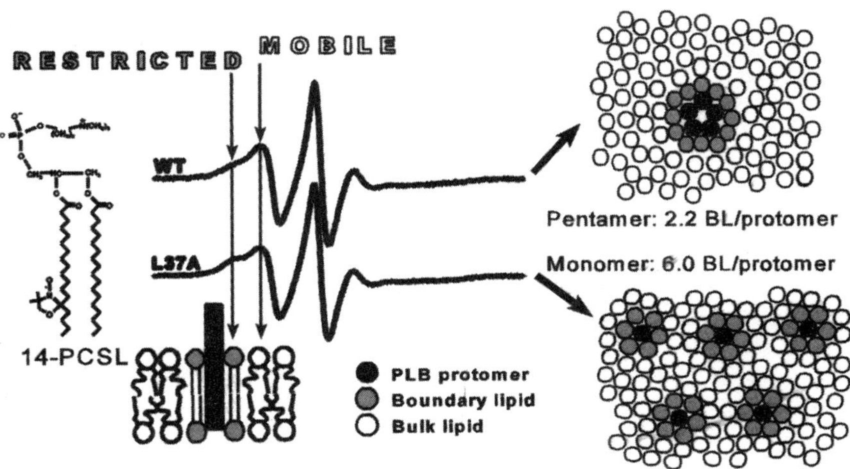

FIGURE 4. Oligomeric state of PLB wild-type (WT) and PLB mutant L37A reconstituted in lipid bilayer membranes, determined by using EPR and a phosphatidylcholine spin label (14-PCSL) to quantitate the number of restricted (boundary) lipids *(gray)* surrounding PLB *(black)*.[17]

number of boundary lipids per PLB protomer was much less than that expected for a monomeric α-helix, indicating that PLB is oligomeric in a lipid bilayer.[17] In contrast, the number of boundary lipids observed for L37A-PLB (a monomer on SDS-PAGE, as shown in FIG. 3, top right) was precisely the number expected for a monomer (FIG. 4). These results indicate that the oligomeric states of these proteins in lipid are similar to those observed on SDS gels[7,9] (FIG. 3). Despite the very different oligomeric states of these proteins, phosphorylation shifts the dynamic monomer-oligomer equilibrium toward oligomers for both proteins in lipid bilayers[17] and causes a similar structural change in the cytoplasmic domain of PLB, as detected by tyrosine fluorescence.[18] Thus the pentameric form does not seem to be required for the key structural changes of PLB. In fact, the monomeric L37A is even more effective than the pentameric wild-type PLB in inhibiting the Ca pump reversibly (FIG. 3, bottom). Thus it seems unlikely that a (presumably oligomeric) PLB channel plays a significant functional role.[1]

EFFECT OF THE Ca PUMP ON OLIGOMERIC INTERACTIONS OF PHOSPHOLAMBAN

Since the EPR boundary lipid method (discussed above) is not applicable in a membrane containing more than one protein, we developed a fluorescence energy transfer method, with probes specifically bound to PLB, to determine the oligomeric state of PLB in the membrane,[19] in the presence and absence of the Ca pump[20] (FIG. 5). In this method, two separate populations of PLB were labeled with fluorescent donors and acceptors, mixed in varying ratios in the absence and presence of the Ca pump, and reconstituted in lipid bilayers (FIG. 2). Quantitative analysis of the energy transfer data showed that PLB is primarily oligomeric in the membrane, but that a small but significant fraction of the PLB protomers is monomeric.[19,20] In the presence of the Ca pump,

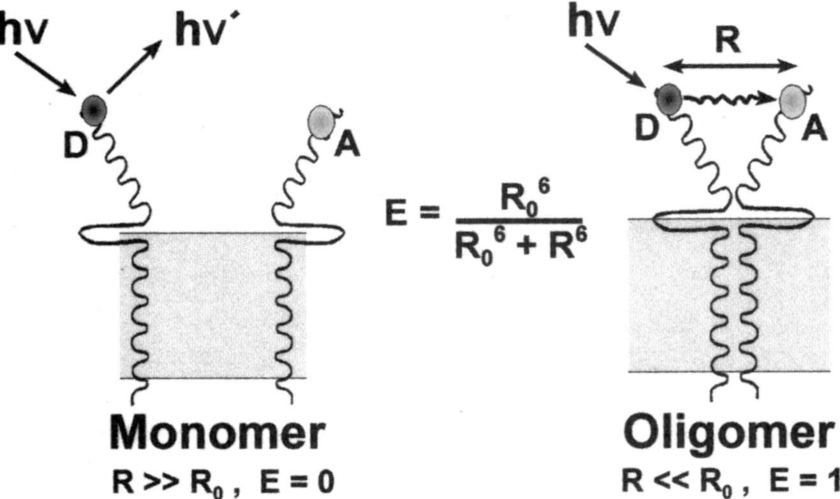

FIGURE 5. Fluorescence energy transfer method of analyzing oligomeric structure of labeled PLB. PLB labeled with donors (D) and acceptors (A) shows no energy transfer in the monomeric state **(left)** but shows complete energy transfer in an oligomer **(right).**[19]

the monomeric fraction substantially increases, indicating that the *Ca pump depolymerizes PLB by binding preferentially to the monomeric form.*[20]

RECIPROCAL AGGREGATION MODEL FOR Ca PUMP REGULATION

The above results support a model in which PLB and the cardiac Ca pump undergo reciprocal changes in oligomeric state in response to PLB phosphorylation, as illustrated in FIGURE 6. In the absence of PLB phosphorylation (top), PLB is in a dynamic equilibrium between monomers and oligomers (probably pentamers), and the Ca pump is inhibited and aggregated due to the binding of PLB monomers. Electrostatic repulsion probably destablizes the PLB oligomer, and electrostatic attraction probably stabilizes pump-PLB interactions, which screen electrostatic repulsion between pump molecules. After phosphorylation, the PLB pentamer becomes stabilized, probably due at least in part to reduced electrostatic repulsion, decreasing the concentration of PLB monomers and thus allowing the pump molecules to become dissociated and activated. The mechanism for the correlation between pump aggregation and inhibition is not known, but may involve the TM domain of PLB binding to the pump and stabilizing the E2 conformation, which correlates with pump aggregation and inhibition.[21]

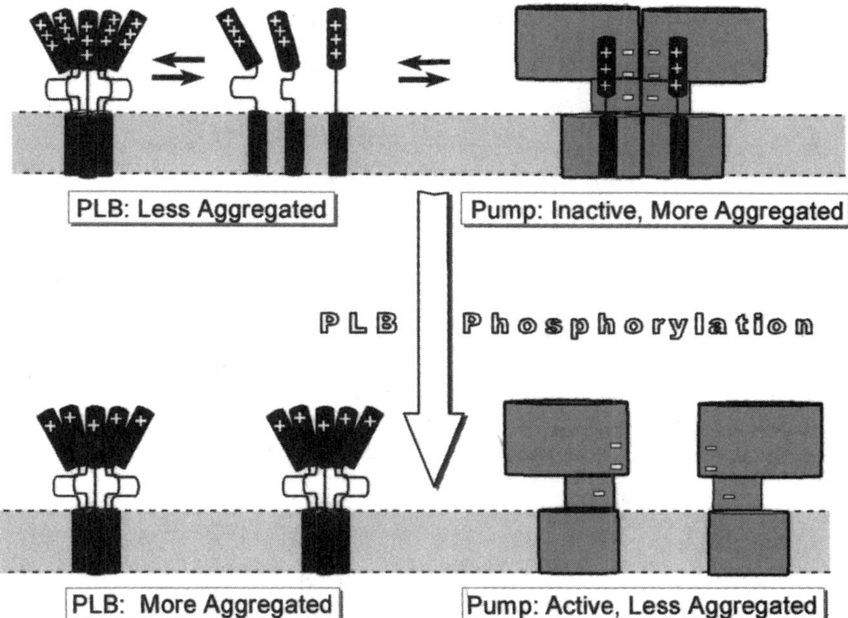

FIGURE 6. Reciprocal aggregation model of Ca pump *(gray)* regulation by PLB *(black)* phosphorylation. Before phosphorylation **(top),** PLB is in a dynamic equilibrium between pentamers and monomers, and the Ca pump is aggregated and inhibited by monomeric PLB. After PLB phosphorylation **(bottom),** PLB pentamers are more stable, reducing the concentration of monomers, disaggregating and activating the Ca pump.

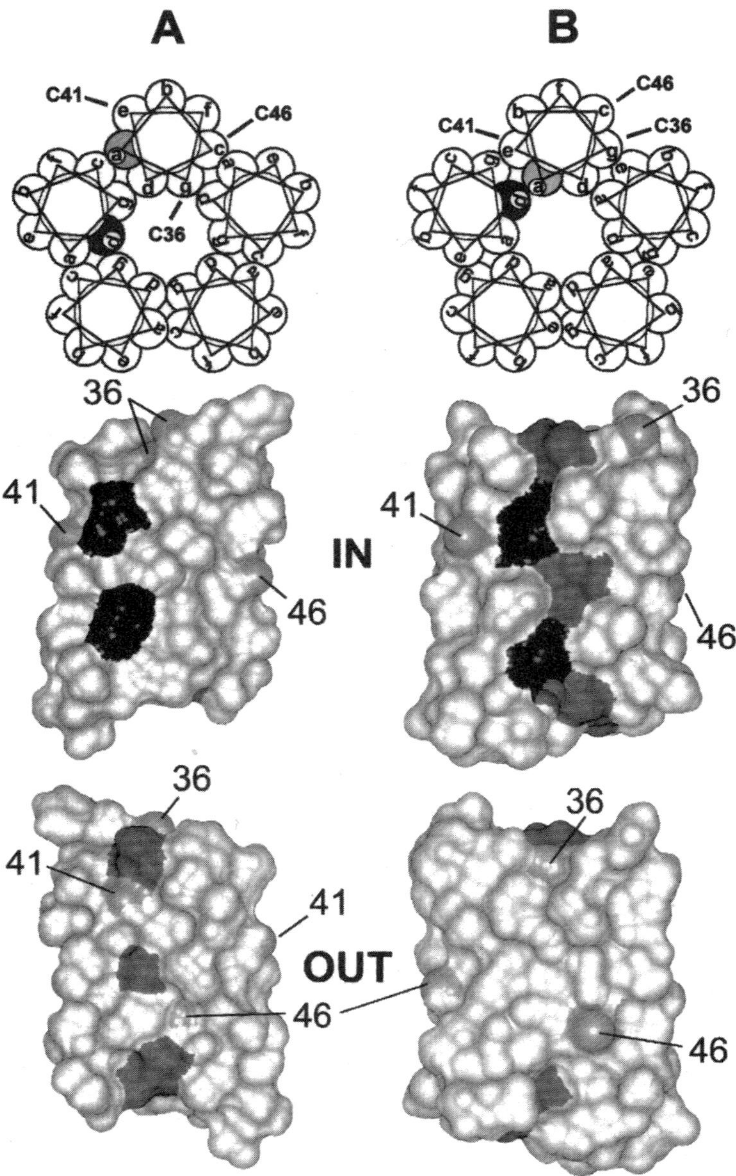

FIGURE 7. Atomic structural models of **(A)** Adams *et al.*[23] and **(B)** Karim *et al.*[22] for the transmembrane domain of the PLB pentamer. **Top:** schematic top view of helix packing in the pentamer, showing the seven helical positions predicted for the packing of helices into a left-handed coiled coil (3.5 residues per turn). **Bottom:** atomic model of two of the helices (side view), showing the view from the inside (IN) and outside (OUT) of the pentamer, highlighting the locations of the three cysteine sulfur atoms (indicated by residue number), and the leucine *(gray)* and isoleucine *(black)* residues that are important for pentamer stability. The two models are energetically equivalent, but model **B** is most consistent with our experimental results.[22]

STRUCTURAL MODEL FOR THE PHOSPHOLAMBAN PENTAMER

We investigated the relative reactivities of the three Cys residues (36, 41, and 46) in the transmembrane domain of PLB and several PLB mutants. We found that Cys 41 is much less reactive than Cys 36 and Cys 46 to sulfhydryl reagents, and that labeling Cys 41 disrupts the PLB pentamer.[22] This suggested that Cys 41 is not accessible to the surface of the PLB pentamer, and that this residue is at or near the interface between helices in the pentamer. This seemed inconsistent with the atomic model proposed previously by Adams *et al.*,[23] based primarily on molecular dynamics simulations (FIG. 7a). In that model, the helices pack together so that helical positions *g* and *d* are in contact, which would make Cys 41 (at helical position *e*) the *most exposed* of the three cysteine residues (FIG. 7A, top), in disagreement with our results.[22] As shown at the bottom of FIGURE 7A, that model also failed to produce the close packing between key leucine side chains (residues 37, 44, and 51, all at helical position *a*) and isoleucine side chains (residues 40 and 47, all at helical position *d*) that had been predicted to form a leucine/isoleucine zipper, on the basis of site-directed mutagenesis.[7] Therefore, we constructed an alternative model (FIG. 7B),[22] refined by molecular dynamics simulation, in which the helical positions *a* and *d* are in contact. The resulting model (FIG. 7B) was energetically equivalent to that of Adams *et al.* (FIG. 7A),[23] but it is more plausible, since it does show clearly the predicted leucine/isoleucine zipper, and it predicts that Cys 41 is the least accessible of the three cysteine residues, in agreement with our experimental results.[22] This work illustrates the importance of experimental constraints in evaluating molecular models for helix packing.

CONCLUSIONS

The dynamic regulation of protein-protein interactions is key to the understanding of Ca pump regulation by phospholamban in the heart. Although much further research is needed to test rigorously the models shown in FIGURES 6 and 7, it is clear that direct measurement of protein dynamics and interactions, using site-specific spectroscopic probes, will continue to be crucial to the elucidation of molecular mechanisms in this and other membrane sysems.

ACKNOWLEDGMENTS

We thank R. Bennett for technical assistance, and H. Kutchai for his contributions to the work on Ca pump oligomeric interactions.

REFERENCES

1. STOKES, D. L. 1997. Keeping calcium in its place: Ca^{2+}-ATPase and phospholamban. Curr. Opin. Struct. Biol. **7:** 550–556.
2. SIMMERMAN, H. K. B., J. H. COLLINS, J. L. THEIBERT, A. D. WEGENER & L. R. JONES. 1986. Sequence analysis of phospholamban. J. Biol. Chem. **261:** 13333–13341.
3. TADA, M. & A. M. KATZ. 1982. Phosphorylation of the sarcoplasmic reticulum and sarcolemma. Annu. Rev. Physiol. **44:** 401–423.
4. VOSS, J., L. R. JONES & D. D. THOMAS. 1994. The physical mechanism of calcium pump regulation in the heart. Biophys. J. **67:** 190–196.
5. REDDY, L. G., L. R. JONES, S. E. CALA, J. J. O'BRIAN, S. A. TATULIAN & D. L. STOKES. 1995. Functional reconstitution of recombinant phospholamban with rabbit skeletal Ca^{2+}ATPase. J. Biol. Chem. **270:** 9390–9397.

6. Reddy, L. G., L. R. Jones, R. C. Pace & D. L. Stokes. 1996. Purified, reconstituted cardiac Ca^{2+}-ATPase is regulated by phospholamban but not by direct phosphorylation with Ca^{++}/calmodulin-dependent protein kinase. J. Biol. Chem. **271:** 14964–14970.
7. Simmerman, H. K. B., Y. M. Kobayashi, J. M. Autry & L. R. Jones. 1996. A leucine zipper stabilizes the pentameric membrane domain of phospholamban and forms a coiled-coil pore structure. J. Biol. Chem. **271:** 5941–5946.
8. Autry, J. M. & L. R. Jones. 1997. Functional co-expression of the canine cardiac Ca^{2+}-pump and phospholamban in Sf21 cells reveals new insights on ATPase regulation. J. Biol. Chem. **272:** 15872–15880.
9. Kimura, Y., M. Kurzydlowski, M. Tada & D. H. MacLennan. 1997. Phospholamban inhibitory function is activated by depolymerization. J. Biol. Chem. **272:** 15061–15064.
10. Squier, T. C., S. E. Hughes & D. D. Thomas. 1988. Rotational dynamics and protein-protein interactions in the Ca-ATPase mechanism. J. Biol. Chem. **263:** 9162–9170.
11. Birmachu, W. & D. D. Thomas. 1990. Rotational dynamics of the Ca-ATPase in sarcoplasmic reticulum studied by time-resolved phosphorescence anisotropy. Biochemistry **29:** 3904–3914.
12. Mahaney, J. E. & D. D. Thomas. 1991. Effects of melittin on molecular dynamics and Ca-ATPase activity in sarcoplasmic reticulum membranes: Electron paramagnetic resonance. Biochemistry **30:** 7171–7180.
13. Voss, J., W. Birmachu, D. M. Hussey & D. D. Thomas. 1991. Effects of melittin on molecular dynamics and Ca-ATPase activity in sarcoplasmic reticulum membranes: Time-resolved optical anisotropy. Biochemistry **30:** 7498–7506.
14. Karon, B. S., J. E. Mahaney & D. D. Thomas. 1994. Halothane and cyclopiazonic acid modulate Ca-ATPase oligomeric state and function in sarcoplasmic reticulum. Biochemistry **33:** 13928–13937.
15. Kutchai, H., J. E. Mahaney, L. M. Geddis & D. D. Thomas. 1994. Hexanol and lidocaine affect the oligomeric state of the Ca-ATPase of sarcoplasmic reticulum. Biochemistry **33:** 13208–13222.
16. Voss, J. C., J. E. Mahaney & D. D. Thomas. 1995. Mechanism of Ca-ATPase inhibition by melittin in skeletal sarcoplasmic reticulum. Biochemistry **34:** 930–939.
17. Cornea, R. L., L. R. Jones, J. M. Autry & D. D. Thomas. 1997. Mutation and phosphorylation change the oligomeric state of phospholamban in lipid bilayers. Biochemistry **36:** 2960–2967.
18. Li, M., R. L. Cornea, J. M. Autry, L. R. Jones & D. D. Thomas. 1998. Phosphorylation-induced structural change in phospholamban and its mutants, detected by intrinsic fluorescence. Biochemistry. In press.
19. Li, M., L. G. Reddy, R. Bennett, D. Silva, L. R. Jones & D. D. Thomas. 1998. Oligomeric structure of phospholamban, studied by fluorescence energy transfer. Biophys. J. Submitted for publication.
20. Reddy, L. G., L. R. Jones & D. D. Thomas. 1998. Depolymerization of phospholamban in the presence of calcium pump: A fluorescence energy transfer study. Biochemistry. Submitted for publication.
21. Shi, Y., B. S. Karon, H. Kutchai & D. D. Thomas. 1996. Phospholamban-dependent effects of C12E8 on calcium transport and molecular dynamics in the heart. Biochemistry **35:** 13393–13399.
22. Karim, C. B., J. D. Stamm, J. Karim, L. R. Jones & D. D. Thomas. 1998. Cysteine reactivity and oligomeric structure of phospholamban and its mutants. Biochemistry. In press.
23. Adams, P. D., I. T. Arkin, D. M. Engelman & A. T. Brünger. 1995. Computational searching and mutagenesis suggest a structure for the pentameric transmembrane domain of phospholamban. Nat. Struct. Biol. **2:** 154–162.

The Sarcoplasmic Reticulum Ca^{2+} Pump: Inhibition by Thapsigargin and Enhancement by Adenovirus-Mediated Gene Transfer[a]

GIUSEPPE INESI, ROBERT WADE, AND TERRY ROGERS

Department of Biochemistry and Molecular Biology, University of Maryland School of Medicine, Baltimore, Maryland 21201, USA

ABSTRACT: The role of the sarcoplasmic reticulum Ca^{2+} pump in the excitation-contraction coupling of cardiac muscle fibers was evaluated in experiments on SR ATPase inhibition with thapsigargin or, alternatively, on Ca^{2+} pump enhancement by SR ATPase transgenic expression. We found that thapsigargin, a highly specific and potent inhibitor of the SR ATPase, produces a strong reduction of cytosolic Ca^{2+} transient and contractile activation in neonatal rat myocytes, in the absence of any other functional effect. On the other hand, Ca^{2+} pump enhancement by ATPase transgenic expression affects dramatically Ca^{2+} transient and twitches, resulting in shorter duration and more rapid decay rates. Of particular interest is gene transfer mediated by recombinant adenovirus vectors under control of a cell-specific promoter, resulting in transgenic expression of all myocytes in culture, and no expression in fibroblasts.

Vesicular fragments of sarcoplasmic reticulum (SR), isolated from skeletal[1,2] and heart[3–5] muscle, were initially referred to as "relaxing factor" since they prevented ATP-dependent activation of myofibrils. It then became apparent that the relaxing effect of SR vesicles is related to its Ca^{2+} pump and to sequestration of cytosolic Ca^{2+}, which can in turn be released for contractile activation of myofibrils. With regard to heart muscle fibers, an important question is related to the contribution of the SR Ca^{2+} pump to cytosolic Ca^{2+} transients, as compared with other Ca^{2+} handling systems such as the plasmalemmal Ca^{2+} pump and the Ca^{2+}/Na^{+} exchanger. The elegant work on regulation by phospholamban[6–8] has shown that activation of the SR Ca^{2+} pump is involved in the physiological mechanism of cardiac response to adrenergic stimuli. On the other hand, we describe here the experimental use of strong perturbations, such as total inhibition of the Ca^{2+} pump by thapsigargin (TG) or its enhancement by transgenic expression of Ca^{2+} ATPase, in order to demonstrate the prominent role of the SR Ca^{2+} pump on contractile activation and relaxation of cardiac myocytes.

INHIBITION BY THAPSIGARGIN

Thapsigargin is a sesquiterpene lactone isolated from the roots of *Thapsia garganica.*[9,10] Its inhibition of sarco- and endoplasmic reticulum Ca^{2+} (SERCA) transport

[a] This work was partially supported by National Institutes of Health Grant P01HL-27867.

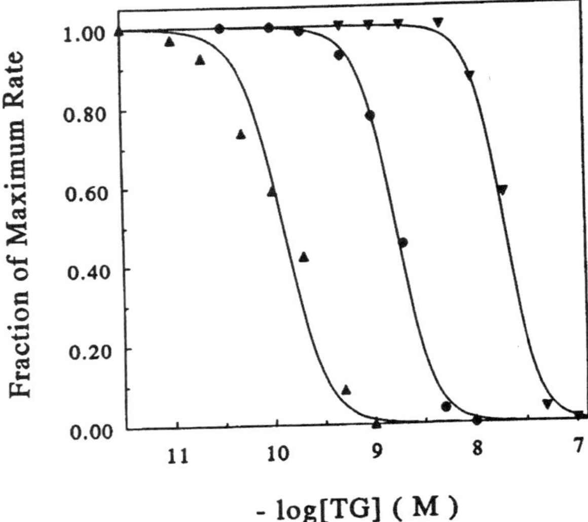

FIGURE 1. Titration of SR ATPase with TG. It is shown that inhibition is produced by amounts of TG stoichiometrically equivalent to the SR ATPase. The three *curves* were obtained with three different concentrations of SR ATPase.[13]

ATPases[11–14] is very potent, and its full effect is obtained at subnanomolar concentrations by stoichiometric titration of ATPase molecules (FIG. 1). The inhibition is also specific inasmuch as the plasmalemmal Ca^{2+} and Na+,K+ ATPases are not affected.[15,16]

Spectroscopic,[17] mutational,18,19 and photolabeling[20] experiments indicate that the thapsigargin binding domain is within or near the membrane-bound region of the SR ATPase, most likely associated with the S3, M3, M4, S3 loop (FIG. 2). Binding of TG yields a TG-ATPase dead-end complex resulting in a "global" effect on the SR ATPase protein, and inhibition of partial reactions occurring at distant domains within the ATPase molecule (i.e., Ca^{2+} binding in the transmembrane region and phosphorylation with Pi in the cytosolic region). The conformation acquired by the ATPase in its dead-end complex with TG favors formation of ordered molecular arrays[21] that are suitable for electron diffraction studies.[22]From the functional point of view, as it relates to excitation-contraction coupling, addition of TG to adult rat heart myocytes main-

→

FIGURE 2. Rabbit skeletal muscle SERCA1 ATPase sequence and its proposed membrane distribution. The diagram is derived from MacLennan *et al.*[25] Tryptic fragment A spans the sequence between Met1 and Arg505 *(triangle)*, and subfragment A1 spans the sequence between Ala199 *(triangle)* and Arg505 *(triangle)*. The *asterisks* indicate the amino (Leu253) and the caboxyl (Arg324) terminals of the segment *(shaded)* of A1, which is labeled with a radioactive azido derivative of TG.[20] This labeled segment includes portions of the S3 and S4 in the stalk, the M3 and M4 transmembrane helices, and the intervening lumenal loop. The residues (Glu309, Glu771, Asn796, Thr799, Asp800, and Glu908) involved in Ca^{2+} binding,[30] and Asp351, involved in formation of the phosphorylated intermediate,[40,41] are denoted by enclosures in *boxes* in the transmembrane and cytosolic regions, respectively.

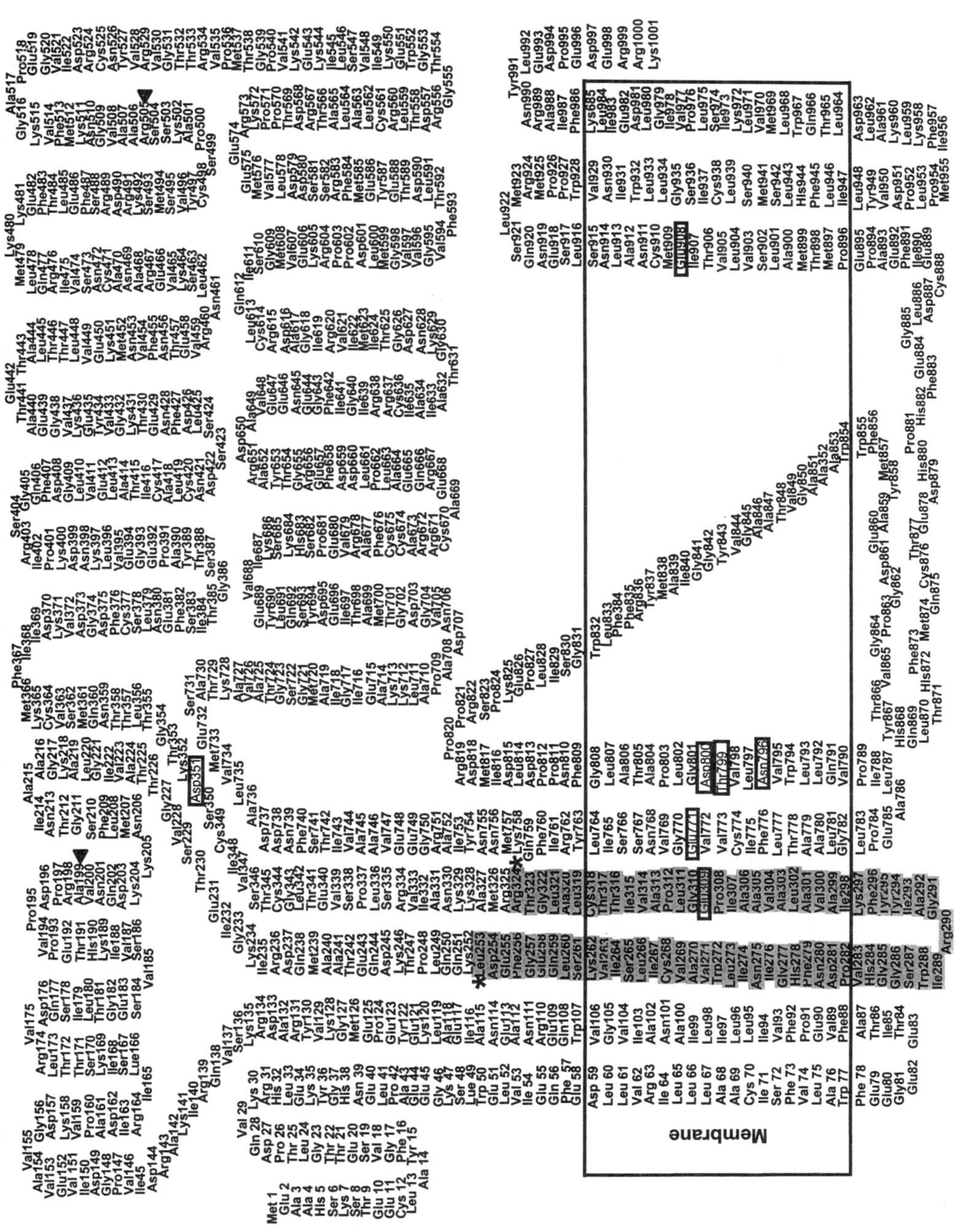
Membrane

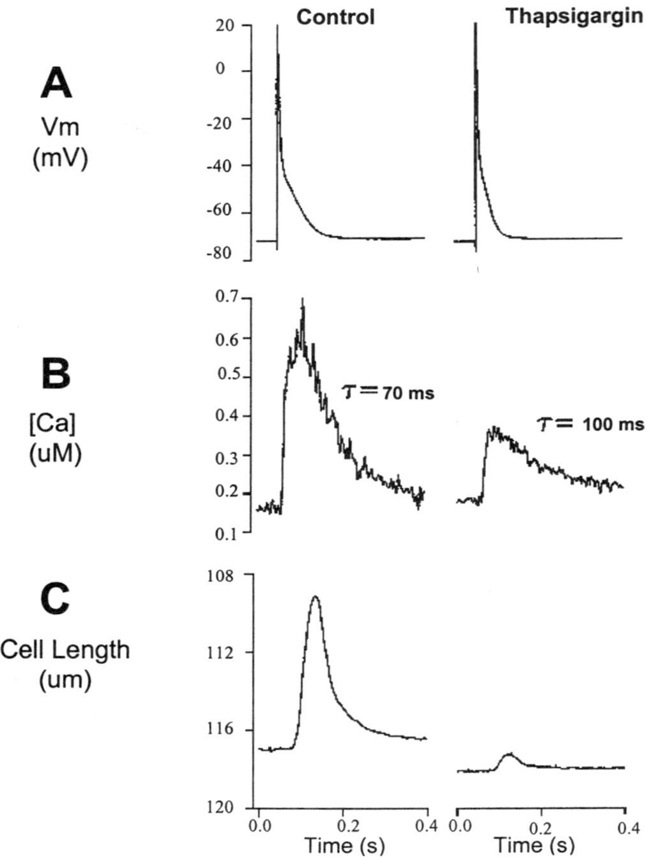

FIGURE 3. Effects of TG on [Ca^{2+}]i transients **(B)** and twitch **(C)** of isolated adult rat cardiac myocytes stimulated to fire action potentials **(A).** The myocyte was held in current clamp mode after a whole-cell patch was established and action potential was elicited at 0.25 Hz by the injection of current pulse at 1.5 threshold. Shown above are the fast time base records of averaged ($n = 3$) action potentials **(A),** [Ca^{2+}]i **(B),** and cell length **(C)** during both control **(left-hand curves)** and 5 minutes after addition of TG **(right-hand curves).**[24]

tained in whole-cell voltage clamp configuration decreases the magnitude of the Ca^{2+} transients and the twitch amplitude by about 80%. It is shown in FIGURE 3 that in addition to a reduction in intensity, the decay rates of Ca^{2+} transients and twitches are prominently slowed down by TG. On the other hand, these effects are not accompanied by significant alterations of the electrical behavior of the sarcolemmal membrane, including the Ca^{2+} currents associated with influx of trigger Ca^{2+}.[23,24] These experiments on specific inhibition of the SR ATPase by TG demonstrate that the SR Ca^{2+} pump plays a prominent role in the amplitude and kinetics of cytosolic Ca^{2+} transients and contractile tension in rat heart myocytes.

TRANSGENIC ATPase EXPRESSION

The availability of cDNA[16,25–28] encoding the SR ATPase isoforms of skeletal (SERCA1) and cardiac (SERCA2A) muscle has rendered possible transgenic expression of the ATPase in cultured cells.[29] This technique has been utilized for mutational analysis of the ATPase, revealing that the ATP binding and phosphorylation sites residue within the cytosolic region of the enzyme, while the Ca^{2+} binding domain resides within the membrane bound region.[30] A peptide segment spanning the M4 transmembrane helix and reaching the phosphorylation site through the S4 stalk segment appears to play an important role in providing a functional linkage between the two distant domains.[31]

We have asked, in general terms, the question of whether it is possible to influence cell functions by transgenic expression of intracellular Ca^{2+} pump. In fact, we were able to develop fibroblast lines in which overexpression of transgenic SERCA1 ATPase resulted in much larger intracellular Ca^{2+} storing capacity, and lower sensitivity to the inhibitory effect of TG on cell proliferation.[32] With regard to the specific function of excitation-contraction coupling in heart muscle, we have then explored methods for cell-specific SR ATPase gene transfer into cardiac myocytes. For this purpose we used recombinant adenovirus vectors[33,34] obtained by cotransfection of 293 cells with a replication-deficient viral plasmid and a shuttle plasmid containing the cDNA of interest under control of a viral or cell-specific promoter. It is known that recombinant adenovirus is a very efficient vector for cardiac myocytes,[35–38] and transfer of heterolo-

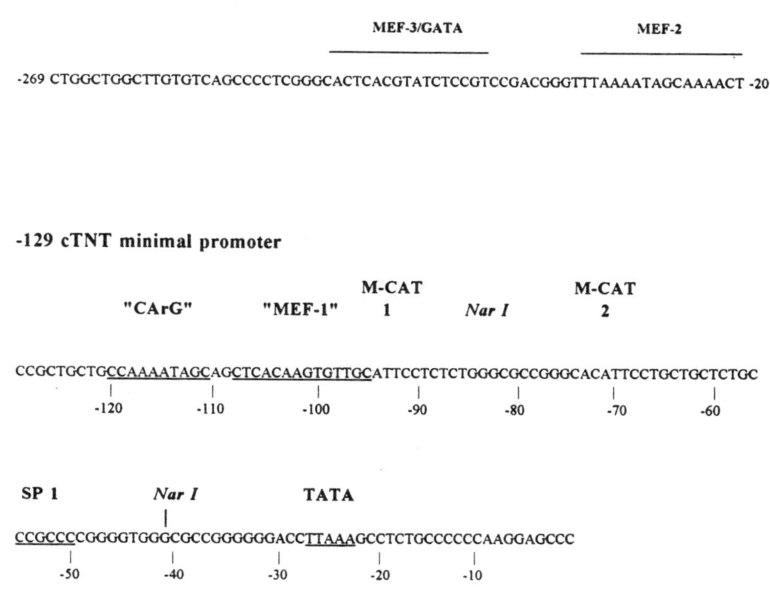

FIGURE 4. Functional elements of the –268 bp segment of the cardiac troponin T (cTnT) promoter. Elements involved in transcription regulation are *underlined.*[42]

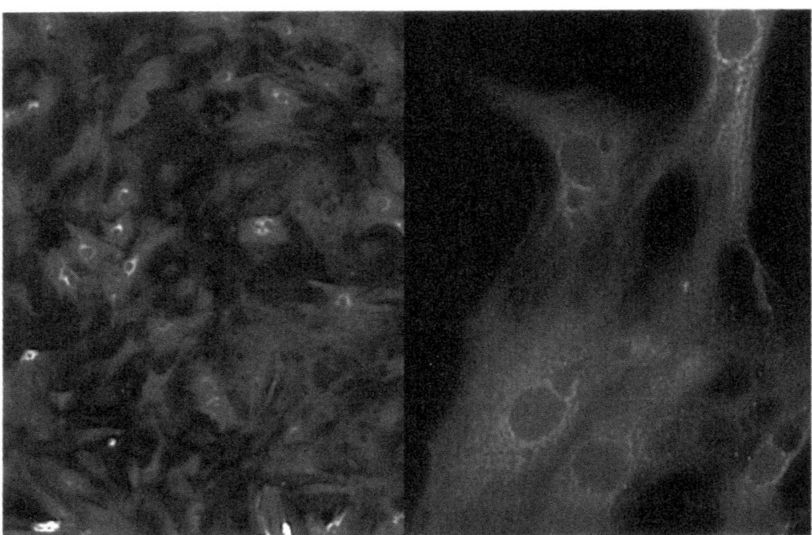

FIGURE 5. Visualization of transgenic SERCA1 expression in chicken embryo cardiac myocytes by immunofluorescent methods. Cultured myocytes were infected with cTnT-SERCA1 recombinant adenovirus (30 pfu per seeded cell). Forty-eight hours following the infection the myocytes were processed for immunofluorescent staining using the SERCA1 specific monoclonal antibody CaF3-5C3.[26] Note, in the large field **(left),** the high number of myocytes expressing transgenic ATPase, and the intracellular membrane targeting of the transgenic ATPase at the higher magnification **(right).**

gous SERCA cDNA in rat cardiac myocytes under control of viral promoters has been reported.[39]

In our laboratory, we have constructed recombinant adenovirus vectors for isomorphic gene transfer of the chicken SERCA1 ATPase into chicken embryo cardiac myocytes, under control of either the constitutive cmv promoter or the cardiac muscle–specific cardiac troponin T (cTnT) promoter (FIG. 4). An advantageous feature of this system is that the transgenic isomorphic SERCA1 ATPase and the endogenous SERCA2A ATPase can be distinguished with monoclonal antibodies that are specifically reactive to either isoform (FIG. 5). We found that while adenovirus-mediated gene transfer under control of a viral (cmv) promoter results in SERCA1 expression in both myocytes and fibroblasts, gene transfer under control of the cTnT promoter results in SERCA1 expression only in myocytes (FIG. 6). Targeting of the transgenic SERCA1 ATPase to intracellular membranes is identical to that of the endogenous SERCA2A ATPase (FIGS. 5 and 7). When we evaluated the Ca^{2+} transport capacity of homogenated myocytes, we found a two–threefold increase of transport rates as a consequence of SERCA1 transgenic expression under control of either viral or cell-specific promoter (FIG. 8).

In a series of experiments, we critically examined the functional significance of the transgene expression of SERCA1 in myocytes. We measured steady state contractions and $[Ca^{2+}]_i$ transients in field-stimulated single-cultured myocytes and compared their

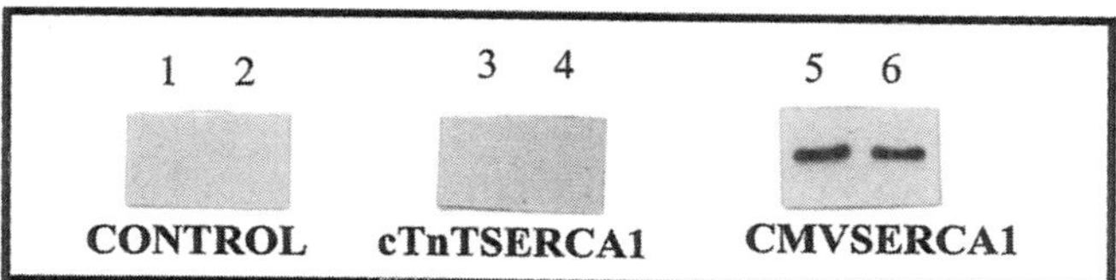

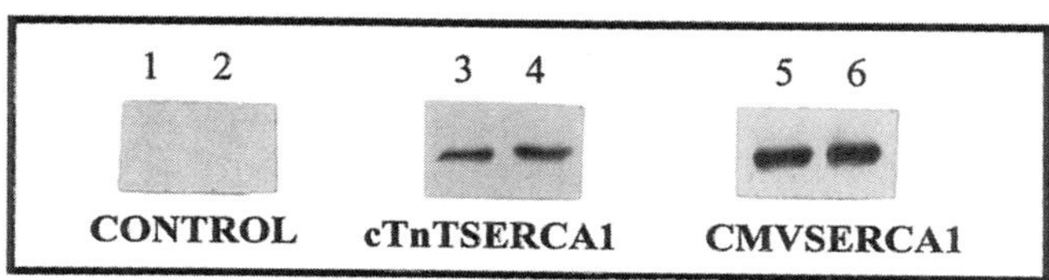

FIGURE 6. Expression of transgenic SERCA1 ATPase in chicken embryo fibroblasts and cardiac myocytes. Cultures of chicken embryo skin fibroblasts or cardiac myocytes were infected with either cTnT-SERCA1 (50 pfu/cell) or cmv-cTnT (10 pfu/cell) recombinant adenovirus, or subjected to a sham procedure. Forty-eight hours following gene transfer the cells were harvested and tested by Western blots, using a SERCA-1 specific monoclonal antibody. Note the occurrence of cmv-SERCA1 expression in both fibroblasts and myocytes, while cTnT-SERCA1 expression occurs only in myocytes.[43]

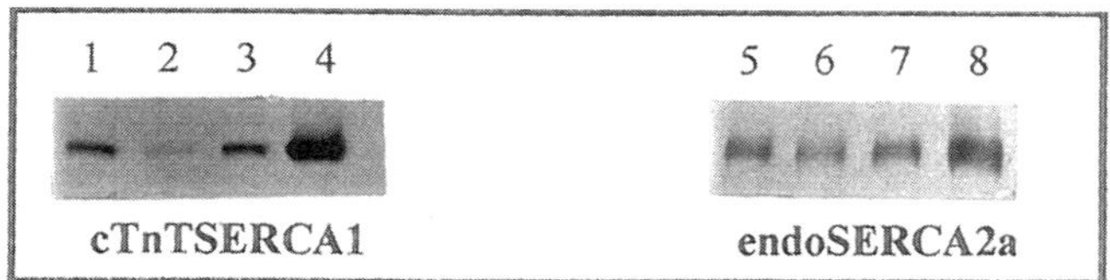

FIGURE 7. Western blots showing the localization of transgenic SERCA1 and endogenous SERCA2A ATPases in subcellular fractions of cardiac myocytes. Cultures of chicken embryo cardiac myocytes were infected with cTnT-SERCA1 recombinant adenovirus (30 pfu/seeded cell). Two days after the infection the cells were harvested, homogenized, and subjected to differential centrifugation. The subcellular fraction was then processed for Western blotting, probing the same samples in parallel with monoclonal antibodies specific for either the transgenic SERCA1 **(left side)** or the endogenous SERCA2A ATPase **(right side).** Samples 1 and 5 refer to the whole homogenate; 2 and 6 to cell membrane and nuclei; 3 and 7 to mitochondria; and 4 and 8 to microsomes. Note the prevalent association of both transgenic and endogenous ATPases with the microsomal fraction (i.e., sarco-endoplasmic reticulum).[43]

properties to those from transfected cells. As shown in FIGURE 9, panel A, transfected cells displayed dramatically shortened twitches, with a decrease in the time to peak and increases in relaxation rate observed. Analysis of the waveforms showed that the peak width at half height decreased from 223 ± 10 msec (n = 24) for control cells to 160 ± 13 ms (n = 15) for cTnT-SERCA1 transfected cells. Panel B shows that SERCA1 ex-

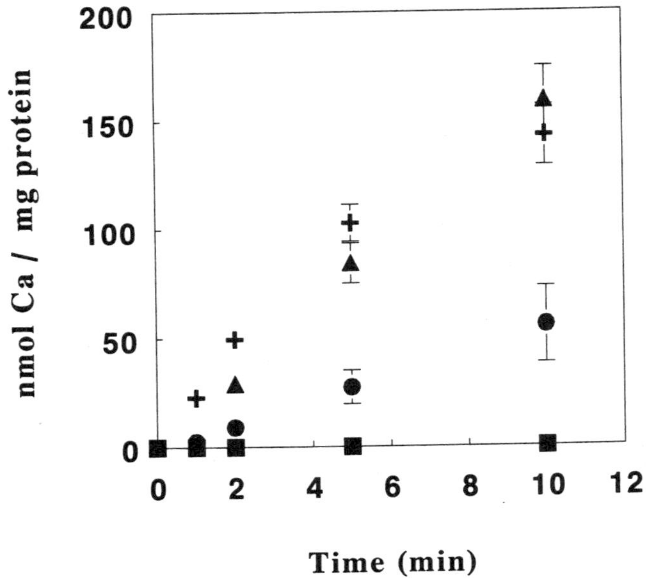

FIGURE 8. ATP-dependent Ca^{2+} uptake in homogenates of chick embryo myocytes. Cultures of chick embryo cardiac myocytes were infected with cTnT-SERCA1 (▲), or cmv-SERCA1 (✚) recombinant adenovirus, with pfu levels of 50 or 10 per seeded cell, respectively. Forty-eight hours following the infection, the myocytes were collected for measurements of ATP-dependent Ca^{2+} uptake (measured by a radioactive isotope and filtration method). Control cultures (●) were subjected to gene transfer procedures without cDNA. Note that Ca^{2+} uptake was totally inhibited by 1 μM TG (■).[43]

pression had a similar effect on the $[Ca^{2+}]_i$ transients. The rate of SR Ca^{2+} reuptake was estimated from the calculation to the first-order time constants (τ) of the decay phase of the $[Ca^{2+}]_i$ transients. This kinetic analysis revealed that SERCA1 expression resulted in a marked increase in the rate of decay as τ decreased by 45%, from 190 ± 18 ms (n = 27) in control to 113 ± 13 ms (n = 15) in cTnT-SERCA1 transfected cells. Taken together these results demonstrate that transgenic expression of isomorphic SERCA1 under control of the cTnT promoter had a significant impact on cardiac cell function.

CONCLUSIONS

Our experiments on specific inhibition and enhancement of the SR ATPase demonstrate that the Ca^{2+} pump of intracellular membranes sustains a very important role in the excitation-contraction coupling of cardiac myocytes. Furthermore, they indicate that it is possible to influence the contractile function of cardiac myocytes by manipulations of the SR Ca^{2+} pump. Finally, we emphasize the importance of cell-specific promoters for selective expression in cardiac myocytes following gene transfer into heterogeneous cell populations.

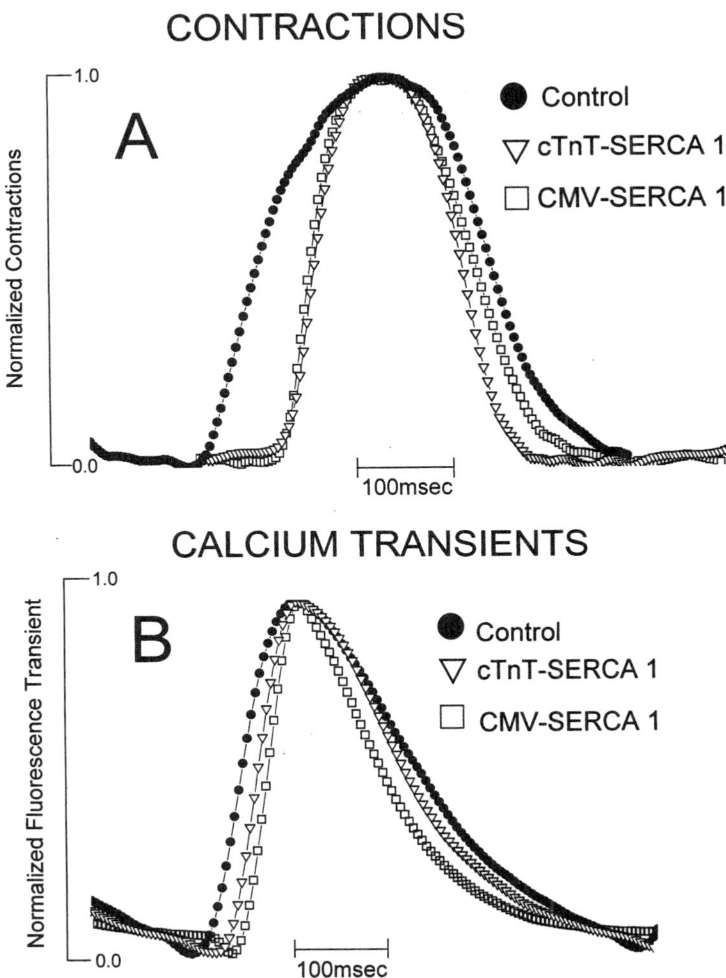

FIGURE 9. Effects of transgenic SERCA1 expression on the contractile behavior and $[Ca^{2+}]i$ transients of chicken embryo cardiac myocytes. In **panel A,** cultured myocytes were field stimulated at 2 Hz and the contractile behavior was recorded with the use of videomicroscopy. Each *curve* represents normalized twitches from three cells that were signal averaged from 20 twitches per cell. In **panel B,** cultured cells were loaded with the Ca^{2+} indicator Fluo-3AM and the resulting fluorescent transients were recorded with an epifluorescence microscope equipped with photomultipliers. The normalized signal average from three cells in each culture is superimposed.

REFERENCES

1. HASSELBACH, W. & M. MAKINOSE. 1961. Die Calciumpumpe der "Erschlaffungsgrana" des Muskels and ihre Abhangigkeit von der ATP-spaltung. Biochem. Z. **333:** 518–528.

2. Ebashi, S. & F. Lippman. 1962. Adenosine triphosphate–linked concentration of calcium ions in a particulate fraction of rabbit muscle. J. Cell Biol. **14:** 389–400.
3. Carsten, M. E. 1964. Cardiac calcium pump. Proc. Natl. Acad. Sci. USA **52:** 1456.
4. Fanburg, B., R. M. Finkel & A. Martonosi. 1964. Role of calcium in the mechanism of relaxation of cardiac muscle. J. Biol. Chem. **239:** 2298.
5. Inesi, G., S. Ebashi & T. Watanabe. 1964. Preparation of vesicular relaxing factor from bovine heart tissue. Am. J. Physiol. **14:** 167–222.
6. Jones, L. R., A. D. Wegener & H. K. Simmerman. 1988. Purification of phospholamban from canine cardiac sarcoplasmic reticulum vesicles by use of sulfhydryl group affinity chromatography. Methods Enzymol. **157:** 360–369.
7. Luo, W., I. L. Grupp, J. Harrer, S. Ponniah, G. Grupp, J. J. Duffy, T. Doetschman & E. G. Kranias. 1994. Targeted ablation of the phospholamban gene is associated with markedly enhanced myocardial contractility and loss of beta-agonist stimulation. Circ. Res. **75:** 401–409.
8. Tada, M., M. Kadoma, M. Inui & J. Fujii. 1988. Regulation of Ca^{2+}-pump form cardiac sarcoplasmic reticulum. Methods Enzymol. **157:** 107–154.
9. Christensen, S. B., I. K. Larsen & U. Rasmussen. 1982. Thapsigargin and thapsigargicin, two histamine liberating sesquiterpene lactones from Thapsia garganica. X-ray analysis of the 7,11-epoxide of thapsigargin. J. Org. Chem. **47:** 649–652.
10. Christensen, S. B. 1988. Interpretation of the NMR and circular dichroic data of the sesquiterpene lactone thapsigargin. Acta Chem. Scand. **B42:** 623–628.
11. Thastrup, O., P. J. Linnebjerg, P. J. Bjerrum, C. M. Knudson & S. B. Christensen. 1987. The inflammatory and tumor-promoting sesquiterpene lactone thapsigargin activates platelets by selective mobilization of calcium as shown by protein phosphorylation. Biochim. Biophys. Acta **927:** 65–73.
12. Thastrup, O., B. Foder & O. Scharff. 1987. The Calcium mobilizing and tumor promoting agent, thapsigargin, elevates the platelet cytoplasmic free calcium concentration to a higher steady state level. A possible mechanism of action for the tumour promotion. Biochem. Biophys. Res. Commun. **142:** 654–660.
13. Sagara, Y. & G. Inesi. 1991. Inhibition of the sarcoplasmic reticulum Ca^{2+} transport ATPase by thapsigargin at subnanomolar concentrations. J. Biol. Chem. **266:** 13503–13506.
14. Kijima, Y., E. Ogunbunmi & S. Fleischer. 1991. Drug action of thapsigargin on the Ca^{2+} pump protein of sarcoplasmic reticulum. J. Biol. Chem. **266:** 22912–22918.
15. Lytton, J., M. Westlin & M. R. Hanley. 1991. Thapsigargin inhibits the sarcoplasmic or endoplasmic reticulum Ca-ATPase family of calcium pumps. J. Biol. Chem. **266:** 17067–17071.
16. Campbell, A. M., P. D. Kessler, Y. Sagara, G. Inesi & D. M. Fambrough. 1991. Nucleotide sequences of avian cardiac and brain SR/ER Ca^{2+}-ATPases and functional comparisons with fast twitch Ca^{2+}-ATPase. Calcium affinities and inhibitor effects. J. Biol. Chem. **266:** 16050–16055.
17. Hua, S., H. Malak, J. R. Lakowicz & G. Inesi. 1995. Synthesis and interaction of fluorescent thapsigargin derivatives with the sarcoplasmic reticulum ATPase membrane-bound region. Biochemistry **34:** 5137–5142.
18. Sumbilla, C., L. Lu, G. Inesi, T. Ishii, K. Takeyasu, Y. Fang & D. M. Fambrough. 1993. Ca^{2+} dependent and thapsigargin-inhibited phosphorylation of Na^{+},K^{+}-ATPase catalytic domain following chimeric recombination with the Ca^{2+}-ATPase. J. Biol. Chem. **268:** 21185–21192.
19. Norregaard, A., B. Vilsen & J. P. Andersen. 1994. Transmembrane segment M3 is essential to thapsigargin sensitivity of the sarcoplasmic reticulum Ca^{2+}-ATPase. J. Biol. Chem. **269:** 26598–26601.
20. Hua, S. & G. Inesi. 1997. Synthesis of a radioactive azido derivative of thapsigargin and photolabeling of the sarcoplasmic reticulum ATPase. Biochemistry **36:** 11865–11872.
21. Sagara, Y., J. B. Wade & G. Inesi. 1992. A conformational mechanism for formation of a dead-end complex by the sarcoplasmic reticulum ATPase with thapsigargin. J. Biol. Chem. **267:** 1286–1292.
22. Stokes, D. L. & J.-J. Lacapère. 1994. Conformation of Ca^{2+}-ATPase in two crystal forms.

Effects of Ca^{2+}, thapsigargin, adenosine 5′-(β,gamma-methylene triphosphate), and chromium(III)-ATP on crystallization. J. Biol. Chem. **269:** 11606–11613.

23. Kirby, M. S., Y. Sagara, S. T. Gaa, G. Inesi, W. J. Lederer, T. B. Rogers. 1992. Thapsigargin inhibits contraction and Ca^{2+} transient cardiac cells by specific inhibition of the sarcoplasmic reticulum Ca^{2+} pump. J. Biol. Chem. **267**(18): 12545–12551.
24. Rogers, T. B., G. Inesi, R. Wade & W. J. Lederer. 1995. Use of thapsigargin to study Ca^{2+} homeostasis in cardiac cells. Bioscience Rep. **15:** 341–349.
25. MacLennan, D. H., C. J. Brandl, B. Korczak & N. M. Green. 1985. Amino-acid sequence of a Ca^{2+}+Mg^{2+} dependent ATPase from rabbit muscle sarcoplasmic reticulum, deduced from its complementary DNA sequence. Nature **316:** 696–700.
26. Karin, N. J., Z. Kaprielian & D. M. Fambrough. 1989. Expression of avian Ca^{2+}-ATPase in cultured mouse myogenic cells. Mol. Cell. Biol. **9:** 1978–1986.
27. Lompre, A. M., F. Lambert, E. G. Lakatta & K. Schwartz. 1991. Expression of sarcoplasmic reticulum Ca^{2+}-ATPase and calsequestrin genes in rat heart during ontogenic development and aging. Circ. Res. **69:** 1380–1388.
28. Wu, K. D. & J. Lytton. 1993. Molecular cloning and quantification of sarcoplasmic reticulum Ca^{2+}-ATPase isoforms in rat muscles. Am. J. Physiol. **264:** C333–C341.
29. Maruyama, K. & D. H. MacLennan. 1988. Mutation of aspartic acid-35, lysine-352 and lysine-515 alters the Ca^{2+} transport activity of the Ca^{2+}-ATPase expressed in COS-1 cells. Proc. Natl. Acad. Sci. USA **85:** 3314–3318.
30. Clarke, D. M., T. W. Loo, G. Inesi & D. H. MacLennan. 1989. Location of high affinity Ca^{2+}-binding sites within the predicted transmembrane domain of the sarcoplasmic reticulum Ca^{2+}-ATPase. Nature **339:** 476–478.
31. Inesi, G., C. Sumbilla & M. E. Kirtley. 1990. Relationships of molecular structure and function in the Ca^{2+} transport ATPase. Physiol. Rev. **70:** 749–760.
32. Hussain, A., C. Garnett, M. G. Klein, J.-J. Tsai-Wu, M. F. Schneider & G. Inesi. 1995. Direct involvement of intracellular Ca^{2+}-transport ATPase in the development of thapsigargin resistance by Chinese hamster lung fibroblasts. J. Biol. Chem. **270:** 12140–12146.
33. Cotten, M., E. Wagner, K. Zatloukal, S. Philips, D. T. Curiel & M. L. Birnstiel. 1992. High efficiency receptor-mediated delivery of small and large gene constructs using the endosome-disruption activity of defective or chemically inactivated adenovirus particles. Proc. Natl. Acad. Sci. USA **89:** 6094–6098.
34. Graham, F. L. & L. Prevec. 1992. Adenovirus based expression vectors and recombinant vaccines. *In* Vaccines: New Approaches to Immunological Problems. R. W. Ellis, Ed.: 363–390. Butterworth. Stoneham, MA.
35. Kass-Eiler, A., E. Falick-Pedersen, M. Alvira, J. Rivera, P. M. Buttrick, B. A. Wittenberg, L. Cipriani & L. A. Leinwand. 1993. Quantitative determination of adenovirus-mediated gene delivery to rat cardiac myocytes in vitro and in vivo. Proc. Natl. Acad. Sci. USA **90:** 11498–11502.
36. Kirschenbaum, L. A., W. R. MacLennan, W. Mazur, B. A. French & M. D. Schneider. 1993. Highly efficient gene transfer into adult ventricular myocytes by recombinant adenovirus. J. Clin. Invest. **92:** 381–387.
37. Schneider, M. D. & B. A. French. 1993. The advent of adenovirus: Gene therapy for cardiovascular disease. Circulation **88:** 1937–1942.
38. Donahue, J. K., K. Kikkawa, D. C. Johns, E. Marban & J. H. Lawrence. 1997. Ultrarapid, highly efficient viral gene transfer to the heart. Proc. Natl. Acad. Sci. USA **94:** 4664–4668.
39. Hajjar, R. J., J. X. Kang, J. K. Gwathmey & A. Rosenzweig. 1997. Physiological effects of adenoviral gene transfer of sarcoplasmic reticulum calcium ATPase in isolated rat myocytes. Circulation **95:** 423–429.
40. Bastide, F., G. Meissner, S. Fleischer & R. L. Post. 1973. Similarity of the active site of phosphorylation of the ATPase for transport of sodium and potassium ions in kidney to that for transport of calcium ion in sarcoplasmic reticulum of muscle. J. Biol. Chem. **248:** 8385–8391.
41. Degani, C. & P. D. Boyer. 1973. A borohydride reduction method for characterization of the acyl phosphate linkage in proteins and its application to sarcoplasmic reticulum adenosine triphosphatase. J. Biol. Chem. **248:** 8222–8226.

42. Mar, J. H., P. B. Antin, T. A. Cooper & C. P. Ordahl. 1988. Analysis of the upstream regions governing expression of the chicken cardiac troponin T gene in embryonic cardiac and skeletal muscle cells. J. Cell Biol. **107:** 573–585.
43. Inesi, G., D. Lewis, C. Sumbilla, A. Nandi, K. W. Huff, T. B. Rogers, D. C. Johns, P. D. Kessler & C. P. Ordahl. 1998. Cell specific Ca^{2+} ATPase isoform expression in cardiac myocytes following gene transfer by recombinant adenovirus vector. Am. J. Physiol. Cell Physiol. **43:** C645–C653.

The Role of Sarcoplasmic Reticulum Proteins in Heart Disease: Introduction

WILLIAM GROSSMAN[a]

Cardiology Division, University of California, San Francisco, Medical Center, Box 0124, 505 Parnassus Avenue, San Francisco, California 94143-0124, USA

The preceding papers have been concerned largely with basic structure and structure-function relations concerning the sarcoplasmic reticular calcium ATPase, phospholamban, and the various ryanodine receptors. This part will focus on how gene expression, function, and structure-function relationships of these active pumps and regulatory proteins are altered in disease states. Of particular interest is the fact that cardiac disease resulting in clinical heart failure is commonly associated with diastolic dysfunction. In up to 40% of patients presenting with clinical congestive heart failure,[1] systolic left ventricular function is normal. It has been well known for nearly 100 years that clinical congestive heart failure may result solely from structural disease that impedes diastolic inflow into the heart; conditions exemplifying this type of heart failure are mitral stenosis, constrictive pericarditis, and restrictive cardiomyopathy. However, it has been recognized over the past 25 years that many patients with congestive heart failure have no obvious structural abnormality, and there has been increasing interest in the possibility that abnormal relaxation of cardiac muscle underlies heart failure in at least some of these patients.

Flash pulmonary edema is a form of acute congestive heart failure commonly seen in the setting of myocardial ischemia. Left ventricular diastolic pressure is increased acutely in the setting of angina pectoris,[2] and although there is some systolic dysfunction in this setting, most studies indicate that impaired relaxation and diastolic dysfunction are the predominant mechanisms for increased diastolic pressure and ultimately, flash pulmonary edema in these patients.[3,4]

Another condition associated primarily with diastolic rather than systolic dysfunction is hypertrophic cardiomyopathy. The diastolic dysfunction in patients with hypertrophic cardiomyopathy is due in part to increased mechanical resistance to diastolic filling associated with a thick-walled left ventricle. However, there is substantial evidence that an important myocardial functional component also contributes to diastolic dysfunction in these patients,[5] and markedly abnormal left ventricular diastolic pressure curves seen in patients with hypertrophic cardiomyopathy can be normalized by administration of a calcium antagonist. Studies in isolated human muscle from patients with hypertrophic cardiomyopathy[6] have demonstrated striking abnormalities of diastolic calcium handling, consistent with dysfunction of the sarcoplasmic reticulum.

Finally, dilated cardiomyopathy, whether due to chronic hypertension, remodeling following a large myocardial infarction, or chronic volume overload, is associated with impairment in both inotropic and lusitropic reserve. This is manifest by failure of the rates of contraction and relaxation to increase in response to heart rate increases in these patients. This lack of positive "Treppe" has long puzzled physiologists and clinicians, but recent evidence indicates that the cause is underlying dysfunction of intra-

[a] Phone: 415-502-8628; fax: 415-476-5875

cellular calcium homeostasis, in large part related to sarcoplasmic reticular dysfunction. In some patients, this abnormality can be compensated for (at least at resting heart rates) by augmented sodium-calcium exchange.[7–9]

Impaired diastolic calcium sequestration due to dysfunction of the sarcoplasmic reticulum may result from inadequate amounts of SERCA-II protein, relative excess of phospholamban, failure to phosphorylate (and thus inactivate) phospholamban, inadequate production or excessive destruction of cyclic AMP, or other as-yet-unspecified mechanisms. Whatever the cause, impaired sarcoplasmic reticular calcium sequestration will inevitably affect not only diastolic relaxation, but also systolic contractility, due to inadequate filling of sarcoplasmic reticular stores with calcium needed for systolic activation. The obligatory relatedness of systole and diastole is well summarized in D. H. Lawrence's poem "Essay on Love" as follows:

> So that the coming together depends on the going apart, the systole depends on the diastole, the flow depends upon the ebb. There can never be love universal and unbroken. The sea can never rise to high tide over all the globe at once. The undisputed of love can never be.
>
> The love between man and woman is the perfect heartbeat of life, systole, diastole.

REFERENCES

1. DOUGHERTY, A. H., G. V. NACCARELLI, E. L. GRAY, C. H. HICKS & R. A. GOLDSTEIN. 1984. Congestive heart failure with normal systolic function. Am. J. Cardiol. **54:** 778–782.
2. BARRY, W. H., J. F. BROOKER, E. L. ALDERMAN & D. C. HARRISON. 1974. Changes in diastolic stiffness and tone of the left ventricle during angina pectoris. Circulation **49:** 255–263.
3. AROESTY, J. M., R. G. MCKAY, G. V. HELLER, H. D. ROYAL, A. V. ALS & W. GROSSMAN. 1985. Simultaneous assessment of left ventricular systolic and diastolic dysfunction during pacing-induced ischemia. Circulation **71:** 889–900.
4. GROSSMAN, W. 1991. Diastolic dysfunction in congestive heart failure. N. Engl. J. Med. **325:** 1557–1564.
5. LORELL, B. H., W. J. PAULUS, W. GROSSMAN, J. WYNNE & P. F. COHN. 1982. Modification of abnormal left ventricular diastolic properties by nifedipine in patients with hypertrophic cardiomyopathy. Circulation **65:** 499–507.
6. GWATHMEY, J. K., S. E. WARREN, G. M. BRIGGS, L. COPELAS, M. D. FELDMAN, P. J. PHILLIPS, M. CALLAHAN, JR., F. J. SCHOEN, W. GROSSMAN & J. P. MORGAN. 1991. Diastolic dysfunction in hypertrophic cardiomyopathy. Effect on active force generation during systole. J. Clin. Invest. **87:** 1023–1031.
7. PIESKE, B., B. KRETSCHMANN, M. MEYER, C. HOLUBARSCH, J. WEIRICH, H. POSIVAL, K. MINAMI, H. JUST & G. HASENFUSS. 1994. Alterations in intracellular calcium handling associated with the inverse force-frequency relation in human dilated cardiomyopathy. Circulation **92:** 1169–1178.
8. MEYER, M., W. SCHILLINGER, B. PIESKE, C. HOLUBARSCH, C. HEILMANN, H. POSIVAL, G. KUWAJIMA, K. MIKOSHIBA, H. JUST & G. HASSENFUSS. 1995. Alterations of sarcoplasmic reticulum proteins in failing human dilated cardiomyopathy. Circulation **92:** 778–784.
9. STUDER, R., H. REINECKE, J. BILGER, T. ESCHENHAGEN, M. BOHM, G. HASENFUSS, H. JUST, J. HOLTZ & H. DREXLER. 1994. Gene expression of the cardiac Na^+-$Ca2^+$ exchanger in end-stage human heart failure. Circ. Res. **75:** 443–453.

Alterations in Heart Failure of Cyclic AMP–Dependent Inotropic and Lusitropic Properties of Cardiac and Skeletal Muscle

AMY BISHOP, KERRY E. TRAVERS, JESSICA GROSSMAN, HEATHER JOHNSON, CYNTHIA PERREAULT, JOHN H. WOOLF, ANTONIO CITTADINI, HUGO GONZALEZ-SERRATOS,[a] AND JAMES P. MORGAN[b]

Charles A. Dana Research Institute and Harvard-Thorndike Laboratory, Department of Medicine, Cardiovascular Division, Beth Israel Deaconess Medical Center and Harvard Medical School, Boston, Massachusetts 02215, USA

[a]*Department of Physiology, University of Maryland, School of Medicine, Baltimore, Maryland 21201-1596, USA*

ABSTRACT: A central working hypothesis in our laboratory is that deficient cellular cyclic AMP concentrations may be responsible, at least in part, for striated muscle dysfunction, both cardiac and skeletal, in heart failure. These results suggest that therapy aimed at restoring cyclic AMP to normal levels may be effective with regard to improving systolic and diastolic function in the heart and may decrease the development of fatigue in skeletal muscle of patients with failure. The use of cyclic AMP–dependent drugs in clinical practice has been limited by side effects associated with raising total cellular content of this cyclic nucleotide. However, evidence suggesting that separate pools of cyclic AMP may exist within the cell raises the possibility that those pools associated with excitation/contraction coupling could serve as more specific therapeutic targets.

The contraction and relaxation of mammalian cardiac and skeletal muscle are complex physiologic processes that are dependent upon the sequential and orderly progression of multiple subcellular events. The cellular regulation of excitation-contraction coupling in the mammalian heart is outlined in FIGURE 1, which divides these processes among four sites: sarcolemma, sarcoplasmic reticulum, regulatory complex, and myofilaments. In normal muscle from various regions of the heart and among different species, differences have been reported in the quantity and composition of these regulatory sites, including receptor and ionic channel types and densities, density and number of ionic pumps and exchangers, particularly those associated with maintaining homeostatic intracellular calcium ($Ca^{2+}{}_i$) levels, and responsiveness.[1–3] The same basic steps of excitation-contraction coupling illustrated in FIGURE 1 also occur in mammalian skeletal muscle, although the cellular composition of these two major types of striated muscle cells differ in some important particulars that adapt them for their own unique function.[2]

For the purposes of this review, the central role played by $Ca^{2+}{}_i$ in modulating the contraction and relaxation of both striated muscle types will be emphasized along with

[b] Address for correspondence: James P. Morgan, M.D., Beth Israel Deaconess Medical Center, 330 Brookline Avenue, Boston, Massachusetts 02215. Phone: 617-667-2191; fax: 617-667-1615.

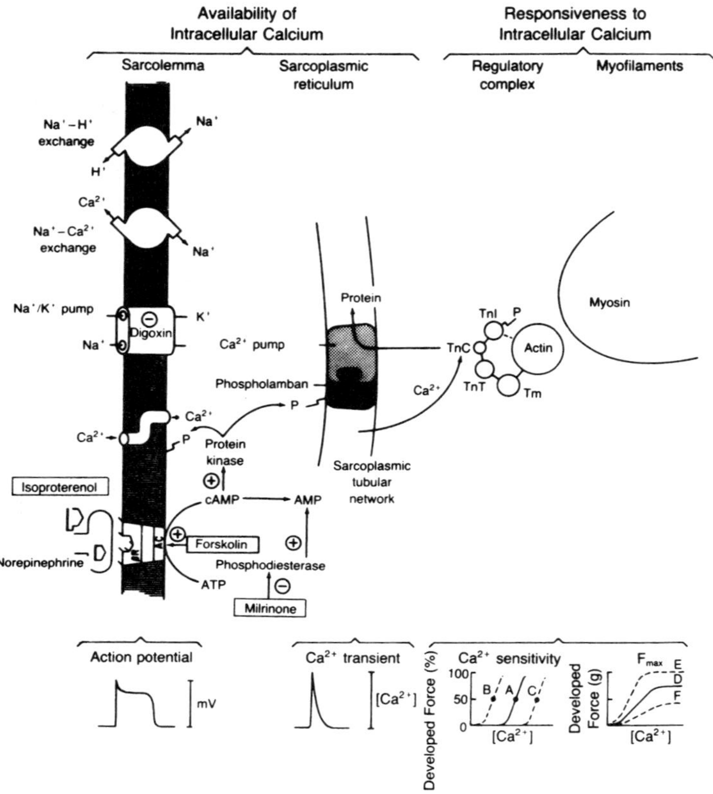

FIGURE 1. Four major cellular sites for the regulation of excitation-contraction coupling in the mammalian heart: sarcolemma, sarcoplasmic reticulum, regulatory complex, and myofilaments. Cardiac contractility may be altered by changing either the availability of intracellular calcium for activation or the responsiveness of the myofilaments to intracellular calcium. Calcium availability is regulated predominantly by sites in the sarcolemma and sarcoplasmic reticulum that can be functionally monitored by means of the action potential and calcium transient, respectively. Responsiveness to intracellular calcium is regulated predominantly by the troponin-tropomyosin complex, attached to actin, and the myofilaments, actin and myosin. These components can be functionally assessed by the calcium sensitivity and maximal calcium-activated force (F_{max}) of fibers rendered hyperpermeable to calcium. See the text for details. The Ca^{2+} transient is the depolarization-induced increase and decrease in the intracellular calcium concentration ($[Ca^{2+}]$); Ca^{2+} sensitivity is the relation between the intracellular calcium concentration and cardiac activation, expressed as a percentage of peak developed force. *Curves* A and D are base-line values of the sensitivity of myofilaments to calcium and F_{max}, respectively. Ca^{2+} sensitivity and F_{max} can change independently of each other. *Curves* B and E show enhancement, and *curves* C and F depression, of Ca^{2+} sensitivity and F_{max}, respectively. TnI denotes troponin I, TnC troponin C, TnT troponin T, Tm Tropomyosin, βR beta-adrenergic receptor, AC adenylate cyclase, cAMP cyclic AMP, and P phosphorylation. (Reprinted with permission from J. P. Morgan.[1])

the important modulatory role on Ca^{2+}_i handling exerted by another second messenger, cyclic adenosine monophosphate (cyclic AMP). We will present evidence supporting the hypothesis that deficient cellular concentrations of cyclic AMP develop in both cardiac and skeletal muscle with the occurrence of heart failure (CHF) and appears to be a major determinant of the abnormal contraction and relaxation of both striated muscle types in this disease state.

CYCLIC AMP AND CARDIAC MUSCLE DYSFUNCTION IN HEART FAILURE

Cyclic AMP is one of several important second messengers in the heart, a group that also includes inositol triphosphate, diacylglyercol, nitric oxide, and the calcium ion itself.[4] Cyclic AMP modulates intracellular Ca^{2+}_i through the activation of protein kinases, which phosphorylate proteins at several subcellular sites, including the sarcolemma, the sarcoplasmic reticulum, and the troponin-tropomyosin regulatory complex on the myofilaments (FIG. 1). Phosphorylation of the voltage-dependent, L-type calcium channels of the sarcolemma increases the intracellular influx of Ca^{2+}, thereby enhancing systolic contraction. Cyclic AMP also enhances relaxation through phosphorylation of sites on the sarcoplasmic reticulum (phospholamban and troponin I on the troponin-tropomyosin complex). Phosphorylation of phospholamban enhances the rate of resequestration of intracellular calcium during diastole; phosphorylation of TnI increases the rate of dissociation of calcium from its binding site on troponin C; and both of these effects result in an enhanced rate of cardiac relaxation.[4]

A variety of cellular abnormalities have been reported to occur in the heart with the onset and progression of failure. Sarcolemmal changes have been reported with regard to the numbers or coupling of adrenergic receptors and voltage-dependent calcium channels. The density of calcium-uptake sites on the sarcoplasmic reticulum has been reported to decrease, and the mechanisms that regulate calcium release appear to be altered. Moreover, the structure of the contractile apparatus and the ability of the mitochondria to supply the ATP necessary to fuel contraction and relaxation may also be impaired. It is, therefore, not surprising that a variety of abnormalities of both systolic and diastolic function have been described in animal models and patients with CHF.[1,5]

Studies with human myocardium are of particular interest and have been reported from several laboratories.[6,7] FIGURE 2 shows intracellular calcium transients, isometric contraction, and action potentials recorded in cardiac muscle from a patient without CHF, a patient without a cardiomyopathy, and a patient with hypertrophic cardiomyopathy. Marked changes from normal can obviously be seen in the calcium signals, action potentials, and tension recordings, both with contraction and relaxation. These sorts of data support the hypothesis that the prolonged contraction of myopathic muscle *in vitro,* as well as the myocardial relaxation abnormalities in patients with dilated cardiomyopathy appear to correlate with changes in intracellular calcium modulation. The details of these alterations have been described elsewhere.[6]

The etiology of the abnormalities described above is undoubtedly complex and involves several different cellular and molecular mechanisms.[5] However, we believe that deficient concentrations of cyclic AMP may play a major role. Evidence to support this hypothesis has been provided by pharmacologic studies with drugs known to increase cellular cyclic AMP concentrations, such as phosphodiesterase inhibitors, which show markedly decreased efficacy in cardiac muscle from patients with heart failure, as illustrated in the bottom panel of FIGURE 3.[8] The resultant prolongation of relaxation that is characteristic of myocardium from animals and patients with failure (middle panel, FIG. 3) can result in incomplete relaxation at higher pacing rates (top panel, FIG.

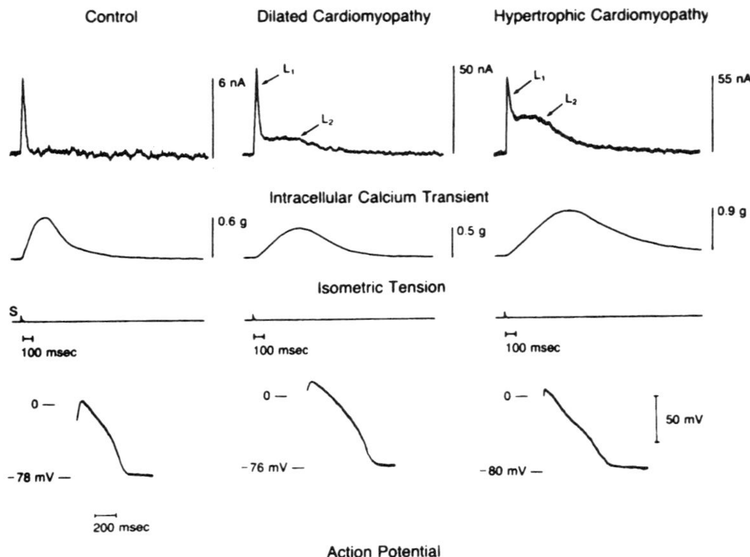

FIGURE 2. Recordings representing intracellular calcium transient (recorded with the bioluminescent indicator aequorin), isometric tension, and stimulus artifact (S) from control and myopathic human *trabeculae carneae,* maintained *in vitro;* and action potentials in different muscles from the same hearts. L_1 and L_2 denote two temporally distinct components of the calcium transients that are typical of failing human muscle. L_2 appears to reflect abnormal Ca^{2+} handling by the sarcoplasmic reticulum and sarcolemma. Note the correlation of L_2 with prolonged action potential duration and delayed relaxation of the isometric contraction. (Reprinted with permission from Gwathmey *et al.*[6])

3). In contrast, the effectiveness of inotropic stimulation with direct adenylate cyclase activators like forskolin appears to be relatively well preserved, and a minimally effective concentration of this agent, given to restore cellular cyclic AMP levels towards normal, also restores the inotropic and lusitropic efficacy of phosphodiesterase inhibitors in myocardium from animals and patients with failure.[9]

These results are consistent with the hypothesis that an abnormality in adenylate cyclase activity, and thus in the production of cyclic AMP, may be a fundamental defect in patients with end-stage heart failure, which would result in decreased cyclic AMP–dependent protein kinase activity, a decrease in the degree of phosphorylation normally present in the cell as a result of this enzymatic activity, and the sarcolemmal, sarcoplasmic reticular, and contractile apparatus dysfunction described above and outlined in FIGURE 1. The precise etiology of this deficiency remains to be determined, but may be related to a relative increase in the ratio of the Gi/Gs proteins that regulate adenylate cyclase activity.[10,11] Moreover, it appears that the degree to which the effectiveness of phosphodiesterase inhibitors is depressed correlates with the severity of heart failure,[12] and that inotropic vs. lusitropic processes may be differentially affected.[13] An un-

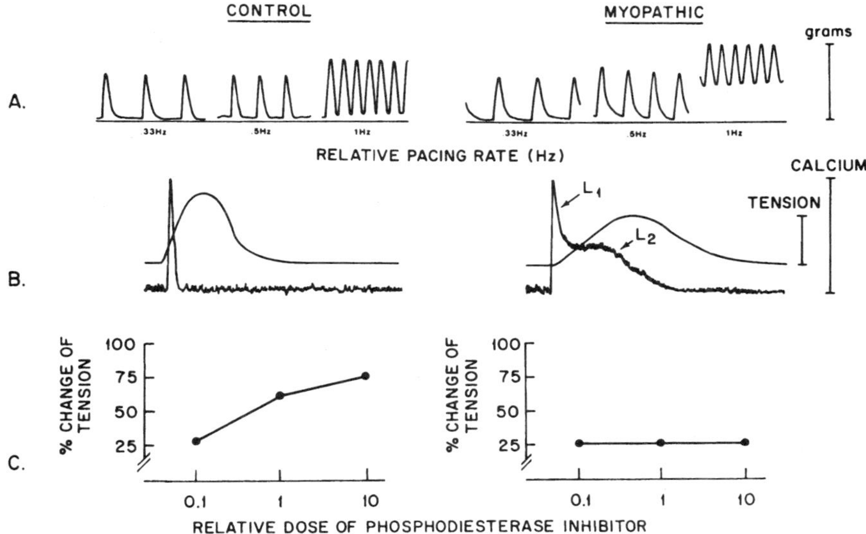

FIGURE 3. Tracings showing signatures of heart failure in isolated human myocardium. **(A)** Reversal of force-frequency relation from positive to negative staircase going from lower to higher pacing frequencies. **(B)** Prolonged $[Ca^{2+}]_i$ transient and twitch; two components, L_1 and L_2, in $[Ca^{2+}]_i$ transient. **(C)** Markedly diminished response to phosphodiesterase inhibitors like milrinone. (Reprinted with permission from Perreault *et al.*[8])

fortunate clinical consequence of this relationship appears to be that cyclic AMP–dependent agents, such as beta adrenergic and phosphodiesterase inhibitors, may be the least effective in the patients who would derive the most benefit from their action—i.e., patients with the most severe degree of systolic and/or diastolic dysfunction.[1]

SKELETAL MUSCLE DYSFUNCTION IN HEART FAILURE AND CYCLIC AMP

Catecholamine effects on skeletal muscle have been specifically related to stimulation of beta-2 adrenergic receptor sites and a consequent elevation in cyclic AMP.[14] A variety of cellular responses to elevation of cyclic AMP have been reported in skeletal muscle, including enhancement of Na^+/H^+ antiporter activity, which has been associated with decreased fatiguability of both fast-twitch and slow-twitch fibers.[15] In addition, Na^+/K^+ ATPase activity appears to be enhanced, decreasing the accumulation of extracellular potassium ions, which have been associated with the development of fatigue.[16,17] These functional effects are attenuated during beta-2 adrenergic receptor down-regulation secondary to *in vivo* treatment with catecholamines.[18,19] Down-regulation of beta-2 receptors on skeletal muscle has also been reported to occur with heart failure, probably due to the high circulating catecholamine levels in this condition.[20,21] Whether this down-regulation is associated with additional changes in G-protein regulation of adenylate cyclase, as has been reported to occur in the heart, remains to be determined.[10,11]

Physiologic concentrations of catecholamines appear to predominantly affect the time course rather than the amplitude of skeletal muscle contraction,[22] although they have been shown to increase force generation in both fast- and slow-twitch skeletal muscle fibers. These effects are associated with changes in cellular cyclic AMP levels in both fast- and slow-twitch muscles.[22,23]

Skeletal muscles from rats with CHF show mechanical dysfunction and abnormal calcium handling, similar to failing myocardium, which may also be due to decreased intracellular cAMP levels. Skeletal muscle from CHF rats have decreased tension development, prolonged calcium transients, and reduced calcium release (see FIG. 4). CHF skeletal muscle also demonstrates enhanced fatigue development and altered calcium signaling during the fatigue cycle. These cellular changes do not appear to be related to disuse atrophy.[24] Studies of amphibian skeletal muscle have demonstrated that fatigue is associated with decreased availability of activator calcium and a transient shift in myofilament calcium sensitivity; the high rate of fatigue development of skeletal muscles in the CHF patient could also be due to a decrease in activator calcium and a change in myofilament Ca^{2+} sensitivity.[25–28] We recently demonstrated that tension development by CHF skeletal muscles can be reversed towards normal with the addition of cyclic AMP.[29] These data, when taken together, indicate that decreased intracellular cAMP levels may be an important mechanism underlying mechanical dysfunction of CHF skeletal muscle, although the precise mechanism of their subcellular effects remains to be determined.

We tested the hypothesis that deficient cellular cyclic AMP is a predominant cause of the mechanical dysfunction of skeletal muscle, as it appears to be in myocardium in CHF. We chose the myocardial infarction model of CHF as a readily reproducible model that appears similar to human CHF in many respects.[30] We established that there is decreased force per unit cross-sectional area and increased fatigue development in CHF muscle, and we sought to restore function of CHF skeletal muscle by elevating intracellular cAMP through the addition of epinephrine. We also measured cyclic AMP levels in CHF skeletal muscle and compared these values to control skeletal muscles. Our data support the hypothesis that decreased cyclic AMP levels are an important cause of skeletal muscle dysfunction in CHF.

For these studies, heart failure was induced by litigation of the coronary artery in Sprague-Dawley rats as previously described.[30] One month after the operation, the animals underwent echocardiography, and the size of the infarct was measured. Only animals certain to develop CHF (i.e., 40–50% infarction) were maintained for the CHF group. Six weeks after surgery, both the sham and infarcted rats were catheterized for hemodynamic measurements. Of the rats with infarctions, only those that showed signs of heart failure with a left ventricular end-diastolic pressure of 20 mm of mercury or more were used. The rats were sacrificed by cardiac excision and the extensor digitorum longus muscles immediately dissected. The muscles were placed in an organ bath, perfused with physiologic salt solution at 22.5 °C, and stimulated with square wave pulses of 0.5 ms duration at 1.5 times the minimum voltage necessary for activation via field electrodes. Muscle lengths were adjusted to the apex of the length-tension curve. Fatigue was induced by repetitive cyclic electric stimulation. Each fatigue cycle was composed of a train of electric shocks delivered at 75 Hz with a train duration of 2 seconds repeated every 3 seconds until fatigue developed. Fatigue was defined as the time required to produce 50% decrease of the initial first tetanic contraction. Epinephrine was added at a concentration of 10^{-7} M to increase diastolic cyclic AMP levels and to determine if altered function of CHF muscles could be restored to normal. Cyclic AMP content was measured in a subset of animals by immunoassay.

FIGURE 5 shows that forces were decreased significantly in CHF skeletal muscles compared with control muscles during twitches and at all tetanic stimulation frequen-

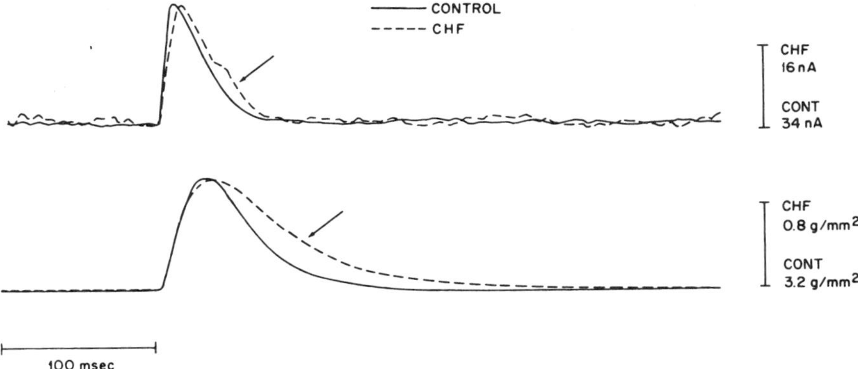

FIGURE 4. Representative aequorin light signals **(top)** and isometric twitches **(bottom)** recorded from an extensor digitorum longus muscle bundle of 100 to 200 cells dissected from control rats (CONT, *solid line*) and rats with chronic heart failure (CHF, *dotted line*). Light and tension responses were electronically adjusted to equal amplitudes and superimposed to illustrate time course differences. Absolute amplitudes of the signals are indicated to the **right** of each panel. Stimulation frequency was 0.33 Hz; pulse duration was 0.5 millisecond. (Reprinted with permission from Perreault *et al.*[24])

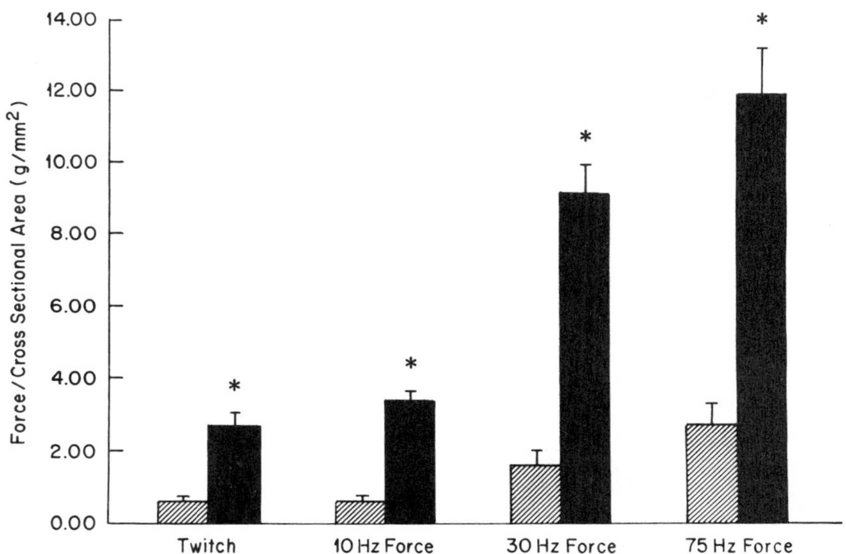

FIGURE 5. Bar graph illustrating mean +/– SEM peak force/cross sectional area at twitch (.33 Hz) and tetani at 10 Hz, 30 Hz, and 75Hz of extensor digitorum longus muscle from rats with CHF and rats with CHF with epinephrine added. $^*p < 0.05$ when compared to control muscles.

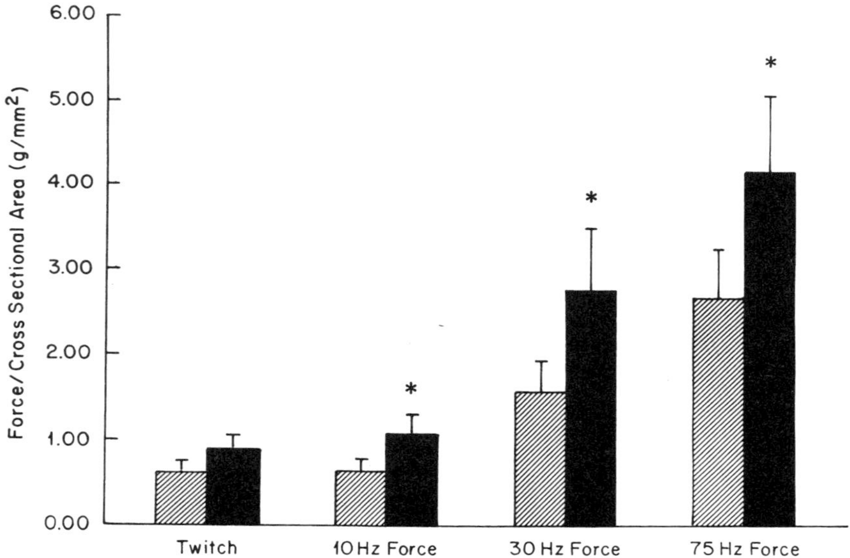

FIGURE 6. Bar graph illustrating mean +/–SEM peak force/cross sectional area at twitch (.33Hz) and tetani at 10Hz, 30 Hz, and 75Hz of extensor digitorum longus muscle from rats with CHF and rats with CHF with epinephrine added. $*p < 0.05$ when compared to muscles with no epinephrine.

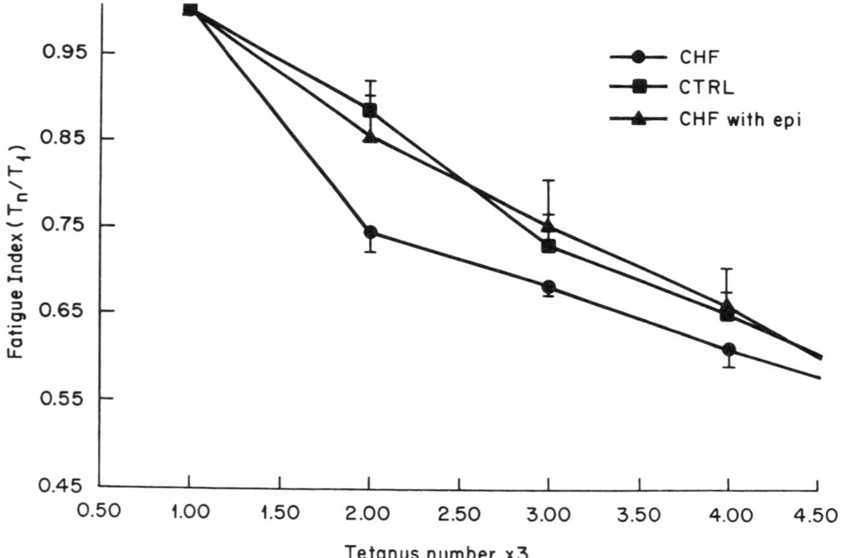

FIGURE 7. Graph illustrating the relation between fatigue index ratio of maximum tetanic tension produced during the nth tetanus output during the first tetanus (Tn/T1) and the number of tetani (n) or time in seconds.

cies. Specific forces of control muscles were not significantly affected by the presence of epinephrine at any of the frequencies used, but in contrast, the specific tension generated by CHF muscles increased significantly at all stimulation frequencies with the addition of 10^{-7} M of epinephrine (FIG. 6). Although CHF muscles responded with an increase in force to maximally effective concentrations of epinephrine, specific forces were not returned to control values at all stimulation frequencies.

We have previously reported that CHF EDL muscles develop fatigue much more rapidly than control muscles.[24] Therefore, we decided to study the effect of epinephrine on fatigue development in control and CHF skeletal muscles. A representative experiment showing the beginning of fatigue development is illustrated in FIGURE 7. In the presence of 10^{-7} epinephrine, not only was the maximum force during the first tetanic stimulation increased towards control values, but also the shape of each individual tetanus was similar to the controls and the development of fatigue was delayed. As shown in FIGURE 7, the fatigue indices were smaller and decreased faster in muscles from CHF animals than in muscles from control rats throughout the period of stimulation. Epinephrine increased the fatigue indices of CHF muscles to control levels. Cellular cyclic AMP levels in the CHF muscles were significantly lower than in the controls (93 +/– 16.5, CHF versus 230 +/– 25.17 pm/g, controls; $p < 0.05$).

SIGNIFICANCE AND LIMITATIONS OF THE DATA

Taken together, the results described above support the unifying hypothesis that dysfunction of both cardiac and skeletal muscle in heart failure is due, at least in part, to deficient cellular cyclic AMP concentrations. While it is extremely unlikely that any single factor can account for all the systolic and diastolic abnormalities that develop with heart failure, our findings suggest that the functional changes that result, may be partially reversible by increasing cellular levels of cyclic AMP in both muscle types. The clinical trials that have appeared to date with catecholamines can be interpreted as support for this hypothesis since, for example, drugs with phosphodiesterase-inhibiting properties increase exercise time, as well as improve systolic and diastolic performance of the heart.[31] Additional studies will be necessary to determine the extent to which these beneficial actions of increasing cyclic AMP are due to direct effects on the skeletal, as well as cardiac, myocytes and to what extent the former is a consequence of the latter. Since fatigue and generalized weakness are among the most disabling symptoms experienced by patients with heart failure, resolution of these questions has potential clinical importance.

The *in vitro* studies described in this review have certain limitations that need to be kept in mind when interpreting the results. Clearly, cyclic AMP is only one of several important second-messenger systems in the heart, and it remains to be shown how it may be related to or interact with nitric oxide, inositol triphosphates, and perhaps other, as yet undescribed, signaling pathways in myocytes. It has been difficult to consistently document decreased cyclic AMP concentrations by quantitative measurement in cardiac muscle samples; this may be due to the heterogeneity of tissue samples studied or, it may, in fact, reflect the existence of different subcellular pools of this cyclic nucleotide that are associated with individual steps in excitation-contraction coupling.[1] For example, a relatively preserved relaxant effect has been associated with cyclic AMP–dependent agents in failing human myocardium, despite significant diminution of their positive inotropic effects.[13] Another important finding that needs to be considered is that addition of cyclic AMP to failing tissue from animal models and patients with heart failure does not completely restore to normal the contractile abnormalities that are present.[24,32] Moreover, many of the same functional abnormalities detectable in failing cardiac muscle are also present in animals and patients with severe left ventricular hypertrophy without failure, thereby raising the possibility that the causative factors are somehow related to the initiation of compensatory hypertrophy in failing hearts. Whether this observation is also true of skeletal muscle remains to be determined. Finally, assuming that the abnormalities present in cardiac and skeletal muscle with heart failure are caused by similar factors, these factors remain unknown at the present time. Leading candidates include the generalized state of hypoxemia that can occur in patients with heart failure, the high-circulating catecholamine levels, or other circulating factors that could exert an action on both cardiac and skeletal muscle.

In summary, the data presented in this review support the hypothesis that skeletal muscle from rats with subacute heart failure induced by myocardial infarction exhibit alterations in excitation-contraction coupling similar to those previously reported in the heart. Functional data support a central role for deficient levels of myoplasmic cyclic AMP concentrations in producing these contractile abnormalities. These findings suggest a unifying hypothesis that deficient cellular cyclic AMP concentrations may be responsible, at least in part, for striated muscle dysfunction both in cardiac and skeletal muscle in heart failure.

REFERENCES

1. Morgan, J. P. 1991. Abnormal intracellular modulation of calcium as a major cause of cardiac contractile dysfunction. N. Engl. J. Med. **325:** 625–632.
2. Katz, A. M. 1992. Physiology of the Heart, 2d edit.: 1–668. Raven Press. New York.
3. Brodde, O.-E., A. Broede, A. Daul, K. Kunde & M. C. Michel. 1992. Receptor systems in the nonfailing human heart. *In* Cellular and Molecular Alterations in the Failing Human Heart. G. Hasenfuss, C. Holubarsch, H. Just & N. R. Alpert, Eds.: 1–4. Steinkoff Verlag. Darmstadt.
4. Katz, A. M. 1983. Cyclic adenosine monophosphate effects on the myocardium: A man who blows hot and cold with one breath. J. Am. Coll. Cardiol. **2:** 143–149.
5. Gaasch, W. H. & M. M. LeWinter, Eds. 1994. Left Ventricular Diastolic Dysfunction and Heart Failure. Lea & Febiger. Philadelphia.
6. Gwathmey, J. K., L. Copelas, R. MacKinnon, *et al.* 1984. Abnormal intracellular calcium handling in myocardium from patients with end-stage heart failure. Circ. Res. **61:** 70–76.
7. Erdmann, E. 1988. The effectiveness of inotropic agents in isolated cardiac preparations from the human heart. Klin. Wochenschr. **66:** 1–6.
8. Perreault, C. L., C. P. Williams & J. P. Morgan. 1993. Cytoplasmic calcium modulation and systolic versus diastolic dysfunction in myocardial hypertrophy and failure. Circulation **87**(Supp. VII): 31–37.
9. Gwathmey, J. K., M. T. Slawsky, R. J. Hajjar, G. M. Briggs & J. P. Morgan. 1990. Role of intracellular calcium handling in force-interval relationships of human ventricular myocardium. J. Clin. Invest. **85:** 1599–1613.
10. Feldman, A. M., A. E. Cates, W. B. Veazey *et al.* 1988. Increase of the 40,000 mol wt. pertussis toxin substrate (G protein) in the failing human heart. J. Clin. Invest. **82:** 189–197.
11. Neumann, J, H. Schmitz, H. Scholz, L. von Meyerinck, V. Doring & P. Kalmar. 1988. Increase in myocardial Gi-proteins in heart failure. Lancet **2:** 936–937.
12. Nabauer, M, M. Bohm, L. Brown *et al.* 1988. Positive inotropic effects in isolated ventricular myocardium from non-failing and terminally failing human hearts. Eur. J. Clin. Invest. **18:** 600–606.
13. Gutstein, D. E., K. Flemmal, E. Bruce, K. E. Travers, J. K. Gwathmey, B. J. Ransil, J. E. Markis, W. Grossman & J. P. Morgan. 1996. Decreased inotropic but relatively preserved relaxation response to cyclic adenosine monophosphate–dependent agents in myopathic human myocardium. J. Cardiac Failure **2:** 285–292.
14. Burr, T., T. Clausen, E. Holmberg, U. Johansson & B. Waldeck. 1982. Desensitization by terbutaline of beta-adrenoceptors in the guinea-pig soleus muscle: Biochemical alterations associated with functional changes. Br. J. Pharmacol. **76:** 313–317.

15. SYME, P. D., F. BRUNOTTE, Y. GREEN, J. K. ARONSON & C. K. RADDA. 1991. The effect of $beta_2$-adrenoceptor stimulation and blockade of L-type calcium channels on in vivo Na^+ H^+ antiporter activity in rat skeletal muscle. Biochem. Biophys. Acta **1093:** 234–240.
16. EVERTS, M. E., K. RETTERSTOL & T. CLAUSEN. 1988. Effects of adrena-line on excitation-induced stimulation of the sodium-potassium pump in rat skeletal muscle. Acta Physiol. Scand. **134:** 189–198.
17. JUEL, C. 1988. The effect of $beta_2$ adrenoceptor activation on ion-shifts and fatigue in mouse soleus muscles stimulated in vitro. Acta Physiol. Scand. **134:** 209–216.
18. HEDBERG, A., H. MATTSON, V. NERME & E. CARLSON. 1984. Effects of in vivo treatment with isoprenaline or prenalterol on beta-adrenoceptor mechanisms in the heart and soleus muscle of the cat. Naunyn-Schmiedeberg's Arch. Pharmacol. **325:** 251–258.
19. ELFELLAH, M. S. & J. L. REID. 1990. Effect of chronic pretreatment of guinea pigs with beta-adrenoceptor agonists on the Na^+, $K(^+)$-pump in skeletal muscle. J. Auton. Pharmacol. **10:** 227–231.
20. FREY, M. J., V. LANOCE, P. B. MOLINOFF & J. R. WILSON. 1989. Skeletal muscle beta-receptors and isoproterenol-stimulated vasodilation in canine heart failure. J. Appl. Physiol. **67:** 2026–2031.
21. BRISTOW, M. R., R. GINSBURG, W. A. MINOBE, R. S. CUBICCIOTTI, W. S. SAGEMAN, K. LURIE, M. E. BILLINGHAM, D. C. HARRISON & E. D. STINSON. 1982. Decrease catecholamine sensitivity and beta-adrenergic receptor density in failing human hearts. N. Engl. J. Med. **307:** 205–211.
22. BOWMAN, W. C. & M. W. NOTT. 1981. Effects of adrenergic activators and inhibitors on the skeletal muscles. Part II. *In* Adrenergic Activators and Inhibitors. L. Szekeres, Ed.: 47–128. Springer-Verlag. New York.
23. BOWMAN, W. C., & M. W. NOTT. 1974. Effects of catecholamines, cyclic nucleotides and phosphodiesterase inhibitors on contractions of skeletal muscles in anaesthetized cats. Clin. Exp. Pharmacol. Physiol. **1:** 309–323.
24. PERREAULT, C. L., H. GONZALEZ-SERRATOS, S. E. LITWIN, X. SUN, C. FRANZINI-ARMSTRONG & J. P. MORGAN. 1993. Alterations in contractility and intracellular Ca^{2+} transients in isolated bundles of skeletal muscle fibers from rats with chronic heart failure. Circ. Res. **73:** 405–412.
25. GODT, R. E., & T. M. NOSEK. 1989. Changes of intracellular milieu with fatigue or hypoxia depress contraction of skinned rabbit skeletal and cardiac muscle. J. Physiol. (Lond.) **412:** 155–180.
26. EBERSTEIN, A, & A. SANDOW. 1963. Fatigue mechanisms in muscle fibers. *In* The Effect of Use and Disuse on Neuromuscular Functions. E. Gutman & P. Hnik, Eds.: 515–526. Elsevier/North Holland Scientific Publisher Ltd. Amsterdam.
27. WESTERBLAD, H., J. A. LEE, A. G. LAMB, S. R. BOLSOVER & D. G. ALLEN. 1990. Spatial gradients of intracellular calcium in skeletal muscle during fatigue. Pfluegers Arch. **415:** 734–740.
28. ROZYCKA, M. & H. GONZALEZ-SERRATOS. 1991. Calcium release imaging of the cross section of isolated skeletal muscle fibers from the frog [abstract]. J. Biophys. **59:** 242a.
29. GROSSMAN, J. D., A. BISHOP, K. E. TRAVERS, C. PERREAULT, J. WOOLF, T. HAMPTON, H. RASGADO-FLORES, H. GONZALEZ-SERRATOS & J. P. MORGAN. 1996. Deficient cellular cyclic AMP may cause both cardiac and skeletal muscle dysfunction in heart failure. J. Cardiac Fail. **2:** S105–S111.
30. LITWIN, S. E. & J. P. MORGAN. 1991. Intracellular Ca^{2+} handling and beta-adrenergic responsiveness of myocardium from rats with large infarctions. Circulation **84:** 11-II-10.
31. LEJEMTEL, T. H., D. GUMBARDO, B. CHADWICK, H. I. RUTMAN & E. H. SONNENBLICK. 1986. Milrinone for long-term therapy of severe heart failure: Clinical experience with special reference to maximal exercise tolerance. Circulation **73:** 213–218.
32. PERREAULT, C. L., R. P. SHANNON, K. KOMAMURA, S. F. VATNER & J. P. MORGAN. 1992. Abnormalities in intracellular calcium regulation and contractile function in myocardium from dogs with pacing-induced heart failure. J. Clin. Invest. **89:** 932–938.

Sarcoplasmic Reticulum Proteins in Heart Failure

STEPHAN E. LEHNART, WOLFGANG SCHILLINGER, BURKERT PIESKE, JÜRGEN PRESTLE, HANJÖRG JUST, AND GERD HASENFUSS[a]

Medizinische Klinik III, Universität Freiburg, 79106 Freiburg, Germany

ABSTRACT: Altered calcium homeostasis may play a key role in the pathophysiology of human heart failure. Levels of sarcoplasmic reticulum (SR) proteins and sarcolemmal Na^+-Ca^{2+} exchanger were analyzed by Western blot in failing and nonfailing human myocardium and related to myocardial function. Levels of the SR calcium release channel and of calcium storage proteins (calsequestrin and calreticulin) were not different in nonfailing and failing hearts. However, proteins involved in calcium removal were significantly altered in the failing human heart: (1) SR-Ca^{2+}-ATPase levels and the ratio of SR-Ca^{2+}-ATPase to its inhibitory protein phospholamban were significantly decreased, and (2) Na^+-Ca^{2+} exchanger levels and the ratio of Na^+-Ca^{2+} exchanger to SR-Ca^{2+}-ATPase were significantly increased. SR-Ca^{2+}-ATPase levels were closely correlated to systolic function as evaluated by frequency potentiation of contractile force. The frequency-dependent rise of diastolic force was inversely correlated with protein levels of Na^+-Ca^{2+} exchanger. These findings indicate that altered expression of SR-Ca^{2+}-ATPase and Na^+-Ca^{2+} exchanger is relevant for altered systolic and diastolic function in human heart failure.

Several studies have indicated that altered calcium cycling may play a dominant role in the disturbed myocardial function in end-stage human heart failure. Myothermal studies have been used to evaluate tension-independent heat in isometrically contracting muscle strip preparations that reflects energy turnover of excitation-contraction-coupling processes. It was observed that the amount and rate of evolution of tension-independent heat is significantly reduced in failing human myocardium at a stimulation rate of 60 beats per minute (37°C). This indicates that the total amount of calcium cycling and the rate of calcium removal are reduced in the failing human myocardium.[1] In accordance with this, systolic free calcium concentration was shown to be reduced when FURA-2 was used to measure free intracellular calcium concentrations in isolated myocytes from failing human hearts.[2] Additionally, it was shown that alteration of calcium transients depends on the frequency of stimulation: using the photoprotein aequorin to evaluate calcium transients in isolated muscle strip preparations, researchers observed that the frequency-dependent rise of the calcium transients is blunted and even that an inversion of the calcium-frequency relation occurs in the majority of ventricular muscle strip preparations from end-stage failing human hearts.[3] Post-rest potentiation of calcium transients was diminished, suggesting decreased sarcoplasmic reticulum calcium accumulation.[4] Regarding diastolic function, studies in isolated my-

[a] Address for correspondence: Gerd Hasenfuss, M.D., Abteilung Kardiologie und Pneumologie, Universität Göttingen, Robert-Koch-Str. 40, 37075 Göttingen, Germany. Phone: 011-49-551-396351; fax: 011-49-551-398918; e-mail: hasenfus@ruf.uni-freiburg.de

ocytes and ventricular muscle strip preparations indicated that diastolic calcium levels are elevated and that calcium transients are prolonged in failing compared to nonfailing human myocardium.[2,5]

There is accumulating evidence that disturbed sarcoplasmic reticulum (SR) function may be an important factor for altered calcium cycling in the failing human heart and that this may be related to altered expression or function of calcium cycling proteins. Knowledge of these changes is a prerequisite for understanding the pathophysiology of myocardial failure and for the development of new strategies to treat patients with heart failure. In the present paper we review data from our own group and from the literature on expression and function of SR proteins as well as the sarcolemmal Na^+-Ca^{2+} exchanger in human heart failure.

SARCOPLASMIC RETICULUM FUNCTION

Calcium release from SR depends on the following components: (a) activation of ryanodine receptors (RyRs) by transsarcolemmal calcium influx; (b) the number of RyRs present in the SR membrane; (c) the functional status of release processes, which includes calcium binding and diffusion within the SR as well as refractoriness of RyRs from previous activation; and (d) SR calcium concentration—i.e., the amount of calcium available for release.

RyRs and SR Calcium Release

The calcium-sensitive RyR, which is located in the immediate vicinity of the L-type calcium channel, is activated by a local increase in calcium concentration subsequent to transsarcolemmal calcium influx.[6] Once activated, the channel opens and releases calcium for activation of contractile proteins.[7,8] This process is termed calcium-induced calcium release.[8] Several groups have studied mRNA expression of the RyR in the failing human heart with inconsistent results (TABLE 1). While Brillantes *et al.* observed decreased mRNA levels in ischemic but not in dilated cardiomyopathy, Go *et al.* described a reduction of RyR mRNA levels in both ischemic and dilated cardiomyopathy.[9,10] In three studies a radioligand binding assay was used. Go *et al.* in a small number of samples (and without any statistical analysis) observed that high-affinity binding sites for [^{3}H]ryanodine were decreased by about 30% in left ventricular myocardium from failing human hearts.[10] Schumacher *et al.* observed no differences in [^{3}H]ryanodine binding between failing and nonfailing hearts.[11] Finally, Sainte Beuve *et al.* observed an increase of RyRs in failing hearts.[12] At the protein level, no change in RyR expression between failing and nonfailing hearts were consistently observed in three different studies.[12–14] From their findings of unchanged protein levels but increased [^{3}H]ryanodine binding in failing hearts, Sainte Beuve *et al.* suggested that ryanodine binding properties may be affected in failing myocardium, which may reflect altered channel activity.[12] Altered function of RyRs was also suggested by D'Agnolo *et al.*[15] They found that the caffeine threshold of the ryanodine receptor was increased, suggesting an impaired gating mechanism of the calcium release channel in dilated cardiomyopathy.[15] Furthermore, Nimer *et al.* reported differences in response to ryanodine between failing and nonfailing myocardium, which may also reflect altered function of the RyRs.[16] In contrast, Holmberg and Williams, who studied the activity of a single RyR under voltage-clamp conditions reported normal basal properties of the RyR from failing human hearts.[17]

TABLE 1. Quantification of SR-Ca^{2+}-Release Channels (RyR) in Human Heart Failure[a]

Quantity	Disease	Method	Reference
28%⇓	ICM	Northern blot	Brillantes *et al.*, 1992[9]
n.s.	DCM	Northern blot	idem
31%⇓	DCM, ICM	Northern blot	Go *et al.*, 1995[10]
Inverse relation with ANF	DCM	Northern blot	Arai *et al.*, 1993[22]
30%⇓	DCM	Northern blot	Sainte Beuve *et al.*, 1997[12]
n.s.	ICM	Northern blot	idem
n.s.	DCM	Western blot	Meyer *et al.*, 1995[13]
n.s.	ICM	Western blot	Schillinger *et al.*, 1996[14]
n.s.	DCM, ICM	Western blot	Sainte Beuve *et al.* 1997[12]
70–114%⇑	DCM, ICM	[^{3}H] ryanodine binding	idem
n.s.	DCM, ICM	[^{3}H] ryanodine binding	Schumacher *et al.* 1995[11]

[a]According to Hasenfuss *et al.*[52]

ABBREVIATIONS: ANF = atrial natriuretic factor; DCM = dilated cardiomyopathy; ICM = ischemic cardiomyopathy; RyR = ryanodine receptor; n.s. = no significant change versus nonfailing human myocardium.

Sarcoplasmic Reticulum Calcium Storage

Calsequestrin and calreticulin are calcium-binding proteins located within the lumen of the SR.[18–20] Calsequestrin, a high-capacity, moderate-affinity calcium-binding protein, is primarily responsible for the calcium storage capacity of the SR in cardiac muscle.[18] Studies in failing human myocardium consistently showed unchanged mRNA and protein levels of calsequestrin as compared to nonfailing myocardium.[13,14,21–23] Similarly, calreticulin protein levels were shown to be unchanged in the failing human heart.[13] This may indicate that the capacity of the SR to bind calcium is unchanged in the failing human myocardium.

Sarcoplasmic Reticulum Calcium Uptake and Accumulation

Calcium transport into the SR occurs by SR-Ca^{2+}-ATPase, which transports two calcium ions per molecule of hydrolyzed ATP against a high ion gradient from a free intracellular calcium concentration between 100 nM and 10 μM to a free calcium concentration inside the SR of ~1 mM.[18,24] The SR competes with the sarcolemmal Na^+-Ca^{2+} exchanger in terms of myoplasmic Ca^{2+} extrusion. Calcium eliminated across the sarcolemma is no longer available for systolic activation of contractile proteins. Of course, regarding calcium elimination from the cytosol and, thus, diastolic function, the SR-Ca^{2+}-ATPase and the Na^+-Ca^{2+} exchanger work in concert. The SR-Ca^{2+}-ATPase is regulated by phospholamban.[18,25,26] Dephosphorylated phospholamban functions as an inhibitor of the SR-Ca^{2+}-ATPase activity. The inhibition has been suggested to involve direct protein interactions followed by conformational changes in the SR-Ca^{2+}-ATPase that result in a decreased affinity of the calcium pump for calcium.[26–28]

Several studies indicated that SR calcium uptake or SR-Ca^{2+}-ATPase activity are reduced in the failing human myocardium.[29–31] This, however, was not observed in another study.[32] In all studies on SR-Ca^{2+}-ATPase mRNA levels published up to now it has been reported that mRNA levels of SR-Ca^{2+}-ATPase are reduced in the failing compared to

TABLE 2. Quantification of SR-Ca^{2+}-ATPase in Human Heart Failure[a]

Quantity	Disease	Method	Reference
45%⇓	DCM, ICM	Northern blot	Mercadier *et al.*, 1990[50]
50%⇓	DCM, ICM	Northern blot	Takahashi *et al.*, 1992[51]
Inverse relation with ANF	DCM	Northern blot	Arai *et al.*, 1993[22]
50%⇓	DCM, ICM	Northern blot	Studer *et al.*, 1994[42]
50–60%⇓	DCM, ICM	Northern blot	Linck *et al.*, 1996[34]
54%⇓	DCM	Northern blot	Schwinger *et al.*, 1995[29]
40%⇓	DCM, ICM	Western blot	Studer *et al.*, 1994[42]
36%⇓	DCM, ICM	Western blot	Hasenfuss *et al.*, 1994[30]
33%⇓	DCM	Western blot	Meyer *et al.*, 1995[13]
n.s.	DCM	Western blot	Movsesian *et al.*, 1994[23]
n.s.	DCM	Western blot	Schwinger *et al.*, 1995[29]
n.s.	DCM, ICM	Western blot	Linck *et al.*, 1996.[34]

[a]According to Hasenfuss *et al.*[52]

ABBREVIATIONS: ANF = atrial natriuretic factor; DCM = dilated cardiomyopathy; ICM = ischemic cardiomyopathy; n.s. = no significant change versus nonfailing human myocardium.

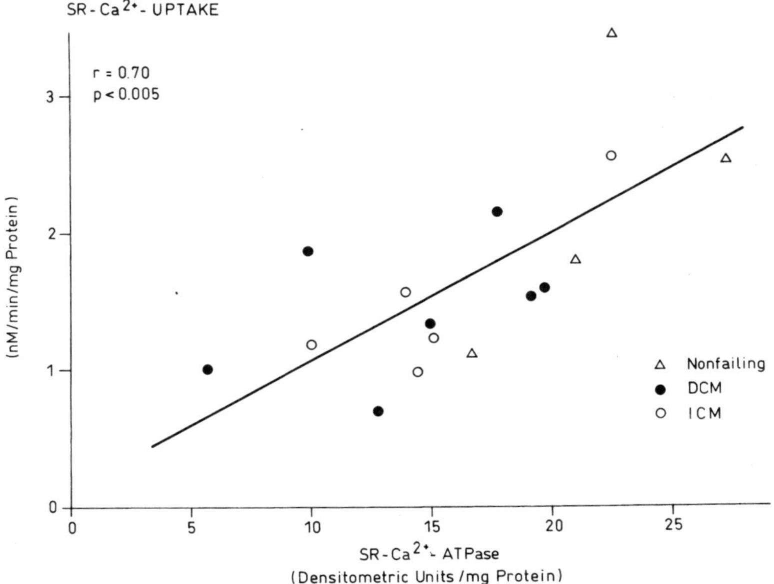

FIGURE 1. Graph showing the relation between sarcoplasmic reticulum calcium uptake measured in myocardial homogenates and protein levels of SR-Ca^{2+}-ATPase, both normalized per total protein. DCM indicates dilated cardiomyopathy; ICM, ischemic cardiomyopathy. (Reprinted from Hasenfuss *et al.*[30] with permission.)

the nonfailing human heart (TABLE 2). However, at the level of protein expression findings have been controversial (TABLE 2). In a study from our group, a significant correlation between SR calcium uptake and SR-Ca^{2+}-ATPase protein levels has been observed (FIG. 1).[30] Furthermore, there was a significant correlation between SR-Ca^{2+}-ATPase protein level and myocardial function, which was assessed by the force-frequency relation (FIG. 2).[30] Also, this analysis indicated that a wide variation exists in protein levels of SR-Ca^{2+}-ATPase within the group of failing hearts (protein levels differed by a factor of four) and that this variation in protein levels matches differences in myocardial function. In other words, in a subgroup of failing hearts SR-Ca^{2+}-ATPase protein levels are similar to those in nonfailing hearts, and this is associated with preserved myocardial systolic function by force-frequency relation.[30]

Regarding phospholamban expression, a decrease in phospholamban mRNA levels has been consistently observed in failing human myocardium (TABLE 3).[23,29,33,34] Only one study showed a small decrease in phospholamban protein levels relative to total protein in failing dilated cardiomyopathy.[13] However, when phospholamban was normalized to calsequestrin, no difference existed between failing and nonfailing myocardium.[13] Interestingly, it was observed by Meyer *et al.* that SR-Ca^{2+}-ATPase protein levels were decreased to a greater proportion than protein levels of phospholamban in the failing myocardium.[13] Accordingly, if we assume that the stoichiometry of phospholamban to SR-Ca^{2+}-ATPase determines the level of SR-Ca^{2+}-ATPase inhibition, this finding indicates that in the basal low phosphorylated state, inhibition of SR-Ca^{2+}-ATPase is more pronounced in the failing compared to nonfailing human myocardium.[35] This could be

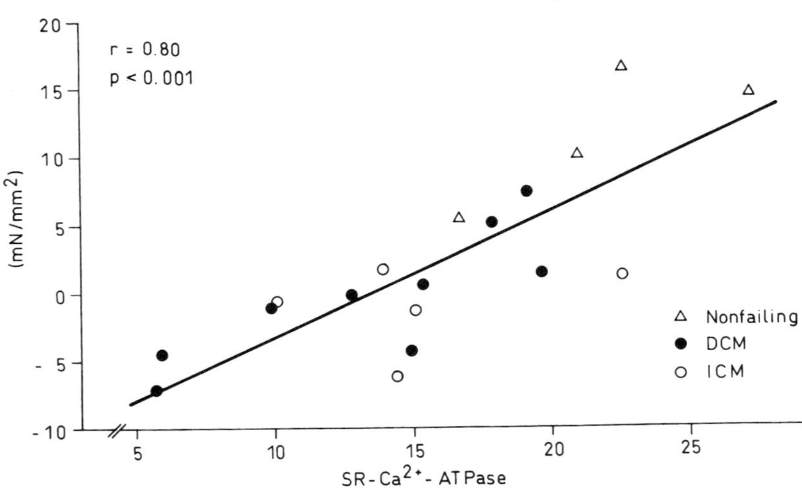

FIGURE 2. Graph showing the relation between change in twitch tension after an increase of the stimulation frequency from 30 to 120 min^{-1} and protein levels of SR-Ca^{2+}-ATPase normalized per total protein. DCM indicates dilated cardiomyopathy; ICM, ischemic cardiomyopathy. (Reprinted from Hasenfuss *et al.*[30] with permission.)

TABLE 3. Quantification of Phospholamban in Human Heart Failure[a]

Quantity	Disease	Method	Reference
⇓	DCM	PCR	Feldman *et al.*, 1991[33]
27–35%⇓	DCM, ICM	Northern blot	Linck *et al.*, 1996.[34]
Inverse relation with ANF	DCM, ICM	Northern blot	Arai *et al.*, 1993[22]
46%⇓	DCM	Northern blot	Schwinger *et al.*, 1995[29]
n.s.	DCM	Western blot	Movsesian *et al.*, 1994[23]
18%⇓	DCM	Western blot	Meyer *et al.*, 1995[13]
n.s.	DCM, ICM	Western blot	Linck *et al.*, 1996[34]
n.s.	DCM	Western blot	Schwinger *et al.*, 1995[29]

[a]According to Hasenfuss *et al.*[52]

ABBREVIATIONS: ANF = atrial natriuretic factor; DCM = dilated cardiomyopathy; ICM = ischemic cardiomyopathy; n.s. = no significant change versus nonfailing human myocardium; PCR = polymerase chain reaction.

one possible explanation of the finding of reduced activity of SR-Ca^{2+}-ATPase in failing compared to nonfailing human myocardium.[29]

In summary, there is considerable evidence that the capacity of the SR calcium pump system to accumulate calcium into the SR is significantly reduced in the failing human heart. In addition, altered expression and function of the Na^+-Ca^{2+} exchanger might further compromise SR calcium accumulation (see below).

TRANSSARCOLEMMAL CALCIUM TRANSPORT

Calcium transport through the sarcolemma is dominated by the activity of the Na^+-Ca^{2+} exchanger, whereas the sarcolemmal Ca^{2+}-ATPase is not considered to contribute quantitatively to calcium elimination and myocardial relaxation on a beat-to-beat basis.[36] The Na^+-Ca^{2+} antiporter extrudes one calcium ion in exchange for three sodium ions using the electrochemical sodium gradient (for review see Refs. 37 and 38). In this mode, it produces a net movement of charge resulting in a net inward current. Also, the Na^+-Ca^{2+} exchanger is voltage dependent and can reverse its mode during the action potential (for review see Refs. 37 and 39). Under experimental conditions with high intracellular sodium levels, the Na^+-Ca^{2+} exchanger can promote calcium influx sufficiently to induce excitation-contraction coupling.[40]

While preliminary data from pooled human heart tissue did not reveal significant changes of Na^+-Ca^{2+} exchanger mRNA levels in failing hearts,[41] Studer *et al.* showed that mRNA as well as protein levels are significantly increased in the failing human heart.[42] This finding was recently confirmed by Flesch *et al.*[43] Accordingly, it was shown that Na^+-Ca^{2+} exchange activity is increased in myocardium from failing hearts.[44] Functional relevance of increased Na^+-Ca^{2+} exchanger expression is evident from a recent study showing that diastolic performance of failing human myocardium correlates inversely with protein levels of Na^+-Ca^{2+} exchanger (FIG. 3).[45]

INTERPRETATION OF THE DATA

At the level of the myocardium, disturbed function of the SR seems to play a central role for the altered systolic and diastolic performance of the failing human heart.

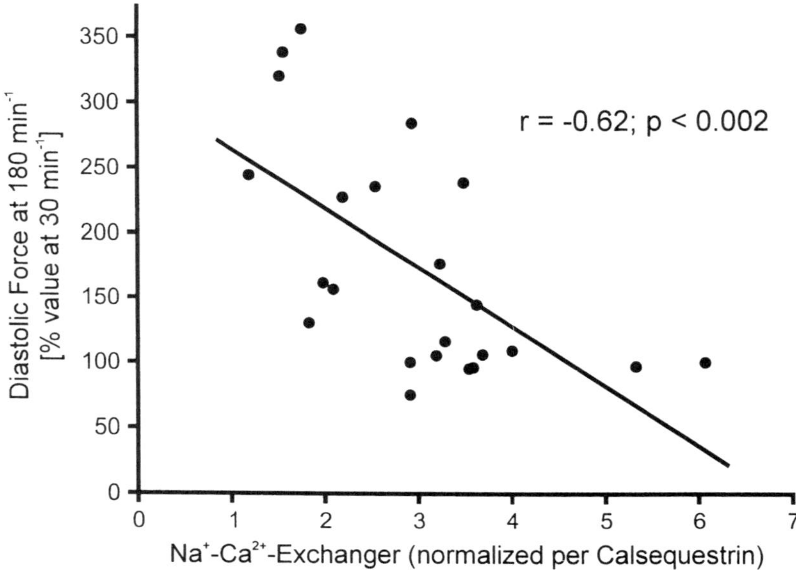

FIGURE 3. Graph showing the relation between the change in diastolic force after an increase of the stimulation frequency from 30 to 180 min^{-1} given in percent of the diastolic force value at 30 min^{-1} and protein levels of the Na^+-Ca^{2+} exchanger. Na^+-Ca^{2+} exchanger protein levels are normalized to calsequestrin protein levels. All data are from end-stage failing human hearts with dilated or ischemic cardiomyopathy.

Under physiological conditions calcium released from the SR is the dominant source for systolic activation of contractile proteins. Diastolic relaxation depends on calcium removal from the cytosol by the SR and the sarcolemmal Na^+-Ca^{2+} exchanger. There is considerable evidence that a major defect of EC-coupling is a decreased capacity of the SR to accumulate calcium. This may result from a decreased number of SR-Ca^{2+}-ATPase pumps,[13,14,30,42] increased inhibition of the SR-Ca^{2+}-ATPase by phospholamban,[13] or decreased activity of the SR-Ca^{2+}-ATPase by other mechanisms.[29] In addition, because the SR-Ca^{2+}-ATPase competes with Na^+-Ca^{2+} exchanger for calcium, increased Na^+-Ca^{2+} exchanger activity may contribute to decreased SR calcium accumulation.[42–44] The decreased capacity of the SR to accumulate calcium may be of minor relevance at low heart rates. However, at higher heart rates—with decreased time available for calcium transport—SR calcium accumulation may become inadequate, calcium release from the SR may decline, and systolic activation of contractile proteins may decrease.[1,2] This is consistent with the findings of an altered force-frequency relation, a frequency-dependent decrease in calcium transients, and a decreased post-rest potentiation in the failing human heart.[3,4,30,46,47] Furthermore, disturbed SR calcium loading at higher heart rates in failing compared to nonfailing human myocardium has been shown by studying rapid cooling contractures.[48] Altered transsarcolemmal calcium influx and in particular attenuation of frequency-dependent up-regulation of L-type calcium current may contribute to the reduced SR calcium load.[49] Furthermore, alterations in the β-adrenoceptor-adenylyl cyclase system with altered cyclic AMP levels may be involved.

A second consequence of decreased SR function is diastolic calcium accumulation, which may result in diastolic activation of contractile proteins and disturbed diastolic function.[45] Because SR-Ca^{2+}-ATPase and Na^+-Ca^{2+} exchanger work in concert regarding removal of calcium from the cytosol, increased activity of the Na^+-Ca^{2+} exchanger may compensate for decreased SR calcium transport and preserve diastolic function. Accordingly, it was shown that in failing human myocardium diastolic function is correlated with protein levels of Na^+-Ca^{2+} exchanger.[45] Of course, calcium eliminated across the sarcolemma by Na^+-Ca^{2+} exchanger is no longer available for systolic activation of contractile proteins. Furthermore, the exchange of one calcium ion for three sodium ions results in an inward current, which may cause altered membrane potential. Therefore, alteration of calcium handling with increased activity of Na^+-Ca^{2+} exchanger relative to SR-Ca^{2+}-ATPase may contribute to disturbed myocardial function as well as to the development of arrhythmias in patients with heart failure.

REFERENCES

1. HASENFUSS, G, L. A. MULIERI, B. J. LEAVITT, P. D. ALLEN, J. R. HAEBERLE & N. R. ALPERT. 1992. Alteration of contractile function and excitation-contraction coupling in dilated cardiomyopathy. Circ. Res. **70:** 1225–1232.
2. BEUCKELMANN, D. J., M. NABAUER & E. ERDMANN. 1992. Intracellular calcium handling in isolated ventricular myocytes from patients with terminal heart failure. Circulation **85:** 1046–1055.
3. PIESKE, B., B. KRETSCHMANN, M. MEYER, C. HOLUBARSCH, J. WEIRICH, H. POSIVAL, K. MINAMI, H. JUST & G. HASENFUSS. 1995. Alterations in intracellular calcium handling associated with the inverse force-frequency relation in human dilated cardiomyopathy. Circulation **92:** 1169–1178.
4. PIESKE, B., M. SUTTERLIN, S. SCHMIDT-SCHWEDA, K. MINAMI, M. MEYER, M. OLSCHEWSKI, C. HOLUBARSCH, H. JUST & G. HASENFUSS. 1996. Diminished post-rest potentiation of contractile force in human dilated cardiomyopathy. Functional evidence for alterations in intracellular Ca^{2+} handling. J. Clin. Invest. **98:** 764–776.
5. GWATHMEY, J. K., L. COPELAS, R. MACKINNON, F. J. SCHOEN, M. D. FELDMANN, W. GROSSMAN & J. P. MORGAN. 1987. Abnormal intracellular calcium handling in myocardium from patients with end-stage heart failure. Circ. Res. **61:** 70–76.
6. CHENG, H., W. J. LEDERER & M. V. CANNELL. 1993. Calcium sparks: Elementary events underlying excitation-contraction coupling in heart muscle. Science **262:** 740–744.
7. BARRY, W. H. & J. H. BRIDGE. 1993. Intracellular calcium homeostasis in cardiac myocytes. Circulation **87:** 1806–1815.
8. FABIATO, A. 1983. Calcium-induced release of calcium from the cardiac sarcoplasmic reticulum. Am. J. Physiol. **245:** C1–C14.
9. BRILLANTES, A. M., P. ALLEN, T. TAKAHASHI, S. IZUMO & A. R. MARKS. 1992. Differences in cardiac calcium release channel (ryanodine receptor) expression in myocardium from patients with end-stage heart failure caused by ischemic versus dilated cardiomyopathy. Circ. Res. **71:** 18–26.
10. GO, L. O., M. C. MOSCHELLA, J. WATRAS, K. K. HANDA, B. S. FYFE & A. R. MARKS. 1995. Differential regulation of two types of intracellular calcium release channels during end-stage heart failure. J. Clin. Invest. **95:** 888–894.
11. SCHUMACHER, C., B. KONIGS, M. SIGMUND, B. KOHNE, F. SCHONDUBE, M. VOB, B. STEIN, J. WEIL & P. HANRATH. 1995. The ryanodine binding sarcoplasmic reticulum calcium release channel in nonfailing and in failing human myocardium. Naunyn-Schmiedeberg's Arch. Pharmakol. **353:** 80–85.
12. SAINTE BEUVE, C., P. D. ALLEN, G. DAMBRIN, F. RANNOU, I. MARTY, P. TROUVE, V. BORS, A. PAVIE, I. GANDGJBAKCH & D. CHARLEMAGNE. 1997. Cardiac calcium release channel

(ryanodine receptor) in control and cardiomyopathic human hearts: mRNA and protein contents are differentially regulated. J. Mol. Cell. Cardiol. **29:** 1237–1246.

13. MEYER, M., W. SCHILLINGER, B. PIESKE, C. HOLUBARSCH, C. HEILMANN, H. POSIVAL, G. KUWAJIMA, K. MIKOSHIBA, H. JUST & G. HASENFUSS. 1995. Alterations of sarcoplasmic reticulum proteins in failing human dilated cardiomyopathy. Circulation **92:** 778–784.
14. SCHILLINGER, W., M. MEYER, G. KUWAJIMA, K. MIKOSHIBA, H. JUST & G. HASENFUSS. 1996. Unaltered ryanodine receptor protein levels in ischemic cardiomyopathy. Mol. Cell. Biochem. **160–161:** 297–302.
15. D'AGNOLO, A., G. B. LUCIANI, A. MAZZUCCO, V. GALLUCCI & G. SALVIATI. 1992. Contractile properties and Ca^{2+} release activity of the sarcoplasmic reticulum in dilated cardiomyopathy. Circulation **85:** 518–525.
16. NIMER, L. R., D. H. NEEDLEMAN, S. L. HAMILTON, J. KRALL & M. A. MOVSESIAN. Effect of ryanodine on sarcoplasmic reticulum Ca^{2+} accumulation in nonfailing and failing human myocardium. Circulation **92:** 2504–2510.
17. HOLMBERG, S. R. & A. J. WILLIAMS. 1989. Single channel recordings from human cardiac sarcoplasmic reticulum. Circ. Res. **65:** 1445–1449.
18. LYTTON, H. & D. H. MACLENNAN. 1991. Sarcoplasmic reticulum. *In* The Heart and Cardiovascular System. H. A. Fozzard, R. B. Hennings, E. Haber & A. M. Katz, Eds.: 1203–1222. Raven Press. New York.
19. MACLENNAN, D. H. & P. T. S. WONG. 1971. Isolation of a calcium-sequestering protein from sarcoplasmic reticulum. Proc. Natl. Acad. Sci. USA **68:** 1231–1235.
20. MICHALAK, M., R. E. MILNER, K. BURNS & M. OPAS. 1992. Calreticulin. Biochem. J. **285:** 681–692.
21. TAKAHASHI, T., P. D. ALLEN, R. V. LACRO, A. R. MARKS, A. R. DENNIS, F. J. SCHOEN, W. GROSSMAN, J. D. MARSH & S. IZUMO. 1992. Expression of dihydropyridine receptor (Ca^{2+} channel) and calsequestrin genes in the myocardium of patients with end-stage heart failure. J. Clin. Invest. **90:** 927–935.
22. ARAI, M., N. R. ALPERT, D. H. MACLENNAN, P. BARTON & M. PERIASAMY. 1993. Alterations in sarcoplasmic reticulum gene expression in human heart failure. A possible mechanism for alterations in systolic and diastolic properties of the failing myocardium. Circ. Res. **72:** 463–469.
23. MOVSESIAN, M. A., M. KARIMI, K. GREEN & L. R. JONES. 1994. Ca^{2+}-transporting ATPase, phospholamban, and calsequestrin levels in nonfailing and failing human myocardium. Circulation **90:** 653–657.
24. BERS, D. M. 1991. Possible sources and sinks of activator calcium. *In* Developments in Cardiovascular Medicine, Vol. 122: Excitation-Contraction Coupling and Cardiac Contractile Force. D. M. Bers, Ed.: 33–48. Kluwer Academic Publishers. Dordrecht.
25. KRANIAS, E. G., J. L. GARVEY, R. D. SRIVASTAVA & R. J. SOLARO. 1985. Phosphorylation and functional modifications of sarcoplasmic reticulum and myofibrils in isolated rabbit hearts stimulated with isoprenaline. Biochem. J. **226:** 113–121.
26. KIM, H. W., N. A. E. STEENAART, D. G. FERGUSON & E. G. KRANIAS. 1990. Functional reconstitution of the cardiac sarcoplasmic reticulum Ca^{2+}-ATPase with phospholamban in phospholipid vesicles. J. Biol. Chem. **265:** 1702–1709.
27. JAMES, P., M. INUI, M. TADA, M. CHIESI & E. CARAFOLI. 1989. Nature and site of phospholamban regulation of the Ca^{2+} pump of sarcoplasmic reticulum. Nature **342:** 90–92.
28. VOSS, J., L. R. JONES & D. D. THOMAS. 1994. The physical mechanism of calcium pump regulation in the heart. Biophys. J. **67:** 190–196.
29. SCHWINGER, R. H., M. BÖHM, U. SCHMIDT, P. KARCZEWSKI, U. BAVENDIEK, M. FLESCH, E. G. KRAUSE & E. ERDMANN. 1995. Unchanged protein levels of SERCA II and phospholamban but reduced Ca^{2+} uptake and Ca^{2+}-ATPase activity of cardiac sarcoplasmic reticulum from dilated cardiomyopathy patients compared with patients with nonfailing hearts. Circulation **92:** 3220–3228.
30. HASENFUSS, G., H. REINECKE, R. STUDER, M. MEYER, B. PIESKE, J. HOLTZ, C. HOLUBARSCH, H. POSIVAL, H. JUST & H. DREXLER. 1994. Relation between myocardial function and expression of sarcoplasmic reticulum Ca^{2+}-ATPase in failing and nonfailing human myocardium. Circ. Res. **75:** 434–442.

31. LIMAS, C. J., M. T. OLIVARI, I. F. GOLDENBERG, T. B. LEVINE, D. G. BENDITT & A. SIMON. 1987. Calcium uptake by cardiac sarcoplasmic reticulum in human dilated cardiomyopathy. Cardiovasc. Res. **21:** 601–605.
32. MOVSESIAN, M. A., M. R. BRISTOW & J. KRALL. 1989. Ca^{2+} uptake by cardiac sarcoplasmic reticulum from patients with idiopathic dilated cardiomyopathy. Circ. Res. **65:** 1141–1144.
33. FELDMAN, A. M., P. E. RAY, C. M. SILAN, J. A. MERCER, W. MINOBE & M. R. BRISTOW. 1991. Selective gene expression in failing human heart. Quantification of steady-state levels of messenger RNA in endomyocardial biopsies using the polymerase chain reaction. Circulation **83:** 1866–1872.
34. LINCK, B., P. BOKNIK, T. ESCHENHAGEN, F. U. MULLER, J. NEUMANN, M. NOSE, L. R. JONES, W. SCHMITZ & H. SCHOLZ. 1996. Messenger RNA expression and immunological quantification of phospholamban and SR-Ca^{2+}-ATPase in failing and nonfailing human hearts. Cardiovasc. Res. **31:** 625–632.
35. KOSS, K. L., I. L. GRUPP & E. G. KRANIAS. 1997. The relative phospholamban and SERCA2 ratio: A critical determinant of myocardial contractility. Basic Res. Cardiol. **92**(Suppl.1): 17–24.
36. BERS, D. M. 1997. Ca transport during contraction and relaxation in mammalian ventricular muscle. Basic Res. Cardiol. **92**(Suppl. 1): 1–10.
37. SCHULZE, D. H. & W. J. LEDERER. 1997. Advances in the molecular characterization of the Na^+/Ca^{2+} exchanger. *In* Molecular Biology of Cardiovascular Disease. A. R. Marks, M. B. Taubman, Eds.: 275–290. Marcel Dekker. New York.
38. PHILIPSON, K. D. 1990. The cardiac Na^+-Ca^{2+}-exchanger. *In* Calcium and the Heart. G. A. Langer, Ed.: 85–108. Raven Press. New York.
39. PHILIPSON, K. D. 1992. Cardiac sodium-calcium exchange research. Trends Cardiovasc. Med. **2:** 12–14.
40. BERS, D. M., D. M. CHRISTENSEN & T. X. NGUYEN. 1988. Can Ca^{2+} entry via the Na^+-Ca^{2+} exchange directly activate cardiac muscle contraction? J. Mol. Cell. Cardiol. **20:** 405–414.
41. KOMURO, I., K. E. WENNINGER, K. D. PHILIPSON & S. IZUMO. 1992. Molecular cloning and characterization of the human cardiac Na^+-Ca^{2+}-exchanger cDNA. Proc. Natl. Acad. Sci. USA **89:** 4769–4773.
42. STUDER, R., H. REINECKE, J. BILGER, T. ESCHENHAGEN, M. BÖHM, G. HASENFUSS, H. JUST, J. HOLTZ & H. DREXLER. 1994. Gene expression of the cardiac Na^+-Ca^{2+}-exchanger in end-stage human heart failure. Circ. Res. **75:** 443–453.
43. FLESCH, M., R. H. G. SCHWINGER, F. SCHIFFER, K. FRANK, M. SUDKAMP, F. KUHN-REGNIER, G. ARNOLD & M. BÖHM. 1996. Evidence for functional relevance of an enhanced expression of the Na^+-Ca^{2+} exchanger in failing human myocardium. Circulation **94:** 992–1002.
44. REINECKE, H., R. STUDER, R. VETTER, J. HOLTZ & H. DREXLER. 1996. Cardiac Na^+-Ca^{2+} exchange activity in patients with end-stage heart failure. Cardiovasc. Res. **31:** 48–54.
45. HASENFUSS, G., M. PREUSS, S. E. LEHNART, J. PRESTLE, M. MEYER & H. JUST. 1996. Relationship between diastolic function and protein levels of sodium-calcium-exchanger in end-stage failing human hearts. Circulation **94**(Suppl. 1): 433.
46. MULIERI, L. A., G. HASENFUSS, B. J. LEAVITT, P. D. ALLEN & N. R. ALPERT. 1992. Altered myocardial force-frequency relation in human heart failure. Circulation **85:** 1743–1750.
47. HASENFUSS, G., C. HOLUBARSCH, H. P. HERMANN, K. ASTHEIMER, B. PIESKE & H. JUST. 1994. Influence of the force-frequency relation on haemodynamics and left ventricular function in patients with non-failing hearts and in patients with dilated cardiomyopathy. Eur. Heart J. **15:** 164–170.
48. PIESKE, B., L. MAIER, T. WEBER, D. M. BERS & G. HASENFUSS. 1997. Alterations in sarcoplasmic reticulum Ca^{2+} content in myocardium from patients with heart failure. Circulation **1996** (Suppl. I): 199.
49. PIOT, C., S. LEMAIRE, B. ALBAT, J. SEGUIN, J. NARGEOT & S. RICHARD. 1996. High frequency-induced upregulation of human cardiac calcium currents. Circulation **93:** 120–128.
50. MERCADIER, J. J., A. M. LOMPRE, P. DUC, K. R. BOHELER, J. B. FRAYSSE, C. WISNEWSKY, P. D. ALLEN, M. KOMAJDA & K. SCHWARTZ. 1990. Altered sarcoplasmic reticulum Ca^{2+}-AT-

Pase gene expression in the human ventricle during end-stage heart failure. J. Clin. Invest. **85:** 305–309.

51. TAKAHASHI, T., P. D. ALLEN & S. IZUMO. 1992. Expression of A-, B-, and C-type natriuretic peptide genes in failing and developing human ventricles. Correlation with expression of the Ca^{2+}-ATPase gene. Circ. Res. **71:** 9–17.
52. HASENFUSS, G. 1998. Alterations of calcium-regulatory proteins in heart failure. Cardiovasc. Res. **37:** 279–289.

cAMP-Mediated Signal Transduction and Sarcoplasmic Reticulum Function in Heart Failure

MATTHEW A. MOVSESIAN[a]

Salt Lake City VA Medical Center and University of Utah School of Medicine, Salt Lake City, Utah 84132, USA

ABSTRACT: There is evidence that the effects of β-adrenergic receptor agonists on myocardial contractility result principally from the phosphorylation of phospholamban by cAMP-dependent protein kinase and the consequent deinhibition of SERCA2 activity and stimulation of sarcoplasmic reticulum Ca^{2+} transport. An impairment in β-adrenergic receptor-stimulated cAMP generation, attributable to down-regulation of β_1-adrenergic receptors and increased activity of Gαi and G protein–coupled receptor kinase, has long been recognized in failing human myocardium. This impairment is associated with a compartment-specific decrease in sarcoplasmic reticulum cAMP content that may selectively reduce phospholamban phosphorylation. Published and preliminary results indicate that two plausible explanations for this compartment-specific decrease—a reduction in sarcoplasmic reticulum–associated cAMP-dependent protein kinase or an increase in sarcoplasmic reticulum–associated cAMP phosphodiesterase—are unlikely. Instead, there is reason to believe that the selective reduction in β_1-adrenergic receptor density in failing myocardium is causally related to this compartment-specific decrease in cAMP content through an as-yet-undetermined mechanism. The fact that the modulation of SERCA2 activity by phospholamban is preserved in failing human myocardium offers an opportunity for improvement in the therapy of heart failure.

THE MODULATION OF CONTRACTION AND RELAXATION BY cAMP

cAMP-mediated signal transduction—a term used in reference to the pathways through which β-adrenergic receptor agonists bind to their G protein–coupled receptors, stimulate adenylate cyclase activity, and thereby increase intracellular cAMP content and the phosphorylation of intracellular proteins by cAMP-dependent protein kinase—is an important means for regulating contraction and relaxation in cardiac myocytes. Identifying the specific molecular mechanism through which this occurs has been problematic, since cAMP-dependent protein kinase phosphorylates a large number of proteins, several of which could potentially be involved in the regulation of contraction and relaxation (FIG. 1). Phosphorylation of L-type Ca^{2+} channels in the sarcolemma, for example, increases their open probability, which could alter intracellular Ca^{2+} homeostasis.[1,2] The same is true of ryanodine-sensitive Ca^{2+} channels in the sarcoplasmic reticulum, which are also substrates for cAMP-dependent protein kinase.[3,4]

[a] Address for correspondence: Cardiology Division, 4A-100 SOM, University of Utah Health Sciences Center, 50 North Medical Drive, Salt Lake City, Utah 84132. Phone: 801-581-7715; fax: 801-581-7735; e-mail: matthew.movsesian@hsc.utah.edu

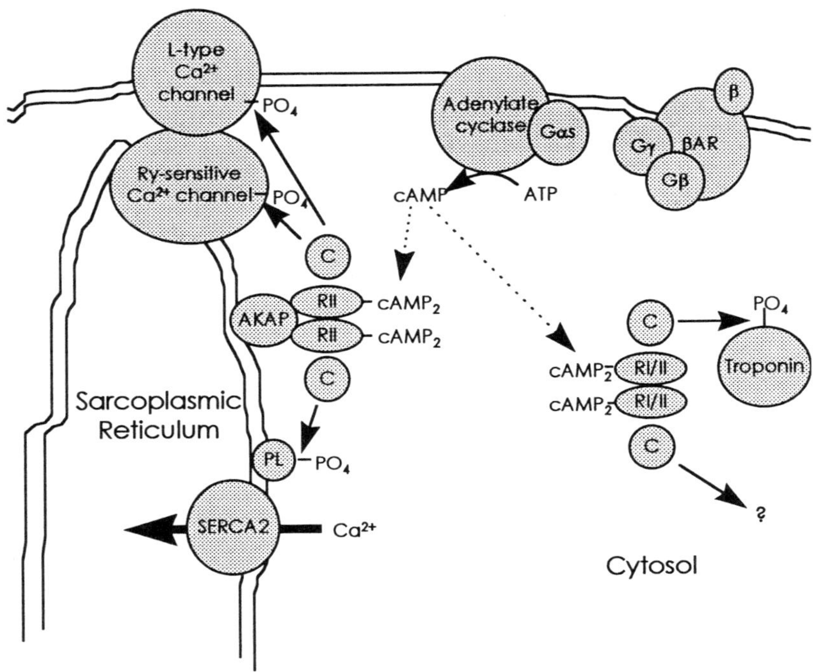

FIGURE 1. Regulation of contraction and relaxation in cardiac myocytes by cAMP-mediated signal transduction. Mechanisms relevant to inotropic and lusitropic responses are shown and explained throughout the text. Abbreviations: βAR, β-adrenergic receptor; Ry, ryanodine; AKAP, A-kinase anchoring protein; C, catalytic subunit of cAMP-dependent protein kinase; RI and RII, regulatory subunits of cAMP-dependent protein kinase; PL, phospholamban. ? refers to unspecified substrates of cAMP-dependent protein kinase.

Phosphorylation of troponin I reduces the apparent affinity of troponin C for Ca^{2+}, altering the Ca^{2+} sensitivity of the contractile elements.[5] Phosphorylation of phospholamban blocks its inhibitory interaction with SERCA2, the Ca^{2+}-transporting ATPase of the sarcoplasmic reticulum, and thereby stimulates ATP-dependent Ca^{2+} sequestration by the sarcoplasmic reticulum during relaxation.[6–8] This latter effect, which increases the speed and degree of relaxation, likely enhances contractility by increasing the difference between intracellular Ca^{2+} concentrations during systole and diastole. The recent observation that inotropic and lusitropic responses to β-adrenergic receptor occupancy are absent from phospholamban-deficient mice—an observation discussed in detail earlier in this volume—suggests (to the extent that these observations are applicable to humans) that phosphorylation of phospholamban by cAMP-dependent protein kinase is the principal event through which agents that increase intracellular cAMP levels elicit inotropic and lusitropic responses in cardiac muscle, and that these responses result from increases in the speed and amplitude of Ca^{2+} sequestration and release by the sarcoplasmic reticulum.[9]

ABNORMAL cAMP GENERATION IN FAILING HUMAN MYOCARDIUM

Alterations in cAMP-mediated signaling are prominently involved in the pathophysiology of heart failure. The best characterized alterations involve the impairment in cAMP generation in failing human myocardium.[10] The principal elements in receptor-mediated cAMP generation are β-adrenergic receptors, G proteins, and adenylate cyclase.[11,12] β_1- and β_2-adrenergic receptors in the plasma membranes of cardiac myocytes associate with Gαs, Gβ, and Gγ. When agonists bind to these receptors, Gαs dissociates and binds to adenylate cyclase, whose conversion of ATP to cAMP is thereby stimulated (FIG. 1). In heart failure, these mechanisms are affected in several ways. There is a 50% reduction in the density of β_1-adrenergic receptors in the plasma membranes of failing myocardium (the density of β_2-adrenergic receptors is essentially unaffected).[13–15] In addition, there are increases in the activity of Gαi,[16,17] which blocks the stimulation of adenylate cyclase by Gαs through a mechanism that remains incompletely understood, and of G protein–coupled receptor kinases,[18] whose phosphorylation of β-adrenergic receptors causes them to bind to β-arrestins.[19,20] Binding to β-arrestins impedes the interaction between β-adrenergic receptors and G proteins, in the process reducing both the affinity of these receptors for their agonists and the stimulation of adenylate cyclase activity upon receptor occupancy. Binding to β-arrestins also results in the reversible intracellular internalization of β-adrenergic receptors, which further uncouples these receptors from adenylate cyclase[21–23] (TABLE 1).

ABNORMAL MODULATION OF SARCOPLASMIC RETICULUM Ca^{2+} SEQUESTRATION IN FAILING HUMAN MYOCARDIUM

Whether there are alterations in the more distal components of this pathway—the phosphorylation of phospholamban by cAMP-dependent protein kinase and the consequent deinhibition of ATP-dependent Ca^{2+} sequestration by the sarcoplasmic reticulum in failing myocardium—has been a matter of controversy. That ATP-dependent Ca^{2+} sequestration by sarcoplasmic reticulum–derived microsomes is impaired in crude tissue homogenates of failing human myocardium seems clear enough,[24–27] but there are unresolved disagreements as to the molecular etiology of this impairment. One group of investigators has reported a ~35% decrease in ATP-dependent Ca^{2+} sequestration in salt-washed sarcoplasmic reticulum–enriched microsomes—i.e., microsomes from which nonintrinsic proteins have been removed—prepared from failing human myocardium, accompanied by comparable decreases in SERCA2 mRNA and protein levels.[25,28,29] Three other groups, however, have reported that ATP-dependent Ca^{2+} sequestration is undiminished in salt-washed sarcoplasmic reticulum–enriched microsomes from failing human myocardium, as are protein levels of SERCA2 and phospholamban.[26,27,30–34] Two of these groups have reported that protein levels for SERCA2 in failing myocardium remain at normal levels despite reductions in SERCA2 mRNA levels.[26,27,35] The other group has reported that the regulation of Ca^{2+} transport by phospholamban phosphorylation is preserved in salt-washed microsomes from failing

TABLE 1. Causes of Impaired cAMP Generation in Failing Human Myocardium

Down-regulation of β_1-adrenergic receptors
Increased activity of Gαi
Increased activity of G protein-coupled receptor kinase

human myocardium, which would suggest that the stoichiometry and coupling of these proteins are unchanged in heart failure.[31]

The preponderance of data seem therefore to suggest that the impairment in Ca^{2+} transport by the sarcoplasmic reticulum in failing human myocardium is not attributable to constitutive changes in the levels of SERCA2 and phospholamban or to a change in their interaction. There is evidence, however—discussed in detail elsewhere in this volume—that the regulation of sarcoplasmic reticulum Ca^{2+} transport by cAMP-dependent protein kinase is altered in this tissue. In crude homogenates of failing human myocardium, the level of phospholamban phosphorylation and the apparent affinity of SERCA2 for Ca^{2+} are reduced relative to the level of phosphorylation of phospholamban and the apparent Ca^{2+} affinity of SERCA2 in preparations from normal hearts.[36] After addition of cAMP-dependent protein kinase catalytic subunit, apparent Ca^{2+} affinity rises to a similar level in both groups. These observations are consistent with a situation in which levels of SERCA2 and phospholamban are undiminished in failing human myocardium, but in which the reduction in cAMP content in this tissue leads to a reduction in phospholamban phosphorylation and a consequent impairment in sarcoplasmic reticulum Ca^{2+} transport.

ALTERED COMPARTMENTATION OF cAMP-MEDIATED SIGNAL TRANSDUCTION IN FAILING HUMAN MYOCARDIUM

It is useful to consider all of this in the context of the intracellular compartmentation of cAMP-mediated signal transduction. cAMP is found both in the cytosol and associated with intracellular membranes of cardiac myocytes, and the content of cAMP in these two compartments can be regulated differentially. Exposure to nonselective β-adrenergic receptor agonists raises both cytosolic and membrane-bound cAMP levels in cardiac myocytes, whereas exposure to prostaglandin E1 (whose receptors, like those of β-adrenergic receptors, are coupled to adenylate cyclase via Gαs[37,38]) increases cytosolic cAMP levels without increasing membrane-bound cAMP levels.[39,40] There is further selectivity at the level of β-adrenergic receptor subtypes. Occupancy of β_1-adrenergic receptors increases both cytosolic and membrane-bound cAMP levels in cardiac myocytes, while occupancy of β_2-adrenergic receptors increases only cytosolic cAMP levels.[41,42] The compartment-selective nature of these effects on intracellular cAMP content are important in the modulation of contraction and relaxation, as the increase in the kinetics of the intracellular $[Ca^{2+}]$ transient and the enhancement of myocardial contractility in response to β-adrenergic receptor agonists correlate closely with increases in membrane-bound cAMP content but not with changes in cytosolic cAMP content.[43] These observations would lead to the prediction that effects on intracellular Ca^{2+} transients and contraction would be preferentially elicited by β_1- rather than β_2-adrenergic receptor agonists, since increases in membrane-bound cAMP content result principally from occupancy of β_1-adrenergic receptors; and this turns out by and large to be the case.[44]

This differential regulation of cytosolic and membrane-associated cAMP content may allow for the differential phosphorylation of cytosolic and membrane-associated substrates of cAMP-dependent protein kinase. This enzyme is itself partitioned between the cytosol and intracellular membranes of cardiac myocytes through mechanisms that are not fully understood.[45] cAMP-dependent protein kinase exists functionally as a tetramer composed of two identical catalytic (C) subunits and two identical regulatory (R) subunits.[46,47] Two principal families of R subunits, designated

RI and RII, have been identified, and the tetrameric enzyme is designated type I or type II based on whether it contains RI or RII subunits. A variety of membrane proteins that bind RII subunits and thereby anchor the type II isoform to intracellular membranes have been identified and designated *A-kinase anchoring proteins* (AKAP's).[48,49] No comparable RI-anchoring proteins have yet been identified, but the type I isoform nevertheless associates with sarcolemmal membranes with high affinity.[50] Both isoforms are also present in the cytosol of cardiac myocytes. Whatever the mechanism underlying the intracellular partitioning of these isoforms, activation of membrane-bound cAMP-dependent protein kinase would be expected to lead predominantly to the phosphorylation of adjacent membrane-bound targets—most notably phospholamban— while activation of cytosolic kinase might have more diffuse effects (FIG. 1).

There is evidence that the compartmentation of cAMP-mediated signal transduction is directly relevant to the regulation of sarcoplasmic reticulum Ca^{2+} sequestration in heart failure. When cytosolic and particulate fractions are prepared from normal and failing human myocardium, there is a marked reduction in cAMP levels in microsomal fractions of failing myocardium, whereas cAMP levels in cytosolic fractions of normal and failing myocardium are essentially indistinguishable.[51] These observations suggest that the impairment in cAMP generation in failing myocardium is somehow associated with a compartment-specific decrease in intracellular cAMP content, and that this compartment-specific decrease is likely to bring about a relatively selective decrease in phospholamban phosphorylation.

That there should be a selective decrease in membrane-associated cAMP content in failing human myocardium is not surprising. As noted earlier, there is evidence from studies in animals that increases in membrane-associated cAMP content are selectively coupled to occupancy of β_1-adrenergic receptors, and that phospholamban phosphorylation itself is specifically coupled to β_1-adrenergic receptor occupancy.[41,42] If these findings are applicable to failing human myocardium, in which there is a selective 50% decrease in β_1-adrenergic receptor density, a selective decrease in membrane-associated cAMP content may be predictable. But the coincidence of a decrease in β_1-adrenergic receptor density and a decrease in membrane-associated cAMP content does not in itself establish a cause-and-effect relationship between these phenomena, and other considerations need to be taken into account. A compartment-specific decrease in membrane-associated cAMP content could occur in the face of a generalized decrease in cAMP generation under two other conditions: There could be a compartment-selective change in cAMP phosphodiesterase activity, such that the rate of hydrolysis of membrane-associated cAMP were higher (relative to the rate of hydrolysis of cytosolic cAMP) in failing human myocardium than in normal myocardium. The evidence that the cytosolic and membrane-associated forms of PDE3, the predominant cAMP hydrolytic enzyme in human myocardium, are separate molecular species would make this possibility seem more plausible.[52] To test this possibility, investigators have examined the level and intracellular distribution of cAMP phosphodiesterase activity in normal and failing human myocardium, and their results indicated that normal and failing human myocardium do not differ in this regard.[53] Alternatively, the selective reduction in membrane-associated cAMP content in failing myocardium could be the result of a reduction in the level of membrane-associated cAMP-dependent protein kinase relative to the level of cytosolic cAMP-dependent protein kinase. To date, however, preliminary reports of experiments in which the level and intracellular distribution of intracellular cAMP-binding sites in normal and failing human myocardium offer no evidence to support this explanation.[54]

FUTURE DIRECTIONS

In summary, it seems that heart failure in humans involves a selective reduction in membrane-associated cAMP content, probably linked to the down-regulation of β_1-adrenergic receptors, that contributes to the impairment of contraction and relaxation by reducing phospholamban phosphorylation and thereby reducing Ca^{2+} sequestration and release by the sarcoplasmic reticulum. We are left, however, with the mystery of *how* membrane-associated cAMP levels are selectively coupled to β_1-adrenergic receptor occupancy—or, to put it another way, how β_2-adrenergic receptor occupancy results in a selective increase in cytosolic cAMP content. The mechanism by which this occurs—and how this mechanism is affected in heart failure—would seem to constitute the most fundamental gap in our understanding of the regulation of sarcoplasmic reticulum function by cAMP.

A consideration regarding the therapeutic implications of these findings seems pertinent. The regulation of SERCA2 activity by phospholamban is an important component in the inotropic and lusitropic responses of human myocardium, and this mechanism appears to be constitutively preserved in failing human myocardium. But current therapy, which is directed at increasing phospholamban phosphorylation in failing human myocardium by increasing intracellular cAMP content, either by stimulating adenylate cyclase or inhibiting cyclic nucleotide phosphodiesterases, suffers from two serious drawbacks. First, both interventions represent attempts to utilize a mechanism—β-adrenergic receptor–stimulated cAMP generation, and more particularly β_1-adrenergic receptor–stimulated cAMP generation—that is constitutively *impaired* in failing myocardium, and this represents a considerable obstacle. Second, the attempt to compensate for a reduction in membrane-associated cAMP content by raising total cAMP content raises the possibility of increasing cAMP levels in a compartment (the cytosol) where the increase may not contribute to contractility but may bring about undesirable side effects. The fact that there is a selective down-regulation of β_1-adrenergic receptors in failing myocardium makes it even more likely that these interventions would result in a disproportionate increase in cytosolic cAMP content, and this may explain the disappointing long-term therapeutic results with phosphodiesterase inhibition in the treatment of heart failure.[55–58] A drug that could bind to phospholamban and cause it to dissociate from SERCA2 might be able to circumvent all of these problems. Whether any such agent will be identified and put to clinical use remains to be seen.

REFERENCES

1. Sculptoreanu, A., E. Rotman, M. Takahashi, T. Scheuer & W. A. Catterall. 1993. Voltage-dependent potentiation of the activity of cardiac L-type calcium channel alpha 1 subunits due to phosphorylation by cAMP-dependent protein kinase. Proc. Natl. Acad. Sci. USA **90:** 10135–10139.
2. De Jongh, K. S., B. J. Murphy, A. A. Colvin, J. W. Hell, M. Takahashi & W. A. Catterall. 1996. Specific phosphorylation of a site in the full-length form of the alpha 1 subunit of the cardiac L-type calcium channel by adenosine 3′,5′-cyclic monophosphate–dependent protein kinase. Biochemistry **35:** 10392–10402.
3. Witcher, D. R., R. J. Kovacs, H. Schulman, D. C. Cefali & L. R. Jones. 1991. Unique phosphorylation site on the cardiac ryanodine receptor regulates calcium channel activity. J. Biol. Chem. **266:** 11144–11152.
4. Hain, J., H. Onoue, M. Mayrleitner, S. Fleischer & H. Schindler. 1995. Phosphorylation modulates the function of the calcium release channel of sarcoplasmic reticulum from cardiac muscle. J. Biol. Chem. **270:** 2074–2081.
5. Solaro, R. J., S. P. Robertson, J. D. Johnson, M. J. Holroyde & J. D. Potter. 1981.

Troponin-I phosphorylation: A unique regulator of the amount of calcium required to activate cardiac myofibrils. Cold Spring Harbor Conf. Cell Proliferation **8:** 901–911.

6. INUI, M., B. K. CHAMBERLAIN, A. SAITO & S. FLEISCHER. 1986. The nature of the modulation of Ca^{2+} transport as studied by reconstitution of cardiac sarcoplasmic reticulum. J. Biol. Chem. **261:** 1794–1800.
7. JAMES, P., M. INUI, M. TADA, M. CHIESI & E. CARAFOLI. 1989. Nature and site of phospholamban regulation of the Ca^{2+} pump of the sarcoplasmic reticulum. Nature **342:** 90–92.
8. SASAKI, T., M. INUI, Y. KIMURA, T. KUZUYA & M. TADA. 1992. Molecular mechanism of regulation of Ca^{2+} pump ATPase by phospholamban in cardiac sarcoplasmic reticulum. Effects of synthetic phospholamban peptides on Ca^{2+} pump ATPase. J. Biol. Chem. **267:** 1674–1679.
9. LUO, W., I. L. GRUPP, J. HARRER, S. PONNIAH, G. GRUPP, J. J. DUFY, T. DOETSCHMAN & E. G. KRANIAS. 1994. Targeted ablation of the phospholamban gene is associated with markedly enhanced myocardial contractility and loss of β-agonist stimulation. Circ. Res. **75:** 401–409.
10. FELDMAN, M. D., L. COPELAS, J. K. GWATHMEY, P. PHILLIPS, S. E. WARREN, F. J. SCHOEN & W. GROSSMAN. 1987. Deficient production of cyclic AMP: Pharmacologic evidence of an important cause of contractile dysfunction in patients with end-stage heart failure. Circulation **75:** 331–339.
11. BENOVIC, J. L., M. BOUVIER, M. G. CARON & R. J. LEFKOWITZ. 1988. Regulation of adenylyl cyclase-coupled β-adrenergic receptors. Annu. Rev. Cell Biol. **4:** 405–428.
12. GOODMAN, A. G. 1995. Nobel Lecture. G proteins and regulation of adenylyl cyclase. Biosci. Rep. **15:** 65–97.
13. BRISTOW, M. R., R. GINSBURG, W. MINOBE, R. S. CUBICCIOTTI, W. S. SAGEMAN, K. LURIE, M. E. BILLINGHAM, D. C. HARRISON & E. B. STINSON. 1982. Decreased catecholamine sensitivity and β-adrenergic-receptor density in failing human hearts. N. Engl. J. Med. **307:** 205–211.
14. BRISTOW, M. R., R. GINSBURG, V. UMANS, M. FOWLER, W. MINOBE, R. RAMUSSEN, P. ZERA, R. MENLOVE, P. SHAH, S. JAMIESON & E. B. STINSON. 1986. β_1- and β_2-adrenergic-receptor subpopulations in nonfailing and failing human ventricular myocardium: Coupling of both receptor subtypes to muscle contraction and selective β_1-receptor down-regulation in heart failure. Circ. Res. **59:** 297–309.
15. BRISTOW, M. R., R. E. HERSHBERGER, J. D. PORT, W. MINOBE & R. RASMUSSEN. 1989. β_1- and β_2-adrenergic receptor–mediated adenylate cyclase stimulation in nonfailing and failing human ventricular myocardium. Mol. Pharmacol. **35:** 295–303.
16. FELDMAN, A. M., A. E. CATES, W. B. VEAZEY, R. E. HERSHBERGER, M. R. BRISTOW, K. L. BAUGHMAN, W. A. BAUMGARTNER & C. VAN DOP. 1988. Increase in the 40,000-mol wt pertussis toxin substrate (G protein) in the failing human heart. J. Clin. Invest. **82:** 189–197.
17. BÖHM, M., P. GIERSCHIK, K. H. JAKOBS, B. PIESKE, P. SCHNABEL, M. UNGERER & E. ERDMANN. 1990. Increase of $G_{i\alpha}$ in human heart with dilated but not ischemic cardiomyopathy. Circulation **82:** 1249–1265.
18. UNGERER, M., M. BÖHM, J. S. ELCE, E. ERDMANN & M. J. LOHSE. 1993. Altered expression of β-adrenergic receptor kinase and β_1-adrenergic receptors in the failing human heart. Circulation **87:** 454–463.
19. LOHSE, M. J., J. L. BENOVIC, A. J. CODIN, M. G. CARON & R. J. LEFKOWITZ. 1990. β-arrestin: A protein that regulates β-adrenergic receptor function. Science **248:** 1547–1550.
20. LEFKOWITZ, R. J., J. INGLESE, W. J. KOCH, J. PITCHER, H. ATTRAMADAL & M. G. CARON. 1992. G-protein-coupled receptors: Regulatory role of receptor kinases and arrestin proteins. Cold Spring Harbor Symp. Quant. Biol. **57:** 127–133.
21. FERGUSON, S. S., W. E. DOWNEY III, A. M. COLAPIETRO, L. S. BARAK, L. MENARD & M. G. CARON. 1996. Role of β-arrestin in mediating agonist-promoted G protein-coupled receptor internalization. Science **271:** 363–366.
22. PIPPIG, S., S. ANDEXINGER & M. J. LOHSE. 1995. Sequestration and recycling of β_2-adrenergic receptors permit receptor resensitization. Mol. Pharmacol. **47:** 666–676.
23. YU, S. S., R. J. OLEFKOWITZ & W. P. HAUSDORFF. 1993. β-adrenergic receptor sequestration. A potential mechanism of receptor resensitization. J. Biol. Chem. **268:** 337–341.
24. LIMAS, C. J., M. T. OLIVAR, I. F. GOLDENBERG, T. B. LEVINE, D. G. BENDITT & A. SIMON.

1987. Calcium uptake by cardiac sarcoplasmic reticulum in human dilated cardiomyopathy. Cardiovasc. Res. **21:** 601–605.

25. Hasenfuss, G., H. Reinecke, R. Studer, M. Meyer, B. Pieske, J. Holtz, C. Holubarsch, H. Posival, H. Just & H. Drexler. 1994. Relation between myocardial function and expression of sarcoplasmic reticulum Ca^{2+}-ATPase in failing and nonfailing human myocardium. Circ. Res. **75:** 434–442.
26. Schwinger, R. H. G., M. Böhm, U. Schmidt, P. Karczewski, U. Bavendiek, M. Flesch, E. G. Krause & E. Erdmann. 1995. Unchanged protein levels of SERCA II and phospholamban but reduced Ca^{2+} uptake and Ca^{2+}-ATPase activity of cardiac sarcoplasmic reticulum from dilated cardiomyopathy patients compared with patients with nonfailing hearts. Circulation **92:** 3220–3228.
27. Flesch, M., R. H. Schwinger, P. Schnabel, F. Schiffer, I. Van Gelder, U. Bavendiek, M. Sudkamp, F. Kuhn-Regnier & M. Böhm. 1996. Sarcoplasmic reticulum Ca^{2+} ATPase and phospholamban mRNA and protein levels in end-stage heart failure due to ischemic or dilated cardiomyopathy. J. Mol. Med. **74:** 321–332.
28. Studer, R., H. Reinecke, J. Bilger, T. Eschenhagen, M. Bohm, G. Hasenfuss, H. Just, J. Holtz & H. Drexler. 1994. Gene expression of the cardiac Na^{+}-Ca^{2+} exchanger in end-stage human heart failure. Circ. Res. **75:** 443–453.
29. Meyer, M., W. Schillinger, B. Pieske, C. Holubarsch, C. Heilmann, H. Posival, G. Kuwajima, K. Mikoshiba, H. Just & G. Hasenfuss. 1995. Alterations of sarcoplasmic reticulum proteins in failing human dilated cardiomyopathy. Circulation **92:** 778–784.
30. Movsesian, M. A., M. B. Bristow & J. Krall. 1989. Calcium uptake by sarcoplasmic reticulum from patients with idiopathic dilated cardiomyopathy. Circ. Res. **65:** 1141–1144.
31. Movsesian, M. A., J. Colyer, J. H. Wang & J. Krall. 1990. Phospholamban-mediated stimulation of Ca^{2+} uptake in sarcoplasmic reticulum from normal and failing hearts. J. Clin. Invest. **85:** 1698–1702.
32. Movsesian, M. A., C. J. Smith, J. Krall, M. R. Bristow & V. C. Manganiello. 1991. Sarcoplasmic reticulum-associated cyclic adenosine 5′-monophosphate phosphodiesterase activity in normal and failing human hearts. J. Clin. Invest. **88:** 15–19.
33. Movsesian, M. A., M. Karimi, K. Green & L. R. Jones. 1994. Ca^{2+}-transporting ATPase, phospholamban and calsequestrin levels in nonfailing and failing human myocardium. Circulation **90:** 653–657.
34. Nimer, L. R., D. H. Needleman, S. L. Hamilton, J. Krall & M. A. Movsesian. 1995. Effect of ryanodine on sarcoplasmic reticulum Ca^{2+} accumulation in nonfailing and failing human myocardium. Circulation **92:** 2504–2510.
35. Linck, B., P. Boknik, T. Eschenhagen, F. U. Müller, J. Neumann, M. Nose, L. R. Jones, W. Schmitz & H. Scholz. 1996. Messenger RNA expression and immunological quantification of phospholamban and SR Ca^{2+}-ATPase in failing and nonfailing human hearts. Cardiovasc. Res. **31:** 625–632.
36. Schwinger, R. H. G., U. Bavendieck, B. Bölck, S. Hörter, S. Hoischen, K. Brixius, P. Karzcewski, E. G. Krause & E. Erdmann. 1996. Phosphorylation of phospholamban influences Ca^{2+}-sensitivity but not maximal Ca^{2+}-ATPase activity of SERCA II in human myocardium. (Abstr.) Circulation **94:** I-673.
37. Ichikawa, A., Y. Sugimoto & M. Negishi. 1996. Molecular aspects of the structures and functions of the prostaglandin E receptors. J. Lipid Mediat. Cell Signal. **14:** 83–87.
38. Negishi, M., A. Irie, Y. Sugimoto, T. Namba & A. Ichikawa. 1995. Selective coupling of prostaglandin E receptor EP3D to Gi and Gs through interaction of alpha-carboxylic acid of agonist and arginine residue of seventh transmembrane domain. J. Biol. Chem. **270:** 16122–16127.
39. Hayes, J. S., L. L. Brunton & S. E. Mayer. 1980. Selective activation of particulate cAMP-dependent protein kinase by isoproterenol and prostaglandin E_1. J. Biol. Chem. **255:** 5113–5119.
40. Buxton, I. L. & L. L. Brunton. 1983. Compartments of cyclic AMP and protein kinase in mammalian cardiomyocytes. J. Biol. Chem. **258:** 10233–10239.
41. Xiao, R. P., C. Hohl, R. Altschuld, L. Jones, B. Livingston, B. Ziman, B. Tantini & E. G. Lakatta. 1994. β_2-adrenergic receptor-stimulated increase in cAMP in rat heart cells

is not coupled to changes in Ca^{2+} dynamics, contractility, or phospholamban phosphorylation. J. Biol. Chem. **269:** 19151–19156.
42. YABANA, H., Y. SASAKI, H. NARITA & T. NAGAO. 1995. Subcellular fractions of cyclic AMP and cyclic AMP–dependent protein kinase and the positive inotropic effects of selective β_1- and β_2-adrenoceptor agonists in guinea pig hearts. J. Cardiovasc. Pharmacol. **26:** 893–898.
43. HOHL, C. M. & Q. LI. 1991. Compartmentation of cAMP in adult canine ventricular myocytes. Relation to single-cell free Ca^{2+} transients. Circulation **69:** 1369–1379.
44. XIAO, R. P. & E. G. LAKATTA. 1993. β_1-adrenoceptor stimulation and β_2-adrenoceptor stimulation differ in their effects on contraction, cytosolic Ca^{2+}, and Ca^{2+} current in single rat ventricular cells. Circ. Res. **73:** 286–300.
45. CORBIN, J. D., P. H. SUGDEN, T. M. LINCOLN & S. L. KEELY. 1977. Compartmentalization of adenosine 3′:5′-monophosphate and adenosine 3′:5′-monophosphate–dependent protein kinase in heart tissue. J. Biol. Chem. **252:** 3854–3861.
46. TAYLOR, S. S., J. A. BUECHLER & W. YONEMOTO. 1990. cAMP-dependent protein kinase: framework for a diverse family of regulatory enzymes. Annu. Rev. Biochem. **59:** 971–1005.
47. SCOTT, J. D. 1991. Cyclic nucleotide-dependent protein kinases. Pharmacol. Ther. **50:** 123–145.
48. LEISER, M., C. S. RUBIN & J. ERLICHMAN. 1986. Differential binding of the regulatory subunits (RII) of cAMP-dependent protein kinase II from bovine brain and muscle to RII-binding proteins. J. Biol. Chem. **261:** 1904–1908.
49. COGHLAN, V. M., S. E. BERGESON, L. LANGEBERG, G. NILAVER & J. D. SCOTT. 1993. A-Kinase anchoring proteins: A key to selective activation of cAMP-responsive events? Mol. Cell. Biochem. **127/128:** 309–319.
50. ROBINSON, M. L., M. A. WALLERT, C. A. REINITZ & J. B. SHABB. 1996. Association of the type I regulatory subunit of cAMP-dependent protein kinase with cardiac myocyte sarcolemma. Arch. Biochem. Biophys. **330:** 181–187.
51. BÖHM, M., B. REIGER, R. H. G. SCHWINGER & E. ERDMANN. 1994. cAMP concentrations, cAMP dependent protein kinase activity, and phospholamban in nonfailing and failing myocardium. Cardiovasc. Res. **28:** 1713–1719.
52. SMITH, C. J., J. KRALL, V. C. MANGANIELLO & M. A. MOVSESIAN. 1993. Cytosolic and sarcoplasmic reticulum–associated low K_m cGMP-inhibited cAMP phosphodiesterase in mammalian myocardium. Biochem. Biophys. Res. Commun. **190:** 516–521.
53. MOVSESIAN, M. A., C. J. SMITH, J. KRALL, M. R. BRISTOW & V. C. MANGANIELLO. 1991. Sarcoplasmic reticulum-associated cyclic adenosine 5′-monophosphate phosphodiesterase activity in normal and failing human hearts. J. Clin. Invest. **88:** 15–19.
54. MOVSESIAN, M. A., J. STAHELI & J. KRALL. 1995. Compartmentation of cAMP-dependent protein kinase in nonfailing and failing human myocardium. (Abstr.) J. Invest. Med. **43:** 357A.
55. MASSIE, B., M. BOURASSA, R. DIBIANCO, M. HESS, M. KONSTAM, M. LIKOFF & M. PACKER. 1985. Long-term oral administration of amrinone for congestive heart failure: Lack of efficacy in a multicenter controlled trial. Circulation **71:** 963–971.
56. DIBIANCO, R., R. SHABETAI, W. KOSTUK, J. MORAN, R. C. SCHLANT & R. WRIGHT. 1989. A comparison of oral milrinone, digoxin, and their combination in the treatment of patients with chronic heart failure. N. Engl. J. Med. **320:** 677–683.
57. URETSKY, B. F., M. JESSUP, M. A. KONSTAM, C. V. DEC, G. W. LEIER, J. BENOTTI, S. MURALLI, H. C. HERRMANN & J. A. SANDBERG. 1990. Multicenter trial of oral enoximone in patients with moderate to moderately severe congestive heart failure. Lack of benefit compared with placebo. Circulation **82:** 774–780.
58. NONY, P., J-P. BOISSEL, M. LIÈVRE, A. LEIZOROVICZ, M. C. HAUGH, S. FAREH, B. DE BREYNE. 1994. Evaluation of the effect of phosphodiesterase inhibitors on mortality in chronic heart failure patients. Eur. J. Clin. Pharmacol. **46:** 191–196.

cAMP-Dependent Protein Kinase A–Stimulated Sarcoplasmic Reticulum Function in Heart Failure[a]

ROBERT H. G. SCHWINGER,[b] BIRGIT BÖLCK, GÖTZ MÜNCH, KLARA BRIXIUS, JOCHEN MÜLLER-EHMSEN, AND ERLAND ERDMANN

Laboratory of Muscle Research and Molecular Cardiology, Clinic III of Internal Medicine University of Cologne, D-50924 Cologne, Germany

ABSTRACT: It is unclear whether decreased protein expression of SERCA2 (SR-Ca^{2+}-ATPase) and phospholamban (PLB), or alterations in the phosphorylation state of PLB leading to increased inhibition of SERCA2 are responsible for the reduced SERCA2 function in failing human myocardium. In crude membrane preparations from patients with terminal heart failure due to idiopathic dilated cardiomyopathy (DCM) and control hearts (NF), SERCA2 activity was measured with a NADH coupled assay. Protein expression of SERCA2 and PLB and the phosphorylation state at the two phosphorylation sites, serine-16-PLB and threonine-17-PLB, were investigated with specific (phosphorylation) antibodies and Western blot technique. In NF, the V_{max} and the Ca^{2+} sensitivity of SERCA2 activity were significantly higher compared to DCM. Protein expression of SERCA2 and PLB were unchanged, whereas the phosphorylation status at both serine-16-PLB and threonine-17-PLB were significantly reduced in DCM. The native phosphorylation status of PLB measured by the back-phosphorylation technique was reduced in DCM as well. After stimulation with protein kinase A only the Ca^{2+} sensitivity, but not V_{max}, increased. The reduced phosphorylation state of PLB may lead to decreased Ca^{2+} sensitivity of SERCA2 in failing human myocardium. The altered regulation of the SR-Ca^{2+}-ATPase in human heart failure may offer an opportunity for an improvement in the therapy of heart failure.

The contraction cycle of the myocyte is closely related to the increase and decrease of intracellular Ca^{2+} availability. Ca^{2+} enters the intracellular compartment via voltage-gated L-type Ca^{2+} channels. Ca^{2+} is stored in the sarcoplasmic reticulum (SR), from which Ca^{2+} can be released by a Ca^{2+}-triggered Ca^{2+} release mechanism via Ca^{2+} release channels. Ca^{2+} accumulation by the cardiac SR occurs through the activity of SERCA2, a 105-kDa Ca^{2+}- and Mg^{2+}-dependent ATPase that transports Ca^{2+} from the cytosol into the lumen of the sarcoplasmic reticulum.[1] The large amounts of Ca^{2+} released from the SR initiate the cross-bridge interaction and thereby an increase in force of contraction. It is important to appreciate, therefore, that SERCA2 activity determines not only the rate and extent of relaxation, but also the rate and amplitude of contraction, since these are determined by the amount of Ca^{2+} sequestered by the sar-

[a] Experimental work was supported by grants to R. H. G. S. from the Deutsche Forschungsgemeinschaft, the Zentrum für Molekulare Medizin Köln (Bundesministeriums für Bildung, Wissenschaft, Forschung und Technologie 1 KS 9501), and Köln Fortune'96/27.

[b] Address for correspondence: Robert H. G. Schwinger, M.D., Clinic III of Internal Medicine, University of Cologne, Joseph-Stelzmann-Str. 9, D-50924 Cologne, Germany. Phone: +0049-221-478-4474; fax: +0049-221-478-6594; e-mail: Robert.Schwinger@medizin.Uni-Koeln.de

coplasmic reticulum and the Ca^{2+} gradient between the sarcoplasmic reticulum and the cytosol at the time that the Ca^{2+} release occurs. The Ca^{2+}-ATPase of the sarcoplasmic reticulum and the Na^{+}-Ca^{2+} exchanger of the sarcolemma seem to be the most important mechanisms to extrude Ca^{2+} from the cytosol during diastole and to lower the high systolic intracellular Ca^{2+} concentrations initiating an effective relaxation.[2] The activity of SERCA2 is modulated through its interaction with phospholamban, a pentamer comprised of five identical 6-kDa (52 amino acids) monomers.[3] In its unphosphorylated form, phospholamban binds to SERCA2 and inhibits Ca^{2+} transport activity, principally by decreasing affinity (increasing K_m) for Ca^{2+}, but also probably by decreasing V_{max}.[4] Phosphorylation of phospholamban by any of several protein kinases—among them are the cAMP-dependent protein kinase, a membrane-associated Ca^{2+}/calmodulin-dependent protein kinase, and protein kinase C—blocks the interaction between phospholamban and SERCA2 and relieves this inhibition.[5–8] While numerous proteins involved in contraction and relaxation are substrates for cAMP-dependent protein kinases, phosphorylation of phospholamban and the resulting de-inhibition of SERCA2 is likely the principal molecular mechanism for the inotropic and lusitropic effects of β-adrenergic receptor agonists. The most convincing evidence comes from experiments comparing myocardial responses to isoprenaline in normal rabbits and in rabbits in which the gene for phospholamban was ablated.[9] After phosphorylation, the inhibitory moiety of phospholamban towards the SERCA2 will be removed, leading to activation of the SERCA2. The contribution of the SR-Ca^{2+}-ATPase and the Na^{+}-Ca^{2+} exchanger in the regulation of the intracellular Ca^{2+} during contraction and relaxation is species dependent. In rat myocardium, the SR-Ca^{2+}-ATPase predominates in the function of lowering intracellular Ca^{2+}, whereas the contribution of the Na^{+}-Ca^{2+} exchanger seems to be negligible. In contrast, in rabbit myocardium Ca^{2+} extrusion via the Na^{+}-Ca^{2+} exchanger contributes more to Ca^{2+} extrusion out of the cytosol than SR-Ca^{2+}-ATPase.[2] The relative contribution of the SR-Ca^{2+}-ATPase to the provision of the Ca^{2+} involved in contractile activation and relaxation in human myocardium is still a matter of debate.

It has been suggested that the contractile apparatus in terminally failing human myocardium maximally increases force development even in the failing heart. However, inotropic stimulation by cAMP-dependent, as well as by cAMP-independent, mechanisms results in an altered diastolic relaxation in papillary muscle strip preparations from patients with dilated cardiomyopathy.[10] During inotropic stimulation, abnormalities in diastolic rather than in systolic contraction become evident. Furthermore, several investigators have demonstrated an altered force-frequency relationship in failing human myocardium.[10–12] In these studies, force of contraction was increased only in nonfailing tissue, but not in diseased human hearts. Similar findings have been reported from *in vivo* measurements after rapid atrial pacing in patients with heart failure.[13] These alterations in contraction coupling have been suggested to be due to altered intracellular Ca^{2+} handling—e.g., the positive force-frequency relationship may be due to changes in the Ca^{2+} content of the sarcoplasmic reticulum.[14] Consistently, differences in intracellular Ca^{2+} handling have been reported in isolated cardiac myocytes from patients with dilated cardiomyopathy in comparison to control cells.[15] Similar findings have been reported by simultaneous measurements of the force of contraction and of the intracellular Ca^{2+} signal using the chemiluminiscent aequorin in intact muscle preparations.[16] If reduced Ca^{2+} loading of the sarcoplasmic reticulum is present in failing human myocardium, diastolic relaxation and frequency-dependent increase in force development are altered. A reduction of SR Ca^{2+} uptake may lead to slower diastolic Ca^{2+} decay and reduced SR Ca^{2+} content, which in turn would cause decreased Ca^{2+} content available for release during the depolarization of the next beat. Because of the dependence of contraction and relaxation upon ATP-dependent Ca^{2+} sequestration by the sarcoplasmic reticulum, the possibility that an impairment in this process might contribute to the pathophysiology of heart failure has been the focus of a large body of research over the past two decades. Thus, special attention has been given to diastolic Ca^{2+} alterations, as it is known that diastolic Ca^{2+} levels are enhanced and that diastolic Ca^{2+} decay is significantly prolonged in cardiomyocytes from patients with terminally heart failure due to dilated cardiomyopathy.[15] These changes could lead to an increase in diastolic tension of the contractile force as well. To study the functional significance of the SERCA2 activity for the contraction cycle in human myocardium the influence of the specific inhibitor of SERCA2, cyclopiazonic acid (CPA), on force generation and on the intracellular Ca^{2+} transient was measured. Cyclopiazonic acid, a mycotoxin produced by various fungi of *Aspergillus* and *Penicillium* species, has been reported to be a selective inhibitor of the SR-Ca^{2+}-ATPase expressed in cardiac muscle.[17] Even at high concentrations, CPA has no effects on Ca^{2+} sensitivity of the contractile apparatus,[17] Ca^{2+} currents,[18] and the Na^+-Ca^{2+} exchanger[19] other than its inhibitory action on the SR-Ca^{2+}-ATPase in cardiac muscle. Because of its low K_D (228 nmol/l), fura 2 is a Ca^{2+} fluorescence indicator more suitable for measuring changes of diastolic Ca^{2+} than aequorin.[20] Furthermore, the fura 2 ratio method[20] has been used as a suitable tool for studying intracellular Ca^{2+} transients and force in isolated muscle strip preparations of rat and human myocardium.[21,22]

It is still a matter of debate whether intracellular Ca^{2+} uptake into the sarcoplasmic reticulum and SR Ca^{2+}-ATPase activity are altered in human dilated cardiomyopathy, possibly due to reduced amount of SERCA2 expression.[14,23,24] As reduced phosphorylation of phospholamban could influence the SERCA2 activity, the phosphorylation state of phospholamban and SERCA2 activity after stimulation with protein kinase A (PKA) were measured. To compare protein expression for SERCA2 and phospholamban, Western blot analysis was performed in the very same preparations. The rationale underlying the experimental approach to this issue and the conclusions that can be drawn from the present experimental findings are examined.

MATERIALS AND METHODS

Preparation of Isolated Human Muscle Strips

Experiments were performed on isolated electrically stimulated right atrial muscle strips from human nonfailing myocardium. Tissue was obtained from patients who had to undergo bypass surgery without clinical signs of heart failure (normal ejection fraction by echographic examination). None of the patients had received Ca^{2+}-channel antagonists within seven days before surgery, or β-adrenoceptor agonists or catecholamines 48 hours before surgery. Drugs used for general anesthesia were flunitrazepam, fentanyl, and pancuronium bromide with isoflurane. The investigation conformed to the principles outlined in the Declaration of Helsinki. Experiments were performed as described previously.[10]

Fura-2 Loading, Ca^{2+} and Force Measurements

Intracellular Ca^{2+} was measured by the fluorescence indicator fura-2.[20] Experiments were performed as previously described.[22,25]

Isolation of Vesicles of Sarcoplasmic Reticulum

The sarcoplasmic reticulum was prepared according to the method of Meissner and Henderson,[26] and Sitsapesan and Williams.[27] Protein content was measured by the method of Lowry.[28] Experiments were performed as described previously.[23]

Measurement of Ca^{2+}-ATPase Activity

The reaction was carried out according to Chu *et al.*[29] and Schwinger *et al.*[23] Ca^{2+}-ATPase activity in cardiac SR was assayed under conditions in which it has previously been shown that *in vitro* preincubation with cAMP and cAMP-dependent protein kinase increased Ca^{2+}-ATPase activity.[30]

Immunoblotting

For determination of SERCA2 and phospholamban in failing and nonfailing human myocardium, immunoblotting techniques were performed as described previously, with slight modifications.[23] SERCA2 and phospholamban were determined in crude membrane preparations from failing and nonfailing myocardium. To identify SERCA2, calsequestrin- and phospholamban-specific commercially available antibodies were used.[31,32]

Back-Phosphorylation

Resuspended membranes (Cardiac SR) were phosphorylated in a medium containing (in mmol/l): histidine/HCl 40, NaCl 100, $MgCl_2$ 10, NaF 15, EGTA 1, C-subunit of cAMP-protein kinase 0.5 * 10^{-3} µg and 43 µg of membrane protein in a final volume of 50 µl, pH 6.8. The samples were preincubated for 2 min at 30 °C. The reaction was initiated by adding 10 µl [γ-^{32}P] ATP 50 µmol/l (2.5×10^6 cpm) and allowed to proceed for 5 min. For termination, 25 µl of an ice-cold stop solution containing 1% SDS, 5% mercaptoethanol, 1 mM EDTA, 10 mM Tris-HCl (pH 8), and 20 µl SDS sample buffer. The samples were immediately boiled in a water bath for 5 min.

Electrophoretic separation was performed in duplicate in a urea/SDS gel system as described by Swank and Munkres,[33] using 12.5% (w/v) acrylamide gels for membrane fractions. Gels were stained with Coomassie Brilliant Blue and destained with methanol/acetic acid/water (3:1:6, by vol.). As molecular mass marker, the test mixture 7 from Biorad (Germany) was used. Autoradiography using X-ray–sensitive film and intensifying screens permitted the detection of ^{32}P-labeled proteins on the gels. The gels were inserted into a film cassette. Densitometric units of the signals were investigated by scanning the whole gel. The band densities were evaluated by densitometric scanning using a computerized imaging system (PDI). Each individual value reported represents the mean of two independent determinations. SERCA2 and PLB levels were normalized against total protein recovered from the myocardium.

Materials

Antibodies used were a monoclonal (mouse) anti-SERCA II-ATPase–IgG1 antibody (Dianova, Hamburg, Germany)[31] and antiphospholamban (mouse)–IgG1 (Biomol, Hamburg, Germany).[32] All other chemicals were of analytical grade or the best grade commercially available. For studies with isolated cardiac preparations, stock solutions were daily prepared in twice-distilled water.

Statistical Analysis

Data shown are mean values with SEM. For comparison within one group, the paired *t*-test was applied. Otherwise, statistical significance was analyzed with Student's *t*-test for unpaired observations or by ANOVA. A value of $p < 0.05$ was considered significant. The statistics was performed according to Wallenstein *et al.*[34]

RESULTS AND DISCUSSION

Protein levels of SERCA2, phospholamban, and calsequestrin, as detected with highly specific antibodies, were unchanged in failing human myocardial tissue compared to controls. Consistent with the results reported herein, Movsesian and coworkers found the immunodetectable levels of SERCA2, phospholamban, and calsequestrin unchanged in the left ventricular myocardium from heart failure patients (dilated cardiomyopathy) as compared to normal controls.[35–37] This contrasts with findings by Studer *et al.*[38] The Ca^{2+}-dependent Ca^{2+} uptake into the sarcoplasmic reticulum as well as the Ca^{2+}-ATPase activity were significantly reduced in crude membrane preparations from terminally failing myocardium compared with nonfailing controls.[23] This is in line with recent reports.[14] However, Movsesian and coworkers found no significant differences between normal hearts and excised failing hearts with respect to V_{max} of SR Ca^{2+} uptake in isolated vesicle preparations (homogenization and differential sedimentation).[36,37,39] Movsesian *et al.* used monoclonal antibodies, which mimic the effects of cAMP-dependent phospholamban phosphorylation, to study the capacity of Ca^{2+} uptake in human cardiac sarcoplasmic reticulum.[39] They observed similar cAMP-dependent phosphorylation and Ca^{2+} uptake in nonfailing and failing myocardium. These findings may be in line with the unchanged protein levels reported.

A decrease in Ca^{2+} uptake in the human failing heart has been also deduced from measurements of intracellular Ca^{2+} movements using intact muscle strip preparations from human failing myocardium.[40] The decreased SERCA2 activity has been shown to contribute to the altered contraction-coupling in failing human myocardium—i.e., altered relaxation and altered force-frequency relationship. FIGURE 1 gives an original tracing of the simultaneous measurements of the intracellular Ca^{2+} transient (fura 2 ratio method) and the twitch of contraction using isolated muscle strips from nonfailing human myocardium to demonstrate the effects of CPA on Ca^{2+} transients. Experiments were performed in the presence of 10 μmol/l and 30 μmol/l CPA as well as under control conditions. In the presence of CPA, the developed tension and the systolic light emission ($R_{340/380}$) were decreased concentration dependently compared to control. CPA increased the diastolic light emission at a concentration of 30 μmol/l. Thus, the activity of SERCA2 influences the contractile twitch and the intracellular Ca^{2+} transient, especially diastolic Ca^{2+} levels, in human myocardium. Beuckelmann and coworkers[15] observed the rate of Ca^{2+} uptake into the sarcoplasmic reticulum to be reduced in isolated myocytes from patients with severe heart failure. These findings may be an indication that the regulation of the SR Ca^{2+} uptake is altered in dilated cardiomyopathy. Therefore, it is not unreasonable to speculate that in the intact heart, differences in regulation of Ca^{2+} uptake into the sarcoplasmic reticulum and in Ca^{2+}-re-

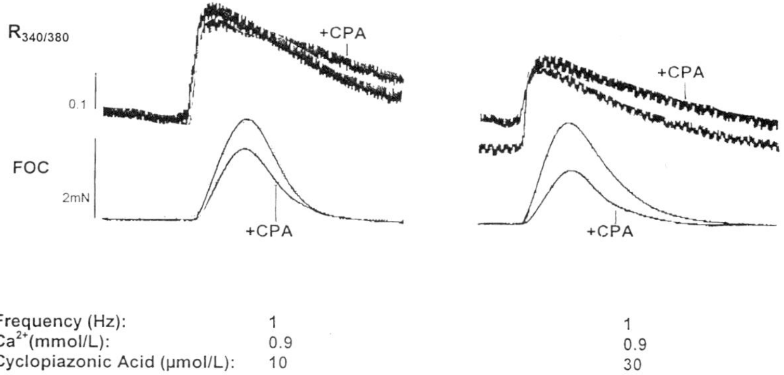

Frequency (Hz):	1	1
Ca^{2+}(mmol/L):	0.9	0.9
Cyclopiazonic Acid (μmol/L):	10	30

FIGURE 1. Original registration of the contractile twitch and the intracellular Ca^{2+} transient of human nonfailing myocardium measured by fura 2. CPA (10, 30 μmol/L) diminished developed tension and systolic light emission. CPA increased diastolic light emission significantly.

lease from the sarcoplasmic reticulum cause the alteration in intracellular Ca^{2+} handling observed by various investigators.

Ca^{2+} uptake is regulated by several factors. Phospholamban is normally a suppressor of the SERCA, but phosphorylation by cAMP-dependent protein kinase A (PKA) (of Ser16) or by Ca^{2+}/calmodulin (CaM)–dependent protein kinase (of Thr17) reverses this effect.[41] (FIG. 2). As the phosphorylation state, and not only the amount, of phospholamban determines activity of SR Ca^{2+}-ATPase, Ca^{2+} uptake–regulating proteins have to be studied functionally. The most likely explanation is a decrease in the phosphorylation of phospholamban in this tissue. As noted earlier, β-adrenergic receptor–mediated cAMP generation is impaired and cAMP levels are diminished in failing human myocardium.[42] A decrease in cAMP-activated phospholamban phosphorylation would result in decreased affinity (increased apparent K_m) for Ca^{2+} and decreased V_{max} of SERCA2 (FIG. 2). As consequences, Ca^{2+} sequestration would be slower and end-diastolic Ca^{2+} accumulation would be less complete, and these effects could contribute to the impaired relaxation, prolonged $[Ca^{2+}]_i$ transient, reduced contractility, and altered force-frequency relationship characteristic of failing human myocardium. This is supported by the finding that in crude membrane preparations the sensitivity towards Ca^{2+} was significantly higher in nonfailing compared to failing myocardium. After preincubation with increasing concentrations of PKA (5–15 μg/ml) the concentration-response curve for Ca^{2+} was shifted significantly to the left for both nonfailing and failing human myocardium, as indicated by reduced EC_{50} (FIG. 3); but the leftward shift was more pronounced in the failing myocardium. However, there was still a significant difference between the V_{max} in failing and nonfailing myocardium. In purified Ca^{2+}-ATPase from canine cardiac sarcoplasmic reticulum co-reconstitution with phospholamban suppressed both Ca^{2+} uptake and Ca^{2+}-ATPase activity. This suppression was fully relieved by a phospholamban monoclonal antibody or by phosphorylation either with cAMP-dependent protein kinase or with Ca^{2+}/calmodulin-dependent protein kinase. This effect is consistent with a change in the Ca^{2+} affinity of the SERCA2 and not with a change in V_{max}.[43] The rate of Ca^{2+} accumulation as a measure of SERCA2 activity was stimulated in proportion with the stoichiometry of phospholamban phosphorylation, irrespective of whether phosphorylation was on Ser16 or Thr17.[41] However, the V_{max} of

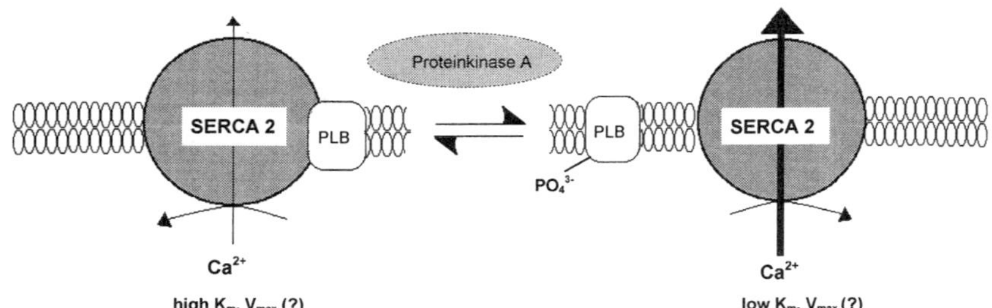

FIGURE 2. SERCA2 activity is regulated by phospholamban. When unphosphorylated, phospholamban binds to SERCA2, raising K_m and possibly lowering V_{max}. Phosphorylation of phospholamban inhibits this interaction and relieves this inhibition.

the SERCA2 may be not altered by phospholamban phosphorylation.[44] In addition, binding of antiphospholamban antibody in human cardiac sarcoplasmic reticulum reduced the K_D of the SERCA2, without affecting V_{max} or n_{Hill}.[35] It has been suggested that the V_{max} is increased via direct phosphorylation of the SERCA2 by a Ca^{2+}/-calmodulin-dependent protein kinase.[45] However, this has yet to be proved in human myocardium.

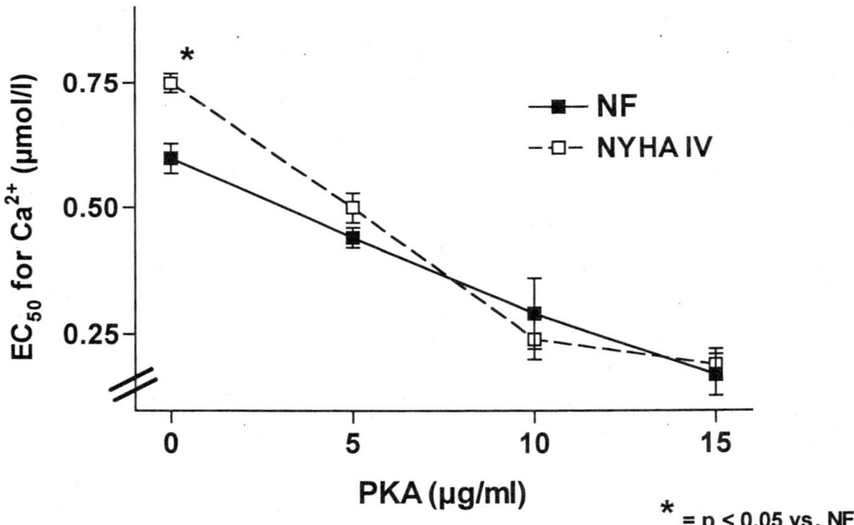

FIGURE 3. Effect of PKA-dependent stimulation on the Ca^{2+} sensitivity of SERCA2 in human failing and nonfailing myocardium. The Ca^{2+} sensitivity of SERCA2 was significantly higher in nonfailing compared to failing myocardium under control conditions. PKA-dependent stimulation reduced the EC_{50} in a concentration-dependent manner in both failing and nonfailing human myocardium.

In both failing and nonfailing human myocardium the Ca^{2+} sensitivity of SERCA2 was increased via cAMP-dependent PKA stimulation in a concentration-dependent manner. These findings provide evidence that stimulation of SR Ca^{2+}-ATPase, mediated by cAMP-dependent phosphorylation of phospholamban, increases the sensitivity of SERCA2 towards Ca^{2+} (FIG. 2). Consistently, the phosphorylation status of phospholamban was higher in nonfailing compared to dilated cardiomyopathic hearts. To study the phosphorylation state of phospholamban the ^{32}P incorporation to phospholamban was measured using a back-phosphorylation technique, as described by Karczewski and coworkers.[46] The PKA-dependent incorporation of ^{32}P to PLB was significantly higher in failing compared to nonfailing myocardium, indicating reduced PLB phosphorylation in left ventricular myocardial tissue of patients suffering from dilated cardiomyopathy (49.7% of nonfailing). FIGURE 4 gives original blots (upper panel) and the amount of ^{32}P incorporation to PLB of nonfailing and failing human myocardium (lower panel). In addition, as measured with specific antibodies against Ser16-P-phospholamban or Thr17-P-phospholamban, the phosphorylation status at both Ser-16-PLB and Thr-17-PLB were significantly reduced in dilated cardiomyopathy.

A paradigm for pathological changes in the abundance and regulation of SERCA2 can be found in the effect of thyroxin on sarcoplasmic reticulum function: chronic exposure to thyroxin increases the level of SERCA2 and decreases the level of phospholamban in cardiac sarcoplasmic reticulum.[47] This combination of effects can explain the

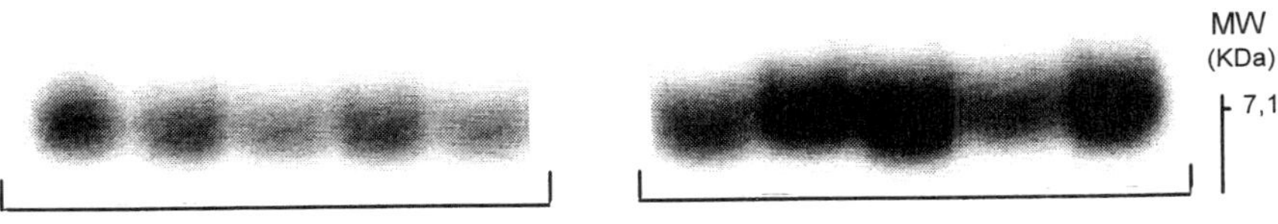

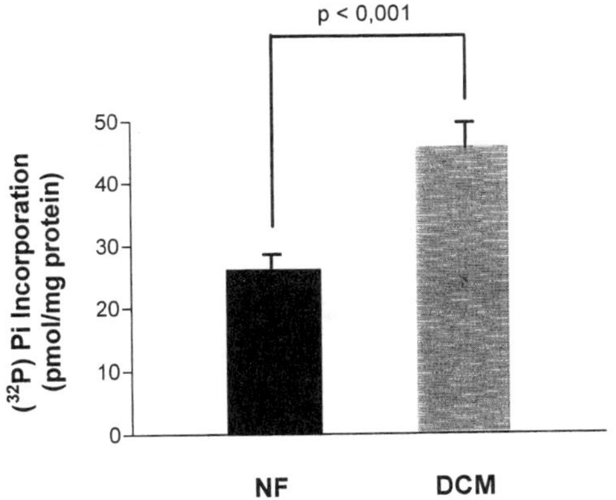

FIGURE 4. 32P incorporation in phospholamban on sarcoplasmic reticulum from human nonfailing (NF) and failing (DCM, dilated cardiomyopathy) myocardium. Phosphor incorporation was significantly lower in nonfailing compared to failing human myocardium.

increase in the basal rate of ATP-dependent Ca^{2+} sequestration in sarcoplasmic reticulum–enriched microsomes isolated from the hearts of hyperthyroid animals as well as the decreased stimulation of Ca^{2+} sequestration by cAMP-dependent protein phosphorylation (and the converse findings in preparations from hypothyroid animals).[48]

The reduced phosphorylation status in terminally failing human myocardium may largely influence the Ca^{2+}-dependent activation of SERCA2. A reduced sensitivity may lead, especially at lower-end diastolic Ca^{2+} concentrations, to slowed Ca^{2+} uptake into the SR and may thereby prolong the contractile twitch. Therefore, reduced cAMP levels in human heart failure could contribute to a decrease in the phosphorylation state of phospholamban and to altered intracellular Ca^{2+} handling as well. The observations that compounds that increase cAMP generation in cardiac myocytes may reverse a negative force-frequency relationship, presumably by increasing phospholamban phosphorylation and thereby stimulating SERCA2 activity;[12] and that specific inhibition of SERCA2 in normal human myocardium converts the positive force-frequency relationship to a negative one and reduces the maximal amplitude of the Ca^{2+} transient (and increases diastolic Ca^{2+}),[25] support this hypothesis. As a result of β-adrenergic receptor down-regulation, increased activity of β-adrenergic receptor kinase, and increased activity of G_i, cAMP generation is impaired, and cAMP levels are reduced in failing human myocardium.[42] In view of the importance of cAMP-dependent phosphorylation of phospholamban and the consequent de-inhibition of SERCA2 activity in normal myocardium, alterations in SERCA2 function and its regulation by phospholamban phosphorylation would be expected to contribute to the molecular pathophysiology of heart failure. However, it is important to point out that the possible contribution of phosphorylation or the lack of other protein kinases has not been explored in this study. In addition, the enhanced activity of phosphatases in human failing myocardium[49] may contribute to the lowered phospholamban phosphorylation and the decreased responsiveness to inotropic agents as well.

In summary, despite unchanged protein levels for SERCA2 and phospholamban in failing and nonfailing human myocardium, SERCA2 activity is reduced in diseased hearts due to altered regulation. In addition to the reduced phospholamban-dependent activation of SERCA2, other regulatory sites may lead to altered SERCA2 activity in failing myocardium as well—e.g., reduced phosphorylation by Ca^{2+}/calmodulin-dependent protein kinase. To elucidate the subcellular mechanisms for altered intracellular Ca^{2+} handling, further studies are required that focus on intracellular regulatory mechanisms.

REFERENCES

1. Movsesian, M. A. *et al.* 1990. Identification and characterization of proteins in sarcoplasmic reticulum from normal and failing human left ventricles. J. Mol. Cell. Cardiol. **22:** 1477–1485.
2. Bassani, J. W. M. *et al.* 1994. Relaxation in rabbit and rat cardiac cells: Species-dependent differences in cellular mechanisms. J. Physiol. **476:** 279–293.
3. Jones, L. R. *et al.* 1985. Purification and characterization of phospholamban from canine cardiac sarcoplasmic reticulum. J. Biol. Chem. **260:** 7721–7730.
4. Sasaki, T. *et al.* 1992. Molecular mechanism of regulation of Ca^{2+} pump ATPase by phospholamban in cardiac sarcoplasmic reticulum. Effects of synthetic phospholamban peptides on Ca^{2+} pump ATPase. J. Biol. Chem. **267:** 1674–1679.
5. Davis, B. A. *et al.* 1983. Regulation of cardiac sarcoplasmic reticulum calcium transport by calcium-calmodulin–dependent phosphorylation. J. Biol. Chem. **258:** 13587–13591.
6. Limas, C. J. 1980. Phosphorylation of cardiac sarcoplasmic reticulum by a calcium-activated, phospholipid-dependent protein kinase. Biochem. Biophys. Res. Commun. **96:** 1378–1383.
7. Tada, M. *et al.* 1979. Mechanism of the stimulation of Ca^{2+}-dependent ATPase of cardiac

sarcoplasmic reticulum by adenosine 3′:5′-monophosphate–dependent protein kinase. J. Biol. Chem. **254:** 319–326.

8. Movsesian, M. A. *et al.* 1984. Phosphorylation of phospholamban by calcium-activated, phospholipid-dependent protein kinase. J. Biol. Chem. **259:** 8029–8032.
9. Luo, W. *et al.* 1994. Targeted ablation of the phospholamban gene is associated with markedly enhanced myocardial contractility and loss of β-agonist stimulation. Circ. Res. **75:** 401–409.
10. Schwinger, R. H. G. *et al.* 1992. Inotropic and lusitropic dysfunction in myocardium from patients with dilated cardiomyopathy. Am. Heart J. **123:** 116–128.
11. Mulieri, L. A. *et al.* 1992. Altered myocardial force-frequency relation in human heart failure. Circulation **85:** 1743–1750.
12. Schwinger, R. H. G. *et al.* 1993. Effect of inotropic stimulation on the negative force-frequency–relationship in the failing human heart. Circulation **88:** 2267–2276.
13. Feldman, M. D. *et al.* 1988. Depression of systolic and diastolic myocardial reserve during atrial pacing tachycardia in patients with dilated cardiomyopathy. J. Clin. Invest. **82:** 1661–1669.
14. Hasenfuss, G. *et al.* 1994. Relation between myocardial function and expression of sarcoplasmic reticulum Ca^{2+}-ATPase in failing and nonfailing human myocardium. Circ. Res. **75:** 434–442.
15. Beuckelmann, D. J. *et al.* 1992. Intracellular calcium handling in isolated ventricular myocytes from patients with terminal heart failure. Circulation **85:** 1046–1055.
16. Gwathmey, J. K. 1990. Role of intracellular calcium handling in force-interval relationships of human ventricular myocardium. J. Clin. Invest. **85:** 1599–1613.
17. Takahashi, S. *et al.* 1995. Effects of cyclopiazonic acid on rat myocardium: Inhibition of calcium uptake into sarcoplasmic reticulum. J. Pharmacol. Exp. Ther. **272:** 1095–1100.
18. Bonnet, V. *et al.* 1994. Potentiation of the twitch responses by inhibitors of sarcoplasmic reticulum Ca^{2+}-ATPase in frog atrial fibres. Eur. J. Pharmacol. **264:** 69–76.
19. Yard, N. J. *et al.* 1994. Effect of cyclopiazonic acid, an inhibitor of sarcoplasmic reticulum Ca^{2+}-ATPase, on the frequency-dependence of the contraction-relaxation cycle of the guinea-pig isolated atrium. Br. J. Pharmacol. **113:** 1001–1007.
20. Grynkiewicz, G. M. *et al.* 1985. A new generation of Ca^{2+} indicators with greatly improved fluorescence properties. J. Biol. Chem. **260:** 3440–3450.
21. Backx, P. H. *et al.* 1995. The relationship between contractile force and intracellular $[Ca^{2+}]$ in intact rat cardiac trabeculae. J. Gen. Physiol. **1:** 1–19.
22. Brixius, K. *et al.* 1997. Effect of inotropic interventions on contraction and Ca^{2+}-transients in the human heart. J. Appl. Physiol. **83:** 652–660.
23. Schwinger, R. H. G. *et al.* 1995. Unchanged protein levels of SERCA II and phospholamban but reduced Ca^{2+}-uptake and Ca^{2+}-ATPase activity of cardiac sarcoplasmic reticulum from patients with dilated cardiomyopathy compared with nonfailing patients. Circulation **92:** 3220–3228.
24. Limas, C. J. *et al.* 1987. Calcium uptake by sarcoplasmic reticulum. Cardiovasc. Res. **21:** 601–605.
25. Schwinger, R. H. G. *et al.* 1997. Effect of CPA on the force-frequency–relationship in human myocardium. J. Pharmacol. Exp. Ther. **283:** 286–292.
26. Meissner, G. & J. S. Henderson. 1987. Rapid calcium release from cardiac sarcoplasmic reticulum vesicles is dependent on Ca^{2+} and is modulated by Mg^{2+}, adenine nucleotide, and calmodulin. J. Biol. Chem. **262:** 3065–3073.
27. Sitsapesan, R. & A. J. Williams. 1990. Mechanisms of caffeine activation of single calcium-release channels of sheep cardiac sarcoplasmic reticulum. J. Physiol. (Lond.) **423:** 425–439.
28. Lowry, O. H. *et al.* 1951. Protein measurements with the folin phenol reagent. J. Biol. Chem. **193:** 265–275.
29. Chu, A. *et al.* 1988. Isolation of sarcoplasmic reticulum fractions referable to longitudinal tubules and junctional terminal cisternae from rabbit skeletal muscle. Methods Enzymol. **157:** 36–46.
30. Lindemann, J. P. *et al.* 1983. β-adrenergic stimulation of phospholamban phosphorylation and Ca^{2+}-ATPase activity in guinea pig ventricles. J. Biol. Chem. **258:** 464–471.

31. JORGENSEN, A. O. *et al.* 1988. A monoclonal antibody to the Ca-ATPase of cardiac sarcoplasmic reticulum cross-reacts with slow type I but not with fast type II canine skeletal muscle fibers: An immunocytochemical and immunochemical study. Cell Motil. Cytoskeleton **9:** 164–174.
32. SUZUKI, T. & J. H. WANG. 1986. Stimulation of bovine cardiac sarcoplasmic reticulum Ca^{2+}-pump and blocking of phospholamban phosphorylation and dephosphorylation by a phospholamban monoclonal antibody. J. Biol. Chem. **261:** 7018–7023.
33. SWANK, R. T. & K. D. MUNKERS. 1971. Molecular weight analysis of oligopeptides by electrophoresis in polyacrylamide gel with sodium dodecyl sulfate. Anal. Biochem. **39:** 462–477.
34. WALLENSTEIN, S. *et al.* 1980. Some statistical methods useful in circulation research. Circ. Res. **47:** 1–9.
35. MOVSESIAN, M. A. *et al.* 1989. Calcium uptake by cardiac sarcoplasmic reticulum from patients with idiopathic dilated cardiomyopathy. Circ. Res. **65:** 1141–1144.
36. MOVSESIAN, M. A. *et al.* 1990. Identification and characterization of proteins in sarcoplasmic reticulum from normal and failing human left ventricles. J. Mol. Cell. Cardiol. **22:** 1477–1485.
37. MOVSESIAN, M. A. *et al.* 1994. Ca^{2+}-transporting ATPase, phospholamban, and calsequestrin levels in nonfailing and failing human myocardium. Circulation **90:** 653–657.
38. STUDER, R. *et al.* 1994. Gene expression of the cardiac Na^{+}-Ca^{2+} exchanger in end-stage human heart failure. Circ. Res. **75:** 443–453.
39. MOVSESIAN, M. *et al.* 1990. Phospholamban-mediated stimulation of Ca^{2+} uptake in sarcoplasmic reticulum from normal and failing hearts. J. Clin Invest. **85:** 1698–1702.
40. GWATHMEY, J. K. *et al.* 1987. Abnormal intracellular calcium handling in myocardium from patients with endstage heart failure. Circ. Res. **61:** 70–76.
41. JACKSON, W. A. & J. COYLER. 1996. Translation of SER16 and Thr17 phosphorylation of phospholamban into Ca^{2+}-pump stimulation. Biochem. J. **316:** 201–207.
42. BRISTOW, M. R. *et al.* 1986. β_1- and β_2-adrenergic-receptor subpopulations in nonfailing and failing human ventricular myocardium: Coupling of both receptor subtypes to muscle contraction and selective β_1-receptor down-regulation in heart failure. Circ. Res. **59:** 297–309.
43. REDDY, L. G. *et al.* 1996. Purified, reconstituted cardiac Ca^{2+}-ATPase is regulated by phospholamban but not by direct phosphorylation with Ca^{2+}/calmodulin dependent protein kinase. J. Biol. Chem. **271:** 14964–14970.
44. ODERMATT, A. *et al.* 1996. The V_{max} of the Ca^{2+}-ATPase of cardiac sarcoplasmic reticulum (SERCA2a) is not altered by Ca^{2+}-calmodulin–dependent phosphorylation or by interaction with phospholamban. J. Biol. Chem. **271:** 14206–14213.
45. XU, A. *et al.* 1993. Phosphorylation and activation of the Ca^{2+}-pumping ATPase of cardiac sarcoplasmic reticulum by Ca^{2+}/calmodulin-dependent protein kinase. J. Biol. Chem. **268:** 8394–8397.
46. KARCZEWSKI, P. *et al.* 1990. Differential sensitivity to isoprenaline of troponin I and phospholamban phosphorylation in isolated rat hearts. Biochem. J. **266:** 115–122.
47. BEEKMAN, R. E. *et al.* 1989. On the mechanism of the reduction by thyroid hormone of β-adrenergic relaxation rate stimulation in rat heart. Biochem. J. **259:** 229–236.
48. SUKO, J. 1971. Alterations of Ca^{2+} uptake and Ca^{2+}-activated ATPase of cardiac sarcoplasmic reticulum in hyper- and hypothyroidism. Biochim. Biophys. Acta **252:** 324–327.
49. NEUMANN, J. *et al.* 1997. Increased expression of cardiac phosphatases in patients with end-stage heart failure. J. Mol. Cell. Cardiol. **29:** 265–272.

Sarco(endo)plasmic Reticulum Ca^{2+} ATPase Isoforms and Their Role in Muscle Physiology and Pathology

EVGENY LOUKIANOV, YONG JI, DEBRA L. BAKER, THOMAS REED, JEGADEESH BABU, TANYA LOUKIANOVA, ADAM GREENE, GARY SHULL, AND MUTHU PERIASAMY[a]

Laboratory of Molecular Cardiology, University of Cincinnati College of Medicine, Cincinnati, Ohio 45267, USA

ABSTRACT: Recent studies suggest that SR Ca^{2+} transport function is altered in hypertrophied and failing myocardium. To understand whether alterations in SR Ca^{2+} ATPase levels affect myocardial contractility, we generated transgenic mice that specifically overexpress SERCA2a or SERCA1 pump in the mouse heart, using the cardiac α-MHC promoter. Analysis of SERCA2a transgenic mice show both an increase in mRNA and protein levels (120–150% of the wild type). Isolated work performing heart preparations revealed that SERCA2a mice have improved myocardial performance. On the other hand, SERCA1 overexpression in the heart resulted in isoform replacement without any change in total SERCA protein. Interestingly, SERCA1 transgenic hearts exhibited super contractility with a significant increase in rates of muscle contraction (+dp/dt) and relaxation (–dp/dT). The time to peak pressure and half-time to relaxation were significantly shorter.

Sarcoplasmic reticulum (SR) is a specialized Ca^{2+} storage membrane system in muscle cells and plays a central role in the contractile function of the muscle by virtue of its ability to regulate intracellular Ca^{2+} concentration.[1,2] Ca^{2+} release from the SR initiates muscle contraction, whereas Ca^{2+} reuptake into the SR membrane vesicle lowers cytosolic calcium, causing muscle relaxation. The events that regulate Ca^{2+} release and removal can affect cytosolic calcium levels and, hence, the rate and extent of muscle contraction and relaxation. The Ca^{2+} reuptake function of the SR is primarily regulated by a Ca^{2+} transport pump, the sarco(endo)plasmic reticulum Ca^{2+} ATPase (SERCA). The SERCA pump is a transmembrane protein of approximately 110 kDa and is expressed at high levels in cardiac, skeletal, and smooth muscle cells.[3]

SR Ca^{2+} ATPase ISOFORMS AND THEIR EXPRESSION PATTERN

Molecular cloning analyses revealed that the SERCA protein isoforms are encoded by a highly conserved family of genes, SERCA1, 2, and 3[4] (TABLE 1). The SERCA1

[a] Address for correspondence: Muthu Periasamy, Ph.D., Director of Molecular Cardiology, University of Cincinnati College of Medicine, 231 Bethesda Avenue, ML0542, Cincinnati, Ohio 45267-0542. Phone: 513-558-3080; fax: 513-558-2002; e-mail: muthu.periasamy@uc.edu

TABLE 1. Protein Isoforms Encoded by and Expression of SERCA1, 2, and 3 Genes

Gene	Isoforms	Tissue Distribution
SERCA1	SERCA1a (8 unique amino acids)	Adult fast-twitch skeletal muscle
	SERCA1b (1 unique amino acid)	Fetal fast-twitch skeletal muscle
SERCA2	SERCA2a (4 unique amino acids)	Cardiac, slow-twitch, and smooth muscle
	SERCA2b (49 unique amino acids)	Ubiquitous, high in smooth muscle
SERCA3	SERCA3a (6 unique amino acids)	Lymphocytes, platelets, epithelial and endothelial cells
	SERCA3b (45 unique amino acids)	

gene encodes two alternatively spliced transcripts, SERCA1a and SERCA1b. SERCA1 proteins are exclusively expressed in the fast-twitch skeletal muscle,[5,6] and differ at the carboxyl end (SERCA1a has eight unique amino acids, whereas SERCA1b has one unique amino acid). SERCA1b is predominantly expressed during the fetal/neonatal stages and represents ~70% of fast-twitch Ca^{2+} ATPase prior to birth. It is gradually replaced by the SERCA1a isoform so that in the adult SERCA1a is the major isoform present in fast-twitch muscle. The SERCA2 gene encodes SERCA2a and SERCA2b isoforms, which differ in the carboxyl terminus (SERCA2a has four unique amino acids, SERCA2b has 49 unique amino acids). SERCA2a is the primary isoform expressed in the atria and ventricle of the heart, and its expression level gradually increases from fetal to adult stage.[7,8] SERCA2a is also expressed abundantly in fetal fast-twitch skeletal muscle and in developing slow-twitch skeletal muscle. However, in adult fast-twitch muscle, it is gradually replaced by SERCA1a isoform postnatally, whereas in slow-twitch muscle SERCA2a continues to be expressed.[5] The SERCA2b isoform is expressed in most cell types, but at high levels in smooth muscle tissues.[9] The SERCA3 gene also encodes two isoforms, SERCA3a and SERCA3b, which are expressed in specialized cell types such as platelets, lymphocytes, and in endothelial and epithelial cells[10] (L. Liu, personal communication).

In adult fast-twitch skeletal muscle SR the SERCA1a isoform is expressed at a three- to fivefold higher level than SERCA2a pump levels in slow-twitch or cardiac muscle SR.[11,12] This difference in pump density may partly account for the different Ca^{2+} uptake capacities of fast- and slow-twitch muscle.[13–15] It has been shown that changes in physiological conditions (and hence changes in necessity for SR Ca^{2+} storage) produce fast-to-slow or slow-to-fast shifts in the SERCA isoform expression in skeletal muscles.[16–18] Fast-twitch fibers can be converted into slowly contracting fibers by chronic low-frequency electrical stimulation.[16] Muscle treated in this way exhibits a switch in Ca^{2+}-ATPase isoform expression from the fast-twitch SERCA1a type to the slow-twitch/cardiac SERCA2a type.[17,18] This is accompanied by slower SR Ca^{2+} uptake and ATPase activity. On the other hand chronically reduced loading of slow-twitch skeletal muscle induces expression of fast SERCA1 mRNA and protein to levels up to half of that reported in control fast-twitch muscle.[19] These studies suggest that differential expression of SERCA isoforms may provide for unique functional properties of different muscles.

REGULATION OF SR Ca^{2+} ATPase EXPRESSION IN CARDIAC HYPERTROPHY AND CONGESTIVE HEART FAILURE

Studies from our laboratory and others have shown that the SR Ca^{2+} ATPase pump level is significantly altered during cardiac adaptation to pressure overload and changes in thyroid hormone level.[20–26] However, there is no switch in the SERCA isoforms during cardiac adaptation to different pathophysiological states. Thyroxine administration in rats and rabbits is associated with increased rates of tension development and enhanced velocity of fiber shortening. The rates of Ca^{2+} uptake and Ca^{2+}-dependent ATP-hydrolysis were increased in hyperthyroid hearts but decreased in hypothyroid hearts.[23] Furthermore, thyroid hormone markedly increases both SR Ca^{2+} ATPase mRNA and protein levels, suggesting that changes in gene expression are primarily responsible for altered SR Ca^{2+} transport function.[20,21,24] Similarly, studies in primate models (baboons) showed that thyroid hormone administration increases SR Ca^{2+} ATPase level and enhances myocardial function.[25,26] On the other hand, chronic pressure overload–induced hypertrophy is associated with decreased SR calcium transport function and levels of SR Ca^{2+} ATPase mRNA and protein.[20,22] Using a guinea pig model, Kiss *et al.*[27] demonstrated that SR Ca^{2+} ATPase protein level was unaltered in hearts with compensated pressure overload hypertrophy, but were reduced significantly in animals with contractile depression and resultant pulmonary congestion. This study indicated that alterations in SR Ca^{2+} ATPase level may be an important determinant of the transition from compensated pressure-overload hypertrophy to congestive heart failure.

Several studies on human hearts also suggest that SR Ca^{2+} transport function is decreased in end-stage heart failure.[28,29] Intracellular Ca^{2+} measurements using Fura-2 showed that Ca^{2+} transients in muscle samples from failing human hearts were markedly prolonged in both Ca^{2+} release and uptake phases.[28,29] Using tissue samples from failing human hearts, we and others have found that the expression level of SR Ca^{2+} ATPase was decreased both at the mRNA[30–33] and the protein levels[34] in end-stage heart failure. The decrease in the levels of SR Ca^{2+} ATPase can be closely correlated with decreased myocardial function.[34] Despite reports to the contrary by some studies,[35,36] the balance of the available data suggest that alterations in SR Ca^{2+} uptake function observed in different models of cardiac hypertrophy and failure can be attributed to changes in the number of Ca^{2+} pump sites.

FUNCTIONAL PROPERTIES OF SERCA ISOFORMS

In recent years the properties of SERCA isoforms have been studied using COS and HEK-293 cell expression systems. These *in vitro* studies revealed that the quantitative properties of SERCA1a, SERCA1b, and SERCA2a when expressed in COS or HEK-293 cells were similar[14,37–41] On the other hand, SERCA2b showed twofold higher Ca^{2+} affinity, twofold lower turnover rates for Ca^{2+} uptake and ATP hydrolysis, and 10-fold lower vanadate sensitivity than SERCA2a.[14,42] SERCA3 displayed a reduced apparent affinity for Ca^{2+}, an increased apparent affinity for vanadate, and an altered pH dependence when compared with other isoforms. These properties of SERCA3 are consistent with an enzyme in which the equilibrium between the E_1 and E_2 conformations is shifted toward the E_2 state.[14] When expressed in COS, HEK-293, or insect cells, the SERCA pump density achieved in microsomes was ~20 times lower compared to cardiac SR[14,15,37–42]; and often a significant fraction of recombinant Ca^{2+} pumps were inactive,[40,42] which may have lead to the loss of pump-pump interaction.[43] These *in vitro* studies should be carefully interpreted, because the nonmuscle cells provide different lipid and protein environments and do not contain natural regulators that are present in cardiac or skeletal muscle SR.[14] Although SERCA1a and SERCA2a isoforms show similar properties when expressed in nonmuscle cells, studies with isolated native SR from cardiac and skeletal muscle reveal that SERCA1a and SERCA2a have different pharmacological properties and diverse response to acidosis.[44,45]

Studies conducted on SR isolated from cardiac and skeletal muscle reveal that the apparent affinity of cardiac SR Ca^{2+} ATPase (SERCA2a) for Ca^{2+} is substantially lower than that of fast-twitch skeletal muscle Ca^{2+} ATPase (SERCA1a) due to the interaction with phospholamban (PLN), a phosphoprotein expressed primarily in cardiac, slow-twitch, and smooth muscle.[14,39,41,46] Unphosphorylated PLN interacts with SERCA2a and decreases its affinity for Ca^{2+}. Phosphorylation of PLN by cAMP-dependent protein kinase in response to β-adrenergic receptor stimulation can displace PLN from the SR Ca^{2+} ATPase and relieve this inhibition.[47]

In vitro experiments suggest that PLN can also interact with other SERCA isoforms. Cross-linking experiments revealed a putative PLN-binding domain that is present in both SERCA1a and SERCA2a.[48–51] Coexpression of PLN with SERCA1a or SERCA2a in HEK-293 cells inhibited Ca^{2+} transport function by lowering the apparent affinity for Ca^{2+}.[39,41,48] Similarly, stable expression of phospholamban in the C_2C_{12} fast-twitch skeletal muscle cell line revealed that SERCA1a can be inhibited by phospholamban.[50] Ectopic expression of phospholamban in mouse fast-twitch skeletal muscle was associated with a decrease in the affinity of SERCA1a for calcium and decreased relaxation rates of the muscle.[52] So the regulation of SERCA by phospholamban is not an inherent property of the cardiac isoform, but rather a consequence of tissue-specific expression of phospholamban.

The role of phospholamban in the heart has been extensively studied using transgenic mouse models. Mice deficient in phospholamban exhibited enhanced myocardial performance associated with an increase in the SERCA2a affinity for Ca^{2+}.[53] Overexpression of phospholamban in the heart resulted in a decrease in SR Ca^{2+} uptake function and depression of cardiac contractile function *in vivo*.[54] These studies suggested that a shift in PLN:SERCA ratio results in a corresponding shift in SERCA affinity for Ca^{2+}, so that an increase in PLN:SERCA ratio leads to decreased Ca^{2+} affinity. However, it should be noted that this conclusion was based on the changes in PLN level only. Further experiments, where the PLN:SERCA ratio is altered by changing SERCA protein level, will clarify the relevance of this parameter.

Recently cDNA encoding sarcolipin (SLN), a low-molecular-weight protein that copurifies with SERCA1, was cloned.[55] SLN mRNA is expressed at high level in fast-twitch skeletal muscle, but at lower level in slow-twitch and cardiac muscle. SLN is homologous to PLN, and it may play an important role in the regulation of SR Ca^{2+} ATPase activity; but the nature of this regulation is not understood at this time

TRANSGENIC ALTERATIONS OF SR Ca^{2+} ATPase EXPRESSION LEVELS

Recent advances in transgenic mouse technology have made it possible to address the significance of SERCA pump isoforms and the physiological relevance of increases or decreases in pump expression. Two major strategies have been used: overexpression or disruption (knockout) of the SERCA genes, as described below.

SERCA2a isoform was overexpressed in the mouse heart, using a hCMV(enhancer)-driven β-actin promoter.[56] This resulted in a 2.6-fold increase in the SERCA2a mRNA level, but in only a 1.2-fold increase in SERCA2a protein. Isolated adult cardiac myocytes obtained from the transgenic mice revealed accelerated calcium transients and significantly faster rates of myocyte shortening and relengthening. In isolated papillary muscle from SERCA2a transgenic mice, the time to half-maximum postrest potentiation was significantly shorter than in nontransgenic littermates. Cardiac function measured *in vivo,* demonstrated significantly accelerated contraction and relaxation in SERCA2a transgenic mice.

To understand the role of SERCA pumps, we have also generated transgenic mouse models that overexpress either SERCA2a or SERCA1a isoform. In our study, we have used the cardiac αMHC promoter to target expression only in the heart muscle. SERCA2a overexpression produced a 4-to 8-fold increase in mRNA level in two independent transgenic (TG) lines; whereas SERCA2a protein level was increased 30% to 50% in transgenic hearts.[57] SERCA2a transgenic hearts demonstrated increased rates of Ca^{2+} uptake and increased myocardial performance, which were proportional to the SERCA2a pump expression levels. On the other hand, ectopic expression of SERCA1a in mouse hearts resulted in a ~2.5-fold increase in the level of total SERCA protein. Interestingly, the level of endogenous SERCA2a pump was decreased to 50% in the transgenic hearts. As a result, the TG hearts contained 80% of SERCA1a, and 20% of SERCA2a. The maximal velocity of Ca^{2+} uptake (V_{max}) and the steady state level of SERCA phosphoenzyme intermediate were considerably higher in SERCA1a TG hearts. Functional analysis of SERCA1a TG hearts revealed that the rates of contraction and relaxation were significantly higher. These findings clearly demonstrate that SERCA overexpression in mammalian heart is associated with significant increases in the cardiac contractile parameters suggesting that SERCA pump level is a critical determinant of myocardial contractility.

The function of SERCA3 isoform is not precisely understood. However, its restricted expression in epithelial and endothelial cells and platelets suggests that it may have unique functional roles in cell signaling. Liu *et al.* have recently mutated the SERCA3 gene in mice.[58] Homozygous mutant mice were viable and fertile, and did not exhibit an overt phenotype. However, acetylcholine-induced endothelium-dependent relaxation of aortas was significantly reduced in mutants. The acetylcholine-induced intracellular Ca^{2+} signal was sharply diminished in SERCA3-deficient cells, and replenishment of acetylcholine-responsive Ca^{2+} stores was severely impaired. These results indicate that SERCA3 plays a critical role in Ca^{2+} signaling events involved in the relaxation of vascular smooth muscle.

PERSPECTIVES AND CONCLUSIONS

Although significant progress has been made towards understanding the enzymatic properties of SR Ca^{2+} ATPase and their role in muscle physiology, there are several important questions that remain to be addressed. What is the functional relevance of each SERCA isoform? Is fast-twitch skeletal muscle isoform SERCA1a functionally distinct from cardiac SERCA2a? Is the PLN:SERCA ratio a true determinant of SERCA affinity for Ca^{2+}? What is the regulatory role of sarcolipin? Are there other modulators of SERCA that remain to be identified? What is the role of SERCA in cardiac pathophysiology? A better understanding of the intrinsic properties of different SERCA isoforms and their regulation by the different modulators will be critical for muscle physiology. This will also enable us to generate new sets of recombinant proteins with improved characteristics for treating disorders of abnormal Ca^{2+} handling/transport using SERCA gene therapy.

REFERENCES

1. SOMMER, J. R. & R. B. JENNINGS. 1992. Ultrastructure of the cardiac muscle. *In* The Heart and Cardiovascular System. H. A. Fozzard, E. Haber, R. B. Jennings, A. M. Katz & H. E. Morgan, Eds.: 3–50. Raven Press. New York.
2. LYTTON, J. & D. H. MACLENNAN. 1992. Sarcoplasmic reticulum. *In* The Heart and Cardiovascular System. H. A. FOZZARD, E. HABER, R. B. JENNINGS, A. M. KATZ & H. E. MORGAN. Eds.: 1203–1222. Raven Press. New York.
3. MACLENNAN, D. H. 1970. Purification and properties of an adenosine triphosphate sarcoplasmic reticulum. J. Biol. Chem. **245:** 4508–4518.
4. ARAI, M., H. MATSUI & M. PERIASAMY. 1994. Sarcoplasmic reticulum gene expression in cardiac hypertrophy and heart failure. Circ. Res. **74:** 555–564.
5. BRANDL, C. J., S. DELEON, D. R. MARTIN & D. H. MACLENNAN. 1987. Adult forms of Ca^{2+}-ATPase of sarcoplasmic reticulum expression in developing skeletal muscle. J. Biol. Chem. **262:** 3768–3774.
6. BRANDL, C. J. N. M. GREEN, B. KORCZAK & D. H. MACLENNAN. 1986. Two Ca^{2+} ATPase genes: Homologies and mechanistic implications of deduced amino acid sequences. Cell **44:** 597–607.
7. MACLENNAN D. H., C. J. BRANDL, B. KORCZAK & N. M. GREEN. 1985. Amino-acid sequence of a $Ca^{2+}Mg^{2+}$-dependent ATPase from rabbit muscle sarcoplasmic reticulum, deduced from its complementary DNA sequence. Nature **316:** 696–700.
8. ZARAIN-HERZBERG, A., D. H. MACLANNAN & M. PERIASAMY. 1990. Characterization of rabbit cardiac sarco(endo)plasmic reticulum Ca^{2+} ATPase gene. J. Biol. Chem. **265:** 4670–4677.
9. LYTTON, J., A. ZARAIN-HERZBERG, M. PERIASAMY & D. H. MACLENNAN. 1989. Molecular cloning of the mammalian smooth muscle sarco(endo)plasmic reticulum Ca^{2+} ATPase. J. Biol. Chem. **264:** 7059–7065.
10. WUYTACK, F., L. DODE, F. BABA-AISSA & L. RAEYMAEKERS. 1995. The SERCA3-type of organellar Ca^{2+} pumps. Biosci. Rep. **15:** 299–306.
11. WU, K. D. & J. LYTTON. 1993. Molecular cloning and quantification of sarcoplasmic reticulum Ca^{2+}-ATPase isoforms in rat muscles. Am. J. Physiol. **264:** C333–C341.
12. ZUBRZYCKA-GAARN, E., B. KORCZAK, H. OSINSKA & M. G. SARSALA. 1982. Studies on sarcoplasmic reticulum from slow-twitch muscle. J. Muscle Res. Cell Motil. **3:** 191–212.
13. BRIGGS, F. N., J. L. POLAND & R. J. SOLARO. 1977. Relative capabilities of sarcoplasmic reticulum in fast and slow mammalian skeletal muscles. J. Physiol. (Lond.) **266:** 587–594.
14. LYTTON, J, M. WESTLIN, S. E. BURKE, G. E. SHULL & D. H. MACLENNAN. 1992. Functional comparisons between isoforms of the sarcoplasmic or endoplasmic reticulum family of calcium pumps. J. Biol. Chem. **267:** 14483–14489.
15. BRIGGS, F. N., K. F. LEE, A. W. WECHSLER & L. R. JONES. 1992. Phospholamban expressed in slow-twitch and chronically stimulated fast-twitch muscles minimally affects calcium affinity of sarcoplasmic reticulum Ca^{2+}-ATPase. J. Biol. Chem. **267:** 26056–26061.
16. SWYNGHEDAUW, B. 1986. Developmental and functional adaptation of contractile proteins in cardiac and skeletal muscles. Physiol. Rev. **66:** 710–771.
17. LEBERER, E., K.-T. HARTNER, C. J. BRANDL, J. FUJII, M. TADA, D. H. MACLENNAN & D. PETTE. 1989. Slow/cardiac sarcoplasmic reticulum Ca^{2+}-ATPase and phospholamban mRNAs are expressed in chronically stimulated rabbit fast-twitch muscle. Eur. J. Biochem. **185:** 51–54.
18. BRIGGS, F. N., K. F. LEE, J. J. FEHER, A. S. WECHSLER, K. OHLENDIECK & K. CAMPBELL. 1990. Ca-ATPase isozyme expression in sarcoplasmic reticulum is altered by chronic stimulation of skeletal muscle. FEBS Lett. **259:** 269–272.
19. SCHULTE, L. M., J. NAVARRO & S. C. KANDARIAN. 1993. Regulation of sarcoplasmic reticulum calcium pump gene expression by hindlimb unweighting. Am. J. Physiol. **264:** C1308–C1315.
20. NAGAI, R., A. Z. HERZBERG, C. J. BRANDL, J. FUJII, M. TADA, D. H. MACLENNAN, N. R. ALPERT & M. PERIASAMY. 1989. Regulation of myocardial Ca^{2+} ATPase and phospholamban mRNA expression in response to pressure overload and thyroid hormone. Proc. Natl. Acad. Sci. USA **86:** 2966–2970.

21. ARAI, M., K. OTSU, D. H. MACLENNAN, N. R. ALPERT & M. PERIASAMY. 1991. Effect of thyroid hormone on the expression of mRNA encoding sarcoplasmic reticulum proteins. Circ. Res. **69:** 266–276.
22. MATSUI, H., D. H. MACLENNAN, N. R. ALPERT & M. PERIASAMY. 1995. Sarcoplasmic reticulum gene expression in pressure overload-induced cardiac hypertrophy in rabbit. Am. J. Physiol. **268:** C252–C258.
23. SUKO, J. 1983. The calcium pump of the cardiac sarcoplasmic reticulum: Functional alterations at different levels of thyroid state in rabbits. J. Physiol.(Lond.) **228:** 563–582.
24. ROHRER, D. K., R. HARTONG & W. H. DILLMANN. 1991. Influence of thyroid hormone and retinoic acid on slow sarcoplasmic reticulum Ca^{2+} ATPase and myosin heavy chain gene expression in cardiac myocytes. J. Biol. Chem. **266:** 8638–8646.
25. KHOURY, S. F., B. D. HOIT, V. DAVE, C. M. PAWLOSKI-DAHM, Y. SHAO, M. GABEL, M. PERIASAMY & R. A. WALSH. 1996. Effects of thyroid hormone on left ventricular performance and regulation of contractile and Ca^{2+}-cycling proteins in the baboon. Circ. Res. **79:** 727–735.
26. HOIT, B. D. C. M. PAWLOSKI-DAHM, Y. SHAO, M. GABEL & R. A. WALSH. 1997. The effects of a thyroid hormone analog on left ventricular performance and contractile and calcium cycling proteins in the baboon. Proc. Am. Assoc. Phys. **109:** 146–153.
27. KISS, E., N. A. BALL, E. G. KRANIAS & R. A. WALSH. 1995. Differential changes in cardiac phospholamban and sarcoplasmic reticular Ca^{2+}-ATPase protein levels. Circ. Res. **77:** 759–764.
28. MORGAN, J. P., R. E. ERNY, P. D. ALLEN, W. GROSSMAN & J. K. GWATHMEY. 1990. Abnormal intracellular calcium handling, a major cause of systolic and diastolic dysfunction in ventricular myocardium from patients with heart failure. Circulation **81**(Suppl. III): III-21–III-32.
29. GWATHMEY, J. K., L. COPELAS, R. MACKINNON, F. J. SCHOEN, M. D. FELDMAN, W. GROSSMAN & J. P. MORGAN. 1987. Abnormal intracellular calcium handling in myocardium from patients with end-stage heart failure. Circ. Res. **61:** 70–76.
30. ARAI, M, N. R. ALPERT, D. H. MACLENNAN, P. BARTON & M. PERIASAMY. 1993. Alterations in sarcoplasmic reticulum gene expression in human heart failure: A possible mechanism for alterations in systolic and diastolic properties of the failing myocardium. Cir. Res. **72:** 463–469.
31. MERCADIER, J-J, A. M. LOMPRE, P. DUC, K. R. BOHELER, J. B. FRAYSSE, C. WISNEWSKY, P. D. ALLEN, M. KOMAJDA & K. SCHWARTZ. 1990. Altered sarcoplasmic reticulum Ca^{2+} ATPase gene expression in the human ventricle during end-stage heart failure. J. Clin. Invest. **85:** 305–309.
32. TAKAHASHI, T., P. D. ALLEN & S. IZUMO. 1992. Expression of A-B- and C-type natriuretic peptide genes in failing and developing human ventricles: Correlation with expression of Ca^{2+} ATPase gene. Circ. Res. **71:** 9–17.
33. STUDER, R., H. REINECKE, J. BILGER, T. ESCHENHAGEN, M. BOHM, G. HASENFUSS, H. JUST & H. DREXLER. 1994. Gene expression of the cardiac $Na^{2+-Ca}2+$ exchanger in end-stage human heart failure. Circ. Res. **75:** 443–453.
34. HASENFUSS, G., H. REINECKE, R. STUDER, M. MEYER, B. PIESKE, J. HOLTZ, C. HOLUBARSCH, H. POSIVAL, H. JUST & H. DREXLER. 1994. Relation between myocardial function and expression of sarcoplasmic reticulum Ca^{2+}-ATPase in failing and nonfailing human myocardium. Circ. Res. **75:** 434–442.
35. MOVSESIAN, M. A., M. KARIMI, K. GREEN & L. R. JONES. 1994. Ca^{2+}-transporting ATPase, phospholamban and calsequestrine levels in nonfailing and failing human myocardium. Circulation **90:** 653–657.
36. MOVSESIAN, M. A., M. R. BRISTOW & J. KRALL. 1989. Ca^{2+} uptake by cardiac sarcoplasmic reticulum from patients with idiopathic dilated cardiomyopathy. Circ. Res. **65:** 1141–1144.
37. CAMPBELL, A. M., P. D. KESSLER, Y. SAGARA, G. INESI & D. M. FAMBROUGH. 1991. Nucleotide sequences of avian cardiac and brain SR/ER Ca^{2+}-ATPases and functional comparisons with fast-twitch Ca^{2+}-ATPase. J. Biol. Chem. **266:** 16050–16055.
38. LYTTON, J., M. WESTLIN & M. R. HANLEY. 1991. Thapsigargin inhibits the sarcoplasmic or endoplasmic reticulum Ca^{2+}-ATPase family of calcium pumps. J. Biol. Chem. **266:** 17067–17071.

39. Kamura, Y., K. Kurzydlowski, M. Tada & D. H. MacLennan. 1996. Phospholamban regulates the Ca^{2+}-ATPase through intermembrane interactions. J. Biol. Chem. **271:** 21726–21731.
40. Maruyama, K. & D. H. MacLennan. 1988. Mutation of aspartic acid-351, lysine-352, and lysine-515 alters the Ca^{2+} transport activity of the Ca^{2+}-ATPase expressed in COS-1 cells. Proc. Natl. Acad. Sci. USA **85:** 3314–3318.
41. Odermatt, A., K. Kurzydlowski & D. H. MacLennan. 1996. The V_{max} of the Ca^{2+}-ATPase of cardiac sarcoplasmic reticulum (SERCA2a) is not altered by Ca^{2+}/calmodulin-dependent phosphorylation or by interaction with phospholamban. J. Biol. Chem. **271:** 14206–14213.
42. Verboomen, H., F. Wuytack, L. Van Den Bosh, L. Mertens & R. Casteels. 1994. The functional importance of the extreme C-terminal tail in the gene 2 organellar Ca^{2+}-transport ATPase (SERCA2a/b). Biochem. J. **303:** 979–984.
43. J. Lytton, & D. H. MacLennan. 1993. ATP-dependent cation pumps of the heart. *In* Molecular Basis of Cardiology. R. Roberts, Ed.: 269–293. Blackwell Scientific Publications. Oxford.
44. Engelender, S. & L. De Meis. 1996. Pharmacological differentiation between intracellular calcium pump isoforms. Mol. Pharmacol. **50:** 1243–1252.
45. Wolosker, H., J. B. Rocha, S. Engelender, R. Panizzutti, J. De Miranda & L. De Meis. 1997. Sarco/endoplasmic reticulum Ca^{2+}-ATPase isoforms: Diverse responses to acidosis. Biochem. J. **321:** 545–550.
46. Autry, J. M. & L. R. Jones. 1997. Functional co-expression of the canine cardiac Ca^{2+} pimp and phospholamban in *Spodoptera frugiperda* (Sf21) cells reveals new insights on ATPase regulation. J. Biol. Chem. **272:** 15872–15880.
47. Koss, K. L. & E. G. Kranias. 1996. Phospholamban: A prominent regulator of myocardial contractility. Circ. Res. **79:** 1059–1063.
48. Fujii, J., K. Maruyama, M. Tada & D. H. MacLennan. 1990. Co-expression of slow-twitch/cardiac muscle Ca^{2+}-ATPase (SERCA2a) and phospholamban. FEBS Lett. **273:** 232–234.
49. Kim, H. W., N. A. E. Steenaart, D. G. Ferguson & E. G. Kranias. 1990. Functional reconstitution of the cardiac sarcoplasmic reticulum Ca^{2+}-ATPase with phospholamban in phospholipid vesicles. J. Biol. Chem. **265:** 1702–1709.
50. Harrer, J. M., S. Ponniah, D. G. Ferguson & E. G. Kranias. 1995. Expression of phospholamban in C_2C_{12} cells and regulation of endogenous SERCA1 activity. Mol. Cell. Biochem. **146:** 13–21.
51. Reedy, L. G., L. R. Jones, S. E. Cala, J. J. O'Brian, S. A. Tatulian & D. L. Stokes. 1995. Functional reconstitution of recombinant phospholamban with rabbit skeletal Ca^{2+}-ATPase. J. Biol. Chem. **270:** 9390–9397.
52. Slack, J., I. L. Grupp, D. G. Ferguson, N. Rosenthal & E. G. Kranias. 1997. Ectopic expression of phospholamban in fast-twitch skeletal muscle alters sarcoplasmic reticulum Ca^{2+} transport and muscle relaxation. J. Biol. Chem. **272:** 18862–18868.
53. W. Luo, I. L. Grupp, J. Harrer, S. Ponniah, G. Grupp, J. J. Duffy, T. Doetschman, E. G. Kranias. 1994. Targeted ablation of the phospholamban gene is associated with markedly enhanced myocardial contractility and loss of β-agonist stimulation. Circ. Res. **75:** 401–409.
54. Kadambi, V. J., S. Ponniah, J. M. Harrer, B. D. Hoit, G. W. Dorn, 2nd, R. A. Walsh & E. G. Kranias. 1997. Cardiac-specific overexpression of phospholamban alters calcium kinetics and resultant cardiomyocyte mechanics in transgenic mice. J. Clin. Invest. **97:** 533–539.
55. Odermatt, A., P. E. M. Taschner, S. W. Scherer, B. Beatty, V. K. Khanna, D. R. Cornblath, V. Chaudhry, W-C. Yee, B. Schrank, G. Karpati, M. H. Breuning, N. Knoers & D. H. MacLennan. 1997. Characterization of the gene encoding human sarcolipin (SLN), a proteolipid associated with SERCA1: Absence of structural mutations in five patients with Brody disease. Genomics **45:** 541–553.
56. He, H., Giordano, F. J. R. Hilal-Dandan, D-J. Choi, H. A. Rockman, P. M. McDonough, W. F. Bluhm, M. Meyer, M. R. Sayen, E. Swanson & W. H. Dillmann. 1997. Overexpression of the rat sarcoplasmic reticulum Ca^{2+} ATPase gene in the heart of trans-

genic mice accelerates calcium transients and cardiac relaxation. J. Clin. Invest. **100:** 380–389.
57. BAKER, D. L., T. REED, I. L. GRUPP, G. GRUPP, A. R. BHAGWAT, B. D. HOIT & R. A. WALSH & M. PERIASAMY. 1997. Overexpression of the cardiac SR Ca^{2+} ATPase increases myocardial performance. Circulation **96:** I-138.
58. LIU, L. H., R. J. PAUL, R. L. SUTLIFF, M. L. MILLER, J. N. LORENZ, R. Y. PUN, J. J. DUFFY, D. H. DOETSCHMAN, Y. KIMURA, D. H. MACLENNAN, J. B. HOYING & G. E. SHULL. 1997. Defective endothelium-dependent relaxation of vascular smooth muscle and endothelial cell Ca^{2+} signaling in mice lacking sarco(endo)plasmic reticulum Ca^{2+}-ATPase isoform 3. J. Biol. Chem. **272:** 30538–30546.

Depletion of Sarcoplasmic Reticulum Calcium Prompts Phosphorylation of Phospholamban to Stimulate Store Refilling[a]

MONINDER SINGH BHOGAL[b] AND JOHN COLYER

School of Biochemistry and Molecular Biology, University of Leeds, Leeds, LS2 9JT, United Kingdom

Store-operated Ca^{2+} entry initiated by retrograde signaling pathways has been described in a wide variety of cell types, including smooth muscle cells and nonmuscle cells.[1–3] However, no such mechanism has been identified in cardiac muscle. We sought to investigate the presence of an analogous phenomenon in cardiac myocytes. The schematic diagram shown in FIGURE 1 describes a simple mechanism by which the myocyte could monitor and regulate lumenal Ca^{2+} load. Phospholamban (PLB) represents a plausible target in this hypothesis; normally an inhibitor of SR Ca^{2+} pump activity, phosphorylation of phospholamban in response to Ca^{2+} store depletion would be expected to accelerate Ca^{2+} uptake by the sarcoplasmic reticulum (SR)[4] and facilitate store refilling. We proposed the presence of a *state of filling* (SOF) kinase—an enzyme capable of sensing lumenal [Ca^{2+}] that will phosphorylate phospholamban in response to changes in lumenal load.

We have observed previously that freshly isolated cardiac myocytes respond to store depletion by phosphorylating phospholamban on Ser^{16}, behavior consistent with the hypothesis outlined above. We have also identified a protein kinase activity associated with the SR. It is active at low [Ca^{2+}] (<3μM), but inhibited by high [Ca^{2+}] (>30μM). This Ca^{2+} sensitivity would preclude regulation of the kinase by cytosolic Ca^{2+}, since cytosolic [Ca^{2+}] rarely reaches levels above 1 μM. However, values of lumenal [Ca^{2+}] seem consistent with the Ca^{2+} sensitivity of the kinase.[6] This evidence, although circumstantial, does imply lumenal control of the identified kinase.

We present here unambiguous evidence that it is lumenal [Ca^{2+}] that regulates the candidate kinase. The kinase is able to monitor the SOF kinase of the SR and respond to changes in SR Ca^{2+} load by phosphorylating phospholamban.

RESULTS AND DISCUSSION

In an effort to establish the means of control of the SOF kinase by Ca^{2+}, we sought to load SR vesicles with Ca^{2+} and determine whether enzyme activity was affected by lumenal Ca^{2+}. SR vesicles were loaded with the membrane-permeant form of Mag fura-5. Substantial lumenal deesterification and therefore loading of the dye was observed. Calcium uptake into Mag fura-5–loaded vesicles was initiated by the addition of Mg.ATP (1.5mM). After an initial increase in lumenal [Ca^{2+}], a steady state loading of ~35 μM was achieved and maintained after 10 minutes (FIG. 2A). Thapsigar-

[a] This work was supported by the British Heart Foundation (PG/96125) and the Medical Research Council (G9428756MA). J. C. is a British Heart Foundation lecturer.

[b] e-mail: M.S.Bhogal@Leeds.ac.uk

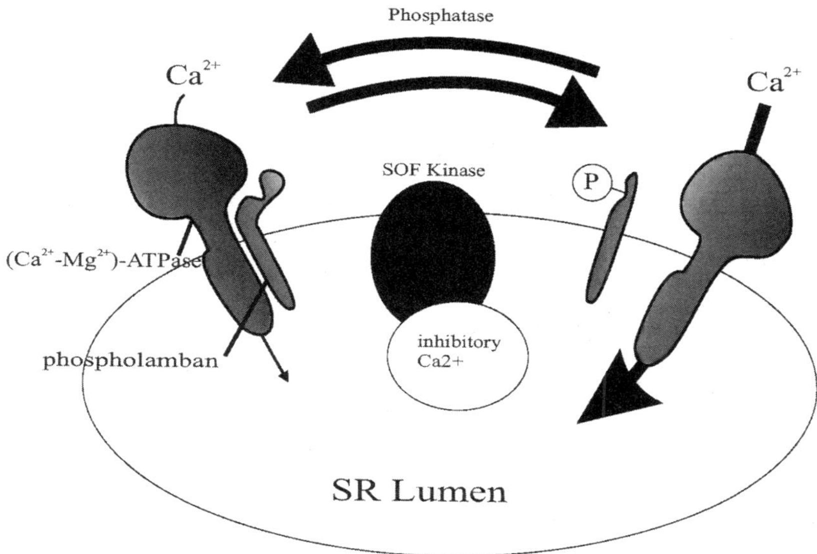

FIGURE 1. A simple mechanism showing the detection and regulation of sarcoplasmic reticulum lumenal Ca^{2+} load. A decrease in $[Ca^{2+}]_L$ would activate the SOF kinase, resulting in a shift in the equilibrium toward phospholamban phosphorylation. This would relieve inhibition of the Ca^{2+}-ATPase and increase the Ca^{2+} pump rate. This response would facilitate Ca^{2+} store refilling.

gin (TG) released ~70% of sequestered Ca^{2+} (FIG. 2Ai) and addition of TG prior to ATP resulted in no significant uptake (FIG. 2Aii), confirming that the majority of Ca^{2+} uptake was into SR vesicles. This represents a situation of 2.5 μM extravesicular $[Ca^{2+}]$ and 35 μM lumenal $[Ca^{2+}]$. If the effect of Ca^{2+} on SOF kinase activity is manifest from the SR lumen, then we would expect some inhibition of SOF kinase activity at this $[Ca^{2+}]_L$ (~35 μM; FIG. 2Ai). FIGURE 2B describes the phosphorylation of phospholamban during the course of Ca^{2+} uptake. The level of phospholamban phosphorylation on Ser^{16} was low prior to the addition of Mg.ATP. On addition of Mg.ATP a burst of phosphorylation was observed, while $[Ca^{2+}]_L$ was low. As steady state Ca^{2+} load was reached (~10 minutes of uptake, 35 μM $[Ca^{2+}]_L$; FIG. 2Ai), a gradual decrease in phospholamban phosphorylation was observed (FIG. 2B, 20 min, 25 min), consistent with an inhibition of kinase action by high lumenal Ca^{2+}. When $[Ca^{2+}]_L$ was reduced to 2.5 μM following introduction of ionomycin, an increase in phospholamban phosphorylation was observed (FIG. 2B, 30 min, 35 min), consistent with activation of the SR kinase (SOF kinase) in response to Ca^{2+} store depletion. Therefore, a direct relationship between $[Ca^{2+}]_L$ and phospholamban phosphorylation has been established, indicating that SOF kinase is regulated by the lumenal concentration of Ca^{2+} in SR.

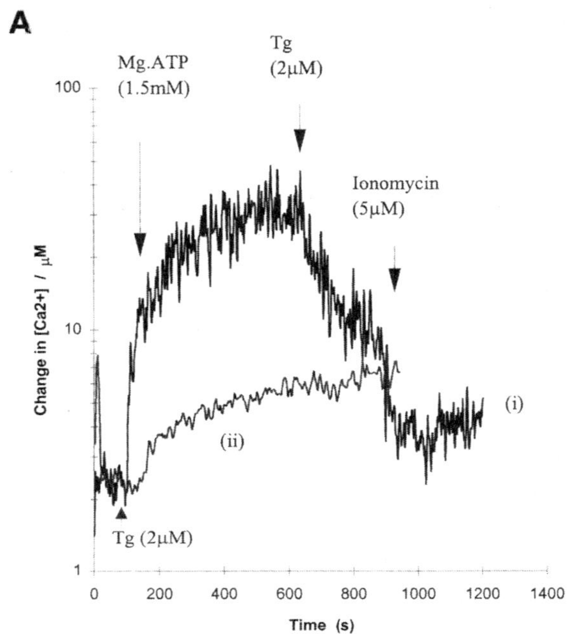

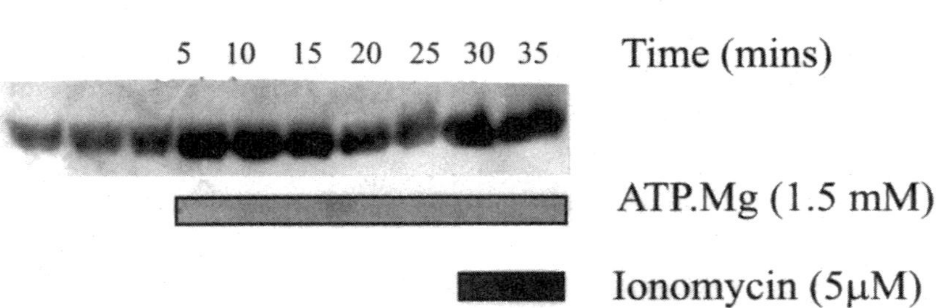

FIGURE 2. Calcium uptake into canine cardiac sarcoplasmic reticulum vesicles: control of phospholamban phosphorylation by luminal [Ca^{2+}]. The fluorescence change of luminal Magfura-5 on addition of Mg.ATP was measured. Conversion of raw fluorescence data by application of an experimentally determined equation shows a steady state loading of ~35 μM Ca^{2+}. **(A)** Trace (i): addition of Mg.ATP (1.5 mM) at 100 s; addition of thapsigargin (TG, 2 μM) at 900 s. Trace(ii): Addition of TG (2 μM) at 30 s; addition of Mg.ATP (1.5 mM) at 100 s. **(B)** In parallel, aliquots of assay medium (7.5 μg protein) were removed at several points before or after the addition of Mg.ATP and quenched using Laemmli sample buffer. Proteins were separated using SDS-PAGE, and phospholamban phosphorylation on Ser^{16} was determined using immunoblotting.

CONCLUSIONS

Loading SR vesicles to steady state (~35 μM) results in inhibition of kinase activity consistent with the Ca^{2+} sensitivity of the SR associated kinase. Collapse of SR load by introduction of ionomycin results in reactivation of kinase activity. The ability to manipulate kinase activity by manipulating $[Ca^{2+}]_L$ indicates lumenal control of SOF kinase. This evidence strongly supports the presence of a novel local feedback mechanism in cardiac SR. Depletion of Ca^{2+} load activates the state of filling kinase, which in turn phosphorylates phospholamban. In its phosphorylated state phospholamban can no longer exert its inhibitory influence on SERCA2a; therefore, an increase in Ca^{2+} pump activity enables the store to refill.

ACKNOWLEDGMENT

We are grateful for the help and advice of Professor Clive H. Orchard throughout these studies and for his provision of myocytes.

REFERENCES

1. Putney, J. W., Jr. 1992. *In* Advances in Second Messenger and Phosphoprotein Research, J. W. Putney, Jr., Ed.: 143–160. Raven. New York.
2. Irvine, R. F. 1992. *In* Advances in Second Messenger and Phosphoprotein Research. J. W. Putney, Jr., Ed.: 161–185. Raven. New York.
3. Fasolato, C., B. Innocenti & T. Pozzan. 1994. TIPS **15:** 77–83.
4. Colyer, J. & J. H. Wang. 1991. J. Biol. Chem. **266:** 17486.
5. Drago, G. A. & J. Colyer. 1994. J. Biol. Chem. **269:** 25073.
6. Bygrave, F. L. & A. Benedetti. 1996 Cell Calcium **19:** 547–551.

Changes in Spatial Arrangement between Individual Ca-ATPase Polypeptide Chains in Response to Phospholamban Phosphorylation

LINDA CHEN, QING YAO, KIMBERLY BRUNGARDT, THOMAS SQUIER, AND DIANA BIGELOW[a]

Department of Biochemistry, University of Kansas, Lawrence, Kansas 66045, USA

We have examined the proximity and spatial grouping of both the cardiac Ca-ATPase and phospholamban (PLB) using steady state anisotropy measurements of fluorescence resonance energy transfer (FRET) between individual molecules of bound fluorescein. Therefore, we have specifically derivatized the Ca-ATPase in cardiac SR with the nucleotide probe fluorescein isothiocyanate (FITC) or with cysteine-reactive iodoacetamidofluorescein (IAF).

FRET MEASUREMENTS BETWEEN Ca-ATPase POLYPEPTIDE CHAINS

The small Stokes shift of fluorescein and its characteristic overlap of emission and absorption spectra as well as its high quantum yield and large extinction coefficient allow fluorescein to serve as both an energy transfer donor and acceptor. Thus two molecules of fluorescein within a critical distance of one another can transfer nonradiative energy (homotransfer) as in the case of different donor and acceptor probes (heterotransfer). With a Förster critical distance (R_0) of 50 Å, homotransfer between fluoresceins has been shown to be capable of providing a sensitive probe of oligomeric associations between proteins.[1–3] Homotransfer strongly depolarizes fluorescence emission as a result of the exchange of nonradiative energy between an initially excited (oriented) fluorophore and one or more nearby randomly oriented fluorophores; thus fluorescence anisotropy is sensitive to homotransfer and dependent upon the number of energy-transferring units within a cluster of nearest neighbors.

For anisotropy measurements cardiac SR membranes were derivatized with progressive amounts of either FITC or IAF. In the case of FITC-modified SR the high degree of initial anisotropy indicates a rigidly bound probe; the anisotropy of bound FITC decreases with increasing probe stoichiometry as a result of FRET between fluorophores on neighboring polypeptide chains, as evidenced by the complete reversal of these decreases upon detergent solubilization with $C_{12}E_8$ (FIG. 1). Likewise bound IAF exhibits FRET-induced depolarization with increasing labeling stoichiometries; however, IAF binds at a site having greater mobility than that of FITC. These data were fit to the model of Weber and Daniels[1] in order to recover both the average distances between fluorophores and the number of fluorophores involved in FRET, which is dependent upon their spatial arrangement (TABLE 1). Activation of calcium transport with cAMP-dependent protein kinase (PKA) results in increased energy transfer between FITCs, indicating their increased proximity (~5 Å). In contrast, bound IAF ex-

[a] Corresponding author. Phone: 785-864-3831; fax: 785-864-5321; e-mail: dbigelow@falcon.cc.ukans.edu

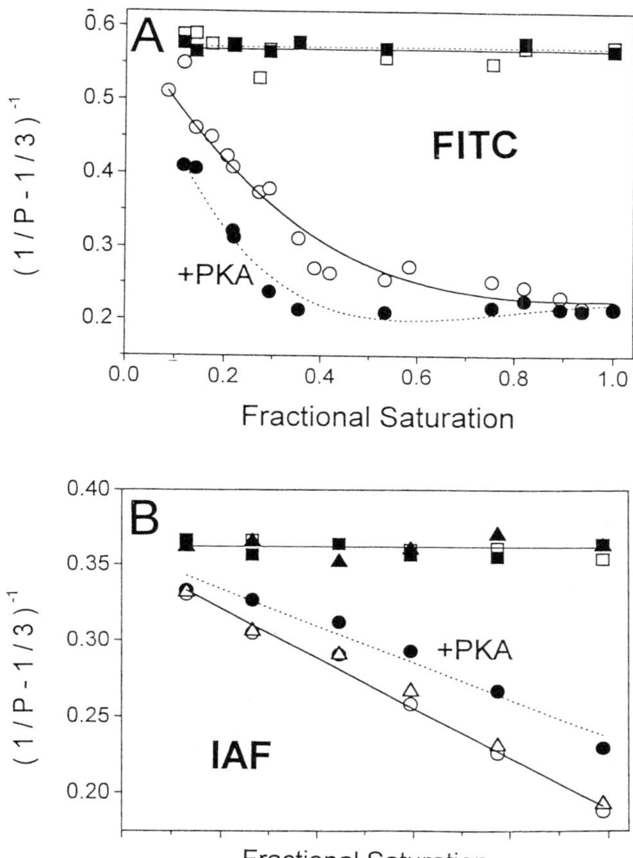

FIGURE 1. Anisotropy $(1/P-1/3)^{-1}$ of FITC- **(panel A)** or IAF- **(panel B)** labeled Ca-ATPase in cardiac SR as a function of fractional saturation of the probe sites. Anisotropy was measured in 0.1 mg SR/ml, 0.1 M KCl, 5 mM $MgCl_2$, i 20 mM MOPS (pH 7.0), 0.1 mM EGTA, and 0.11 mM $CaCl_2$ (Ca_{free} = 0.50 μM) and in the absence *(open symbols)* and presence *(closed symbols)* of 80 μg/ml PK A, 1 μM cAMP, and 0.1 mM ATP. Subsequent solubilization of SR with 6 mM $C_{12}E_8$ (□, ■, ▲) demonstrates that the anisotropy loss of native membranes with fractional saturation is due to FRET.

hibits decreased energy transfer with PKA activation, indicating that IAF sites move farther apart (~9Å). These spectral changes are reversible upon subsequent treatment of SR with alkaline phosphatase. Thus these results suggest a reorientation of individual Ca-ATPase polypeptide chains with respect to one another as a result of changes in the phosphorylation state of PLB. The functional significance of these structural changes can be appreciated from the inactivation profile resulting from FITC modification, which is first order for nonactivated SR and second order for PKA-activated membranes, and suggests monomeric and dimeric functional units, respectively.

TABLE 1. Recovered Values from the Best Fit of Anisotropy Data to Theory[a]

Sample	r_{av} (Å)[b]	θ_{av} (degrees)[c]
FITC-Ca-ATPase		
Nonactivated	24.0 (±1)	40 (±2)
PKA-activated	18.7 (±2)	39 (±1)
IAF-Ca-ATPase		
Nonactivated	31 (±2)	38.5 (±2)
PKA-activated	40 (±3)	35.0 (±3)

[a] As previously described by Weber & Daniel.[1]
[b] Average donor-acceptor distance.
[c] Average angle between absorption and emission dipoles.

FRET BETWEEN PLB POLYPEPTIDES

A similar approach was taken with PLB, taking advantage of the single lysine (Lys3) within the PLB sequence. In this instance PLB was purified from cardiac SR and labeled with FITC before reconstitution with varying amounts of unlabeled PLB and affinity-purified Ca-ATPase into liposomes (at a PLB:Ca-ATPase ratio of 5:1). Activation by calcium or cAMP-dependent protein kinase (PKA) of these membranes is comparable to that observed for native cardiac SR membranes (V_{max} 25 °C: 2.2 IU), demonstrating that substantial populations of both Ca-ATPase and PLB are asymmetrically oriented and conformationally competent to allow the functional interactions and the structural transitions required for increased calcium transport in response to the phosphorylation of PLB. Concomitant with the increased labeling of PLB by FITC is the loss of the ability of PKA to activate the Ca-ATPase (FIG. 1B). The progressive loss of activation induced by FITC modification exhibits a second-order pattern indicating that activation of the Ca-ATPase involves two interacting PLB molecules. FRET measurements indicate a spatial grouping of five or more in these proteoliposomes assuming a homogeneous population. Further work will involve explicit consideration of multiple populations of spatial groupings with variation of the molar ratios of PLB:Ca-ATPase in reconstituted proteoliposomes.

REFERENCES

1. WEBER, G. & E. DANIEL. 1966. Cooperative effects in binding by bovine serum albumin. II. The binding of 1-anilino-8-naphthalenesulfonate. Polarization of the ligand fluorescence and quenching of the protein fluorescence. Biochemistry **5:** 1900–1907.
2. HIGHSMITH, S. & J. A. COHEN. 1987. Spatial organization of CaATPase molecules in sarcoplasmic reticulum vesicles. Biochemistry **26:** 154–190.
3. RUNNELS, L. W. & S. SCARLATA. 1995. Theory and application of fluorescence homotransfer to melittin oligomerization. Biophys. J. **69:** 1569–1583.

Nucleotide Mimetics Reverse Phospholamban Regulation in Cardiac Sarcoplasmic Reticulum

KATHLEEN E. COLL, ROBERT G. JOHNSON, JR., AND EDWARD McKENNA[a]

Merck Research Laboratories, WP44-B124, West Point, Pennsylvania 19486, USA

Plant-derived polyphenolic nucleotide mimetics, quercetin,[1] ellagic acid, and tannin exert inhibitory effects on a variety of ATP-requiring enzymes. Surprisingly, at low concentrations, these compounds appear to stimulate cardiac sarcoplasmic reticulum (SR) Ca^{2+}ATPase activity; only at higher concentrations are the inhibitory effects seen. The stimulation appears to be caused by the loss of inhibition by phospholamban (PLB) and not a direct stimulatory effect. The stimulatory effect exhibits a strong MgATP dependency,[1] implying that they interact with Ca^{2+}ATPase and not PLB.

RESULTS

Low micromolar concentrations of tannin ($EC_{50} \approx 3$ µM) and ellagic acid ($EC_{50} \approx 5$ µM) stimulate the rate of calcium uptake (FIG. 1) into cardiac SR at low free Ca^{2+} (pCa 7.0). The stimulatory action of ellagic acid remains at higher concentrations, while the stimulatory action of tannin rapidly wanes and complete inhibition is observed at 10 µM. At a high free Ca^{2+} (pCa 5.5), the stimulatory effect is absent, while the inhibitory effect of tannin remains. In skeletal muscle SR (lacking phospholamban) ellagic acid had virtually no effect, and only the inhibitory activity of tannin is present regardless of the free Ca^{2+} (data not shown). The stimulation of Ca^{2+}ATPase activity is equivalent to the effect of anti-PLB monoclonal antibody 1D11. Furthermore, stimulation is additive with submaximal amounts of mAb 1D11, and hydrophilic PLB (1–25 and 1–30) peptides, even at 50 µM, cannot reverse the stimulatory effect (data not shown).

The calcium sensitivity of SR Ca^{2+}ATPase increases, like that observed with mAb 1D11, in the presence of optimal stimulatory concentration of tannin and ellagic acid (FIG. 2). The data suggest that the observed stimulation by tannin and ellagic acid represents a reversal of PLB's inhibitory effect on cardiac SR Ca^{2+}ATPase and not a direct stimulatory action.

CONCLUSIONS

Compounds interacting with the nucleotide binding site (NBS) of cardiac SR Ca^{2+}ATPase cause the loss of PLB inhibition. No evidence for a direct interaction as previously purported for tannin[2] or ellagic acid[3] with PLB was found. We postulate that

[a] Corresponding author. Phone: 215-652-2128; fax: 215-652-1658; e-mail: Edward_mckenna @merck.com

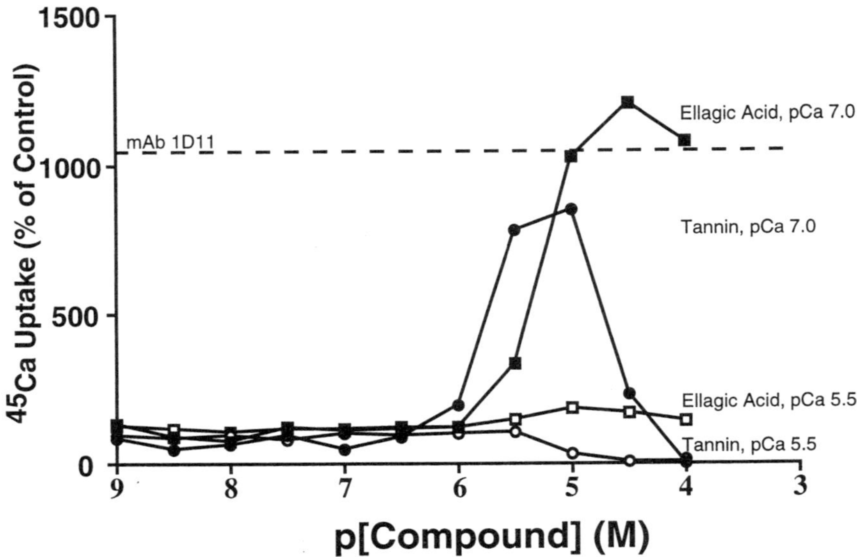

FIGURE 1. Concentration dependence of the effects of ellagic acid and tannin on calcium uptake into cardiac SR at pCa 7.0 and pCa 5.5. The reaction media consisted of 20 mM imidazole, pH 7.1, 109.7 mM KCl, 5 mM K_2oxalate, 5 mM NaN_3, 1.09 mM $MgCl_2$, 0.5 mM EGTA, 3.75 mM MgATP, 100 μg/ml SR protein, and 1 % DMSO. The data were normalized to the basal $^{45}Ca^{2+}$ uptake rate of 6.59 nmole/mg/min at 25 °C. The means of triplicate measurements are shown.

both stimulation and inhibition result from action on the NBS within Ca^{2+}ATPase. While the NBS has been extensively probed, the definitive structure and oligomeric state have not been solved. Two interacting NBS (we believe to be a Ca^{2+}ATPase dimer, but only one monomer can form phosphoenzyme) with dual roles for MgATP—a high-affinity (K_d = 2–4 μM) catalytic site resulting in a phosphoenzyme intermediate; and a low-affinity (K_d ~ 1 mM) regulatory site that occurs after phosphoenzyme formation and causes an accelerated turnover of phosphoenzyme—have often been described in the literature.[4] However, in the absence of Mg or at acid pH, ATP exhibits a single intermediate binding affinity of 20 μM. Nucleotide mimetics, also, have intermediate binding affinities and do not discriminate between the two sites. However, since they lack a high-energy phosphate, they cannot interact with the catalytic site. Thus, low mimetic concentrations mimic the effect of nucleotide at the regulatory site to eliminate PLB inhibition. Higher concentrations prevent MgATP from binding to provide the high-energy phosphate for catalysis. Phospholamban has previously been suggested[5] to interfere with the accelerative effect of MgATP binding to the regulatory nucleotide site. This report offers the converse—that nucleotide mimetics binding to the regulatory NBS interfere with PLB regulation. The precise mechanism, such as reducing the PLB binding affinity, occlusion of the PLB binding site, or change in the oligomeric composition, is not known. We suggest that PLB may act like a wedge between the dimer Ca^{2+}ATPase complex. The binding of nucleotide mimetic to one of the Ca^{2+}ATPase molecules would cause a conformational change, restoring the negative cooperativity between the two NBS as well as relieving the stabilizing effect of PLB.

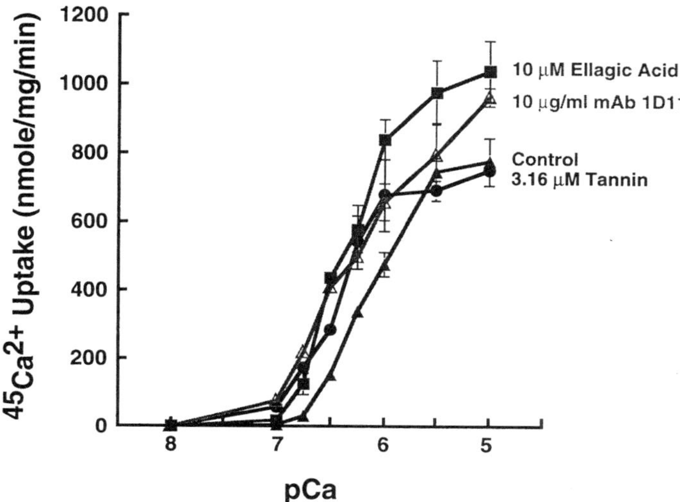

FIGURE 2. Effects of optimal stimulatory concentrations of ellagic acid and tannin on the calcium dependence of the rate of calcium uptake into cardiac SR. Measurements were made at 37 °C as described in the legend to FIGURE 1 over a range of free Ca^{2+}. The curves were fitted to the equation $V = V_{max}/[1 + K_m/[Ca^{2+}])^{n_H}]$, where n_H is the Hill coefficient, and the fitted lines are shown. The results of the fit are summarized below:

Treatment	V_{max} (nmole/mg/min)	$K_{m(Ca)}$ (μM)	n_H
Cardiac SR	786.0 ± 22.6	0.724 ± 0.048	1.81 ± 0.18
+ mAb 1D11	953.9 ± 56.6	0.371 ± 0.086	1.44 ± 0.19
+ 10 μM ellagic acid	1023.0 ± 38.0	0.443 ± 0.038	1.83 ± 0.24
+ 3.16 μM tannin	734.7 ± 22.3	0.355 ± 0.025	2.03 ± 0.24

REFERENCES

1. McKenna, E., J. S. Smith, K. E. Coll, E. K. Mazack, E. J. Mayer, J. A. Antanavage, R. T. Wiedmann & R. G. Johnson. 1996. Dissociation of phospholamban regulation of cardiac sarcoplasmic reticulum Ca^{2+}ATPase by quercetin. J. Biol. Chem. **271:** 24517–24525.
2. Chiesi, M. & R. Schwaller. 1994. Reversal of phospholamban-induced inhibition of cardiac sarcoplasmic reticulum Ca^{2+}ATPase by tannin. Biochem. Biophys. Res. Comm. **202:** 1668–1673.
3. Berrebi-Bertrand, I., P. Lahouratate, V. Lahouratate, J. C. Camelin, J. Guibert & A. Bril. 1997. Mechanism of action of sarcoplasmic reticulum calcium-uptake activators. Eur. J. Biochem. **247:** 801–809.
4. Dupont, Y., R. Pougeois, M. Ronjat & S. Verjovsky-Almeida. 1985. Two distinct classes of nucleotide binding sites in sarcoplasmic reticulum Ca-ATPase revealed by 2′,3′-O-(2,4,6-trinitrocyclohexadienylidene)-ATP. J. Biol. Chem. **260:** 7241–7249.
5. Lu, Y. Z., Z. C. Xu & M. A. Kirchberger. 1993. Evidence for an effect of phospholamban on the regulatory role of ATP in calcium uptake by the calcium pump of cardiac sarcoplasmic reticulum. Biochemistry **32:** 3105–3111.

Reduced Contractile Function Characteristic of Hibernating Human Heart Is Not Mediated by Phospholamban

ELISABETH DEINDL,[a] ELFRIEDE NEUBAUER, ALBRECHT ELSÄSSER, RENÉ ZIMMERMANN, AND WOLFGANG SCHAPER

Max-Planck-Institute for Physiological and Clinical Research, W. G. Kerckhoff-Institute, Department of Experimental Cardiology, Benekestrasse 2, D-61231 Bad Nauheim, Germany

The term *hibernating myocardium* was first defined by Rahimtoola. It refers to chronically impaired left ventricular function, due to reduced blood supply, that is completely restored upon reperfusion.[1,2] Cardiac contraction and relaxation are modulated by Ca^{2+} fluxes regulated by the sarcoplasmic reticulum, in particular by the Ca^{2+}-ATPase (SERCA2), which itself is regulated by the phosphoprotein phospholamban (PLB).[3] PLB in the dephosphorylated state is an inhibitor of SERCA2, and phosphorylation relieves this inhibition.[4] It is therefore conceivable that increased levels of PLB or decreased levels of SERCA2 are responsible for the reduced contractile function in the hibernating human heart. To address this point we analyzed the expression of PLB and SERCA2 on protein and mRNA level in biopsies taken in hibernating regions from patients.

MATERIALS AND METHODS

Biopsies taken from hibernating regions of 14 patients (previously diagnosed on the basis of dobutamine echocardiography) during coronary bypass surgery were frozen immediately in liquid nitrogen. For control, tissue from ASD (atrial-septal defect) or healthy hearts (which could not be transplanted due to technical reasons) were taken. RNA isolation using a RNeasy Total RNA Purification Kit (Qiagen) was done according to the manufacturer's protocol; protein extraction, slot blot and Western blot according to standard procedures.[5] For protein detection an ECL Western Blotting detection system (Amershan) was used. Signals for PLB mRNA and SERCA2 mRNA were normalized to Poly $(A)^+$-RNA. Quantification of signals was performed by laser-densitometry or via a PhosphorImager (Molecular Dynamics). The oligonucleotides used for hybridization were complementary to PLB mRNA (GAGCGAGTGAG-GTATTGGAC, pos. 210–191), to SERCA2 mRNA (CCAGCACCTCCTCCAC-CGTC, pos. 43–24), or to the Poly $(A)^+$-tail of total mRNA (oligo dT, 30mer). For detection of desmin we used a monoclonal antibody (Sigma, product No. D-1033, dilution 1:3000); of SERCA2 a monoclonal antibody (BIOMOL, Catalog No. SA-209, dilution 1:3000); of PLB a monoclonal antibody (A1, dilution 1:5000, a generous

[a] Corresponding author. Phone: +49(0)6032705404; fax: +49(0)6032705419; e-mail: edeindl @kerckhoff.mpg.de

gift from M. Tada, Osaka[6]). The secondary antibody was a anti-mouse IgG (Santa Cruz Biotechnology, dilution 1:3000).

RESULTS

To analyze whether the reduced contractile function of hibernating human myocytes is mediated by the SERCA2/PLB system, we analyzed the mRNA expression level of both transcripts in biopsies taken from 11 patients via slot blot. Results revealed in seven biopsies a sizable reduction of PLB mRNA (up to more than 80%) and only a mild reduction of SERCA2 mRNA (in some cases less than 10%) compared to tissue from patients with an ASD that showed normal cardiac function before elective cardiac surgery. In four biopsies neither PLB mRNA nor SERCA2 mRNA could be detected (TABLE 1). The ratio PLB mRNA from ASD versus PLB mRNA from hibernating myocardium was <0.001; that of SERCA2 mRNA was <0.05. To determine the protein abundance we performed quantitative Western blot analysis. All biopsies taken from three individual patients exhibited—compared to healthy control heart—increased protein amounts of SERCA2 (1.3 of control), decreased levels of PLB (0.7 of control), and unchanged amounts of desmin (data not shown), which was analyzed for reasons of control (FIG. 1).

DISCUSSION

To analyze the role of the SERCA2/PLB system in hibernating human myocardium we investigated the expression of both genes on mRNA and protein level. For PLB we found markedly reduced mRNA levels, which were reflected by a slight reduction in protein level. Western blot results revealed for PLB amounts of about 0.7 compared to healthy control heart. The slot blot result displayed for SERCA2 mRNA in most cases only a mild reduction in biopsies taken from hibernating regions of patients, but Western blot showed an increased level of this protein compared to control. As decreased levels of PLB should increase active Ca^{2+} transport by augmenting the turnover rate of the SERCA2, our data indicate that on the molecular level an effort is made to compensate for the reduced contractility via enhancing the activity of SERCA2. This effort, which is enhanced by the increased amount of SERCA2, fails be-

TABLE 1. Amount of PLB and SERCA2 mRNA from Hibernating Human Heart as Percent of the Value Obtained from Control Tissue (ASD)

Human Biopsy	PLB	SERCA2
A	16%	80%
B	33%	96%
C	—	—
D	42%	91%
E	—	—
F	—	—
G	—	—
H	75%	92%
I	32%	64%
J	18%	58%
K	3%	8%

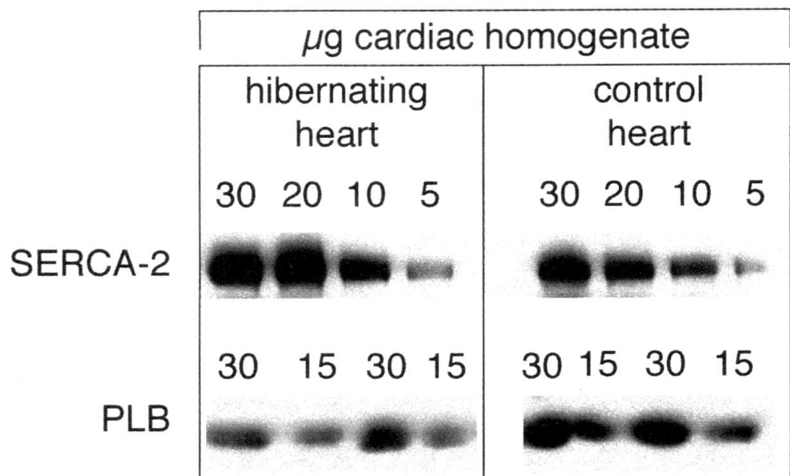

FIGURE 1. Western blot analysis of SERCA2 and PLB in hibernating human heart and healthy control heart. The linear range as shown for SERCA2 was used to determine relative changes in protein level.

cause of the reduced oxygen supply. We therefore conclude that hibernating myocardium does not represent a regulated mechanism to adapt for reduced oxygen supply, controlled by the SERCA2/PLB system. Patients with the diagnosis of hibernating myocardium should therefore undergo coronary bypass surgery without delay.

REFERENCES

1. Rahimtoola, S. H. 1989. The hibernating myocardium. Am. Heart J. **117**(1): 211–221.
2. Rahimtoola, S. H. 1993. The hibernating myocardium in ischaemia and congestive heart failure. Eur. Heart. J.: 212–220.
3. Tada, M. & M. Inui. 1983. Regulation of calcium transport by the ATPase-phospholamban system. J. Mol. Cell. Cardiol. **15:** 565–575.
4. Kim, H. W., A. E. Steenaart, D. G. Ferguson & E. G. Krainas. 1990. Functional reconstitution of the cardiac sarcoplasmic reticulum Ca^{2+}-ATPase with phospholamban in phospholipid vesicles. J. Biol. Chem. **265**(3): 1702–1709.
5. Sambrook, J., E. F. Fritsch & T. Maniatis. 1989. Molecular Cloning: A Laboratory Mannual. Cold Spring Harbor Laboratory Press. Cold Spring Harbor, NY.
6. Suzuki, T. & J. H. Wang. 1986. Stimulation of bovine cardiac sarcoplasmic reticulum Ca^{2+} pump and blocking of phospholamban phosphorylation and dephosphorylation by a phospholamban monoclonal antibody. J. Biol. Chem. **261**(15): 7018–7023.

Immunofluorescence Localization of SERCA2a and the Phosphorylated Forms of Phospholamban in Intact Rat Cardiac Ventricular Myocytes[a]

G. A. DRAGO,[b,c] J. COLYER,[c] AND W. J. LEDERER[d]

[c]*The School of Biochemistry and Molecular Biology, University of Leeds, Leeds, LS2 9JT, United Kingdom*

[d]*Departments of Molecular Biology and Biophysics, and of Physiology, Medical Biotechnology Center, University of Maryland School of Medicine, 725 West Lombard Street, Baltimore, Maryland 21201, USA*

Contractile, electrical, and metabolic function of heart muscle is regulated to a large extent by intracellular calcium. The steady state of intracellular Ca^{2+} concentration ($[Ca^{2+}]_i$) is dependent on the balance of Ca^{2+} influx and extrusion across the sarcolemmal membrane, while the $[Ca^{2+}]_i$ transient depends on those Ca^{2+} fluxes and also on the Ca^{2+} released and reaccumulated by intracellular stores. In this study we investigate the subcellular distribution of two important proteins that regulate the uptake of Ca^{2+} into the major intracellular Ca^{2+} store of the cardiac myocyte, the sarcoplasmic reticulum (SR): (1) SR Ca^{2+} ATPase (SERCA2a) and (2) phospholamban (PLB). SERCA2a and PLB are both integral membrane proteins found in the SR membrane. In the unphosphorylated state, PLB interacts directly with SERCA2a to inhibit its transport of Ca^{2+} from the cytosol to the SR lumen, and thus the Ca^{2+}-ATPase activity is inhibited. However, activation of β-adrenergic receptors on the sarcolemma of the cardiac cell induced by increased levels of circulating catecholamines leads to the phosphorylation of PLB at the Ser16 (PLB-16P) and Thr17 (PLB-17P) sites, via the cAMP-dependent kinase (PKA) and Ca^{2+}/calmodulin-dependent kinase (CaMKII) signaling pathways, respectively. This phosphorylation of PLB relieves the inhibition of SERCA2a by PLB and thus leads to increased Ca^{2+} ATPase activity and increased Ca^{2+} transport into the SR.

Recent studies showing that spatially distinct signaling enzymes can exist in cardiac cells and are correlated with spatially distinct functional heterogeneity[1,2] prompted us to examine the subcellular distribution of PLB. The following question was investigated: is there any evidence that PLB-16P and PLB-17P serve different purposes? This immunofluorescence confocal examination of heart cells investigates this question using distinct antibodies, each of which could recognize a distinct phosphorylated form of PLB (see below and Ref. 3). Here we report that there are distinct subcellular distributions of PLB-16P and of PLB-17P and speculate on their functional significance.

[a] This work was funded by the British Heart Foundation (grant number FS/96068), the National Heart and Research Fund, and the National Institutes of Health.

[b] Corresponding author: Dr. Guido A. Drago, The School of Biochemistry and Molecular Biology, The University of Leeds, Leeds LS2 9JT, United Kingdom. Phone: +44 113 233 3178; fax: +44 113 233 3167; e-mail: G.A.Drago@Leeds.ac.uk

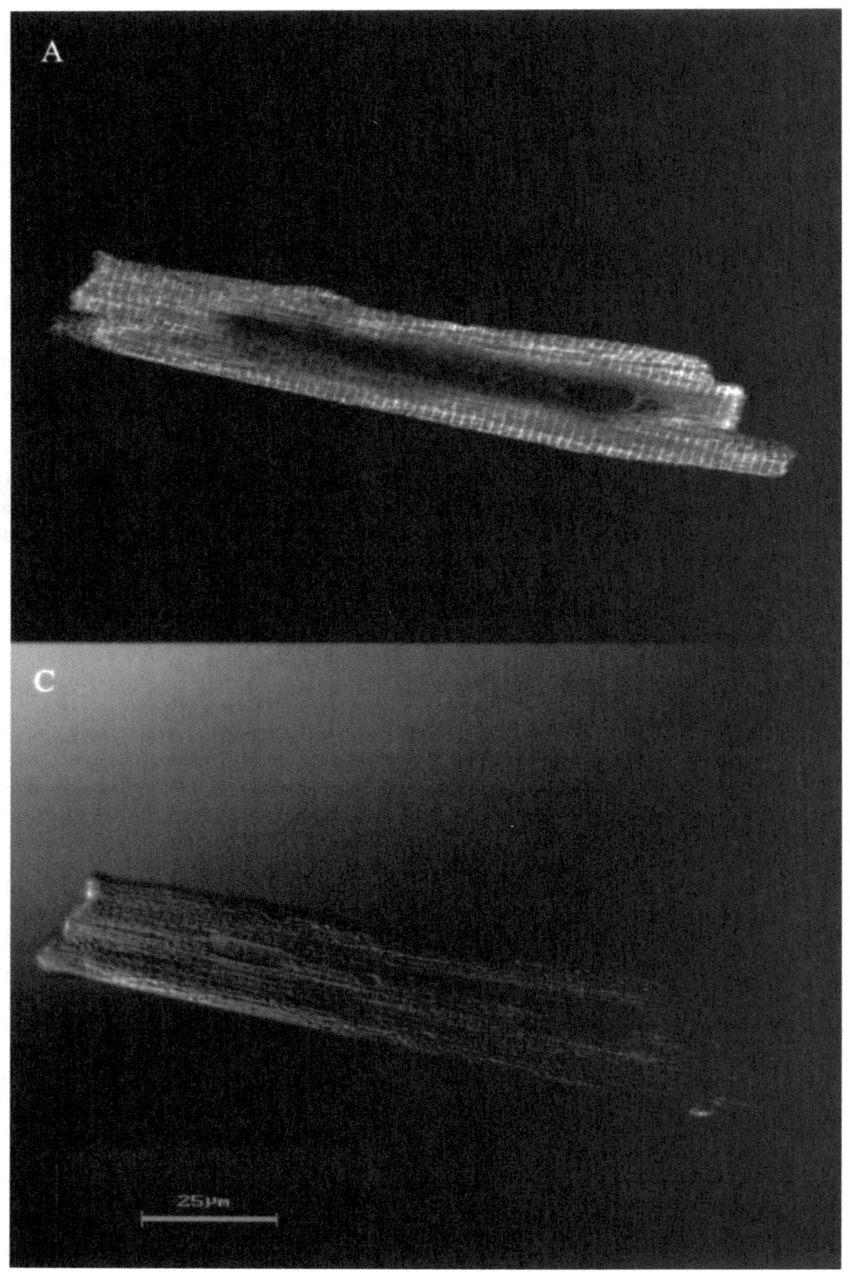
A
C
25μm

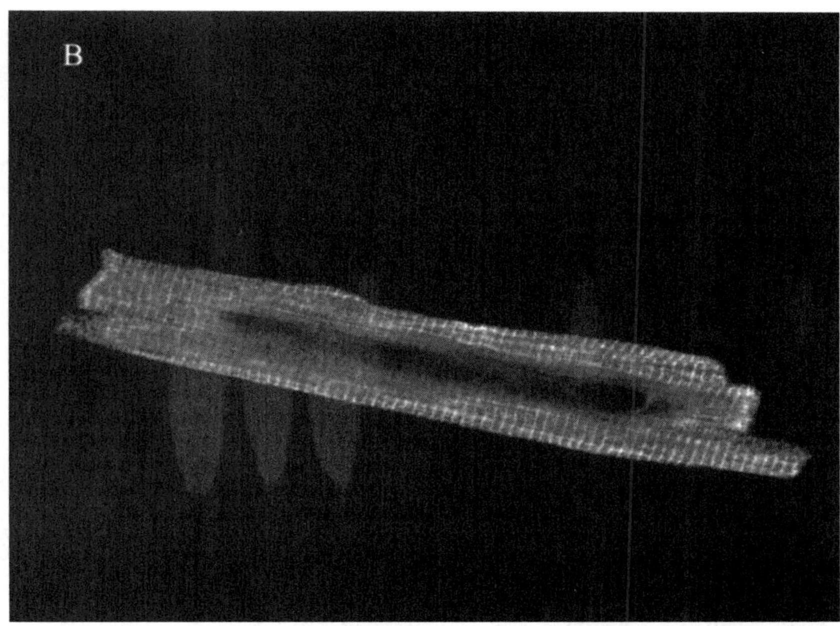

FIGURE 1 *(above and facing page).* Immunolocalization of SERCA2a and PLB in the intact rat cardiac ventricular myocyte. Confocal images of single heart cells show three views of one cell. **A.** The immunofluorescence of PLB probed with the monoclonal antibody A1, raised to the complete PLB protein sequence, and revealed with a goat anti-mouse CY5-linked secondary antibody. **B.** The immunofluorescence of SERCA2a probed with the rabbit "CLEP" antibody, raised to the C-terminal 8 residues of SERCA2a, and revealed with a goat anti-rabbit FITC-linked secondary antibody. **C.** A DIC image of the cell. The cells used in this image were quiescent, and fixed and premeabilized with *no* PKA activation.

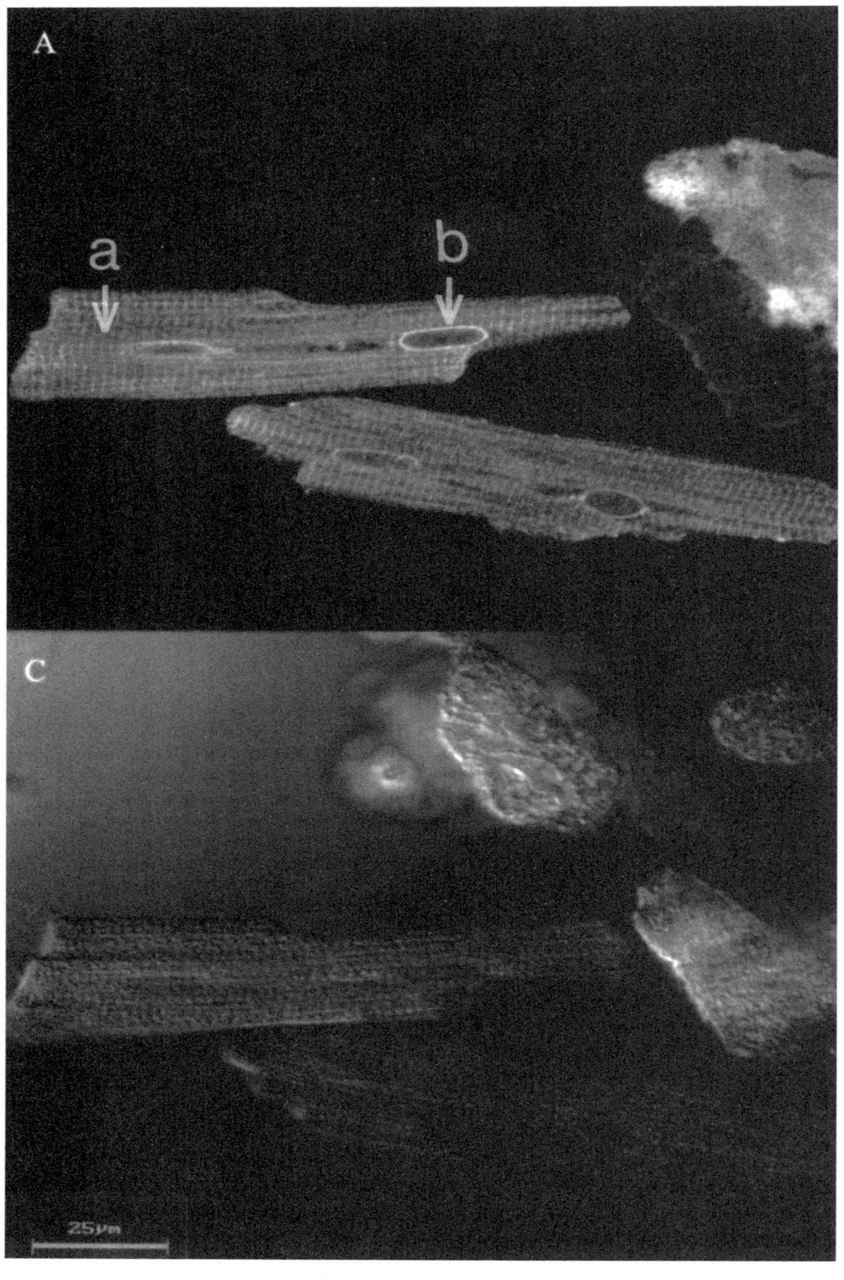
A
a
b
C
25μm

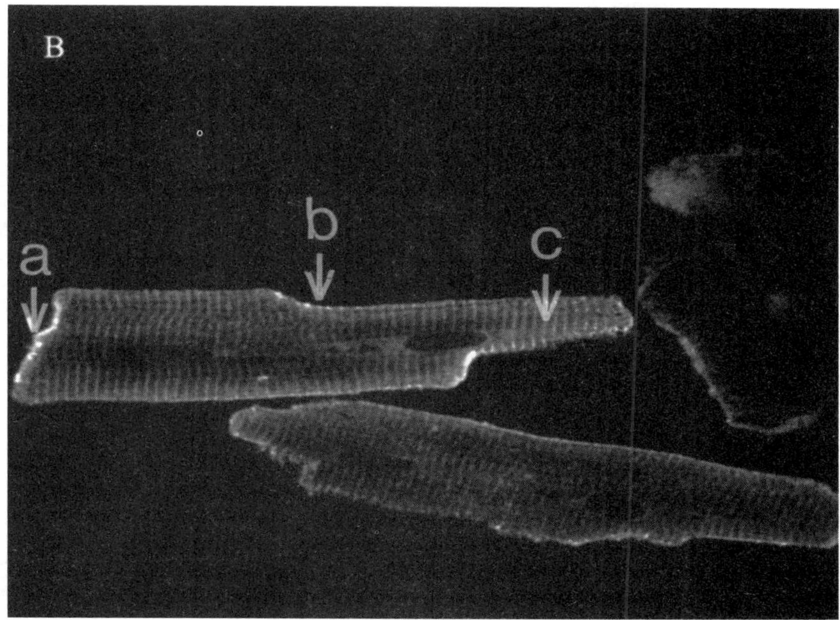

FIGURE 2 *(above and facing page).* Immunolocalization of PLB phosphorylated at Ser16 (PLB-16P) and of PLB phosphorylated at Thr17 (PLB-17P) in intact rat cardiac ventricular myocytes. Confocal images of heart cells reveal three views. **A.** Immunofluorescence of PLB-16P. The Z-lines and the perinuclear region are bright, indicating that abundant PLB-16P is found in these regions (indicated by *arrows* a and b, respectively). In contrast, there is little immunofluorescence in the intercalated disk region and along the external surface membrane region. The rabbit PLB-16P antibody was labeled with CY5-linked Fab monovalent secondary antibody. **B.** Immunofluorescence of PLB-17P. The intercalated disks and the external surface membrane and the Z-line region are bright, indicating that abundant PLB-17P is found in these regions (indicated by *arrows* a, b, and c, respectively). In contrast, there is little immunofluorescence in the perinuclear region. The PLB-17P antibody was labeled with FITC-linked Fab monovalent secondary antibody. **C.** A DIC image of the cells. The cardiac myocytes used in this image were stimulated at 0.1 Hz by external shocks and were exposed to 1 μM isoprenaline in HEPES-buffered physiological saline (pH 7.3).

METHODS

Rat cardiac ventricular myocytes were prepared by Langendorff perfusion and either processed immediately for immunofluorescence microscopy or subjected to stimulation at 0.1Hz plus 1μM isoprenaline for 5 minutes in HEPES based physiological saline (pH 7.3). Cells were subsequently fixed and permeabilized in 100% ethanol at –20 °C for 15 minutes and washed four times in PBS containing 5% normal goat serum (NGS) and 3% bovine serum albumin (BSA) for a duration of 15 minutes each. The cells were incubated with a 1:50 dilution of monoclonal and polyclonal rabbit antisera to specific cardiac protein targets in 5% NGS/3% BSA in PBS overnight at 4 °C on a rocking platform. Cells were washed as before and incubated with a 1:200 dilution of goat anti-mouse and anti-rabbit secondary antibodies conjugated with either fluorescein isothiocyanate (FITC) or indodicarbocyanaine (CY5) in NGS/BSA/PBS for 2 hours at room temperature with rocking. Following four further washes, 20 μl of myocyte suspension was mounted on a microscope slide with an equal volume of Slowfade-Light Anti-Fade Reagent in glycerol buffer. The labeling of cells with secondary antibodies alone was carried out as a negative control.

In the event of using primary antibodies from the same species, cells were probed with a primary antisera to the first target (1:100), followed by incubation with an excess of monovalent FITC- or CY5-labeled secondary antiserum raised to the Fab fragment of the immunoglobulin molecule (1:50). This was followed by incubation with an excess of unconjugated Fab monovalent secondary antiserum (1:50). This was followed by incubation with a primary antiserum to a second target (1:50) and the normal secondary antiserum conjugated either to FITC or CY5 (1:200).[4] Appropriate control incubations were processed in the same manner. The immunocytochemical staining of the intact ventricular myocytes was visualized by excitation at 488 nm for FITC and 674 nm for CY5, with emission spectra detected between 515–565 nm and 670–810 nm, respectively, using a Zeiss Laser Scanning Confocal Microscope (LSCM). Differential interference contrast images (DIC) were also collected.

RESULTS

FIGURE 1 shows the complete complete colocalization of SERCA2a and PLB staining in the intact cardiac ventricular myocyte following staining with the A1 (PLB) (panel A) and the CLEP (SERCA2a) (panel B) antisera, respectively. The characteristic striated staining pattern was observed as previously reported.[5] The Z-lines of the sarcomere are brightest on the immunofluorescence images. This region of the sarcomere is rich in junctional and corbular SR. There is only modest but measurable immunofluorescence between the Z-lines. These observations are consistent with the findings and interpretations of Jorgensen and Jones.[5] While they noted that the density of PLB was greater along the longitudinal SR (found between the Z-lines), there is much less membrane per volume viewed. The net result is greater immunofluorescence along the Z-line. Here we also report the presence of SERCA2a and PLB in the perinuclear region of the cardiac cell, although the immunofluorescence is weaker than that seen along the Z-lines. Note also that PLB staining (panel A) is observed to be significantly stronger than that noted for SERCA2a (panel B).

We used the phosphorylation site-specific antisera to the Ser16P and Thr17P forms of PLB to examine the degree of overlap and the unique staining pattern displayed by these antisera compared with those revealed by the A1 PLB antibody. PLB Ser16P staining is strong at the Z-line (FIG. 2, panel A, arrow a) and in the perinuclear region (arrow b). Immunofluorescence is weak between the Z-lines, weak at the intercalated disk region and along the external surface membrane. PLB Thr17P staining is noted to be strong in the intercalated disk region of the cell (FIG. 2, panel B, arrow a) along the external sarcolemmal membrane (arrow b) and along the Z-lines (arrow c).

DISCUSSION

Because of the function of PLB to modulate the SR Ca^{2+} ATPase, we expect PLB to be colocalized with SERCA2a. Our observation is consistent with this expectation and with the findings of Jorgensen and Jones.[5] We have found that the nature of the phosphorylation of PLB is different in different regions of the cell. The PLB-17P is found in the regions known to be important for EC coupling. In contrast the PLB-16P appears to be colocalized along the Z-lines with PLB-17P but is also found in the perinuclear region and the regions rich in ER. This is the first clear demonstration of spatially resolved differences in the phosphorylated species of PLB, but the importance of these features at a functional level must await further examination.

ACKNOWLEDGMENTS

We would like to thank Ceci Neubauer, Keith Dilly, Fernando Santana, and Paul Luther for their advice and technical support.

REFERENCES

1. GASSER, J. *et al.* 1988. Heterogeneous distribution of calmodulin- and cAMP-dependent regulation of Ca^{2+} uptake in cardiac sarcoplasmic reticulum subfractions. Eur. J. Biochem. **176:** 535–541.
2. XIAO, R-P. *et al.* 1994. Dual regulation of Ca^{2+}/calmodulin-dependent kinase II activity by membrane voltage influx. Proc. Natl. Acad. Sci. USA **91:** 9659–9663.
3. DRAGO, G. A. & J. COLYER. 1994. Discrimination between two sites of phosphorylation on adjacent amino acids by phosphorylation specific antibodies to phospholamban. J. Biol. Chem. **269:** 25073–25077.
4. WESSEL, G. M. & D. R. MCCLAY. 1986. Two embryonic, tissue-specific molecules identified by a double-label immunofluorescence technique for monoclonal antibodies. J. Histochem. Cytochem. **34:** 703–706.
5. JORGENSEN, A. O. & L. R. JONES. 1987. Immunoelectron microscopical localization of phospholamban in adult canine ventricular muscle. J. Cell. Biol. **104:** 1343–1352.

Phosphorylation of the Thr[17] Residue of Phospholamban

New Insights into the Physiological Role of the CaMK-II Pathway of Phospholamban Phosphorylation

ALICIA MATTIAZZI,[a,b] LETICIA VITTONE,[a] CECILIA MUNDIÑA-WEILENMANN,[a] AND MATILDE SAID

Centro de Investigaciones Cardiovasculares, Facultad de Ciencias Médicas, Universidad Nacional de La Plata, 60 y 120, (1900) La Plata, Argentina.

Phospholamban (PHL) can be phosphorylated by either cAMP-dependent protein kinase (PKA) or Ca^{2+}-calmodulin–dependent protein kinase (CaMKII) at two different sites: Ser[16] and Thr[17], respectively, both *in vitro* and in the intact heart.[1–3] In the intact heart, whereas the physiological role of the PKA-dependent pathway of PHL phosphorylation has strong experimental support, the functional meaning of the CaMKII-dependent pathway remains unclear, particularly in the absence of β-adrenoceptor stimulation. In fact, several attempts to activate the CaMKII pathway of PHL phosphorylation in the absence of high cAMP levels have failed.[4,5] The present experiments were undertaken to gain further insight into the physiological role of Thr[17] phosphorylation of PHL. With this purpose experiments were designed in the isolated functioning heart in an attempt to know whether simultaneous activation of CaMKII and inhibition of PHL phosphatase produced an increase in Thr[17] phosphorylation in the absence of β-adrenoceptor stimulation and if the increase in Thr[17] phosphorylation that occurred was associated with a positive lusitropic effect, both in the presence and in the absence of β-adrenoceptor stimulation.

METHODS

Experiments were performed in isolated hearts from Wistar rats. Perfusion of the hearts, quantification of ^{32}P incorporation into PHL and detection of site-specific phosphorylated PHL were performed as previously described.[3,5]

RESULTS AND DISCUSSION

FIGURE 1 shows overall results of PHL phosphorylation, immunodetection of site-specific phosphorylated PHL, and decrease in half–relaxation time ($t_{1/2}$) of experiments performed in the absence and presence of 30 nM isoproterenol given simultaneously with different interventions that gradually decreased the Ca^{2+} supply to the cell. The de-

[a] Established Investigators of Consejo Nacional de Investigaciones Científicas y Técnicas (CONICET, Argentina).

[b] Corresponding author. Phone: 54-21-834833; fax: 54-21-25-5861; e-mail: cicme@isis.unlp.edu.ar

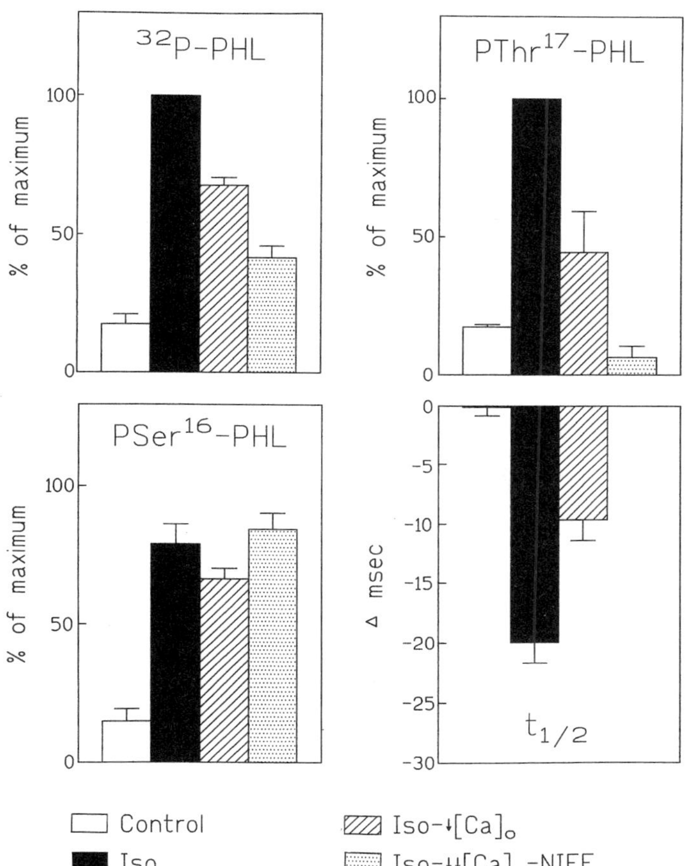

FIGURE 1. Overall results of ^{32}P incorporation into PHL ($n = 3$) and of the immunodetection of the site-specific phosphorylated PHL (PSer^{16}-PHL and PThr^{17}-PHL) ($n = 3$) obtained from hearts perfused in the absence and presence of 30 nM isoproterenol (Iso), isoproterenol + low $[Ca]_o$ (0.25mM), and isoproterenol + low $[Ca]_o$ (0.07mM) + the calcium channel blocker nifedipine (400 nM). Results are expressed as percentage of the maximal signal achieved in each experimental series. The **lower right panel** shows mean ± SEM of half–relaxation time ($t_{1/2}$), expressed as differences with respect to control values, obtained from the same hearts used in the immunodetection experiments.

crease in Ca^{2+} supply to the cell decreased PHL phosphorylation. This decrease was due exclusively to a decrease in Thr^{17} phosphorylation and was associated with a significant reduction of the positive lusitropic effect evoked by β-adrenoceptor stimulation. The $t_{1/2}$ decreased by 20 ±1.8 ms after isoproterenol administration and only 9.7 ± 1.7 ms after administration of isoproterenol at low $[Ca]_o$. FIGURE 2 shows the overall results of the experiments in which $[Ca]_o$ was increased in the absence and presence of the phosphatase inhibitor okadaic acid. Immunodetection of site-specific phosphorylated

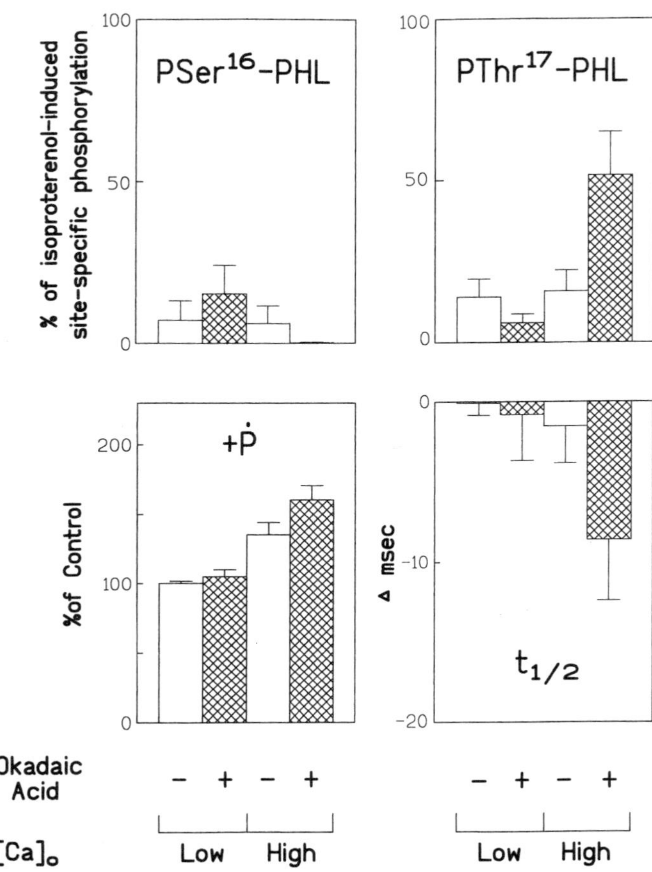

FIGURE 2. Overall results of the experiments in which $[Ca]_o$ was increased in the absence and presence of the phosphatase inhibitor okadaic acid. **Upper panels:** Mean ± SEM values of the immunodetected phosphorylated sites (P-Ser^{16} and P-Thr^{17}) of PHL obtained after the densitometric analysis of the signal of four immunoblots. Results are expressed as percentage of the Iso-induced site-specific phosphorylation, run in parallel. **Lower panels:** Mechanical parameters (maximal rate of pressure development, $+\dot{P}$) and $t_{1/2}$ of the same experimental series.

PHL (upper panel) showed that increasing $[Ca]_o$ increased Thr^{17} phosphorylation only when okadaic acid was present. This increase in Thr^{17} phosphorylation was associated with a positive lusitropic effect (decrease in $t_{1/2}$, lower right panel). The increase in maximal rate of pressure development ($+\dot{P}$) produced by increasing $[Ca]_o$ (lower left panel) was slightly greater in the presence of okadaic acid than in its absence. However, this difference did not attain significant levels. Similar results were obtained when $[Ca]_o$ was increased in the presence of other interventions, such as acidosis, known to produce a type-1 phosphatase inhibition.[6] The results indicate (1) that Thr^{17} phosphorylation may be detected in the absence of β-adrenoceptor stimulation when PHL phosphatases are inhibited; (2) phosphorylation of Thr^{17} was associated with a positive lusitropic effect both in the presence and absence of isoproterenol. The experiments provide evidence supporting the idea that phosphorylation of Thr^{17} of phospholamban relies on a basic mechanism underlying any phosphorylation process—i.e., the relative degree of protein kinase and phosphatase activities. The reported inhibition of PP1 by a PKA-dependent mechanism[7] gives a possible clue to explain why CaMKII-dependent PHL phosphorylation had previously been detected only in the presence of high intracellular cAMP levels.[4,5]

REFERENCES

1. SIMMERMAN, H. K. *et al.* 1986. Sequence analysis of phospholamban: Identification of phosphorylation sites and two major structural domains. J. Biol. Chem. **261:** 13333–13341.
2. WEGENER, A. D. *et al.* 1989. Phospholamban phosphorylation in intact ventricles: Phosphorylation of serine 16 and threonine 17 in response to beta-adrenergic stimulation. J. Biol. Chem. **264:** 11468–11474.
3. MUNDIÑA-WEILENMANN, C. *et al.* 1996. Immunodetection of phosphorylation sites gives new insights into the mechanisms underlying phospholamban phosphorylation in the intact heart. J. Biol. Chem. **271:** 33561–33567.
4. LINDENMANN, J. P. & A. M. WATANABE. 1985. Phosphorylation of phospholamban in the intact myocardium. Role of Ca^{2+}-calmodulin-dependent mechanisms. J. Biol. Chem. **260:** 4516–4525.
5. VITTONE, L. *et al.* 1990. cAMP and calcium-dependent mechanisms of phospholamban phosphorylation in the intact hearts. Am. J. Physiol. **258:** H318–H325.
6. MUNDIÑA-WEILENMANN, C. *et al.* 1996. Effects of acidosis on phosphorylation of phospholamban and troponin I in rat cardiac muscle. Am. J. Physiol. **270:** C107–C114.
7. COHEN, P. & P. T. W. COHEN. 1989. Protein phosphatases come of age. J. Biol. Chem. **264:** 21435–21438.

A Quantitative Immunoassay for the Measurement of Phospholamban Levels and Phosphorylation States

Measurement of Phospholamban Levels in Transgenic Mouse Hearts

ERNEST J. MAYER,[a] GEORGE M. SAVAGE, AND ROBERT G. JOHNSON, JR.

Merck Research Laboratories, WP 38T-1, West Point, Pennsylvania 19486, USA

Phospholamban (PLB) plays a critical role in cardiac function by regulating calcium uptake via inhibition of the calcium ATPase, which is reversed by phosphorylation. Two critical factors affecting regulation are the stoichiometry between calcium ATPase and PLB protein levels and the percentage of PLB that is phosphorylated.[1] Together these parameters are critical determinants of cardiac contractility. However, the relationship between these parameters and the abnormal cardiac contraction and relaxation observed in patients with heart failure is not understood. To address this question it is necessary to accurately measure the levels of calcium ATPase and PLB along with the phosphorylation state of PLB from human clinical biopsies from early- to end-stage heart failure. To achieve these goals, dot blot (DB) and Western blot (WB) assays are being developed to quantitate the level of PLB in failing hearts and to ultimately determine the effect of heart failure on PLB's basal phosphorylation state. While WBs have the advantage of separating the desired protein from contaminating components in crude cardiac homogenates, DBs allow greater throughput, accuracy, and precision. In addition, quantitation is not complicated by PLB's multiple oligomeric forms. To distinguish between phosphorylated and nonphosphorylated PLB, two antibodies were used: mAb 1D11,[2] which recognizes an epitope within PLB 7-17 and has affinity toward PLB regardless of its phosphorylation state, and Ab 285 (generated against PLB 9-19Y Ser-PO_4), which selectively binds to PLB when it is phosphorylated at Ser^{16}. PLB protein levels were measured in crude cardiac homogenates from wild-type, transgenic PLB-knockout and PLB-overexpressing (OE) mice[3] using mAb 1D11 to calibrate the assays.

RESULTS

When phosphorylated and nonphosphorylated synthetic PLB (standardized by amino acid analysis) was used as the standard, signals of equivalent intensity were obtained on DB (FIG. 1(a)) and WB (FIG. 1(b)) when probed with mAb 1D11. Of note, synthetic PLB$\pm PO_4$, unlike native PLB found in cardiac sarcoplasmic reticulum (SR), forms a ladder of high-order protein aggregates that do not dissociate even upon boil-

[a] Corresponding author. Phone: 215-652-3761; fax: 215-652-9275; e-mail: ernie__mayer@merck.com

ing. Preliminary experiments suggest that these differences may possibly be due to the absence of endogeneous lipids, since synthetic PLB does not form a ladder of aggregates when coelectrophoresed with skeletal muscle SR (data not shown). In addition, phosphorylated PLB has a slightly slower mobility on SDS-PAGE gels,[4] which is exaggerated by the higher molecular-weight aggregates. Polyclonal Ab 285 exhibited a specificity of greater than 100-fold toward phosphorylated PLB versus nonphosphorylated PLB (FIG. 1(a)). In fact, nonphosphorylated PLB is not detectable on the WB when Ab 285 is used. Interestingly, Ab 285 does recognize a small amount of PLB in the canine cardiac SR preparation, which runs at a slightly higher molecular mass, suggesting that some phosphorylated PLB is present despite the absence of phosphatase inhibitors during its preparation.

To test the ability to distinguish between small differences in PLB expression levels,

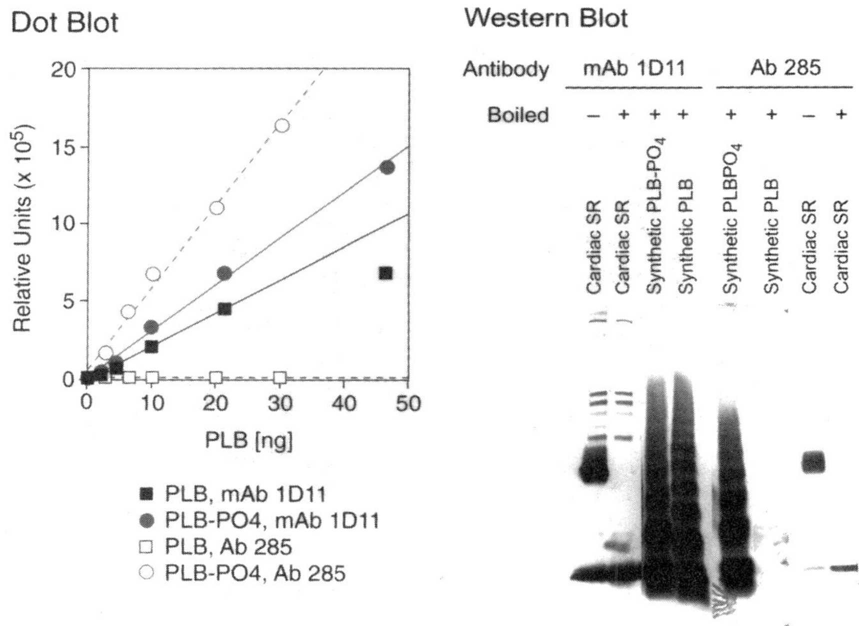

FIGURE 1. Left: Dot blot quantification of synthetic PLB±PO_4. Samples of synthetic PLB±PO_4 (0–100 ng/70 µl) were loaded in triplicate onto 0.05 µm nitrocellulose membranes in a Bio-Rad DB apparatus. Vacuum was applied at 5 inches Hg and the membrane rinsed with 100 µL 20 mM tris/HCl pH 7.4, 150 mM NaCl (TBS)/well. Membranes were blocked overnight with 3% BSA in TBS, then rinsed two times with TBS/0.05% Tween 20. Membranes were incubated with mAb 1D11 or Ab 285 for 3 h at room temperature in 3% BSA/TBS and then rinsed three times with TBS/Tween. Each membrane was incubated with 10 µCi ^{125}I-Protein A for 2 h, rinsed four times with TBS/Tween, dried, exposed to a Phosphoimager screen overnight, and analyzed with Microsoft Excel. **Right:** Western blot analysis of synthetic PLB±PO_4 and canine cardiac SR. Cardiac sarcoplasmic reticulum (1 µg) or synthetic PLB±PO_4 (30 ng) before and after boiling was run on a 10–20% Tricine mini-gel, then transferred to a nitrocellulose membrane. Protein was visualized by the same protocol as used in the dot blot.

TABLE 1. Levels (ng PLB/μg Protein) of Total PLB in Transgenic Mouse Cardiac Samples[a]

	Knock Out	Wild-Type	Hetero. OE	Homo. OE
Dot blot	0.00	0.97±0.13	3.99±0.75	8.80±1.39
Western blot	0.00	1.11	2.93	5.46

[a] Mouse hearts were excised, freeze clamped, homogenized in solubilization buffer (50 mM $NaPO_4$, pH 7.0, 10 mM NaEDTA, 10 mM NaF, 50 mM *n*-octyl-β-D glucopyranoside, 1 mM AEBSF, and 1 mM DTT) under liquid N_2 and then thawed prior to centrifugation in a microfuge for 5 minutes to remove insoluble material. Protein levels were quantitated using an Amido black assay with BSA as a standard. Samples were measured at several protein concentrations in the linear range of the synthetic PLB standard curve (0.5–2.0 μg protein/well). PLB was detected using ^{125}I-mAb 1D11, which significantly reduced but did not eliminate nonspecific binding that was observed when mAb 1D11 followed by ^{125}I-protein A was used.

crude cardiac homogenates prepared from wild-type, PLB knockout and PLB overexpressing mice were analyzed. Since PLB runs as multiple oligomeric species on WBs and the number of sample wells is limited, the DB was selected for quantitation. For comparative purposes a representative sample using WB was analyzed. Results, summarized in TABLE 1, were normalized so that the level of PLB in cardiac homogenates from knockout mice was zero. A low background signal is present and is thought to result from nonspecific binding of ^{125}I-mAb 1D11 to the nitrocellulose membrane. PLB levels in knockout mice were set to zero since (1) these mice lack the PLB gene, (2) homogenates run on WBs did not exhibit a band at the appropriate molecular weight, and (3) rabbit skeletal muscle SR homogenates also exhibited this low-level background on DBs. Results from these experiments indicate wild-type mouse hearts contain 0.16 nmoles PLB/mg protein, which represents approximately 0.1% of total protein. The relative expression of PLB (compared to wild-type) in transgenic mouse hearts was similar to previous values;[3] PLB-knockout (0); wild-type (1X); heterozygous OE (2X); and homozygous OE (4X) (Kranias, personal communication). These results represent the first quantitation of PLB levels in transgenic mice.

CONCLUSIONS

PLB levels were determined using synthetic PLB as a standard in crude cardiac homogenates from wild-type and transgenic mice using mAb 1D11 in immunoblot assays. The phosphorylation-specific antibody 285 exhibited a high level of selectivity on WBs and DBs and will enable this work to be extended to include the determination of PLB phosphorylation levels. Finally, these techniques can be used to simultaneously quantitative calcium ATPase to provide an accurate measure of protein stochiometry and allow an assessment of the interrelationship between pertinent proteins of cardiac contractility. In summary, these assays provide a framework for quantitating PLB expression levels and its phosphorylation state.

ACKNOWLEDGMENTS

We thank Dr. Bo Pan for his assistance in the preparation of the mouse hearts and Dr. William Hucke for his assistance in preparation of Ab 285.

REFERENCES

1. Hasenfuss, G. *et al.* 1997. Calcium handling proteins in the failing heart. Basic Res. Cardiol. **92** (Suppl. 1): 87–93.
2. Mayer, E. J. *et al.* 1996. Biochemical and biophysical comparison of native and chemically synthesized phospholamban and a monomeric phospholamban analog. Biol. Chem. **271:** 1669–1667.
3. Kadambi, V. J. *et al.* 1997. Cardiac-specific overexpression of phospholamban alters calcium kinetics and resultant cardiomyocyte mechanics in transgenic mice. J. Clin. Invest. **97:** 533–539.
4. Cuifeng, L. *et al.* 1990. Immunological detection of phospholamban phosphorylation states facilitates the description of the mechanism of phosphorylation and dephosphorylation. Biochem. **29:** 4535–4540.

Cytosolic Domain of Phospholamban Remains Associated with the Ca-ATPase Following Phosphorylation by cAMP-dependent Protein Kinase[a]

SEWITE NEGASH, HONGYE SUN, QING YAO, SWEE YONG GOH, DIANA J. BIGELOW, AND THOMAS C. SQUIER[b]

Department of Biochemistry, Cell, and Molecular Biology, University of Kansas, Lawrence, Kansas 66045-2106, USA

The calcium transport activity of the Ca-ATPase in cardiac sarcoplasmic reticulum (SR) membranes is regulated by phospholamban (PLB), which represents a major target of the β-adrenergic cascade in the heart. Upon phosphorylation of PLB by cAMP-dependent protein kinase (PKA), the calcium-dependent ATPase activity is enhanced at submicromolar calcium concentrations. The inhibition of ATPase activity by PLB involves direct contact interactions between PLB and the Ca-ATPase, since the cytosolic domain of PLB has previously been shown to directly interact with a sequence near the nucleotide binding cleft of the Ca-ATPase.[1–3] Furthermore, it has been suggested that the phosphorylation of PLB may result in the dissociation of its cytosolic domain from the Ca-ATPase.[1] There are, however, no direct measurements in biological membranes containing the Ca-ATPase of the structural alterations in the cytosolic domain of PLB upon phosphorylation by PKA.

To investigate possible alterations in the physical relationship between PLB and the Ca-ATPase that correlate with the phosphorylation of PLB in biological membranes, we have coreconstituted purified preparations of the Ca-ATPase and PLB in liposomes composed of SR lipids. The calcium-dependence of the ATPase activity of the Ca-ATPase reconstituted in the presence of PLB is analogous to that observed in native cardiac SR membranes (FIG. 1). Likewise, subsequent to the phosphorylation of PLB by PKA one observes a similar activation of the Ca-ATPase in both native cardiac and reconstituted preparations, indicating that the inhibitory interaction between PLB and the Ca-ATPase in these reconstituted preparations is physiologically relevant. To directly monitor the structural coupling between PLB and the Ca-ATPase, we have reconstituted a fluorescently labeled PLB containing dansyl-chloride at Lys_3 in either SR lipids only or in the presence of the Ca-ATPase. Dansyl-chloride was chosen, since its large Stokes shift precludes homotransfer between chromophores located on adjacent PLB monomers, and allows an unambiguous measurement of the rotational dynamics of PLB in these functionally reconstituted membranes. This fluorescent derivative of PLB inhibits the Ca-ATPase in an analogous manner to that observed in cardiac SR membranes (FIG. 1), indicating that dansyl-chloride does not interfere with either spe-

[a] This work was supported by Grant GM46837 from the National Institutes of Health.

[b] Corresponding author. Phone: 785-864-4008; fax: 785-864-5321; e-mail: TCSQUIER@KUHUB.CC.UKANS.ED

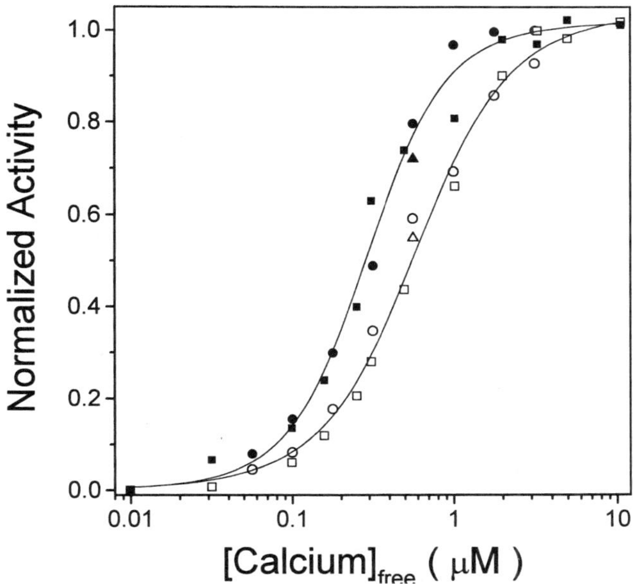

FIGURE 1. Functional Reconstitution of PLB with the Ca-ATPase. Calcium-dependent ATPase activity of cardiac SR Ca-ATPase (□, ■) and Ca-ATPase purified from skeletal SR and coreconstituted with PLB (○, ●) or with PLB labeled with dansyl chloride (Δ, ▲) in the absence (□, ○, Δ) or presence (■, ○, ▲) of PKA. ATP hydrolysis activity was determined in a solution containing 0.1 M KCl, 1 mM EGTA, 5 mM $MgCl_2$, 1 μM CCCP, 2 μM valinomycin, 2 μM A23187, 50 mM MOPS (pH 7.0), and sufficient calcium to yield the indicated concentration. Protein concentration was 10 μg/mL. Activation of the Ca-ATPase involved the addition of 10 μg/mL PKA and 1 μM cAMP. Following incubation of the mixture for 10 min at 25°C, 5 mM ATP was added to start the reaction. Maximal ATPase activities were 1.0 ± 0.1 μmol P_i mg^{-1} min^{-1} for cardiac SR Ca-ATPase (□,■) and 3.9 ± 0.1 μmol P_i mg^{-1} min^{-1} for the Ca-ATPase coreconstituted with PLB (○,●).

cific functional interactions between PLB and the Ca-ATPase or with the binding and phosphorylation of PLB by PKA.

We have used frequency-domain fluorescence spectroscopy to investigate the functional interaction between the cytosolic domain of PLB and the Ca-ATPase, and possible alterations in their association subsequent to the phosphorylation of PLB by PKA. The average fluorescence lifetime ($\bar{\tau}$) of dansyl-chloride in PLB reconstituted in SR lipids ($\bar{\tau}$= 5.3 ± 0.1 ns) is much smaller than that of PLB coreconstituted with the Ca-ATPase ($\bar{\tau}$= 7.4 ± 0.2 ns), suggesting that the amino-terminus of PLB is in a structurally different environment when PLB binds to the Ca-ATPase. Upon phosphorylation of PLB coreconstituted with the Ca-ATPase we observe a large decrease in $\bar{\tau}$, suggesting that there are substantial alterations in the polarity in the environment surrounding dansyl-chloride. In contrast, $\bar{\tau}$ is insensitive to the phosphorylation of PLB by PKA when PLB is reconstituted only with SR lipids. These latter results indicate that there are structural changes in the vicinity of Lys_3 upon phosphorylation of Ser_{16} that correspond to alterations in the structural coupling between PLB and the Ca-

ATPase, and that phosphorylation itself does not significantly alter the polarity in the vicinity of dansyl-chloride at Lys_3 in PLB.

Complementary measurements of the fluorescence anisotropy of dansyl-chloride permit the resolution of possible alterations in the interaction between PLB and the Ca-ATPase. We have therefore measured the modulated anisotropy and differential phase between 2 MHz and 100 MHz of dansyl-chloride either coreconstituted with the Ca-ATPase or in the presence of SR lipids only. We find that the rotational correlation times of PLB are similar, irrespective of whether PLB is reconstituted in the presence of SR lipids only or coreconstituted with the Ca-ATPase (TABLE 1), suggesting that the structures of the cytosolic domain are very similar in both preparations. Likewise, there is a significant residual anisotropy (r_∞) associated with PLB in both preparations, indicating that the rotational dynamics of the amino-terminal domain of PLB is highly restricted. These latter results suggest that the amino-terminus of PLB is structurally coupled to the transmembrane domain through stable secondary structural elements. The larger residual anisotropy observed when PLB is reconstituted in the presence of the Ca-ATPase relative to that observed for PLB in lipids suggests that contact interactions between PLB and the Ca-ATPase further restrict the rotational mobility of the amino-terminal domain of PLB. These latter results are consistent with previous measurements that indicate a direct structural interaction between PLB and the Ca-ATPase.[1]

Consistent with earlier proposals that suggest that the phosphorylation of PLB may either modify the secondary structure of PLB or alter oligomeric associations between PLB monomers,[4,5] we find that the phosphorylation of PLB reconstituted in SR lipids only by PKA results in a substantial reduction in r_∞. In contrast, phosphorylation of PLB coreconstituted with the Ca-ATPase by PKA does not significantly alter either the rotational dynamics or residual anisotropy of PLB. These latter results indicate that the cytoplasmic domain of PLB remains tightly associated with the Ca-ATPase subsequent to its phosphorylation, and the corresponding activation of the transport activity of the Ca-ATPase is not the result of the dissociation of PLB from

TABLE 1. Rotational Dynamics of PLB Reconstituted in SR Lipids[a]

Sample	Conditions	$g_1 \times r_0$	ϕ_1 (ns)	$g_2 \times r_0$	ϕ_2 (ns)	r_∞
PLB	Control	0.119 (0.001)	0.8 (0.1)	0.094 (0.003)	7.8 (0.4)	**0.043 (0.003)**
	+PKA	0.104 (0.003)	1.2 (0.1)	0.098 (0.003)	9.0 (0.6)	**0.028 (0.002)**
PLB + CaATPase	Control	0.102 (0.009)	1.2 (0.1)	0.091 (0.005)	7.7 (0.3)	**0.083 (0.001)**
	+PKA	0.097 (0.011)	1.1 (0.3)	0.090 (0.008)	8.3 (0.3)	**0.082 (0.001)**

[a]Frequency-domain fluorescence anisotropy measurements of the rotational dynamics of dansyl-chloride bound to Lys_3 in PLB either reconstituted with SR lipids or in the presence of the Ca-ATPase. The reported correlation times (ϕ_1 and ϕ_2), their associated amplitudes ($g_1 \times r_0$ and $g_2 \times r_0$), and the residual anisotropy (r_∞) are obtained from a multiexponential fit to the experimental data using frequency-independent errors of 0.2° and 0.005 for the differential phase and modulated anisotropy, respectively. *Experimental conditions:* 0.1 M KCl, 5 mM $MgCl_2$, 100 μM EGTA, 103 μM $CaCl_2$, 50 mM MOPS (pH 7.0), and 5 mM ATP and when indicated subsequent to the addition of 40 μg/mL PKA and 1 μM cAMP. In all cases the free calcium concentration was 0.5 μM. Samples contain 50 μg mL^{-1} reconstituted sample. Temperature was 25°C.

the Ca-ATPase. These results indicate that the reduced lifetime of dansyl-PLB reconstituted with the Ca-ATPase upon phosphorylation by PKA (see earlier) is the result of alterations in the local environment around Lys_3 in PLB that results from the altered conformation of PLB bound to the Ca-ATPase.

REFERENCES

1. James, P., M. Inui, M. Tada, M. Chiesi & E. Carafoli. 1989. Nature and site of phospholamban regulation of hte Ca^{2+} pump of sarcoplasmic reticulum. Nature **342:** 90–92.
2. Toyofuku, T., K. Kurzydlowski, M. Tada & D. H. MacLennan. 1994. Amino acids Lys-Asp-Asp-Lys-Pro-Val402 in the Ca^{2+}-ATPase of cardiac sarcoplasmic reticulum are critical for functional association with phospholamban. J. Biol. Chem. **269:** 22929–22932.
3. Negash, S., L. T. Chen, D. J. Bigelow & T. C. Squier. 1996. Phosphorylation of phospholamban by cAMP-dependent protein kinase enhances interactions between Ca-ATPase polypeptide chains in cardiac sarcoplasmic reticulum membranes. Biochemistry **35:** 11247–11259.
4. Mayer, E. J., E. McKenna, V. M. Garsky, C. J. Burke, H. Mach, C. R. Middaugh, M. Sardana, J. S. Smith & R. G. Johnson. 1996. Biochemical and biophysical comparison of native and chemically synthesized phospholamban and a monomeric phospholamban analog. J. Biol. Chem. **271:** 1669–1677.
5. Cornea, R. L., L. R. Jones, J. M. Autry & D. D. Thomas. 1997. Mutation and phosphorylation change the oligomeric structure of phospholamban in lipid bilayers. Biochemistry **36:** 2960–2967.

Immunodetection of Phosphorylation Sites of Phospholamban in Aortic Smooth Muscle

Effects of Sodium Nitroprusside

LETICIA VITTONE,[a,c,d] CECILIA MUNDIÑA-WEILENMANN,[a,d] MATILDE SAID,[a] G. RINALDI,[b,d] GLADYS CHIAPPE DE CINGOLANI,[a,d] AND ALICIA MATTIAZZI[a,d]

[a]*Centro de Investigaciones Cardiovasculares, Facultad de Ciencias Médicas, Universidad Nacional de La Plata, La Plata, Argentina*
[b]*Cátedra de Fisiología, Departamento de Ciencias Biológicas, Facultad de Ciencias Exactas, Universidad Nacional de La Plata, La Plata, Argentina*

The importance of phospholamban (PHL) phosphorylation in the regulation of cardiac contractility and relaxation is well established. PHL also has been shown to be present in smooth muscle.[1,2] The role of PHL in the function of this type of muscle is, however, less well defined. Some evidence suggests that activation of cGMP-dependent protein kinase (PKG) in vascular smooth muscle has a pivotal role in the decrease of $[Ca]_i$ caused by activation of the sarcoplasmic-endoplasmic reticulum Ca^{2+} ATPase (SERCA2) by phosphorylation of PHL.[1-3] More recent experiments in PHL-deficient mice have emphasized the role of PHL in the regulation of smooth muscle contractility. In these experiments, however, the effect of PHL on relaxation was less clear.[4] In the present experiments, specific antibodies to PHL and to Ser^{16}- and Thr^{17}-phosphorylated PHL peptides were used in cat aorta to determine (1) the presence of PHL and (2) the effect of administration of nitroprusside (NP) to activate the PKG-dependent pathway on phosphorylation of Ser^{16} and Thr^{17} residues of PHL. The effect of NP on mechanical relaxation was also studied. It will be shown that NP produced a dose-dependent phosphorylation of Ser^{16} residue of PHL and that this phosphorylation was associated with its relaxant effect on the cat aorta.

METHODS

Experiments were performed in aortas isolated from adult cats. Mechanical behavior was measured as previously described.[5] Isolation of SR membranes was performed for smooth muscle according to Levitsky *et al.*,[6] and as previously described in our own laboratory,[7] for cardiac muscle. Specific antibodies to PHL and to Ser^{16}- and Thr^{17}-phosphorylated PHL peptides were used using the technique previously described.[7]

[c] Address for correspondence: Dr. L. Vittone, Centro de Investigaciones Cardiovasculares, 60, 120, 1900, La Plata, Argentina. Phone: 54-21-83-4833; fax: 54-21-25-5861; e-mail: cicme@isis.unlp.edu.ar

[d] Established Investigators of Consejo National de Investigaciones Cientificas y Técnicas (CONICET, Argentina).

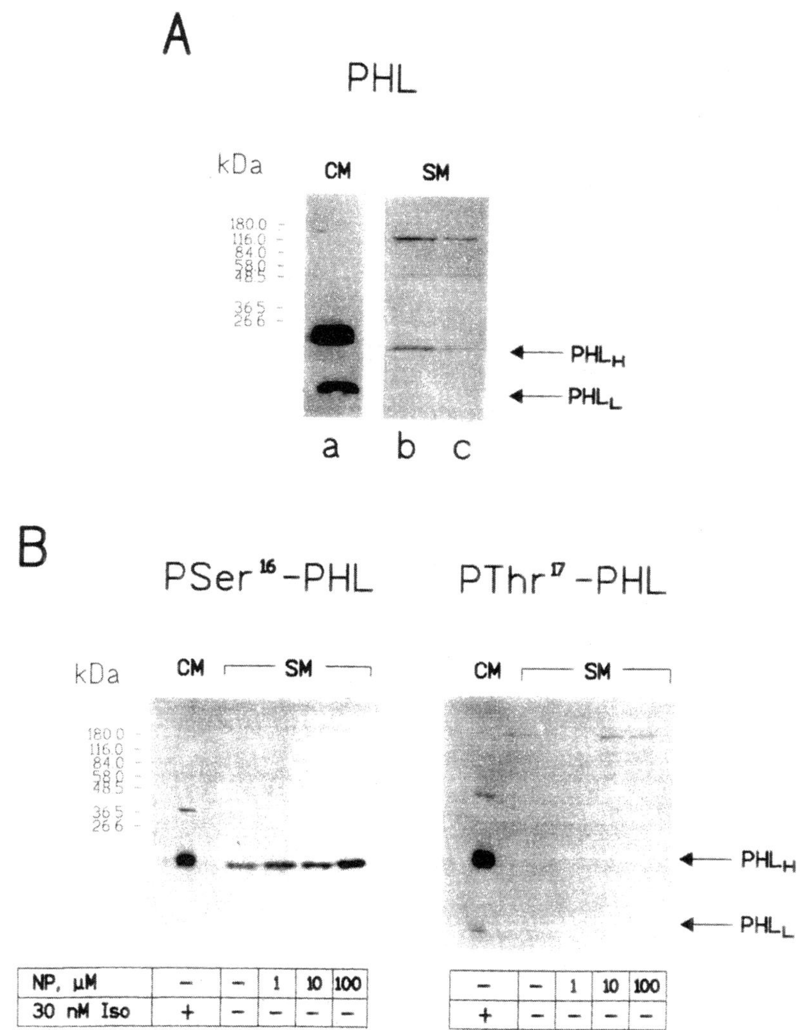

NP, µM	–	–	1	10	100
30 nM Iso	+	–	–	–	–

–	–	1	10	100
+	–	–	–	–

FIGURE 1. Panel A. Immunoblots of microsomes prepared from rat heart or cat aorta. Twenty µg of cardiac microsomes (CM, *lane a*) were electrophoresed simultaneously with 50 µg *(lane b)* and 25 µg *(lane c)* of vascular smooth muscle (SM) microsomes in order to compare the relative amounts of phospholamban (PHL) in both tissues. Proteins were transferred to PVDF membranes, and blots were probed with the monoclonal antibody to PHL (1:5000). Antibody binding was visualized using a chemiluminescence detection kit. **Panel B.** Effects of increasing sodium nitroprusside (NP) concentrations on Ser^{16} and Thr^{17} phosphorylation of PHL in smooth muscle.

Fifty µg of SM microsomes were electrophoresed and transferred to PVDF membranes. Blots were probed with polyclonal antibodies to Ser^{16} and Thr^{17} phosphorylated PHL phosphopeptides (1:5000). Antibody binding was visualized as in Panel A. NP produced a dose-dependent increase in Ser^{16} phosphorylation without affecting the phosphorylation of Thr^{17}. In the first lane of each blot, isoproterenol-induced phosphorylation of Ser^{16} and Thr^{17} in CM microsomes is shown for comparison.

TABLE 1. Overall Results of the Mechanical and Biochemical Experiments[a]

	Relaxation % of Control	PSer^{16}-PHL % of Control
1 μM NP	51.5 ± 9.5 $n = 4$	172.3 ± 1.3 $n = 2$
10 μM NP	74.3 ± 9.0 $n = 4$	268.2 ± 44.1 $n = 4$
100 μM NP	81.2 ± 7.3 $n = 4$	250.4 ± 56.8 $n = 4$

[a] The results are expressed as percent of control. For the mechanical data, control was the difference between the maximal force in response to KCl 80 mM and the force remaining after repeated washings at the end of the experiments. For the biochemical data the control for PSer^{16}-PHL phosphorylation was the value of PSer^{16}-PHL of the sample not treated with NP, which was run in parallel with the samples treated with the different NP concentrations in each experiment.

RESULTS AND DISCUSSION

Immunoblots of SR membranes probed with the monoclonal antibody to PHL, showing the presence of PHL in cat aortic rings, are depicted in panel A of FIGURE 1. Panel B shows immunoblots of SR membrane vesicles obtained from aortic rings superfused with different NP concentrations to stimulate the PKG cascade of PHL phosphorylation. NP induced a dose-dependent phosphorylation of Ser^{16} residue of PHL without affecting Thr^{17} phosphorylation. The increase in Ser^{16} phosphorylation was associated with the relaxant effect of NP on aortic rings (TABLE 1).

In vitro studies of bovine pulmonary artery have suggested that both PKA and PKG phosphorylated PHL at the same Ser^{16} residue. This conclusion was drawn from the discovery that the stimulatory effect of both kinases on SERCA2 was not additive.[3] The availability of specific antibodies against the phosphorylated Ser^{16} and Thr^{17} phosphopeptides of PHL allowed us to determine that stimulation of the PKG-cascade of PHL phosphorylation evoked an increase in Ser^{16} phosphorylation. This increase appeared to be associated with a significant relaxant effect on the aortic rings. To our knowledge this is the first direct evidence of phosphorylation of a Ser^{16} site by stimulation of the PKG-cascade and of its association with a relaxant effect in an *in vivo* preparation.

REFERENCES

1. CORNWELL, T. L., K. B. PRYZWANSKY, T. A. WYATT & T. M. LINCOLN. 1991. Regulation of sarcoplasmic reticulum protein phosphorylation by localized cyclic GMP–dependent protein kinase in vascular smooth muscle cells. Mol. Pharmacol. **40:** 923–931.
2. KARCZEWSKI, P., M. KELM, M. HARTMANN & J. SCHRADER. 1992. Role of phospholamban in NO/EDRF-induced relaxation in rat aorta. Life Sci. **51:** 1205–1210.
3. RAEYMAEKERS, L., F. HOFMANN & R. CASTEELS. 1988. Cyclic GMP-dependent protein kinase phosphorylates phospholamban in isolated sarcoplasmic reticulum from cardiac and smooth muscle. Biochem. J. **252:** 269–273.
4. LALLI, J., J. HARRER, W. LUO, E. KRANIAS & R. PAUL. 1997. Targeted ablation of the phospholamban gene is associated with a marked decrease in sensitivity in aortic smooth muscle. Circ. Res. **80:** 506–513.

5. RINALDI, G. J. & H. E. CINGOLANI. 1983. The effect of substituted sydnonimines on coronary smooth muscle relaxation and cyclic guanosine monophosphate levels. Circulation **68:** 1315–1320.
6. LEVITSKY, D. O., M. CLERGUE, F. LAMBERT, M. V. SOUPONITSKAYA, T. H. LE JEMTEL, Y. LECARPENTIER & A. LOMPRÉ. 1993. Sarcoplasmic reticulum calcium transport and Ca^{2+}-ATPase gene expression in thoracic and abdominal aortas of normotensive and spontaneously hypertensive rats. J. Biol. Chem. **268:** 8325–8331.
7. MUNDIÑA-WEILENMANN, C., L. VITTONE, M. ORTALE, G. CHIAPPE DE CINGOLANI & A. MATTIAZZI. 1996. Immunodetection of phosphorylation sites gives new insights into the mechanisms underlying phospholamban phosphorylation in the intact heart. J. Biol. Chem. **271:** 33561–33567.

Phospholamban Gene Dosage Effects in Chemically Permeabilized Mouse Cardiac Muscle

RICHARD T. WIEDMANN,[a,b] BO-SHENG PAN,[a] EVANGELIA G. KRANIAS,[c] SHERRI MOTZEL,[d] AND ROBERT G. JOHNSON, JR.[a]

Departments of [a]Pharmacology and [d]Laboratory Animal Resources, Merck Research Laboratories, West Point, Pennsylvania 19486, USA

[c]Department of Pharmacology and Cell Biophysics, University of Cincinnati, College of Medicine, Cincinnati, Ohio 45267, USA

Phospholamban (PLB) regulates cardiac sarcoplasmic reticulum (SR) Ca^{2+} pump activity by decreasing the apparent Ca^{2+} sensitivity of the pump. An increased ratio of PLB to SR Ca^{2+} pump has been implicated in the reduced rate of Ca^{2+} uptake by SR isolated from failing human hearts.[1] Results from studies using mice with genetically altered levels of PLB suggest that the ratio of PLB to cardiac SR Ca^{2+} pump affects the Ca^{2+} sensitivity of the pump as measured by the rate of Ca^{2+} uptake into SR vesicles in cardiac homogenates.[2–4] We studied PLB gene dosage effects on the activity of the cardiac SR Ca^{2+} pump *in situ* by using saponin-permeabilized cardiac muscle from wild-type (WT), PLB-deficient, and transgenic PLB-overexpressing (PLB-OE) mice.

METHODS

The methods used to generate the PLB-deficient mice have been described previously.[2] The PLB-OE mice were generated by inbreeding an existing transgenic line that expresses twice the amount of PLB compared to WT mice.[3] The relative levels of PLB and SR Ca^{2+} pump protein in cardiac homogenates from WT, PLB-deficient, and PLB-OE mice were determined by Western blot analysis. Cardiac right-ventricular trabeculae were isolated from WT, PLB-deficient, and PLB-OE mice and treated either with 50 μg/mL of saponin to permeabilize the sarcolemmae, but leave the SR and myofilaments functional, or with 1% Triton X-100 to permeabilize all of the membranes and leave only the myofilaments functional. The SR of the saponin-permeabilized trabeculae were allowed to load (i.e., accumulate) Ca^{2+} at a pCa of 7.2 for various durations in the following "loading" solution: 10 mM EGTA, 1.31 mM $CaCl_2$, 5.4 mM Na_2ATP, 15 mM Na_2creatine phosphate, 8.2 mM $MgCl_2$, 47.3 mM KCl, 30 mM imidazole, 1 mM dithiothreitol, 1 mM sodium azide, 10 μM leupeptin, and pH=7.0. Caffeine was then used to induce SR Ca^{2+} release by transferring the trabeculae to a "releasing" solution that had the same composition as the loading solution, but with the following exceptions: 0.1 mM EGTA, 7.6 mM $MgCl_2$, 77.1 mM KCl, 50 mM caffeine, and no added $CaCl_2$. The peak amplitudes of the resulting caffeine-induced tension transients, which

[b]Address for correspondence: Richard T. Wiedmann, Merck Research Laboratories, WP44-B122, West Point, Pennsylvania 19486. Phone: 215-652-3880; fax: 215-652-1658.

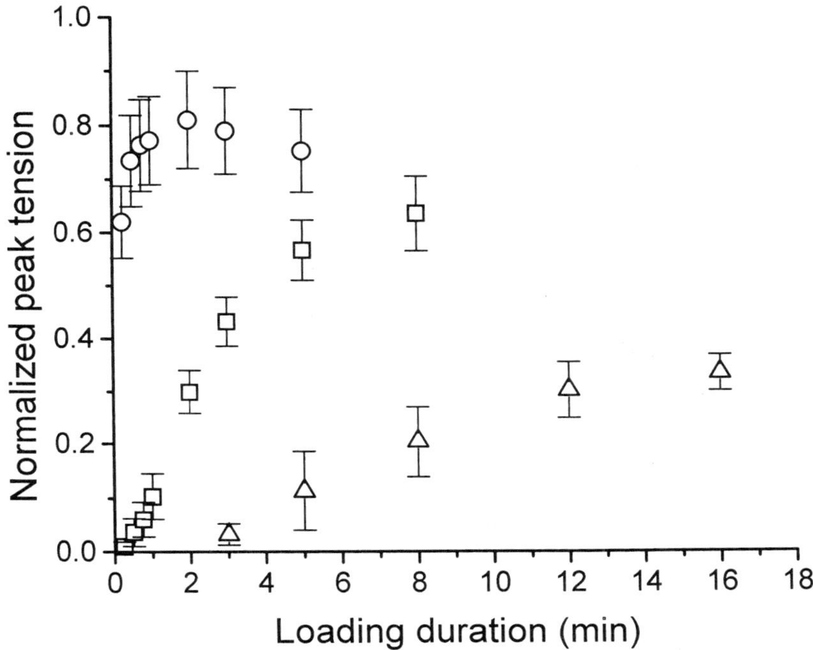

FIGURE 1. Relationship between normalized peak tension of caffeine-induced tension transients and duration of SR Ca^{2+} loading at a pCa of 7.2 for saponin-permeabilized wild-type (□), phospholamban-deficient (○), and phospholamban-overexpressing (Δ) mouse cardiac right ventricular trabeculae. Peak tension in response to 50 mM caffeine following each loading duration was normalized to the maximum Ca^{2+}-induced tension at a pCa of 4.6. Each symbol represents the mean ± SEM from 6 wild-type, 6 phospholamban-deficient, or 4 phospholamban-overexpressing trabeculae.

were used as indirect measures of the releasable SR Ca^{2+} load, were normalized to the maximum Ca^{2+}-induced tension in the loading solution at a pCa of 4.6 with 50 mM caffeine added. Myofilament Ca^{2+} sensitivity was assessed by determining the tension-pCa relationships of the Triton-permeabilized trabeculae in the aforementioned loading solution but with 50 mM caffeine added and at increasing pCa values. Peak tension at each pCa was normalized to the maximum Ca^{2+}-induced tension generated by each trabecula and the data from each muscle type were fit to the Hill equation: normalized peak tension = $[Ca^{2+}]^n/([Ca^{2+}]^n + K^n)$, where K is the free Ca^{2+} concentration ($[Ca^{2+}]$) yielding half-maximal normalized peak tension and n is the Hill coefficient. All of the experiments were conducted at 22–25°C.

RESULTS AND CONCLUSIONS

Western blot analysis of the cardiac homogenates from the WT, PLB-deficient, and PLB-OE mice revealed a PLB protein ratio of 1:0:4, respectively, with no significant dif-

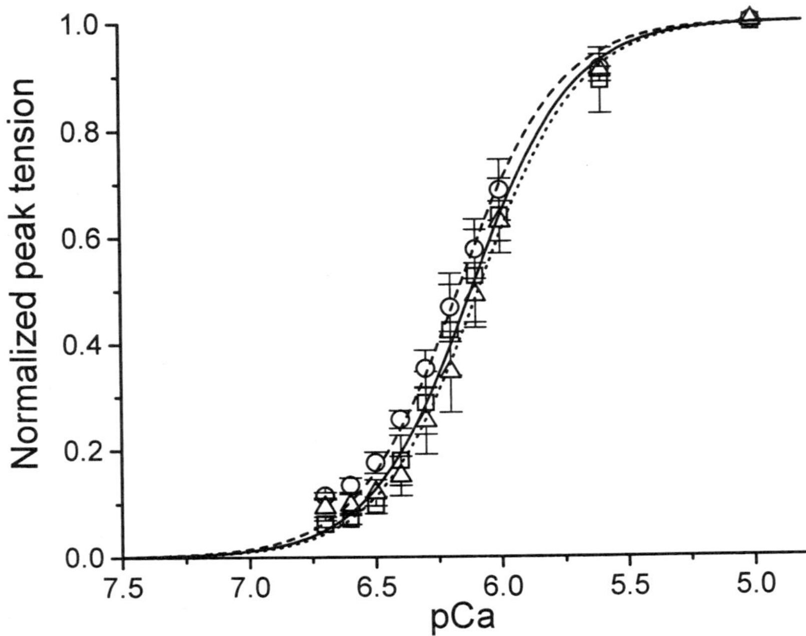

FIGURE 2. Normalized peak tension-pCa relationships of Triton-permeabilized wild-type (□, ____), phospholamban-deficient (○, -----), and phospholamban-overexpressing (Δ, ...) mouse cardiac right ventricular trabeculae. Peak tension at each pCa was normalized to the maximum Ca^{2+}-induced tension for each trabecula. Each *symbol* represents the mean ± SEM from 4 trabeculae and each *curve* is the least-squares fit of each set of data to the Hill equation. The pCa_{50} values (i.e., the pCa value at which normalized tension was half-maximal) were determined to be 5.92, 6.00, and 6.04 for the wild-type, phospholamban-deficient, and phospholamban-overexpressing trabeculae, respectively, and were not statisically different..

ferences in the relative amounts of SR Ca^{2+} pump protein (data not shown). The time-dependence of SR Ca^{2+} loading at a pCa of 7.2 was clearly different for the WT, PLB-deficient, and PLB-OE cardiac muscle (FIG. 1). There was an inverse relationship between the relative level of PLB and the SR Ca^{2+} loading rate, as reflected by the relationship between the loading duration and the normalized peak amplitude of the caffeine-induced tension transients for the three types of cardiac muscle. The nearly identical normalized peak tension-pCa relationships for the Triton-permeabilized trabeculae from the WT, PLB-deficient, and PLB-OE mice as shown in FIGURE 2, indicate that the observed differences in the peak amplitudes of the caffeine-induced tension transients cannot be attributed to differences in myofilament Ca^{2+} sensitivity between the three types of cardiac muscle. The inverse relationship between SR Ca^{2+} loading rate and PLB level in the WT, PLB-deficient, and PLB-OE cardiac muscle is consistent with previous reports of an inverse relationship between the Ca^{2+}-dependence of SR Ca^{2+} uptake rate and the ratio of PLB to SR Ca^{2+} pump[2–4] and supports the hypothesis that an increased PLB to SR Ca^{2+} pump ratio contributes to the diminished SR Ca^{2+} pump activity that reportedly occurs in failing human hearts.[1]

REFERENCES

1. HASENFUSS, G., M. MEYER, W. SCHILLINGER, M. PREUSS, B. PIESKE & H. JUST. 1997. Calcium handling proteins in the failing human heart. Basic Res. Cardiol. **92** (Suppl. 1): 87–93.
2. LUO, W., I. L. GRUPP, J. HARRER, S. PONNIAH, G. GRUPP, J. J. DUFFY, T. DOETSCHMAN & E. G. KRANIAS. 1994. Targeted ablation of the phospholamban gene is associated with markedly enhanced myocardial contractility and loss of β-agonist stimulation. Circ. Res. **75:** 401–409.
3. KADAMBI, V. J., S. PONNIAH, J. M. HARRER, B. D. HOIT, G. W. DORN II, R. A. WALSH & E. G. KRANIAS. 1996. Cardiac-specific overexpression of phospholamban alters calcium kinetics and resultant cardiomyocyte mechanics in transgenic mice. J. Clin. Invest. **97:** 533–539.
4. LUO, W., B. M. WOLSKA, I. L. GRUPP, J. M. HARRER, K. HAGHIGHI, D. G. FERGUSON, J. P. SLACK, G. GRUPP, T. DOETSCHMAN, R. J. SOLARO & E. G. KRANIAS. 1996. Phospholamban gene dosage effects in the mammalian heart. Circ. Res. **78:** 839–847.

Fatigue Conditions Alter Sarcoplasmic Reticulum Function of Striated Muscle

MARK ANTHONY W. ANDREWS[a,c] AND THOMAS M. NOSEK[b]

[a]*Department of Medical Physiology, New York College of Osteopathic Medicine of NYIT, Old Westbury, New York 11568-8000, USA*

[b]*Department of Physiology and Endocrinology, Medical College of Georgia, Augusta, Georgia 30912-3000, USA*

The decline in muscle function that occurs with repeated stimulation and under hypoxic and/or ischemic conditions (fatigue) results from decreases in maximal Ca^{2+}-activated force generation (F_{max}) and Ca^{2+} sensitivity of the contractile apparatus, along with alterations in Ca^{2+} uptake and release by the sarcoplasmic reticulum (SR).[1] These effects are thought to be due to a number of factors, including the accumulation of metabolic products generated within the cells. While a number of putative metabolic factors, for example, inorganic orthophosphate, and H^+, have been under investigation for some time,[2] it is becoming increasingly evident that the accumulation of lactate has significant deleterious effects on striated muscle function, independent of pH.[3]

L(+)-Lactate (LL) accumulates in skeletal muscle and in the myocardium, as the aerobic pathways of ATP regeneration cannot keep pace with the rate of ATP utilization, primarily due to a limited oxygen availability. Under these conditions, ATP production becomes increasingly dependent upon anaerobic glycolysis, and concentrations of LL rapidly increase from 1–2 mM (at rest) to 20 mM or more.[1,3] We have demonstrated that such concentrations of LL significantly decrease F_{max} in striated muscle independent of pH changes.[3] In experiments presented here, we have furthered our investigations, attempting to determine whether or not LL alters Ca^{2+} uptake by Ca^{2+}-induced Ca^{2+} release (CICR) from the SR of striated muscle cells at a constant pH.

METHODS

All experiments were carried out at room temperature (22°C) on single muscle fibers of fast-twitch extensor digitorum longus (EDL) muscles taken from mature male rats. All solution compositions were formulated by solving the set of simultaneous equations describing the multiple equilibria of ions in solution.[4] The control bathing solution (REL), upon which all experimental solutions were also based, contained (in mM): 1.0 Mg^{2+}, 5.0 MgATP, 15 phosphocreatine, 140 mM potassium methanesulfonate, 5 imidazole, and 10 EGTA (differences from these levels are noted in parentheses), with a final ionic strength of 170 mM, pH of 7.0, and a pCa ($-\log[Ca^{2+}]$) > 8.5 (no added Ca^{2+})

[c] Corresponding author: Phone: 516-686-3776; fax: 516-686-3832; e-mail: mawandrews@compuserve.com

unless otherwise noted. Appropriate amounts of potassium L(+)-lactate were added as required.

Fiber preparations involved excision of the EDL from a euthanized rat, rinsing the muscle with REL, and immediate dissection of the muscle into small fiber bundles. These bundles were then stored overnight at 4°C (to stabilize the function of the muscle fibers) in REL containing (in mM) 0.1 mM phenylmethylsulfonyl fluoride, 0.1 leupeptin, 1.0 benzamidine, 0.01 μM aprotinin, and 1 dithiothreitol (to inhibit proteolysis). The following day, fiber bundles were taken and the sarcolemma and *t*-tubules were permeabilized by immersion of the fibers in REL plus 25 μg/mL saponin for 30 min, leaving the SR intact.[5] Single fibers were then dissected in REL and mounted on an optoelectric force transducer apparatus (Scientific Instruments Gmbh, Heidelberg, Germany).

Ca^{2+} loading and release from the SR involved five steps:[5] (1) initial depletion of SR Ca^{2+} by immersion in REL plus 25 mM caffeine for one minute; (2) washing in REL to remove any caffeine; (3) loading with Ca^{2+} for 15 s in REL (pCa = 6.6) containing 0, 10, 20, or 30 mM LL (15 SR loading at 0 mM LL yielded 90% of the maximal Ca^{2+} loading achieved in 60 s); (4) washing in REL (0.05 EGTA, 0.1 Mg^{2+}) for 45 s; and (5) emptying the SR of Ca^{2+} by exposure to REL (0.05 EGTA, 0.02 Mg^{2+}) containing 25 mM caffeine. The magnitude of the contractile response in step 5 functioned as the assay for Ca^{2+} content of the SR.

CICR was determined by following steps 1–3, then blocking further Ca^{2+} uptake by immersion of the fiber in a rigor solution[5] (pCa > 8.5, 5 EGTA, 0 ATP for 2 min). CICR was then induced by exposure of the fiber to REL, or to REL containing 10 μM Ca^{2+} (pCa = 5), for 30 s. The release process was then terminated by placing the fiber in REL with 10 mM procaine for 30 s. The amount of Ca^{2+} remaining in the SR was determined by processing the fibers through steps 4 and 5.

Throughout all experiments, each fiber was exposed to all conditions and served as its own control with all conditions randomized and all results normalized to the maximum caffeine-induced contracture at the control condition noted. Hypotheses were tested at an α-value of 0.05 by one-way ANOVA with multiple comparisons.

RESULTS

As indicated in FIGURE 1, Ca^{2+} loading of the SR for 15 s (but not for 60 s) was significantly decreased to 81 ± 6%, 87 ± 4%, and 92 ± 4% ($n = 12$) of 15-s control loading by 10, 20, and 30 mM LL, respectively. Furthermore, FIGURE 2 illustrates that, following control loading of the SR for 15 s, a 30-s release period in REL (pCa = 5) caused the SR to release 15 ± 2% ($n = 26$) of its Ca^{2+} content, while CICR increased to 27 ± 3%, 33 ± 3%, and 37 ± 7%, in LL concentrations of 10, 20, and 30 mM, respectively ($n = 6$). A 30-s release period in REL, in the absence or presence of LL (not shown), did not cause significant Ca^{2+} release from the SR.

DISCUSSION

These results indicate that, in the presence of LL, there is a decrease in the rate at which SR Ca^{2+} uptake occurs (possibly related to a decrease in the rate of the Ca^{2+}-ATPase, unpublished results), but no alteration of maximal uptake when sufficient time is allowed (60 s). As can be noted in FIGURE 1, the decrease in SR loading is greatest at 10 mM, recovering slightly as LL concentration was increased to 20 mM and 30 mM.

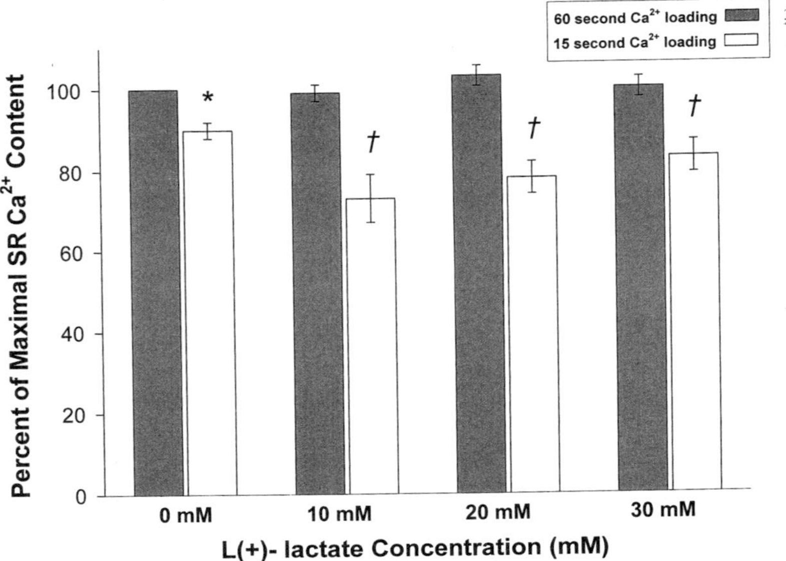

FIGURE 1. Effect of L(+)-lactate on calcium loading: Ca^{2+} uptake is significantly inhibited when fibers are loaded for 15 s (to approximately 90% of maximum) in the presence of 10, 20, and 30 mM L(+)-lactate ($n = 12$), with no effect of L(+)-lactate on Ca^{2+} uptake at a loading time of 60 s ($n = 6$). Data are presented as the mean amount of Ca^{2+} loaded into the SR ± SEM. Data for each fiber were normalized to the maximal level of Ca^{2+} uptake in the absence of L(+)-lactate with 60 s Ca^{2+} loading. *Indicates that there is a significant difference ($p < 0.05$) between that condition and 60 s Ca^{2+} loading at 0 L(+)-lactate; †indicates that there is significant difference ($p < 0.05$) between that condition and both 60- and 15-s Ca^{2+} loading at 0 L(+)-lactate.

The presence of a possible biphasic effect here is of interest because a biphasic alteration had been noted in F_{max} as LL was increased.[3] However, the mechanism of such a biphasic response in F_{max}, or in the present case, remains undetermined.

Given the rapid nature of SR loading *in vivo,* any decrease in Ca^{2+} loading of the SR by LL could result in a greater amount of Ca^{2+} remaining in the cytoplasm between repeated activations and explain, at least in part,[3] the slowing of skeletal muscle relaxation noted during periods of repeated activations.[6] With regard to cardiac muscle, all other factors remaining constant, such a decrease in the rate of Ca^{2+} loading of the SR could result in both a decreased Ca^{2+} content of the SR and elimination of the Ca^{2+} not loaded into the SR, by sarcolemmal Ca^{2+} ATPases. This would result in decreased contractile force on consequent beats (a "reverse treppe" effect). Such decreases in SR Ca^{2+} content might be ameliorated, or overcome, by other functional alterations of the myocardium, such as increased opening of sarcolemmal Ca^{2+} channels (known to occur); however, reduced Ca^{2+} loading of the SR might still decrease the total amount of Ca^{2+} available to the contractile apparatus and, in turn, decrease force generation. Present results also indicate that LL does not affect the "leakiness" of the SR, but does increase CICR (FIG. 2). The preceding effects were all shown to be reversible when LL was eliminated from the solutions.

Thus it is evident that L(+)-lactate not only affects F_{max} of striated muscle,[3] but also

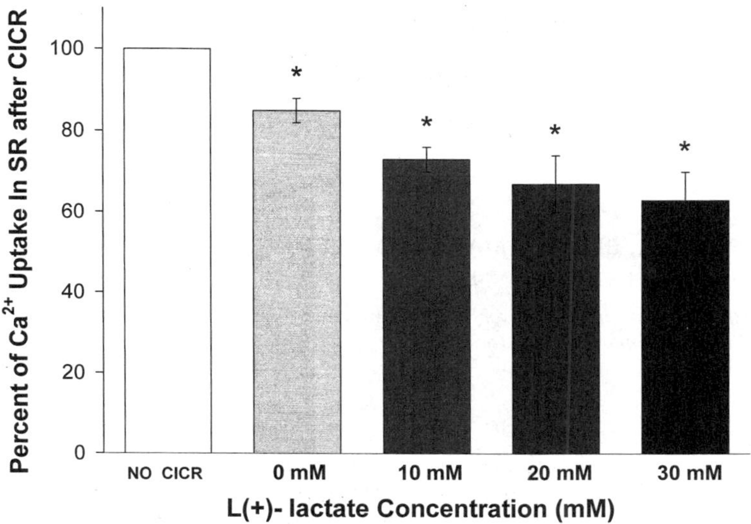

FIGURE 2. Effect of lactate on Ca^{2+}-induced Ca^{2+} release (CICR) from the SR: when the releasing solution contained a Ca^{2+} concentration of pCa 5, a 30-s exposure caused a significant CICR in the absence of L(+)-lactate. This CICR increased as L(+)-lactate concentration of the releasing solution was increased to 10, 20, and 30 mM. There was no significant effect of LL on the Ca^{2+} content of the SR when the releasing solution had a pCa > 8.5. Data are presented as the mean amount of Ca^{2+} remaining in the SR ± SEM. Data for each fiber were normalized to the SR Ca^{2+} content before exposure to releasing solution. *Indicates that there is a significant difference ($p <$ 0.05) between that condition and 15-s Ca^{2+} loading at 0 L(+)-lactate (with no consequent CICR).

alters the capacity of the SR to handle Ca^{2+}, as it slows Ca^{2+} uptake by the SR and increases CICR from the SR at L(+)-lactate concentrations generated *in vivo.* These effects of L(+)-lactate on the SR are larger in magnitude than the previously determined effects of LL on the contractile apparatus.[3]

REFERENCES

1. Fitts, R. H. 1994. Cellular mechanisms of muscle fatigue. Physiol. Rev. **74:** 49–94.
2. Godt, R. E. & T. M. Nosek. 1989. Changes of intracellular milieu with fatigue or hypoxia depress contraction of skinned rabbit skeletal and cardiac muscle. J. Physiol. **412:** 155–180.
3. Andrews, M. A. W., R. E. Godt & T. M. Nosek. 1996. The influence of physiological L(+)-lactate pevels on contractility of skinned striated muscle of rabbit. J. Appl. Physiol. **80:** 2060–2065.
4. Andrews, M. A. W., D. W. Maughan, T. M. Nosek & R. E. Godt. 1991. Ion-specific and general ionic effects on contraction of skinned fast-twitch skeletal muscle from the rabbit. J. Gen. Physiol. **98:** 1105–1125.
5. Zhu, Y. & T. M. Nosek. 1991. Inositol triphosphate enhances Ca2+ oscillations but not Ca2+-enduced Ca2+ release from cardiac sarcoplasmic reticulum. Pflügers Arch. **418:** 1–6.
6. Westerblad, H. & J. Lannergren. 1991. Slowing of relaxation during fatigue in single mouse muscle fibres. J. Physiol. **434:** 323–336.

Postrest Potentiation of Active Force in Mouse Papillary Muscles Is Greatly Accelerated by Increased Stimulus Frequency

WOLFGANG F. BLUHM,[a] MARKUS MEYER, ERIC A. SWANSON, AND WOLFGANG H. DILLMANN

Department of Medicine, University of California at San Diego, 9500 Gilman Drive, La Jolla, California 92093-0618, USA

Postrest contractions are an important experimental tool for investigating cardiac excitation-contraction coupling.[1] Recently, we were able to document postrest potentiation of active force in papillary muscles from mice.[2] The speed of postrest potentiation may be indicative of the activity of the sarcoplasmic reticulum (SR) Ca^{2+}-ATPase (SERCA2a), since overexpression of SERCA2a accelerated postrest potentiation.[2] The activity of SERCA2a is regulated through phosphorylation of the inhibitory protein phospholamban.[3] Here we show that the speed of postrest potentiation in mouse papillary muscles increases sharply with the rate of stimulation, suggesting that phosphorylation of phospholamban may be involved in the frequency-dependent regulation of active force.

METHODS

We used our recently developed method[2] to measure force development in left ventricular papillary muscles from six wild-type mice and six mice expressing a rat SERCA2a transgene. Briefly, hearts were removed from mice anesthetized with ketamine and xylazine. Papillary muscles were excised under oxygenated Tyrode solution containing 30 mM 2,3-butanedione monoxime, inserted into Ω-shaped clamps made from strips of platinum foil, tied with 6.0 braided silk suture, and mounted on hooks of platinum wire in a muscle chamber.

Muscles were perfused with 2.5 mM Ca^{2+} Tyrode solution at 37 °C and stimulated at 2 Hz and 6 Hz through the platinum clamps. Muscles were stretched to L_{max}, and force was measured with an isometric force transducer and recorded on a strip chart recorder. Forces (in mN) were normalized by the muscle cross-sectional areas to yield stresses (in mN/mm^2).

Postrest potentiation was studied by stopping stimulation for intervals ranging from 0.5 s to 15 s and resuming regular stimulation. The stress of the first postrest contraction reached a maximum after rest intervals of 5 to 15 s. The time to half-maximum postrest potentiation (half-time) was the rest interval after which the stress of the first

[a] Corresponding author. Phone: 619-534-9937; fax: 619-534-9932; e-mail: bluhm@bioeng.ucsd.edu

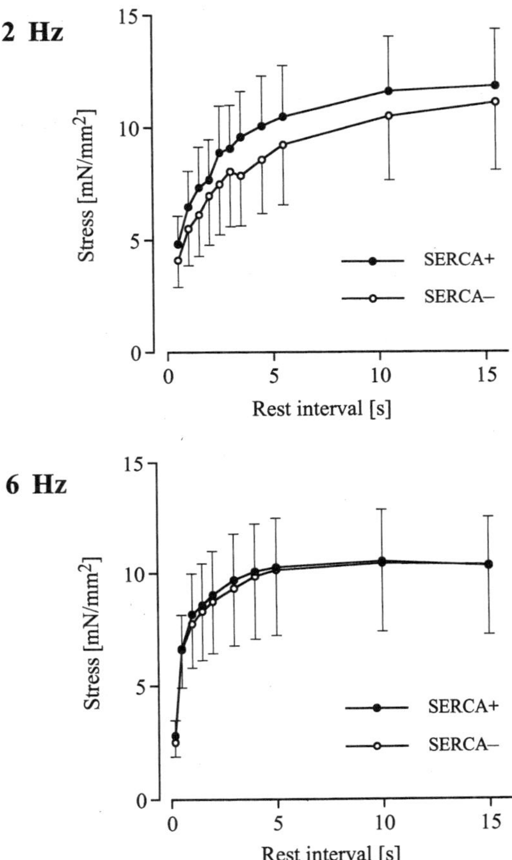

FIGURE 1. Time courses of postrest potentiation for papillary muscles at 2-Hz and 6-Hz stimulus frequency. SERCA–: wild-type mice, SERCA+: mice expressing a rat SERCA2a transgene.

postrest contraction was closest to the average stress of the steady state contraction and the maximum postrest contraction. Linear interpolation between data points was used to determine the fast half-times at 6 Hz.

Data are expressed as mean ± SEM. Statistical comparisons were made by unpaired or paired Student's *t*-tests.

RESULTS

The 12 papillary muscles had a length of 2.1 ± 0.1 mm and a cross-sectional area of 0.43 ± 0.03 mm^2, with no significant differences between groups.

At 2-Hz stimulation, papillary muscles from wild-type mice developed an active force of 4.1 ± 1.2 mN/mm^2 under steady state conditions (0.5 s interval) (FIG. 1, top).

With increasing rest intervals, the active force of the first postrest contraction gradually increased and reached a maximum of 11.1 ± 3.0 mN/mm^2 after 15 s. The half-time of this postrest potentiation was 3.3 ± 0.2 s (FIG. 2). In muscles from SERCA2a transgenic mice, this postrest half-time was significantly reduced to 2.4 ± 0.1 s ($p = 0.001$). While the active forces developed after each rest interval were slightly larger in SERCA2a transgenic muscles than in wild-type muscles, these differences were not statistically significant.

At 6-Hz stimulation, the postrest behavior was markedly different (FIG. 1, bottom). In muscles from both wild-type and transgenic mice, the half-time of postrest potentiation was sharply reduced to about 0.5 s ($p < 0.0001$, compared to 2 Hz). In addition, half-times were not significantly different between wild-type and transgenic muscles ($p = 0.74$). At steady state stimulation (0.16-s interval), active force decreased significantly in both wild-type and transgenic muscles compared to 2 Hz ($p < 0.05$), reflecting a negative force-frequency relation. However, the maximum forces reached during postrest potentiation following stimulation at either 2 or 6 Hz were not significantly different.

DISCUSSION

We have shown that the speed of postrest potentiation in mouse papillary muscles depends markedly on the frequency of stimulation. Although postrest potentiation of active force in the rodent may occur without increased SR Ca^{2+} content,[4] the accelerated postrest potentiation is most likely indicative of increased SERCA2a activity.[2] Therefore, our data strongly suggests an influence of stimulus frequency on the efficiency of SR Ca^{2+} pumping.

The two most potent regulators of SERCA2a activity are phospholamban and the cytoplasmic Ca^{2+} concentration. The increased speed of potentiation does not appear

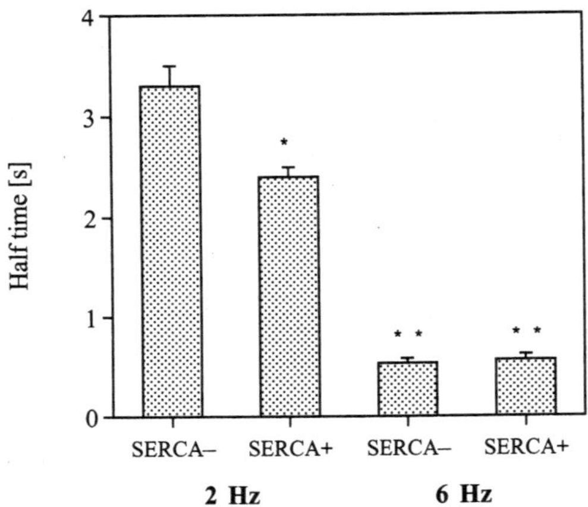

FIGURE 2. Half-times of postrest potentiation for papillary muscles at 2-Hz and 6-Hz stimulus frequency. SERCA–: wild-type mice, SERCA+: mice expressing a rat SERCA2a transgene, *: $p = 0.001$ when compared to wild-type (unpaired), **: $p < 0.0001$ when compared to 2 Hz (paired).

to be mediated by changes in Ca^{2+} concentration, since no change in passive force and rather a decrease in active force were observed at the higher stimulation rate.

Our data may therefore suggest a frequency-dependent interaction of SERCA2a and phospholamban. We hypothesize that at low frequencies phospholamban may be predominantly unphosphorylated and hence inhibit most endogenous SERCA2a. Additional SERCA2a transgene would then increase Ca^{2+} pumping significantly, as indicated by the decreased postrest half-time of SERCA2a transgenic muscles. At higher frequencies, increased phosphorylation of phospholamban and reduced inhibition of SERCA2a could explain the greatly accelerated postrest potentiation. Furthermore, the SERCA2a transgene would have a smaller effect when added to a pool of mostly uninhibited endogenous SERCA2a, which would help to explain that at 6 Hz there was no difference in half-times between wild-type and transgenic muscles.

In summary, our data suggests the new and intriguing hypothesis of a frequency-dependent interaction of SERCA2a and phospholamban, which may have important implications for the mechanisms of the cardiac force-frequency relation.

REFERENCES

1. BERS, D. M. 1985. Ca influx and sarcoplasmic reticulum Ca release in cardiac muscle activation during postrest recovery. Am. J. Physiol. **248:** H366–H381.
2. HE, H. *et al.* 1997. Overexpression of the rat sarcoplasmic reticulum (SR) Ca^{2+} ATPase gene in the heart of transgenic mice accelerates calcium transients and cardiac relaxation. J. Clin. Invest. **100:** 380–389.
3. KOSS, K. L., & E. G. KRANIAS. 1996. Phospholamban: A prominent regulator of myocardial contractility. Circ. Res. **79:** 1059–1063.
4. BERS, D. M. *et al.* 1993. Paradoxical twitch potentiation after rest in cardiac muscle: Increased fractional release of SR calcium. J. Mol. Cell. Cardiol. **25:** 1047–1057.

Metabolic Inotropy and Calcium Transients in Isolated Rat Cardiomyocytes

ROBERT D. LASLEY,[a,b,c] BRADLEY J. MARTIN,[a] HECTOR H. VALDIVIA,[a] ROBERT M. MENTZER, JR.,[a,b] AND ROLF BÜNGER[d]

[a]*Departments of Surgery and Physiology, University of Wisconsin, Madison, Wisconsin, USA*
[d]*Uniformed Services University of the Health Sciences, Bethesda, Maryland, USA*

The administration of supraphysiologic concentrations of pyruvate, an intermediary metabolite, to *in vitro*[1] and *in vivo*[2] myocardium induces a rapid positive inotropic effect. It is currently thought that pyruvate's inotropic effect is related to its ability to increase myocardial energetics, i.e., myocardial phosphorylation potential. The exact link between pyruvate's metabolic and contractile effects is not known, but it has been hypothesized that increased phosphorylation potential provides a greater driving force for energy-dependent sarcoplasmic reticulum (SR) Ca^{2+}-ATPase activity.[3] Pyruvate also increases the cytosolic $NAD^+/NADH$ ratio and cytosolic oxidation potential, which may modulate the sensitivity of the SR calcium release channel/ryanodine receptor. The purpose of this study was to determine whether pyruvate increases contractility and intracellular calcium in ventricular myocytes.

METHODOLOGY

Calcium-tolerant ventricular myocytes were isolated from male, adult Wistar rats using standard enzymatic dispersion techniques.[4] Cells were isolated and studied with a physiologic HEPES (N-[2-hydroxyethyl]piperazine-*N′*-[2-ethanesulfonic acid]) buffer containing 11.0 mM glucose and 1.0 mM $CaCl_2$ (37° C, pH 7.0) gassed with 100% oxygen. Cell length and myocyte shortening were measured with a video system and edge detection software. Intracellular calcium was measured in myocytes preloaded with the fluorescent calcium indicator fura 2-acetoxymethylester (AM) at a concentration of 2 μM (10 minutes at 37° C). Studies were performed at 37° C during field stimulation at 0.5 Hz. The free cytosolic calcium concentration ($[Ca^{2+}]_i$) was calculated according to the method of Grynkiewicz and colleagues.[5] All cells were superfused with standard HEPES buffer (pH 7.4) containing 11 mM glucose (Control) to record baseline measurements. Cells ($N \geq 5$ per group) were then treated with either 5 mM pyruvate, 100 nM isoproterenol, 5 mM acetate, 5 mM lactate, or 250 μM alpha-cyano-4-hydroxycinnamate. The hydroxycinnamate-treated cells were subsequently exposed to either 5 mM pyruvate or 5 mM acetate. Hydroxycinnamate is a non-competitive inhibitor of both the mitochondrial and sarcolemmal monocarboxylate transporter, however at the concentration used in the present study it has been shown to inhibit mitochondrial pyruvate uptake, without significantly affecting sarcolemmal pyruvate transport.[6] All data are presented

[b] Present address: Department of Surgery, University of Kentucky College of Medicine, Room MN 273 Chandler Medical Center, 800 Rose Street, Lexington, Kentucky 40536-0084.
[c] Corresponding author. Phone: 606-323-3372; fax: 606-323-8141; e-mail: rlasley@pop.uky.edu

as mean ± SEM. Data were analyzed using a one-way analysis of variance (ANOVA) and Scheffe multiple comparison confidence intervals to detect group differences. Differences were deemed significant when p values < 0.05 were indicated.

RESULTS

The results are shown in TABLE 1. Exposure to pyruvate (5 mM) for 10 minutes increased systolic $[Ca^{2+}]_i$ by 42 ± 6% compared to baseline systolic values in the presence of glucose alone. This increase in calcium was associated with a 33 ± 5% increase in twitch amplitude. The metabolic-induced effects of pyruvate compared favorably to the β-adrenergic receptor–induced effects of isoproterenol. Acetate had no significant effect on either twitch amplitude or intracellular calcium. Results similar to those obtained with acetate were obtained with another mitochondrial substrate, octanoate (0.2 mM). The responses to pyruvate were blocked significantly by the monocarboxylate transport inhibitor alpha-cyano-4-hydroxycinnamate, as cell shortening and systolic $[Ca^{2+}]_i$ were reduced 58 ± 4 and 72 ± 7%, respectively, compared to pyruvate alone.

A comparison of the effects of pyruvate and lactate is illustrated in FIGURE 1. Although 5 mM lactate significantly increased twitch amplitude and systolic $[Ca^{2+}]_i$, these effects were less than those induced by the same concentration of pyruvate. The differences between pyruvate and lactate were more pronounced at the concentration of 20 mM, where pyruvate's positive effects persisted, but the effects of lactate dissipated.

DISCUSSION

The results of this study indicate that the positive inotropic effect of pyruvate in ventricular myocardium is associated with an increase in the intracellular calcium transient. Based on the blockade of these effects with a dose of the monocarboxylate transport inhibitor, alpha-cyano-4-hydroxycinnamate, which is thought to be selective for mitochondrial transport, these results suggest that pyruvate's effects are mediated by mito-

TABLE 1. Cell Shortening and Intracellular Calcium Results

	Cell Short (% Baseline)	Sys $[Ca^{2+}]$ (nM)
Control	—	397 ± 6
PYR	133 ± 5*	552 ± 12*
ISO	163 ± 5*	703 ± 25*
ACET	111 ± 6	399 ± 4
OCT	103 ± 3	413 ± 3
HC	67 ± 5*	291 ± 10*
PYR + HC	81 ± 3*#	324 ± 4#
ACET + HC	106 ± 1	389 ± 10

NOTE: Data are expressed as mean ± SEM, $N \geq 5$ per group. Measurements were taken after 10 minutes' superfusion with each agent, with the exception of isoproterenol (ISO, 100 nM), in which data were collected after 2 minutes' exposure. Cell shortening (Cell Short) is expressed as percentage of baseline values recorded with control HEPES (11 mM glucose). Systolic calcium concentration (Sys [Ca]) is expressed as nM. PYR, pyruvate (5 mM); ACET, acetate (5 mM); OCT, octanoate (0.2 mM); HC, alpha-cyano-4-hydroxycinnamate (250 μM).

*$p < 0.05$ vs. control.

#$p < 0.05$ vs. PYR.

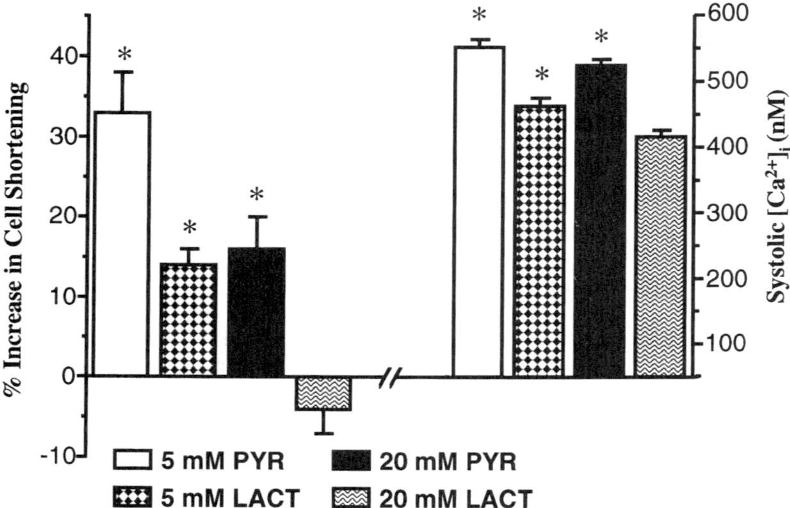

FIGURE 1. A comparison of the effects of equivalent doses (5 and 20 mM) of pyruvate (PYR) and lactate (LACT) on cell shortening (*left ordinate*) and intracellular calcium ($[Ca^{2+}]_i$; *right ordinate*). Values are expressed as mean ± SEM. $*p < 0.05$ vs. control. All studies were performed at 37°C. Since neither agent altered diastolic $[Ca^{2+}]_i$, only systolic calcium values are shown. The changes in cell shortening are referenced to % shortening values obtained in myocytes superfused initially with HEPES containing only 11 mM glucose. Basal systolic $[Ca^{2+}]_i$ values were 384 ± 9 nM.

chondrial metabolism. Other mitochondrial substrates, acetate and octanoate, did not alter contractility or intracellular calcium. Although myocardial energetics were not measured in this study, similar doses of pyruvate have been shown to increase phosphorylation potential in intact myocardium.[1,2] Since pyruvate's effects were neither completely blocked by hydroxycinnamate nor mimicked by lactate, pyruvate-induced increases in the cytosolic redox potential may also be involved, albeit to a substantially lesser degree. These results provide strong circumstantial evidence that cardiac contractility and function may be sensitive to "energetic modulation" of intracellular calcium.

REFERENCES

1. Zhou, Z., R. D. Lasley, J. O. Hegge, R. Bünger & R. M. Mentzer. 1995. Myocardial stunning: A therapeutic conundrum. J. Thorac. Cardiovasc. Surg. **110:** 1391–1401.
2. Bünger, R., R. T. Mallet, & D. A. Hartman. 1988. Pyruvate-enhanced phosphorylation potential and inotropism in normoxic and postischemic isolated working heart. Eur. J. Biochem. **180:** 221–233.
3. Mallet, R. T. & R. Bünger. 1994. Energetic modulation of cardiac inotropism and sarcoplasmic reticular calcium uptake. Biochim. Biophys. Acta. **1224:** 22–32.
4. Haworth, R. A., D. R. Hunter & H. A. Berkhoff. 1980. The isolation of calcium-resistant myocytes from the adult rat. J. Mol. Cell. Card. **12:** 715–723.
5. Grynkiewitz, G., M. Poenie & R. Y. Tsien. 1985. A new generation of Ca^{2+} indicators with greatly improved fluorescence properties. J. Biol. Chem. **260:** 3340–3347.
6. Wang, X., A. J. Levi & A. P. Halestrap. 1996. Substrate and inhibitor specificities of the monocarboxylate transporters of single rat heart cells. Am. J. Physiol. **39:** H476–H484.

Endothelial Protective Effect of Verapamil against Acute Myocardial Contractile Dysfunction in Isolated Working Rat Hearts Subjected to Global Ischemia

PERICLE DI NAPOLI,[a] ATTILIO DI CRECCHIO, GAETANO CONTEGIACOMO, PAOLO TILOCA, ALFONSO ANTONIO TACCARDI, ALESSANDRO MAGGI, MARCELLO DI MUZIO,[b] AND ANTONIO BARSOTTI

Department of Cardiology and Cardiac Surgery, and [b]Department of Oncology and Neuroscience, University of Chieti, Chieti, Italy

Ischemia and reperfusion (I/R) may result in injury to cellular components of the hearts. In addition to damaging myocytes and their contractile capability, I/R may inflict early and severe injury on the vasculature that, in turn, may further compromise the return of normal coronary perfusion and the survival of cardiomyocytes.[1] Several studies[2,3] suggest that calcium antagonists (CA) may reduce mechanical dysfunction and ultrastructural damage of ischemic and reperfused myocardium; nonetheless, the effects of CA against postischemic microvasculature damage are still not well understood. In this study we evaluated (1) the effect of verapamil administration before ischemia against the postischemic permeability changes of microvascular endothelium and (2) the consequence of nitric oxide (NO) synthesis inhibition on endothelial effect of CA and coronary microcirculation.

MATERIAL AND METHODS

Experiments were carried out in 52 Wistar rats (250–300 g) isolated and perfused according to working heart technique. The hearts were divided into four groups: (A) control hearts perfused with modified Krebs-Henseleit buffer (KH, N=10); (B) hearts perfused with KH containing 0.25 μM verapamil (N=10); (C) 0.50 μM verapamil (N=10), and (D) 1 μM verapamil (N=10). After a 20-min stabilization, hearts were subjected to 15 min global ischemia and 60 min reperfusion (N=7/group). The drug was added to the perfusion buffer at the beginning of experiments. We measured hemodynamic parameters (aortic and coronary flows, aortic pressure, heart rate, pressure-rate product, and coronary resistance calculated as aortic pressure/coronary flow), creatine kinase (CK) release in coronary effluent, heart weight changes (myocardial edema index), microvascular permeability [using fluorescein isothiocyanate albumin (FITC-albumin) as a macromolecular tracer] and ultrastructural morphometry.[4] FITC-albumin was dissolved in KH (250 mg/200 ml) and administered (N=3/group) during the 20 min after

[a] Address for communication: Dr. Pericle Di Napoli, Istituto di Clinica Cardiovascolare—Università di Chieti, Ospedale S. Camillo de Lellis, Via Forlanini 50, 66100 Chieti, Italy. Phone/fax: 39 871 41512; e-mail: dinapoli@unich.it

ischemia. The FITC-albumin extravasation was quantified with computer-assisted image analysis on the basis of integrated optical intensity (IOI) measurements.[5] Moreover, in order to test the hypothesis of a relationship between verapamil-induced cardioprotection and NO synthesis, in additional rat hearts (N=12; 3/group) we performed the same experiments adding to KH 30 μM L-NAME (N^{ω}-nitro-L-arginine methyl ester), a specific inhibitor of NO synthesis.

RESULTS

In groups C and D we observed a significant decline of ventricular function associated with a significant increase of CK release (FIG. 1) with respect to controls during post-ischemic reperfusion. In Group B, a significant reduction of post-ischemic mechanical dysfunction (systolic aortic pressure at 50 min for Group B, 85 ± 4.7, and Group A, 66 ± 5.1 mmHg, p<0.001) was detected associated with a reduction of CK release (at 50 min. for Group A, 25 ± 6.1; for Group B, 7.3 ± 3.8 IU/g wet weight, p<0.001). Additionally in groups A, C, and D, a significant increase of coronary resistances (CR, FIG. 1) with respect to basal levels was noted, while in group B post-ischemic CR didn't changed with respect to pre-ischemic values. These data agree with heart weight changes (A, 24 ± 3.7; B, 9 ± 2, p<0.001 vs. A and C, 18 ± 5.5 and D, 21 ± 6%). Vascular permeability changes are reported in FIGURE 1. In 0.25 μM verapamil-treated hearts a significant reduction of post-ischemic FITC-albumin extravasation was detected. In control hearts and at higher verapamil concentrations (0.50 and 1 μM) L-NAME treatment didn't significantly changed pre- and post-ischemic hemodynamic performance, CK release, and heart weight changes. Conversely, in 0.25 μM verapamil-treated hearts, a significant reduction of the cardioprotection against mechanical dysfunction and CK release was evidenced associated with a significant myocardial edema and FITC-albumin extravasation (FIG. 2). The reduction of endothelial and myocytic damage in Group B and its increase after L-NAME treatment was also confirmed by electron microscopy evaluation.

DISCUSSION

Results from the present study suggest that low-doses of verapamil, administered before ischemia, can provide (1) endothelial protection against I/R injury in isolated working rat hearts, (2) improvement of coronary microcirculation by modulating coronary resistances and ischemia-induced microvascular hyperpermeability, and (3) this endothelial protection is, at least in part, mediated by NO synthesis. Previous studies[1,6] reported that microvascular permeability changes and their main consequence, as interstitial edema, significantly modulate I/R damage and coronary perfusion. The mechanisms involved in the regulation of basal and postischemic fluid exchange within the interstitium (endothelium-extracellular matrix-myocytes) are various and not well understood. Local hemodynamic, osmotic and oncotic pressures, endothelial permeability, endothelium integrity and interendothelial cell gaps, adhesion molecules expression, and inflammatory reaction modulation represent the main physiopathogenic factors.[7,8] In this process intracellular Ca^{2+} is actively involved. In fact, Ca^{2+} modulates vascular tone and gap formation between endothelial cells and reduces phospholipases and protein kinase C activity, platelet-activating factor release, and inflammatory reaction (vascular cell adhesion molecules expression, endothelins, and oxygen free-radicals production).

The role of NO is still unclear. The physiological release of small quantities of NO

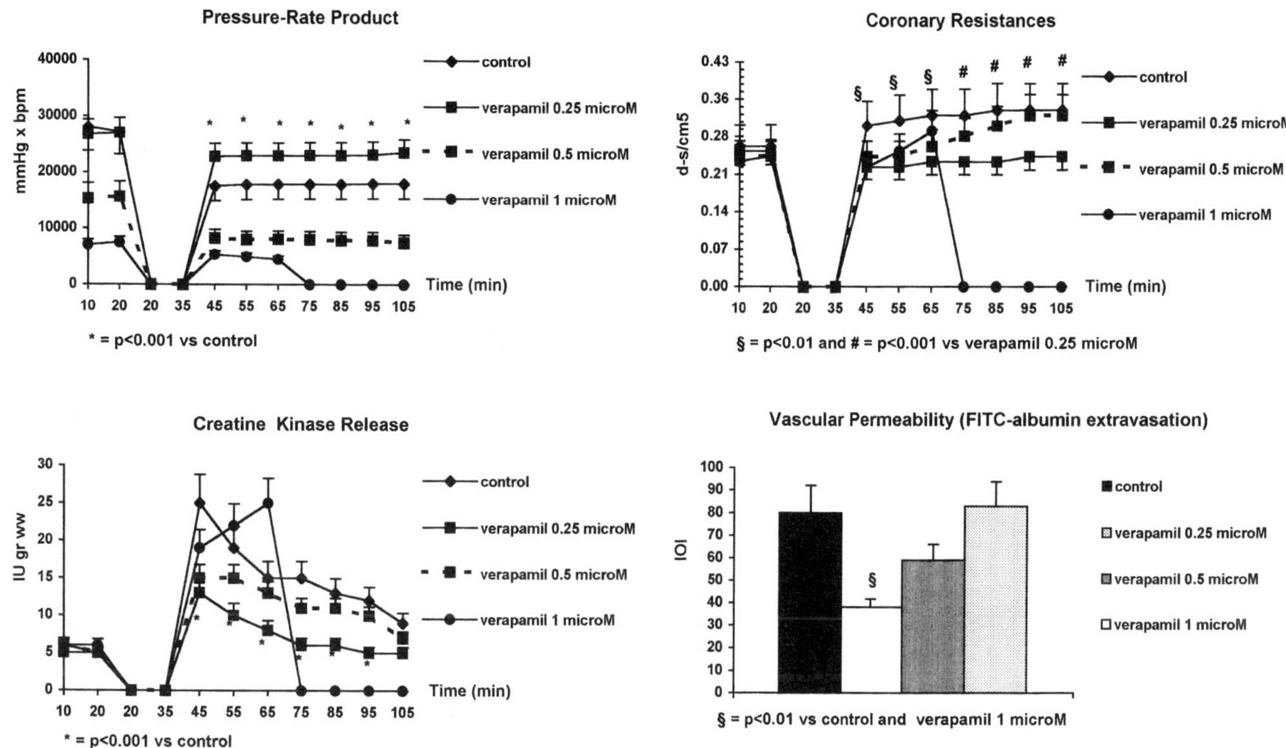

FIGURE 1. Time course of pressure-rate product (mm Hg × ml × min^{-1}); coronary vascular resistances (dynes-sec/cm^{-5}); creatine kinase release in coronary effluent (IU × g wet weight); and FITC-albumin extravasation (Integrated Optical Intensity units). Data are expressed as mean ± SD.

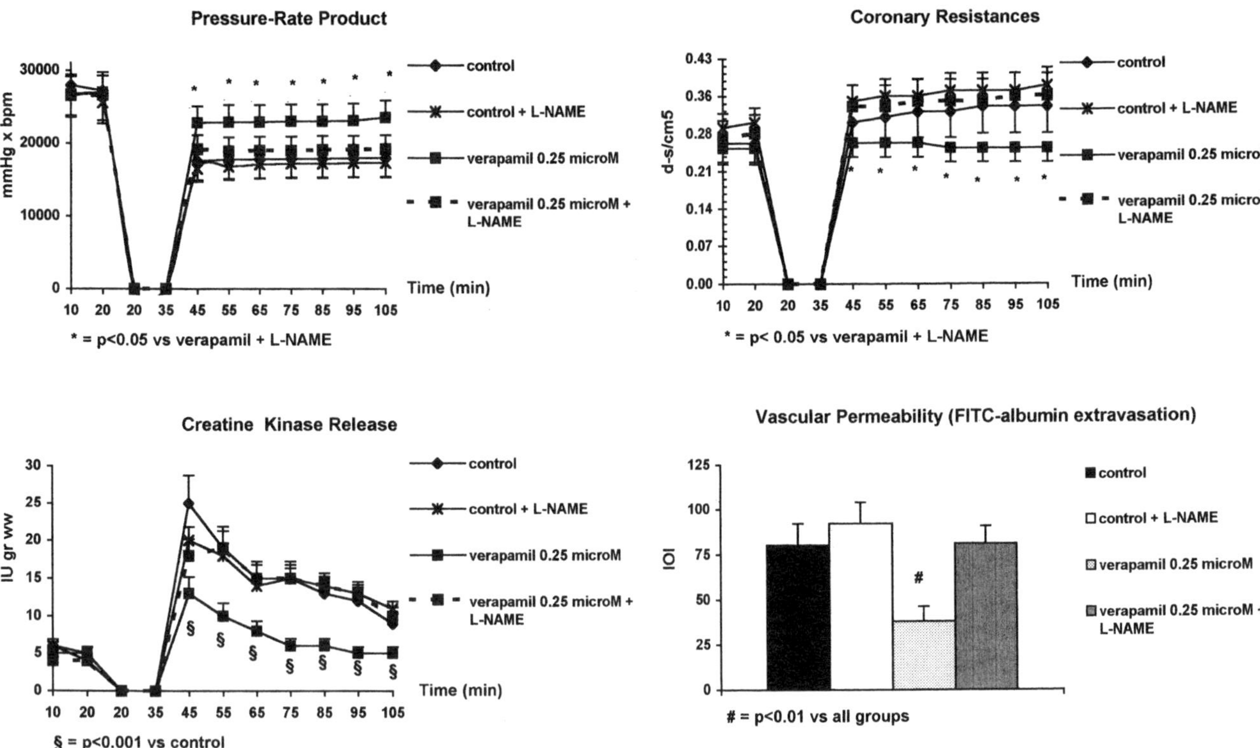

FIGURE 2. Effect of L-NAME administration in control and 0.25 μM verapamil groups. Time course of pressure-rate product (mm Hg × ml × min^{-1}); coronary vascular resistances (dynes-sec/cm^{-5}); creatine kinase release in coronary effluent (IU × g wet weight); and FITC-albumin extravasation (Integrated Optical Intensity units). Data are expressed as mean ± SD.

provides for the maintenance of coronary vasodilator tone, inhibition of platelet aggregation, and the adhesion of neutrophils and platelets to the vascular endothelium. Furthermore, NO has direct negative inotropic and chronotropic effects. In cardiac pathology, its role remains unclear and various studies reported the negative effects of an excessive NO production after I/R.[9] In our experiments we noted that NO synthesis inhibition with L-NAME does not affect preischemic ventricular function. On the other hand, NO synthesis inhibition does not reduce I/R injury and does induce a significant reduction of verapamil cardioprotection. This finding suggests that the effects of verapamil on coronary microcirculation (endothelial permeability and vascular resistances) may depend on a modulation of intracellular calcium homeostasis and endothelial NO synthesis. Whether this apparent synergistic action between Ca^{2+} and NO synthesis is a consequence of the decreased endothelial damage due to the reduction of Ca^{2+} overload or is the result of a direct interaction between intracellular Ca^{2+} and NO synthase activity remains unclear and may be a subject of further investigation.

REFERENCES

1. Hearse, D. J., L. Maxwell *et al.* 1993. The myocardial vasculature during ischemia and reperfusion: a target for injury and protection. J. Mol. Cell. Cardiol. **25:** 739–800.
2. Kloner, R. A. & E. Braunwald. 1987. Effect of calcium antagonists on infarcting myocardium. Am. J. Cardiol. **59:** 84B–94B.
3. Dagenais, F., R. Cartier *et al.* 1997. Calcium-channel blockers preserve coronary endothelial reactivity after ischemia-reperfusion. Ann. Thorac. Surg. **63:** 1050–1056.
4. Di Napoli, P., M. Di Muzio *et al.* 1997. Precondizionamento ischemico del miocardio: Ruolo delle alterazioni della permeabilità del microcircolo coronarico. Cardiologia **1:** 59–67.
5. Ramirez, M. M. & S. M. Quardt *et al.* 1995. Platelet activating factor modulates microvascular permeability through nitric oxide synthesis. Microvasc. Res. **50:** 223–234.
6. Di Napoli, & A. Di Crecchio *et al.* 1997. Endothelial permeability as factor affecting reperfusion damage. Int. Med. **5:** 1–7.
7. Oshiro, H. & I. Kobayashi *et al.* 1995: L-Type calcium channel blockers modulate the microvascular hyperpermeability induced by platelet-activating factor in vivo. J. Vasc. Surg. **22:** 732–741.
8. Yamaguchi, M. & H. Suwa *et al.* 1997. Selective inhibition of vascular cell adhesion molecule-1 expression by verapamil in human vascular endothelial cells. Transplantation **63:** 759–764.
9. Schulz, R. & R. Wambolt. 1995. Inhibition of nitric oxide synthesis protects the isolated working rabbit heart from ischemia-reperfusion injury. Cardiovasc. Res. **30:** 432–439.

Cardiac Responses to Calcium Sensitizers and Isoproterenol in Intact Guinea Pig Hearts

Effects on Cyclic AMP Levels, Protein Phosphorylation, Myoplasmic Calcium Concentration, and Left Ventricular Function

EVA KRISTOF, GYULA SZIGETI,[a] ZOLTAN PAPP, ANNAMARIA BODI, ANDREA FACSKO,[b] LASZLO KOVACS,[a] JULIUS G. PAPP,[c] EVANGELIA G. KRANIAS,[d] AND ISTVAN EDES[e]

Departments of Heart and Lung Diseases, [a]Physiology, and [b]Ophthalmology, University Medical School of Debrecen, Debrecen, Hungary

[c]Department of Pharmacology, Albert Szent-Gyorgyi Medical University, Szeged, Hungary

[d]Department of Pharmacology and Cell Biophysics, University of Cincinnati, Cincinnati, Ohio, USA

The new class of positive inotropic agents, the Ca^{2+} sensitizers (Pimobendan, EMD 53998, Levosimendan, and OR-1896) have been the subject of extensive experimental and clinical research in recent years. A typical feature of these agents is that increases in the inotropic state may occur with little or no increase in the Ca^{2+} transient. An interesting, but poorly understood, feature of the above-mentioned Ca^{2+} sensitizing agents is that they all have phosphodiesterase (PDE) inhibitory activities as well.[1,2] Consequently, in intact preparations, the mechanism of the positive inotropic action may be related to both Ca^{2+} sensitization as well as cyclic AMP (cAMP)-mediated protein phosphorylation. The present study in guinea pig hearts examines the dose-dependent effects of different Ca^{2+} sensitizers on (1) cardiac function (measured as left ventricular contractility, +dP/dt), (2) Ca^{2+} transients (Fura-2 fluorescence ratio, assayed from Fura-2 loaded, beating hearts), (3) phosphorylation of key intracellular phosphoproteins *in situ* (measured from ^{32}P-perfused hearts), and (4) myocardial cAMP levels. This integrative approach enabled us to study the Ca^{2+} sensitizing and PDE inhibitory potentials of the different compounds and address the question of whether their Ca^{2+} sensitizing properties are important *in situ.*

RESULTS AND DISCUSSION

Perfusion of the hearts with increasing concentrations of Levosimendan, OR-1896, Pimobendan, and EMD 53998 resulted in dose-dependent elevations in +dP/dt and peak fluorescent ratio values (FIG. 1). Analysis of the functional responses revealed that Levosimendan and OR-1896 were the only compounds, at a low concentration (0.03

[e] Address for communication: Istvan Edes, Department of Heart and Lung Diseases, University Medical School of Debrecen, 4004 Debrecen, P.O.B. 1, Hungary. E-mail: edes@lib.dote.hu

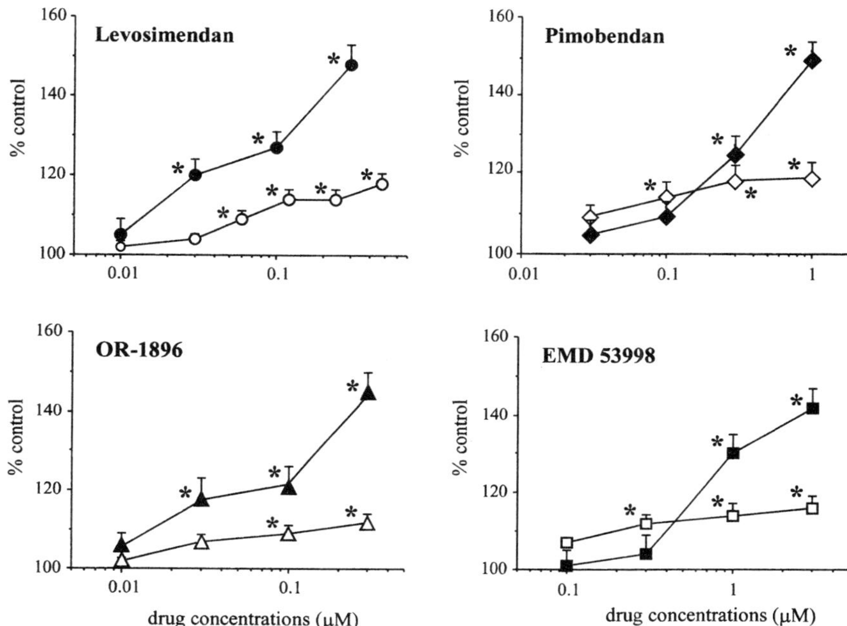

FIGURE 1. Dose-response relations of Levosimendan (●, **top left**); OR-1896 (▲, **bottom left**); Pimobendan (◆, **top right**); and EMD 53998 (■, **bottom right**) on +dP/dt *(closed symbols)* and peak Ca^{2+} ratio values *(open symbols)*. Hearts were perfused with the different Ca^{2+} sensitizers for 6 minutes. The basal value, obtained in the absence of any positive inotropic agents, was regarded as 100%, and the increases in contractility and peak Ca^{2+} ratio following the administration of the different agents are expressed in percentages. Each value represents the mean ± SEM of at least 3 different hearts. *Asterisks* denote $p < 0.05$ when compared to basal values.

μM), to increase myocardial contractility without affecting the myoplasmic Ca^{2+} transient significantly. In contrast, administration of low concentrations of Pimobendan or EMD 53998 were associated with more pronounced increases in peak calcium levels (in percentage) compared to those of +dP/dt (FIG. 1). Exposure of the hearts to 0.03 μM Levosimendan or OR-1896 did not appear to alter the tissue cAMP level and the ^{32}P-incorporation into troponin I or C protein, while a slight, but significant, increase was noted for phospholamban (TABLE 1). In the case of the EMD 53998- and Pimobendan-perfused hearts, the dose-dependent increase in the cardiac function (+dP/dt) was always associated with the simultaneous increase in tissue cAMP levels and phosphorylation of cardiac phosphoproteins (TABLE 1).

Our results demonstrate that the recently developed Ca^{2+} sensitizers (Levosimendan, OR-1896, Pimobendan, and EMD 53998) all possess a PDE inhibitory potential in perfused beating heart preparations. However, at low concentrations Levosimendan and its derivative, OR-1896 acted preferably as Ca^{2+} sensitizers, since they elicited increases in inotropy without any changes in lusitropy, chronotropy (data not shown), and tissue cAMP levels. Moreover, in the same hearts, no increase was noted in the phosphorylation of myofibrillar proteins as compared to control values. In support of this hy-

TABLE 1. The Effect of Ca^{2+} Sensitizers on Myocardial Protein Phosphorylation and Tissue cAMP Levels

	Phospholamban (^{32}P/mg protein)	Troponin I (^{32}P/mg protein)	C Protein (^{32}P/mg protein)	cAMP (pmol/mg protein)
Control (*N*=7)	91±5	118±7	111±9	4.3±0.3
Levosimendan				
0.03 μM (*N*=6)	133±6*	122±9	125±9	5.6±0.7
0.1 μM (*N*=6)	182±6*	175±9*	179±8*	7.0±0.5*
0.3 μM (*N*=6)	187±6*	195±9*	188±8*	8.0±0.5*
OR-1896				
0.03 μM (*N*=4)	155±4*	132±7	125±10	5.2±0.5
0.1 μM (*N*=3)	197±8*	169±8*	157±10*	6.1±0.4*
0.3 μM (*N*=3)	238±10*	189±8*	160±12*	7.3±0.6*
EMD 53998				
0.3 μM (*N*=3)	96±7	102±6	121±10	5.7±0.5
1 μM (*N*=5)	142±5*	142±8*	160±9*	7.3±0.5*
3 μM (*N*=4)	169±8*	172±10*	175±13*	8.9±0.6*
Pimobendan				
0.1 μM (*N*=3)	99±8	111±8	124±11	5.8±0.6
0.3 μM (*N*=5)	130±6*	163±9*	172±12*	7.5±0.5*

NOTE: ^{32}P-perfused guinea pig hearts were exposed to the indicated agent and freeze-clamped as described in METHODS. Control hearts were perfused with Krebs buffer only, under identical conditions. Results are mean±SEM of *N* hearts.

*$p < 0.05$ when compared with control values.

pothesis, Ca^{2+} measurement experiments indicated that the increases in contractile function by 0.03 μM Levosimendan or OR-1896 were not accompanied by any significant increases in the peak fluorescent ratios. In contrast, increasing concentrations of Pimobendan and EMD 53998 appeared to elevate the peak Ca^{2+} levels first, followed by increases in contractility at higher concentrations. This finding is in agreement with the results of Ishisu and colleagues,[3] who were also unable to demonstrate the calcium-sensitizing effect of EMD 53998 on isolated guinea pig hearts studied under similar conditions. Interestingly in our preparations, perfusion with 0.03 μM Levosimendan or OR-1896 was associated with a slight, but significant, phosphorylation of phospholamban. These findings are in agreement with previously published observations,[1] and probably reflect the relative selectivity of the PDE-inhibitory potential of Levosimendan and OR-1896 on the sarcoplasmic reticular (SR) compartment. Phosphorylation of phospholamban was reported to be associated with increased SR Ca^{2+} uptake due to higher affinity of the SR Ca^{2+}-ATPase for Ca^{2+}.[4] This increased Ca^{2+} uptake may override the negative lusitropic effect of Ca^{2+} sensitization on myofibrils and may explain the lack of changes on the relaxation parameters in these hearts. In conclusion, it appears that low concentrations of Levosimendan and OR-1896 preferably act by increasing the response of the myofilaments to Ca^{2+}, confirmed by the combined determination of myoplasmic Ca^{2+} transients, tissue cAMP levels, and phosphorylation of key myofibrillar phosphoproteins. In the cases of all concentrations of Pimobendan and EMD 53998 and the higher doses of Levosimendan and OR-1896, the increases in contractility were always associated with PDE inhibition–mediated responses (elevations in Ca^{2+} transients, tissue cAMP levels, and phosphorylation of key myocardial phosphoproteins).

REFERENCES

1. EDES, I. *et al.* 1995. Effects of Levosimendan, a cardiotonic agent targeted to troponin C, on cardiac function and on phosphorylation and Ca^{2+} sensitivity of cardiac myofibrils and sarcoplasmic reticulum in guinea pig heart. Circ. Res. **77:** 107–113.
2. SOLARO, R. J. 1996. Calcium sensitizers and molecular mechanism of altered response of cardiac myofilaments to calcium. *In* Molecular and Cellular Mechanisms of Cardiovascular Regulation. M. Endoh *et al.,* Ed.: 363–372. Springer-Verlag, Tokyo, Japan.
3. ISHISU, R. *et al.* 1996. Differential effects of EMD-53998 on calcium-pressure relationship in normal and ischemic guinea pig heart. Am. J. Physiol. **271:** H311–H319.
4. EDES, I. & E. G. KRANIAS. 1995. Ca^{2+}-ATPases. *In* Cell Physiology Source Book. N. Sperelakis, Ed.: 156–165. Academic Press. New York, NY.

Cyclosporin A Induces Alteration of Ca Release Channel in Cardiac Sarcoplasmic Reticulum[a]

D. H. KIM,[b] K. S. PARK, E. H. LEE, T. K. KIM, AND C.-S. PARK

Department of Life Science, Kwangju Institute of Science and Technology (K-JIST), Kwangju 506-712, Korea

Cyclosporin A (CsA) is a powerful immunosuppressant widely used to prevent organ rejection.[1] The clinical application of CsA is limited by various toxic side effects, such as nephrotoxicity and cardiotoxicity. Mechanical changes of rat heart were reported to occur by chronic treatment with CsA.[1] For this study, experiments were performed to test the hypothesis that the CsA-mediated mechanical alterations[1] are caused by molecular alterations of Ca release channels (CRC) in sarcoplasmic reticulum (SR).

Male Sprague-Dawley (SD) rats were treated with CsA for 3 weeks by subcutaneous injection.[1] Preparations of whole homogenates, SR vesicles, equilibrium ryanodine binding, Ca flux measurements, and Western blot analysis were performed, as described previously.[2–4]

To examine whether CsA treatment alters the characteristics of CRC in the SR of rat heart, ryanodine binding to whole homogenates was measured at various [^{3}H]ryanodine concentrations. The densities of CRC, as determined by maximal ryanodine binding to the receptor (B_{max}), was significantly lower in CsA-treated than in control animals (29%) (TABLE 1). The lower density of CRC in CsA-treated animals was further confirmed by oxalate-supported Ca uptake and Western blot analysis that showed a significant decrease in CRC amounts in the SR (TABLE 1). The dissociation constant of ryanodine to CRC (K_d) was significantly higher in CsA-treated rats (TABLE 1), indicating that the affinity to ryanodine is lower in CsA-treated rats.

To investigate the effect of CsA treatment on agonist sensitivity of cardiac CRC, ryanodine binding with various caffeine concentrations was measured at 0.03 μM Ca. EC_{50} of caffeine for activation of ryanodine binding in CsA-treated animals was significantly lower than in the controls (3.00± 0.10 vs. 3.56± 0.17 mM, $p<0.05$). This higher caffeine sensitivity was further supported by single channel and Ca flux data showing that mean open probability (P_o) of CRC and the amounts of Ca release from SR increased significantly in the presence of caffeine (TABLE 1). The increased P_o appeared to be due to the increased mean open time of CRC (TABLE 1). These results suggest that the underlying mechanisms for caffeine-mediated gating of CRC may be altered by CsA treatment. On the other hand, Ca sensitivity of ryanodine binding was not affected by CsA.

Ruthenium red (RR) is an effective CRC blocker. To examine the effects of RR on CRC of control and CsA-treated rat hearts, ryanodine binding in the presence of RR was determined at 3.16 μM Ca. IC_{50} of ruthenium red to inhibit ryanodine binding was significantly higher in CsA-treated rat hearts than in control heart (5.36 ± 0.70 vs. 2.88 ± 0.50 μM, $p<0.05$), suggesting that the mechanisms responsible for RR inhibition are altered by CsA treatment. Since RR and ryanodine may share the same binding site, it

[a]This work was supported by "Star Project" from the Korean Ministry of Science and Technology and Genetic Engineering and a research grant from the Korean Ministry of Education.

[b]Address for communication: Dr. Do Han Kim, Kwangju Institute of Science and Technology (K-JIST), Department of Life Science, 572 Sangam-dong, Kwangsan-ku, Kwangju 506-712, Korea. Phone: 82-62-970-2485; fax: 82-62-970-2484; e-mail: dhkim@eunhasu.kjist.ac.kr

TABLE 1. Effects of Chronic Treatment with CsA on Rat Cardiac SR

Experiment	Material	Parameter	CsA Effect
Ryanodine binding	WH	B_{max}	Decrease
		K_m	Increase
		EC_{50}(Ca)	No change
		EC_{50}(caffeine)	Decrease
		IC_{50}(RR)	Increase
Ca uptake (+oxalate)	WH	Uptake rate	No change
		Ryanodine-sensitive uptake	Decrease
Planar lipid bilayer	SR vesicles	Slope conductance	Decrease
		P_o (+caffeine)	Increase
		EC_{50}(caffeine)	Decrease
		Mean open time	Increase
		Mean closed time	No change
		Ryanodine-sensitivity	Decrease
Ca release by caffeine	SR vesicles	Release amount	Increase
		EC_{50}(caffeine)	Decrease
Western blot	SR vesicles	CRC density	Decrease
		Ca-ATPase density	No change

ABBREVIATIONS: WH, whole homogenates; EC_{50}, drug concentration for half-maximal activation; IC_{50}, drug concentration for half-maximal inhibition; and P_o, channel open probability.

is tempting to speculate that the ryanodine/RR binding site(s) is altered in CsA-treated animal heart. In contrast to the CsA effects on CRC, the activity and the density of Ca-ATPase were not altered by CsA (TABLE 1).

The underlying molecular mechanisms for the modification of the characteristics of CRC by CsA are not yet known. It is known that the tetrameric structure of CRC is stabilized by the channel-associated FKBP. Functional studies have shown that FK506 or rapamycin, which dissociate FKBP from CRC, increases the open probability and reduces the current amplitude of CRC.[4] The chronic modification of the CRC and the lack of direct effect of CsA suggest that the immunosuppressive properties of this agent may not directly cause the modification. Thus, it is tempting to speculate that CsA could cause molecular changes of CRC or associated protein(s). Elucidation of the molecular mechanisms for the altered CRC activities in CsA-treated animals must await further studies such as molecular characterization of the CRC.

REFERENCES

1. BANIJAMALI, H.S., M.H. TER KEURS, L.C. PAUL & H.E. TER KEURS. 1993. Excitation-contraction coupling in rat heart: Influence of cyclosporin A. Cardiovasc. Res. **27:** 1845–1854.
2. KIM, D. H., F. MKPARU, C.-R. KIM & R. F. CAROLL. 1994. Alteration of Ca release channel function in sarcoplasmic reticulum of pressure-overload-induced hypertrophic rat heart. Mol. Cell. Cardiol. **26:** 1505–1512.
3. VALDIVIA, C., D. VAUGHAN, B. V. L. POTTER & R. CORONADO. 1992. Fast release of ^{45}Ca induced by inositol 1,4,5-trisphosphate and Ca in the sarcoplasmic reticulum of rabbit skeletal muscle: evidence for two types of Ca release channels. Biophy. J. **61:** 1184–1193.
4. MARKS, A. R. 1997. Intracellular calcium-release channels: Regulators of cell life and death. Am. J. Physiol. **272:** H597–H605.

Thermodynamic Limitation for the Sarcoplasmic Reticulum Ca^{2+}-ATPase Contributes to Impaired Contractile Reserve in Hearts[a]

RONG TIAN[b]

NMR Laboratory for Physiological Chemistry, Department of Medicine, Brigham & Women's Hospital and Harvard Medical School, 221 Longwood Avenue, Boston, Massachusetts 02115, USA

Contraction and relaxation of cardiac myocytes requires rapid cycling of Ca^{2+} into and out of the cytosol. This process utilizes a high level of free energy from ATP hydrolysis ($|\Delta G{\sim}p|$).[1,2] One reason for this high energy requirement is the high concentration gradient of Ca^{2+} (~10,000-fold) between the cytosol and the sarcoplasmic reticulum (SR), the primary source of Ca^{2+} during contraction.[1,2] This gradient is maintained by the SR Ca^{2+}-ATPase reaction, which pumps Ca^{2+} back into the SR during relaxation. The thermodynamic driving force ($\Delta G_{SRCa\text{-}ATPase}$) required to maintain the Ca^{2+} gradient across the SR membrane can be estimated by the formula below assuming there is no electrical gradient across the SR membrane:

$$\Delta G_{SRCa\text{-}ATPase} = -2RT\ln[Ca^{2+}]_{SR\ lumen}/[Ca^{2+}]_{cytosol},$$

where R is the gas constant and T is the absolute temperature. It has been reported that for the magnitude of the Ca^{2+} gradient under physiological conditions, the SR Ca^{2+}-ATPase reaction requires a $|\Delta G|$ of at least 52 kJ/mol, ~90% of the free energy released from ATP hydrolysis under physiological conditions ($|\Delta G{\sim}p|$, 59–60 kJ/mol).[2] Thus, $|\Delta G_{SRCa\text{-}ATPase}| \approx 0.9\ |\Delta G{\sim}p|$. This limited thermodynamic reserve may render the SR Ca^{2+} loading highly vulnerable to a decrease in $|\Delta G{\sim}p|$. It should be mentioned that the requirement for the SR Ca^{2+}-ATPase is substantially higher than that of two other key ATPases in cardiac myocytes, namely, Na^+/K^+ ATPase (46 kJ/mol) and the actomyosin ATPase (45–50 kJ/mol).[4] Therefore, a small decrease in $|\Delta G{\sim}p|$ could affect SR Ca^{2+}-ATPase reaction without altering the function of other ATPases.

We hypothesize that a decrease in the reserve of $\Delta G{\sim}p$ depletes contractile reserve by limiting the availability of intracellular Ca^{2+} during inotropic stimulation. To test this, we performed two parallel experiments in isolated perfused rat hearts: in the first we monitored left ventricular function simultaneously with myocardial energetics using ^{31}P NMR spectroscopy; in the second, we monitored left ventricular function simultaneously with cytosolic Ca^{2+} concentration ($[Ca^{2+}]_c$) using indo-1 fluorescence. Results obtained from these experiments will be presented and discussed in the following two sections. In these experiments, $|\Delta G{\sim}p|$ was decreased by acutely and selectively inhibiting the creatine kinase (CK) activity (by > 95%) using a low dose of iodoacetamide (IA, 90–120 μmol), a sulfhydryl modifier, without affecting the major ATP synthesis

[a] This work supported by the National Institutes of Health Heart Failure SCOR Grant (HL 52350).

[b] Phone: 617-732-6995; fax: 617-732-6990; e-mail: rong@bustoff.bwh.harvard.edu

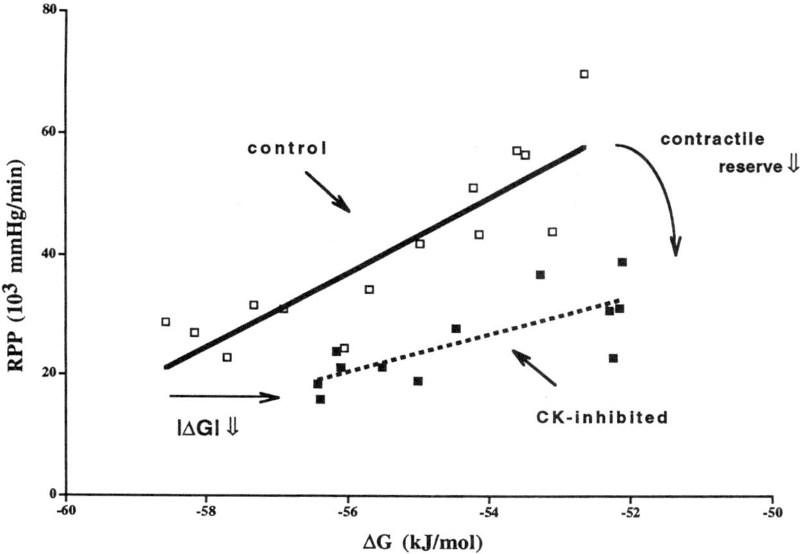

FIGURE 1. The relationship between ΔG~p and RPP in control and CK-inhibited hearts. (Adapted from Tian.[3])

and utilization pathways.[3–5] Inhibiting the CK reaction (PCr + ADP + H^+ <==> ATP + Cr) causes a ~twofold increase in [ADP] (in μM range) without altering [ATP] and [Pi] (both in mM range), resulting in a significant decrease in |ΔG~p| (|ΔG~p| = |ΔG° – RTln([ATP]/[Pi][ADP]|).[3,4]

$\Delta G_{\sim p}$ AND CONTRACTILE FUNCTION

FIGURE 1 shows the results obtained from concurrent measurement of |ΔG~p| and cardiac performance during baseline (perfusate [Ca^{2+}] = 1.2 mM) and high Ca^{2+} perfusion (perfusate [Ca^{2+}] = 3.3 mM) in control and CK-inhibited hearts.[3] Left ventricular (LV) function, estimated as the product of heart rate and LV developed pressure (RPP), is plotted against ΔG~p calculated using measurements from ^{31}P NMR spectroscopy and biochemical assays in the same hearts. Baseline RPP is unaltered in CK-inhibited hearts, but |ΔG~p| was reduced from 58 to 56 kJ/mol. The increase in RPP during high Ca^{2+} perfusion is accompanied by a decreased in |ΔG~p| in both groups. Interestingly, both group achieve the maximal RPPs at the |ΔG~p| of 52 kJ/mol, the level required by the SR Ca^{2+}-ATPase. However, for the CK-inhibited hearts, even a small increase in workload resulted in a marked increase of [ADP] (because the buffering function of the CK reaction is lost) and a rapid reduction in |ΔG~p|.[3] Importantly, contractile reserve, defined as the ability to increase RPP in response to high Ca^{2+} perfusion, was impaired in CK-inhibited hearts (FIG. 1).[3,4] Thus, a moderate decrease in |ΔG~p| does not alter baseline contraction but limited the recruitment of contractile reserve.

$\Delta G_{\sim p}$ AND $[Ca^{2+}]_c$

$[Ca^{2+}]_c$ was measured using indo-1 fluorescence in isolated perfused hearts for both control and CK-inhibited groups during baseline and high Ca^{2+} perfusion using the same protocol as described above.[6] Increasing perfusate $[Ca^{2+}]$ causes a marked increase of peak systolic $[Ca^{2+}]_c$ (from 561±61 to 872±160 nM, $p<0.05$) and $[Ca^{2+}]_c$ transient in control hearts. In contrast, no increase in systolic $[Ca^{2+}]_c$ is observed during high Ca^{2+} perfusion in CK-inhibited hearts (from 451±29 to 461±45 nM, p=ns). Similarly, RPP increases by 76% during high Ca^{2+} perfusion in control hearts while no change is observed in CK-inhibited hearts.[6] Thus, in these hearts, the inability to increase contractile function in response to high Ca^{2+} perfusion is associated with an inability to increase $[Ca^{2+}]_c$.

Taken together, results shown here support the hypothesis that a decrease in $|\Delta G{\sim}p|$ impairs Ca^{2+} handling, thereby limiting contractile reserve. Although the underlying mechanism for imparied Ca^{2+} homeostasis in CK-inhibited hearts may be multifactorial, a thermodynamic limitation of the SR Ca^{2+}-ATPase reaction is likely to be a major mechanism. Because of the limited reserve in $\Delta G{\sim}p$ for the SR Ca^{2+}-ATPase reaction, even a moderate decrease in $|\Delta G{\sim}p|$ may result in a mismatch between $\Delta G{\sim}p$ and $\Delta G_{SRCa\text{-}ATPase}$ causing impaired SR loading. Decreased net SR Ca^{2+} accumulation may reduce contractility and systolic $[Ca^{2+}]_c$ in two ways: first, less SR Ca^{2+} available for release and second, a lower fractional release of Ca^{2+} at a lower SR Ca^{2+} content.[7]

ACKNOWLEDGMENTS

I would like to thank Drs. S. Albert Camacho, Vincent M. Figueredo, Jessica M. Halow, and Joanne S. Ingwall for their contributions in this study.

REFERENCES

1. HASSELBACH, W. 1983. Energetics and electrogenicity of the sarcoplasmic reticulum calcium pump. Annu. Rev. Physiol. **45:** 325–339.
2. KAMMERMEIER, H. 1987. High energy phosphate of the myocardium: concentration versus free energy change. Basic Res. Cardiol. **82**(suppl 2): 31–36.
3. TIAN, R. *et al.* 1996. Energetic basis for reduced contractile reserve in isolated rat hearts. Am. J. Physiol. **270:** H1207–H1216.
4. HAMMAN, B. L. *et al.* 1995. Inhibition of creatine kinase reaction decreases the contractile reserve of isolated rat hearts. Am. J. Physiol. **269:** H1030–H1036.
5. TIAN, R. *et al.* 1997. Role of MgADP in the development of diastolic dysfunction in the intact beating rat heart. J. Clin. Invest. **99:** 745–751.
6. TIAN, R. *et al.* 1996. Inhibition of creatine kinase limits contractile reserve by blunting the increase of cytosolic calcium. Circulation **94:** I-420.
7. BASSANI, J.W.M. *et al.* 1995. Fractional SR Ca release is regulated by trigger Ca and SR Ca content in cardiac myocytes. Am. J. Physiol. **268:** C1313–C1329.

Sarcoplasmic Reticulum Calcium ATPase Over-expression Induces Cellular Calcium Overload and Cell Death[a]

TONY S. MA[b]

Baylor College of Medicine and Veterans Affairs Medical Center, 2002 Holcombe Boulevard, Research 151, Houston, Texas 77030, USA

Cell growth and signal transduction depend on precise balances in ionic milieu. The sequestration process in response to an elevated intracellular calcium concentration is thought to be mediated primarily by an SR calcium-ATPase.[1] In the heart, this is represented by SERCA2A,[2] representing one of three genes in the SERCA isogene group. We have designed a series of rabbit SERCA2A cDNA expression constructs for *in vitro* expression in COS cells and, using adenovirus technology for gene delivery, begun to study the functional consequence of SERCA2A overexpression.

SR CALCIUM TRANSPORT ACTIVITY WAS DIRECTLY CORRELATED TO SERCA TRANSGENE mRNA AND PROTEIN LEVEL

We have improved transient transfection efficiency greater than fivefold by co-transduction with Adenovirus F2, which is a transgeneless virus containing a CMV promoter. Transgene expression of SERCA2A of different constructs showed that a positive linear correlation was present between the level of SERCA2A mRNA and that of SERCA2A protein (FIG. 1E) and between SERCA2A protein level and calcium uptake capacity of the cell homogenate (FIG. 1F). The epitope-tagged constructs (pJL9ET and pJL12ET) showed marked attenuation of the SERCA2A activity as compared to other constructs.

SERCA OVEREXPRESSION WAS ASSOCIATED WITH CELLULAR CALCIUM OVERLOAD, DNA FRAGMENTATION, AND CELL DEATH

The pJL7 expression construct was rescued into an adenovirus vector[3] and used for subsequent functional analysis. This viral construct was designated AD.JL7. The calcium uptake rate was 7.5 ± 2.0 nmole/mg protein/10 min for control Ad.LacZ transduced cells and was significantly different from the value of 704.4 ± 21.2 nmole/mg protein/10 min for the Ad.JL7 transduced cells ($p = 0.01$, $N = 5$). Cytopathic changes were evident at 48–60 hours following Ad.JL7 viral transduction. An elevated level of cellular calcium level, as reflected by an increase of resting Fluo-3 signal, was seen in

[a] This research was supported by a Veterans Administration Merit Review Grant, a Grant-in-Aid from the American Heart Foundation (96011550), and by the Bugher Foundation.

[b] Phone: 713-791-1414; fax: 713-794-7770; e-mail: tma@tmc.bcm.edu

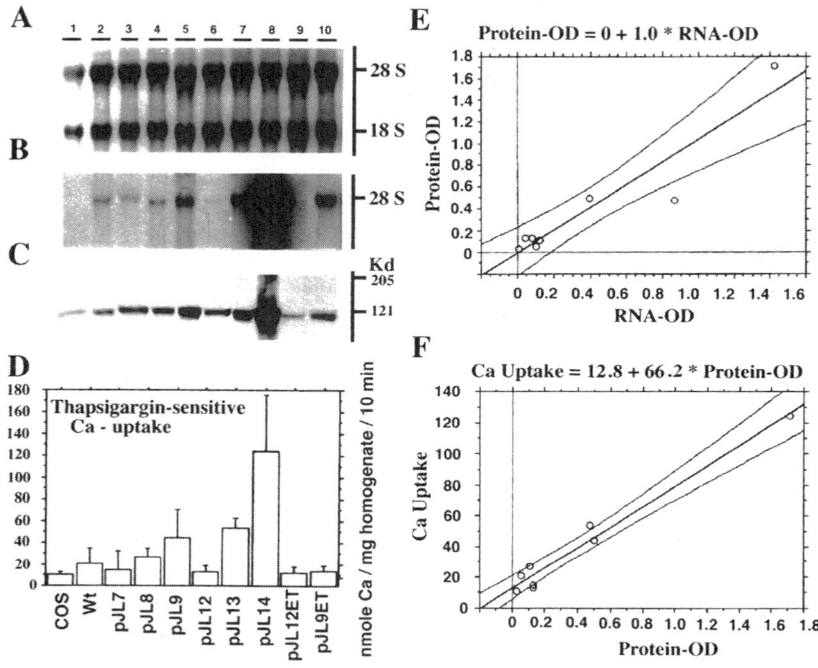

FIGURE 1. Adenovirus-facilitated transient transfection in COS cells. Transient transfection with SERCA2A expression constructs in COS cells were performed using the DEAE-dextran method, with the addition of adenovirus F2 at a concentration of 1E10 (1×10^{10} virus /ml). The clone pJG1 contains the full-length SERCA2A cDNA under the control of CMV promoter. Plasmid pJL7 contains an added human growth hormone poly-A signal. Plasmid pJL8 has the 5′ untranslated region removed by double-stranded site-directed mutagenesis using the Mutagene system (Clontech). The plasmid pJL9 has both deletion of 5′ untranslated and addition of exogenous poly-A signal. Plasmic pJL12 is driven by a RSV promoter. Plasmid pJL13 has an added β-globin intron. Plasmic pJL14 is driven by SV40 promoter. Plasmic pJL9-ET and pJL12-ET have a FLAG epitope (Eastman Kodak) inserted into the carboxy-terminus of the cDNAs. The cells were analyzed 60 hours following transfection. **(A)** Ethidium bromide–stained total COS RNA following formaldehyde gel electrophoresis. **(B** and **C)** Respectively, the Northern and Western blot analysis of the total RNA and protein. **(D)** Thapsigargin-sensitive $^{45}Ca^{2+}$-uptake capacity of COS cell homogenate of three separate experiment (mean ± SD, $N = 3$): *Lane* 1, mock transfection; *lanes* 2–10 different SERCA2A constructs. **(E)** Regression analysis between the SERCA2A mRNA and protein levels as determined by optical scanning of the autoradiograms. **(F)** Regression analysis between the SERCA2A protein level and the cell homogenate $^{45}Ca^{2+}$-uptake (mean of three experiments). The epitope-tagged constructs with altered calcium transport activities were not included in the regression analysis.

Ad.JL7 transduced cells (FIG. 2A). SERCA overexpression was associated with changes in nuclear morphology at light microscopy level, including nuclear condensation and fragmentation. Ad.JL7 transduction produced cellular genomic DNA fragmentation as compared to transduction by control AD.LacZ (FIG. 2B). This effect was also reflected in the total amount of DNA that was recovered per dish (FIG. 2C). DNA nicking was

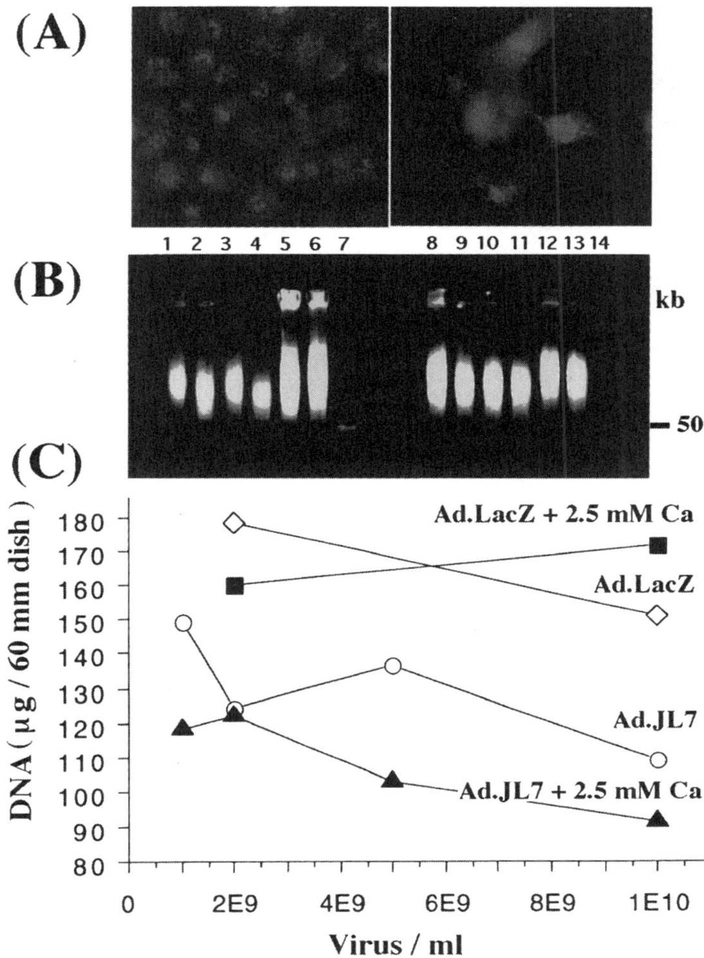

FIGURE 2. Fluo-3 fluorescence microscopy and pulsed-field gel electrophoresis of genomic DNA following AD.JL7 transduction. COS cells were transduced with control virus Ad.LacZ (**A,** *left panel*) or with SERCA virus Ad.JL7 (**A,** *right panel*) at a dose of 5E9 and analyzed 60 hours later using Fluo-3. DNA was also purified and subjected to pulsed-field gel electrophoresis from cells refed with DMEM (**B;** *lanes* 1–6) or with DMEM with an additional 2.5 mM calcium (**B;** *lanes* 8–13). The different lanes are as follows: Ad.JL7 at 1E9 (*lanes* 1&8), Ad.JL7 at 2E9 (*lanes* 2&9), Ad.JL7 at 5E9 (*lanes* 3&10), Ad.JL7 at 1E10 (*lanes* 4&11), Ad.LacZ at 2E9 (*lanes* 5&12), Ad.LacZ at 1E10 (*lanes* 6&13), and lambda DNA marker of molecular weight of 50 kb (*lanes* 7&14). DNA of the cultured cells around 200–500 kb in size was isolated by the standard technique.[7] Pulsed-field gel electrophoresis with 1% agarose was performed using 350 mA at 60-s pulses for 12 h followed by 370 mA at 90 s for 6 h (Geneline II, Beckman) using 1 × TAE. Total DNA recovered per plate was plotted as a function of viral doses **(C).**

confirmed with TUNEL assay (Boehringer) and cell death was confirmed by Live/Death Cell Assay (Molecular Probes).

Down-regulation of SERCA has been postulated to be functionally linked to the generation, maintenance, and/or the progression of some cardiac diseases.[4–6] The present data suggest that the participation of SERCA in cellular calcium metabolism may be more complicated then this simple model has stipulated, and that an uncoordinated and strong up-regulation of SERCA may be associated instead with pathologic entities. Furthermore, a primary down-regulation of SERCA in some disease states may not be simply maladaptive as previously suggested.

ACKNOWLEDGMENT

We appreciate the gift of the adenovirus shuttle vector and adenoviral LacZ reporter from Dr. F. L. Graham.

REFERENCES

1. HASSELBACH, W. 1964. Relaxing factor and the relaxation of muscle. Prog. Biophys. Mol. Biol. **14:** 169–222.
2. MACLENNAN, D. H., C. J. BRANDL, B. KORCZAK & N. M. GREEN. 1985. Amino-acid sequence of a Ca $^{2+}$ + Mg $^{2+}$-dependent ATPase from rabbit muscle sarcoplasmic reticulum, deduced from its complementary DNA sequence. Nature(Lond.) **316:** 696–700.
3. GRAHAM, F.L. & I. PREVEC. 1991. Manipulation of adenovirus vectors. *In* Methods in Molecular Biology, vol. 7: Gene transfer and expression protocols. E.J. MURRAY, Ed.: 109–128. The Humana Press Inc., Clifton, NJ.
4. DE LA BLASTIE, D., D. LEVITSKY, I. RAPPAPORT, J-J. MERCADIER, F. MAROTTE, C. WISNEWSKY, V. BROVKOVICH, K. SCHWARTZ & A-M. LOMPRE. 1990. Function of the sarcoplasmic reticulum and expression of its Ca $^{2+}$-ATPase gene in pressure overload-induced cardiac hypertrophy in the rat. Circ. Res. **66:** 554–564.
5. STUDER, R., H. REINECKE, J. BILGER, T. ESCHENHAGEN, M. BOJM, G. HASENFUB, H. JUST, J. HOLTZ & H. DREXLER. 1994. Gene expression of the cardiac Na $^{+}$-Ca $^{2+}$ exchanger in end-stage human heart failure. Circ. Res. **75:** 443–453.
6. ARAI, M., H. MATSUI & M. PERIASAMY. 1994. Sarcoplasmic reticulum gene expression in cardiac hypertrophy and heart failure. Circ. Res. **74:** 555–564.
7. SAMBROOK, J., E. F. FRITSCH & T. MANIATIS. 1992. *In* Molecular cloning: A laboratory manual. 2nd edit. Cold Spring Harbor Laboratory Press. Plainview, New York.

Pressure Overload Induces Overexpression of Annexins II and V in Aortic-Banded Rats

ION I. MORARU,[a] SERGEI SYRBU, KATERINA MICHAELS,[b] DO HAN KIM,[b,c] DIANA MALCHOFF, AND JAMES WATRAS[b]

Departments of Surgery and [b]Medicine, University of Connecticut School of Medicine, Farmington, Connecticut 06030, USA

Chronic pressure overload of the heart induces cardiac hypertrophy and frequently leads to a gradual transition to heart failure.[1] Changes in myocardial gene expression may be in part responsible for the observed alterations in myocardial contraction and relaxation during overload. Differential gene display is a new approach to directly identify specific changes in gene expression.[2] We analyzed mRNA from left ventricles of rats subjected to chronic pressure overload induced by aortic banding and found increased expression of the annexin II gene. Annexin II protein forms a heterotetramer (two annexin II molecules and two molecules of p11) that was previously named calpactin I and lipocortin II.[3] Annexin II is a member of a supergene family of non-EF-hand Ca^{2+}- and phospholipid-binding proteins that includes annexin V and VI, the major cardiac annexins.[4] Here we report that these three annexins are regulated differently in the heart of rats subjected to chronic pressure overload.

METHODS

Young (175–200 g weight) male Sprague-Dawley rats (N=24) were subjected to banding of the descending aorta and sacrificed at 7 days and 8 weeks post-surgery.[5] Separately, sham-operated control animals were subjected to the same surgical procedure except that the ligature around the aorta was left untied. Total RNA was purified from frozen ventricular tissue fragments by a modification of the acid guanidinium thiocyanate method and mRNA extracted using paramagnetic particles (PolyAtract™; Promega Corp., Madison, WI). Aliquots containing 10 ng mRNA were reverse-transcribed and amplified based on the method described by Ralph and colleagues.[6] Reverse-transcription was performed using oligo$(dT)_{15}$ as primer and 2 µl of a 1:5 dilution of the cDNA was used in 20 µl PCR amplification reactions with primers ZF-8 and ZF-9; negative controls were done by omitting reverse transcriptase from the first reaction. After separation on a 6% polyacrylamide/urea sequencing gel, the amplified fragments that showed differential expression were re-amplified by high-stringency PCR with the appropriate primer, subcloned into the pCR II vector (TA Cloning®; Invitrogen, Carlsbad, CA), and sequenced by the dideoxy chain termination method. Northern blottings were performed using random-primed ^{32}P-labeled probes and an

[a] Address for correspondence: Ion I. Moraru, M.D., Ph.D., Surgical Research Center, University of Connecticut Health Center, Farmington, Connecticut 06030-1110. Phone: 860-679-2908; fax: 860-679-2451; e-mail: moraru@panda.uchc.edu

[c] Present address: Department of Life Science, Kwangju Institute of Science and Technology, Kwangju, Korea.

aqueous exclusion hybridization rate-enhancing solution (QuickHyb®; Stratagene, La Jolla, CA) according to manufacturer's protocols. Signal quantification was done by radiometric scanning with a Phosphorimager™ SI (Molecular Dynamics, Sunnyvale, CA). Results were calibrated by re-probing for glyceraldehyde-3-phosphate dehydrogenase mRNA levels.

RESULTS

Chronic aortic banding (8 weeks) resulted in cardiac hypertrophy as shown by a 37±5.6% increase in heart/body weight ratios compared to sham-operated controls. Frozen left ventricular fragments from banded and sham-operated animals were used for differential display analysis of mRNA levels. Screening with two primers of the circularly permutated 20-primer set described by Ralph and colleagues revealed seven fragments that showed a change in expression in the hypertrophied hearts. One of these fragments was identified by sequencing to be part of the annexin II gene. Quantitative Northern hybridization was performed to estimate changes in myocardial mRNA levels for annexin II as well as for annexin V and annexin VI, the most abundant annexins in cardiac tissue.[4] FIGURE 1(A) shows that both annexin II and V were overexpressed in the hypertrophied hearts while no significant changes were detected in annexin VI mRNA. When experiments were performed on a separate group of rats sacrificed at 7 days after aortic banding surgery a similar overexpression of annexin II and V was observed (FIG. 1,B) without significant change in annexin VI mRNA. Thus, the expression of annexins II and V appears to be an early and persistent effect of pressure overload.

DISCUSSION

In the present study, differential display PCR identified annexin II as a specifically up-regulated gene in hypertrophied rat hearts. To test whether this is a selective induction of annexin II expression or part of a more general pattern of changes in annexin gene expression, determinations of mRNA levels for annexins V and VI, which have a significant constitutive expression in cardiomyocytes, were also performed. In contrast to annexins II and V, annexin VI mRNA appeared unchanged in the hypertrophied hearts. In addition, annexin II up-regulation was greater at 8 weeks pressure overload than at one week, whereas annexin V expression showed no significant difference in the degree of up-regulation at these two time points. These results suggest that the different members of the annexin family are individually regulated during the development of cardiac hypertrophy.

Although annexins are Ca^{2+} binding proteins and Ca^{2+} is a major regulator of cardiomyocyte function, the role of these proteins in the heart is not known. Annexin II has been identified in non-cardiomyocyte cells in normal hearts and has been shown to play an important role in the mechanism of exocytosis in secretory cells.[7] Whether the observed up-regulation of annexin II could be related to the re-induction in ventricular cardiomyocytes of atrial natriuretic factor gene expression and secretion that occurs in hypertrophied and failing hearts[8] remains to be determined. Annexin V is present in significant amount in normal cardiomyocytes and its increase after pressure overload may be related to the altered intracellular Ca^{2+} homeostasis that characterizes hypertrophied and failing myocardium. This hypothesis is further supported by our recent experiments showing that an antibody to annexin V can block the ATPase activity of the sarcoplasmic reticulum Ca^{2+} pump in human failing hearts.[9]

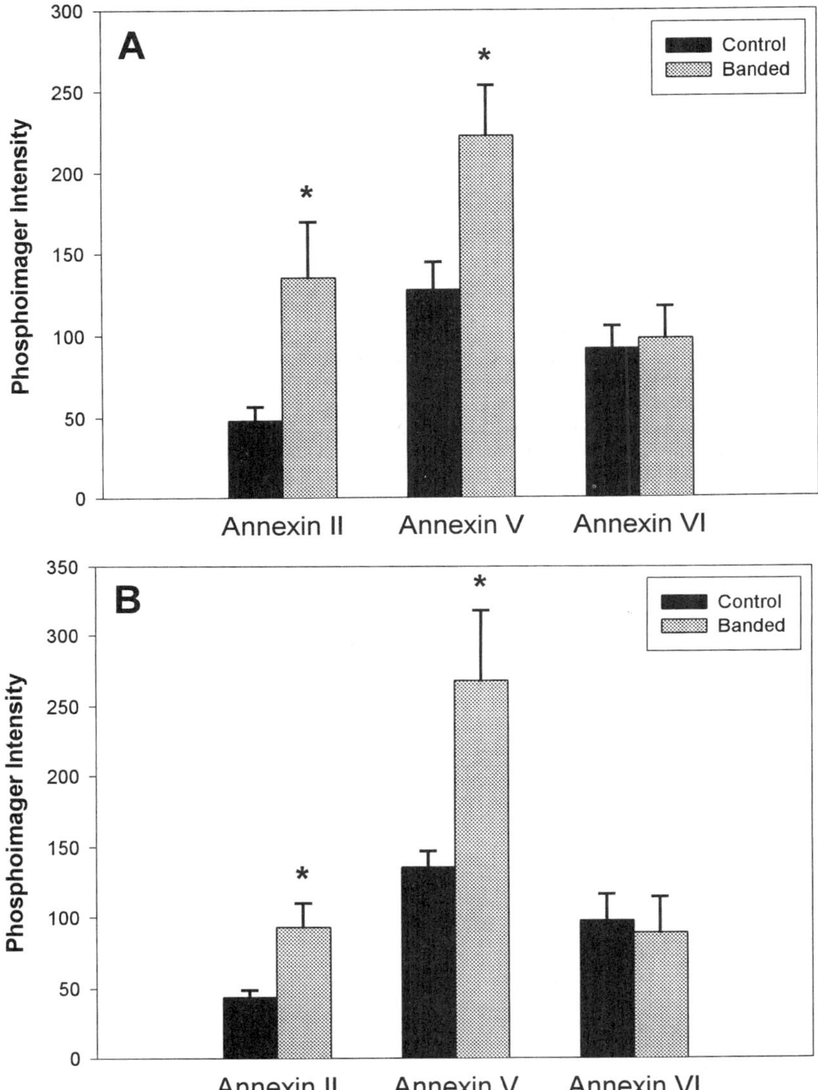

FIGURE 1. Northern blot analysis of annexins II, V, and VI mRNA in rat hearts 8 weeks after aortic banding **(A)** or 7 days after aortic banding **(B),** compared to age-matched sham-operated rats. The intensities of the bands in the Northern blots were quantitated (in arbitrary units) using a Phosphorimager™ SI and calibrated by reprobing for a housekeeping gene mRNA (GAPDH), with data presented as mean intensity ± SD for 6 hearts in each group. A statistically significant change ($p < 0.05$) in signal intensity in hearts from aortic-banded rats (compared to sham-operated rats) is indicated by an *asterisk.*

In summary, pressure overload–induced hypertrophy is associated with an increased expression of annexins II and V. We hypothesize that annexin V up-regulation may contribute to the altered Ca^{2+} transport in failing hearts.

REFERENCES

1. Katz, A. M. 1994. The cardiomyopathy of overload: An unnatural growth response in the hypertrophied heart. Ann. Intern. Med. **121 (5):** 363–371.
2. McClelland, M., F. Mathieu-Daude & J. Welsh. 1995. RNA fingerprinting and differential display using arbitrarily primed PCR. Trends Genet. **11 (6):** 242–246.
3. Raynal, P., & H. B. Pollard. 1994. Annexins: the problem of assessing the biological role for a gene family of multifunctional calcium- and phospholipid-binding proteins. Biochim. Biophys. Acta **1197 (1):** 63–93.
4. Doubell, A. F., C. Lazure, C. Charbonneau & G. Thibault. 1993. Identification and immunolocalisation of annexins V and VI, the major cardiac annexins, in rat heart. Cardiovasc. Res. **27 (7):** 1359–1367.
5. Michaels, K., C. H. Cho, I. Moraru, N. Spoerel & D. H. Kim. 1996. Quantitation of Ca^{2+} release channel mRNA in pressure-overload induced hypertrophic rat heart by competitive reverse transcription and competitive polymerase chain reaction. Mol. Cells. **6 (5):** 528–533.
6. Ralph, D., M. McClelland & J. Welsh. 1993. RNA fingerprinting using arbitrarily primed PCR identifies differentially regulated RNAs in mink lung (Mv1Lu) cells growth arrested by transforming growth factor beta 1. Proc. Natl. Acad. Sci. USA **90 (22):** 10710–10714.
7. Creutz, C. E. 1992. The annexins and exocytosis. Science **258 (5084):** 924–931.
8. Feldman, A. M., E. O. Weinberg, P. E. Ray & B. H. Lorell. 1993. Selective changes in cardiac gene expression during compensated hypertrophy and the transition to cardiac decompensation in rats with chronic aortic banding. Circ. Res. **73 (1):** 184–192.
9. Moraru, I. I., S. Syrbu, N. Zecevic, W. D. Hager, J. Watras & F. Messineo. 1998. An antibody to annexin V blocks Ca^{2+}-dependent ATPase activity of sarcoplasmic reticulum in human failing hearts. Ann. N.Y. Acad. Sci.: **853.** This volume.

An Antibody to Annexin V Blocks Ca^{2+}-Dependent ATPase Activity of Sarcoplasmic Reticulum in Human Failing Hearts

ION I. MORARU,[a] SERGEI SYRBU,[b] NADA ZECEVIC,[b] W. DAVID HAGER,[b] JAMES WATRAS,[b] AND FRANK MESSINEO[b,c]

Departments of Surgery and [b]Medicine, University of Connecticut School of Medicine, Farmington, Connecticut 06030, USA

Annexins are found in a variety of cell types and are members of a multigene family of non-EF-hand Ca^{2+} binding proteins.[1] A total of 13 annexins have been identified, though only 10 of these annexins are found in mammals.[1] Annexin V is up-regulated in rat hearts following pressure overload–induced hypertrophy[2] and in failing human hearts,[3,4] though the intracellular localization of the up-regulated annexin V is unclear. The possibility exists that the up-regulated annexin V binds nonspecifically to the sarcolemma and intracellular membranes of cardiomyocytes in the presence of Ca^{2+}. Alternatively, a fraction of the up-regulated annexin V may be integrated into a particular membrane such as the sarcoplasmic reticulum (SR). The present study uses an antibody to annexin V to study the interaction of this molecule with the cardiac SR. The results demonstrate that a pool of annexin V is closely associated with the SR Ca^{2+}-ATPase (SERCA2) in the human failing heart, raising the possibility that annexin V may modulate SR Ca^{2+} transport.

METHODS

Explanted hearts from patients with congestive heart failure were obtained at the time of heart transplantation. The freshly explanted heart was rinsed with ice-cold lactate Ringer's solution, then the left ventricular free wall was cut into small pieces, immediately frozen in liquid nitrogen, and stored at –80°C until use. Highly purified SR vesicles were prepared from pieces of the frozen explanted hearts by a combination of differential centrifugation and sucrose step-gradient centrifugation, with SR vesicles collected at the 30/40% sucrose interface. Alternatively, a modification of the calcium-oxalate loading technique was employed to obtain highly purified SR vesicles.[5,6] These highly purified SR fractions were incubated (15 min at 37°C) with an anti-annexin V monoclonal antibody or with non-immune mouse IgG (control) and then assayed for Ca^{2+}-dependent ATPase activity using γ-^{32}P–labeled ATP. To calculate Ca^{2+}-dependent ATPase activity, Ca^{2+}-independent ATPase activity (measured in the presence of 1 mM EGTA, with no added $CaCl_2$) was subtracted from total ATPase activity (measured in the presence of 5 μM free Ca^{2+}).

[a] Address for correspondence: Ion I. Moraru, M.D., Ph.D., Surgical Research Center, University of Connecticut Health Center, Farmington, Connecticut 06030-1110. Phone: 860-679-2908; fax: 860-679-2451; e-mail: moraru@panda.uchc.edu

[c] Present address: Department of Cardiology, New York Hospital, Queens, New York.

In immunoprecipitation experiments, microsomes isolated by differential centrifugation from the left ventricular free wall of failing human hearts were solubilized in 1% Triton X-100, then precleared with protein G-sepharose. After 45-min incubation of the supernatant with excess anti-annexin V monoclonal antibody, protein G-sepharose was added and the resulting precipitate was subjected to ECL Western blot analysis (Amersham Corp., Arlington Heights, IL) using antibody probes as indicated in the figure legend.

RESULTS

Immunoblotting using an antiserum to annexin V indicated the presence of annexin V in the highly purified SR fractions isolated from the left ventricular free wall of failing human hearts. When SR vesicles were preincubated with an anti-annexin V monoclonal antibody, the Ca^{2+}-dependent ATPase activity of the SR vesicles decreased by more than 90% (FIG. 1). The antibody did not influence the Ca^{2+}-independent ATPase activity of the vesicles (FIG. 1). These results were obtained using SR vesicles

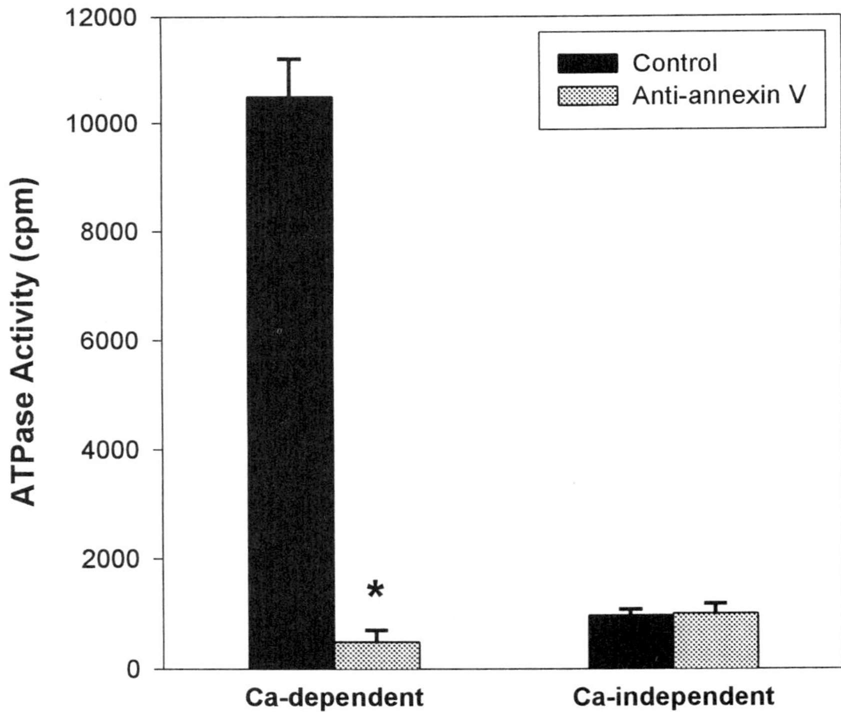

FIGURE 1. ATPase activity of purified SR vesicles in the absence (control) and presence of an antibody to annexin V. Ca^{2+}-dependent ATPase and Ca^{2+}-independent ATPase activities were calculated as described in METHODS. Data are means ± SE ($N = 6$), with statistically significant changes ($p < 0.05$) in ATPase activity indicated by an *asterisk*.

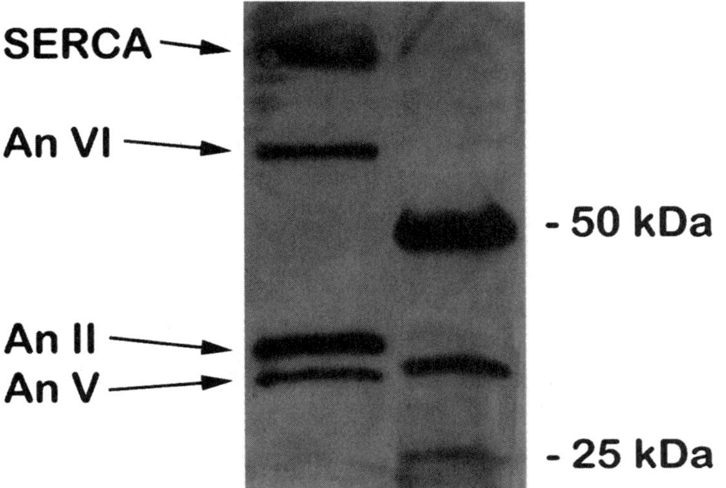

FIGURE 2. Immunoprecipitation of annexin V from failing human heart microsomes. Western blots of solubilized microsomes from left ventricular myocardium *(left lane)* and the immunoprecipitate obtained using a monoclonal antibody to annexin V *(right lane)* were probed with antibodies to annexin II, annexin V, annexin VI, and SERCA2. The bands at 50 kDa and 25 kDa represent the IgG heavy and light chains, respectively, of the anti-annexin V antibody used in the immunoprecipitation. There was no evidence of SERCA2 in the anti-annexin V immunoprecipitate.

isolated by sucrose gradient centrifugation. Similar results, however, were also obtained using the calcium-oxalate purified SR vesicles. All ATPase activities were determined during the linear phase of ATP hydrolysis.

We used immunoprecipitation and immunoblotting experiments to determine if the anti-annexin V monoclonal antibody that was used in the ATPase assays cross-reacted with SERCA2. There was no evidence of any interaction between the anti-annexin V monoclonal antibody and SERCA2 in Western blots of SR proteins (data not shown). Additionally, no evidence of interaction was seen under nondenaturing conditions (FIG. 2). The left lane in FIGURE 2 shows that the crude microsomal preparation used contains SERCA2, annexin II, annexin V, and annexin VI. The right lane in FIGURE 2 shows that upon solubilization of this microsomal fraction using a non-ionic detergent, the antibody to annexin V precipitated only annexin V. These results suggest that inhibition of the SR Ca^{2+}-ATPase activity by the anti-annexin V monoclonal antibody was not due to nonspecific interaction of the antibody with SERCA2 or with other annexins.

DISCUSSION

Annexins have been well characterized in terms of protein structure, although their intracellular functions remain poorly understood.[7] Annexin V has been shown to form channels in artificial planar lipid bilayers,[8] and to be present in cardiomyocytes.[9] We have previously reported that annexin V is up-regulated in the hypertrophied and failing heart.[2,4] Up-regulation of annexin V in the SR may therefore impair the ability of the SR to sequester Ca^{2+} by increasing SR Ca^{2+} efflux. No direct evidence of Ca^{2+} fluxes due to the presence of endogenous annexin V in cellular membranes, however, has been reported. In the present study, we show that an antibody to annexin V can inhibit SR Ca^{2+}-ATPase activity, which may reflect a close association of annexin V with SERCA2. While the degree of inhibition depends on the amount of anti-annexin V antibody, the ability of the antibody to almost completely inhibit SERCA2 activity is particularly interesting, since the level of SERCA2 probably exceeds the level of annexin V in the cardiomyocyte. As indicated in the *Results* section, we have ruled out the possible artifact of nonspecific interaction of the antibody with SERCA2, since we have been unable to detect cross-reactivity between the antibody and SERCA2 using either Western blotting or immunoprecipitation. It has recently been shown that aggregation of SERCA2 in the SR inhibits SERCA2 activity,[10,11] raising the possibility that annexin V (perhaps in combination with annexin V antibody) may promote aggregation of SERCA2, such that a low ratio of annexin V to SERCA2 may be sufficient for complete inhibition of ATPase activity. Direct studies (aimed at assessing aggregation of SERCA2 and determining the ratio of annexin V to SERCA2) are needed to directly test this hypothesis.

In summary, the present study shows that an antibody to annexin V can markedly inhibit the Ca^{2+}-dependent ATPase activity of SR isolated from failing human myocardium. This effect may reflect a close association of annexin V with SERCA2. In view of our recent observation that up-regulation of annexin V in rat cardiomyocytes is associated with a decrease in SERCA2 activity (manuscript submitted for publication), we hypothesize that the observed up-regulation of annexin V in the failing human heart may contribute to the slowed myocardial relaxation seen in heart failure patients.

REFERENCES

1. Smith, P. D., & S. E. Moss. 1994. Structural evolution of the annexin supergene family. Trends Genet. **10 (7):** 241–246.
2. Moraru, I. I., S. Syrbu, K. Michaels, D. H. Kim, D. Malchoff, & J. Watras. 1997. Pressure overload induces overexpression of annexins II and V in aortic-banded rats. Ann. N.Y. Acad. Sci.: **853.** This volume.
3. Song, G., C. M. Pawloski-Dahm, D. Kirkpatrick, W. L. E., & R. A. Walsh. 1996. Cardiac annexins are differentially regulated in human end-stage heart failure. Circulation **94** (8SI): I-725–I-726.
4. Syrbu, S., J. Watras, N. Zecevic & I. I. Moraru. 1996. Functional association of annexin V with the sarcoplasmic reticulum Ca^{2+}-ATPase of human failing heart. Presented at the Conference on the Molecular Biology of the Normal, Hypertrophied, and Failing Heart. Salt Lake City, UT.
5. Jones, L. R. & S. E. Cala. 1981. Biochemical evidence for functional heterogeneity of cardiac sarcoplasmic reticulum vesicles. J. Biol. Chem. **256 (22):** 11809–11818.
6. Chamberlain, B. K., D. O. Levitsky & S. Fleischer. 1983. Isolation and characterization of canine cardiac sarcoplasmic reticulum with improved Ca^{2+} transport properties. J. Biol. Chem. **258 (10):** 6602–6609.
7. Raynal, P., & H. B. Pollard. 1994. Annexins: the problem of assessing the biological role for a gene family of multifunctional calcium- and phospholipid-binding proteins. Biochim. Biophys. Acta **1197 (1):** 63–93.
8. Berendes, R., D. Voges, P. Demange, R. Huber & A. Burger. 1993. Structure-function analysis of the ion channel selectivity filter in human annexin V. Science **262 (5132):** 427–430.

9. Doubell, A. F., C. Lazure, C. Charbonneau & G. Thibault. 1993. Identification and immunolocalisation of annexins V and VI, the major cardiac annexins, in rat heart. Cardiovasc. Res. **27 (7):** 1359–1367.
10. Mersol, J. V., H. Kutchai, J. E. Mahaney & D. D. Thomas. 1995. Self-association accompanies inhibition of Ca-ATPase by thapsigargin. Biophys. J. **68 (1):** 208–215.
11. Shi, Y., B. S. Karon, H. Kutchai & D. D. Thomas. 1996. Phospholamban-dependent effects of C12E8 on calcium transport and molecular dynamics in cardiac sarcoplasmic reticulum. Biochemistry **35 (41):** 13393–13399.

Reduced Sarcoplasmic Reticulum Ca^{2+} Release in Rabbits with Left Ventricular Dysfunction

PAUL NEARY,[a,b] STUART M. COBBE,[c] AND GODFREY L. SMITH[b]

[b]*Clinical Research Initiative in Heart Failure University of Glasgow, University of Glasgow, Glasgow G12 8QQ, United Kingdom*

[c]*Department of Cardiology, Glasgow Royal Infirmary, Glasgow, United Kingdom*

Heart failure is a clinical syndrome characterized by impaired left ventricular function. The pathophysiology of heart failure is complex and multifactorial, but abnormal contractile function of cardiac myocytes is central to ventricular dysfunction.[1] Abnormalities of Ca^{2+} homeostasis are thought to contribute to contractile dysfunction in ventricular myocytes in heart failure (see Gwathmey and colleagues[2] for review) with a prolongation of the intracellular Ca^{2+} transient, and a possible reduction of the systolic amplitude of the Ca^{2+} transient. The findings of abnormal expression of sarcoplasmic reticulum (SR) proteins in heart failure[3] suggested that SR dysfunction may contribute to alterations in the Ca^{2+} transient, but these findings have been disputed by some authors.[4] In addition, a number of cellular factors are altered in heart failure that may directly depress the Ca^{2+} content of the SR, including sarcolemmal Ca^{2+} currents,[5] cardiac phosphate metabolism,[6] and intracellular pH.[6] Preparation of SR vesicles allows complete control of the intracellular conditions but markedly disrupts the geometry of the SR. The purpose of this study was therefore to investigate SR function in heart failure in isolation from changes in other cellular factors, while retaining the structural integrity of the SR.

METHODS

Left ventricular dysfunction was induced in adult male New Zealand White rabbits (3.1–4.2 kg) by ligation of the marginal branch of the left circumflex artery. Cardiac remodelling was allowed to progress for 8 weeks after which the degree of dysfunction was confirmed and quantified by echocardiography prior to sacrifice.

Single myocytes were isolated by Langendorff perfusion of rabbit heart with protease and collagenase solutions. Isolated cells were placed into the chamber of a perfusion bath (300 µl volume), on an inverted Nikon microscope, and perfused with an EGTA-buffered solution to mimic intracellular conditions (EGTA 0.1 mM; ATP 5 mM; Phosphocreatine 15 mM; HEPES 25 mM; KCl 120 mM; $MgCl_2$ 5.6 mM; free Ca^{2+} approximately 20 nM). Fluorescence at 340 nm and 380 nm was measured using a spinning wheel system and Cairn spectrophotometer. Single cells were anchored using a blunt, sealed, glass microelectrode coated in "cell-tak" to improve holding, and perfused at 0.5 ml per minute at room temperature. Cells were permeabilized by brief exposure to β-escin (100 µg per ml), a saponin-like molecule that removes cholesterol moieties from the sarcolemma.

[a] Address for correspondence: Paul Neary, Clinical Research Fellow, Clinical Research Initiative in Heart Failure, West Medical Building, Glasgow University, Glasgow G12 8QQ, United Kingdom. Phone: 44-141 339 8855 (ext.2508); fax: 44-141 330 4612; e-mail: P.Neary@bio.gla.ac.uk

Ca^{2+} release from SR was monitored by including Fura-2 acid (10 μM solution) in the perfusate. Cellular contraction was simultaneously monitored using real-time video recording. Ca^{2+} release and cell contraction was stimulated by the rapid injection of caffeine (20 mM) close to the cell or by raising cytosolic [Ca^{2+}] until spontaneous release occurred. The amplitude of caffeine-induced and spontaneous Ca^{2+} release were compared in cells from control and experimental rabbits.

RESULTS

Mean ejection fractions (± SEM) for control and experimental animals were 73.8% (± 1.9) and 48.1% (± 2.9), respectively. TABLE 1 shows mean data for caffeine-induced and spontaneous SR Ca^{2+} release at cytosolic [Ca^{2+}] 50–250μM. The amplitude of caffeine-induced SR Ca^{2+} release was significantly lower at 50–100μM cytosolic [Ca^{2+}] ($p<0.05$), and spontaneous SR Ca^{2+} release was significantly lower at 150–250μM cytosolic [Ca^{2+}] ($p<0.01$). This is shown in FIGURE 1.

DISCUSSION

Abnormal Ca^{2+} homeostasis has previously been shown in preparations from patients with terminal heart failure, but these results in this model of compensated left ventricular dysfunction confirm that abnormalities of Ca^{2+} handling are present in the early stages of ventricular remodelling (8 weeks post-infarct). This β-escin–permeabilized cardiac cell preparation allowed the study of the Ca^{2+} accumulating ability of the SR in isolation from any changes in sarcolemmal Ca^{2+} transport and cardiac metabolism, whilst the SR structure remains undisturbed. The consequences of a reduced ability of the SR to accumulate Ca^{2+} in heart failure would be a reduction in the amplitude of systolic Ca^{2+} release, and hence a reduction in the force of contraction.

Given that the amplitude of both spontaneous and caffeine-induced SR Ca^{2+} release are reduced, it is likely that this reflects impaired SR Ca^{2+} loading, rather than impaired release per se, since caffeine-induced Ca^{2+} release is thought to maximally stimulate Ca^{2+}-induced Ca^{2+} release. This is in keeping with previous reports of a reduction in protein levels of the SERCA-2 (SR Ca^{2+}-ATPase pump). This does not however exclude the presence of additional direct abnormalities of SR Ca^{2+} release, and further ex-

TABLE 1. Caffeine-Induced and Spontaneous Ca^{2+} Release in Sham and LVD Rabbits

	Caffeine-Induced Release			Spontaneous Release		
Cytosolic [Ca^{2+}]	LVD	Sham	*p*	LVD	Sham	*p*
50nM	20.2±3.4	36.8±3.5	<0.05	—	—	—
100 nM	44.3±6.1	64.3±6.1	<0.05	—	—	—
150 nM	45.3±8.1	69.8±9.9	>0.05	37.5±4.3	81.5±9.5	<0.01
200 nM	—	—	—	51.9±4.4	103.3±12.8	<0.01
250 nM	—	—	—	75.5±7.1	153.7±15.1	<0.01

NOTE: LVD rabbits were subjected to induced left ventricular dysfunction. Experimental details in text. Ca^{2+} release shown in nM ± SEM.

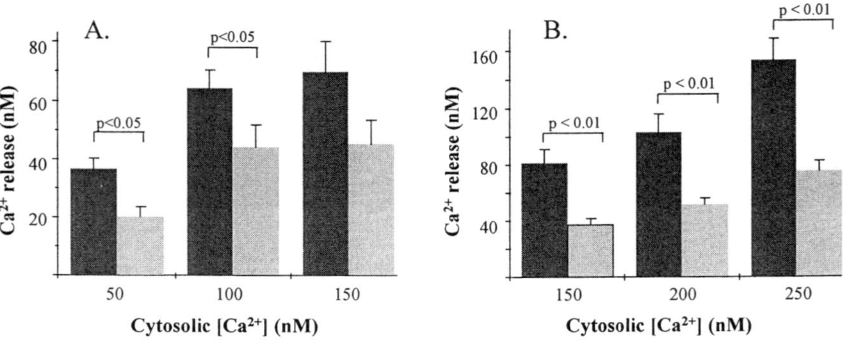

FIGURE 1. Plot of cytosolic [Ca^{2+}] against amplitude of SR Ca^{2+} release. **(A)** Caffeine-induced. **(B)** Spontaneous.

periments are needed to investigate the function of the Ca^{2+} release channel (the ryanodine receptor) in heart failure.

REFERENCES

1. Del Monte, F. *et al.* 1995. Cell geometry and contractile abnormalities of myocytes from failing human left ventricle. Cardiovasc. Res. **30:** 281–290.
2. Gwathmey, J.K. *et al.* 1995. Basic pathophysiology of heart failure. Cardiol. Revs. **3:** 282–291.
3. Movsesian, M. A. *et al.* 1990. Identification and characterization of proteins in sarcoplasmic reticulum from normal and failing human left ventricles. J. Mol. Cell. Cardiol. **22:** 1477–1485.
4. Schwinger, R. H. G. *et al.* 1995. Unchanged protein-levels of serca-ii and phospholamban but reduced Ca^{2+} uptake and Ca^{2+}-ATPase activity of cardiac sarcoplasmic-reticulum from dilated cardiomyopathy patients compared with patients with nonfailing hearts. Circulation **92:** 3220–3228.
5. Ouadid, H. *et al.* 1995. Calcium currents in diseased human cardiac cells. J. Cardiovasc. Pharmacol. **25:** 282–291.
6. Elliott, A. C. *et al.* 1992. Metabolic changes during ischaemia and their role in contractile failure in isolated ferret hearts. J. Physiol. **454:** 467–490.

Structural Proximity of Mitochondria to Calcium Release Units in Rat Ventricular Myocardium May Suggest a Role in Ca^{2+} Sequestration

V. RAMESH,[a] V. K. SHARMA,[b] S-S. SHEU,[b] AND C. FRANZINI-ARMSTRONG[c,d]

[a]*Division of Cardiology, Children's Hospital of Philadelphia, Philadelphia, Pennsylvania, USA*
[c]*Department of Cell and Developmental Biology, University of Pennsylvania, Philadelphia, Pennsylvania 19104, USA*
[b]*Department of Pharmacology and Physiology, University of Rochester, Rochester, New York 14642, USA*

There has been significant controversy[1,2] about whether or not mitochondria are capable of transiently sequestering Ca^{2+}. This question is of special importance in cardiac muscle, where mitochondria occupy a large portion of the cell volume. Isolated mitochondria have relatively low affinity[3] for Ca^{2+}—i.e., K_m of 2 to 30 μM—and thus they are not expected to compete successfully with the Ca^{2+} ATPase of the sarcoplasmic reticulum (SR). Electron microprobe analysis experiments have indicated a low steady state content of calcium $[Ca]_m$ in liver mitochondria, and either no changes or an increase in $[Ca]_m$ upon activation of cardiac muscle.[1] A transient increase in $[Ca]_m$ has also been detected *in vivo* using a recombinant chimeric aequorin targeted to the mitochondria in pancreatic β-cells,[4] hepatocytes[5] and isolated cardiomyocytes[6]; and *in vitro,*[7] affecting the rate of relaxation in red skeletal muscle fibers, by decreasing the clearing time for cytoplasmic Ca^{2+}. Geometrical factors play a major role in determining the time course of local Ca^{2+} gradients within the cytoplasm. In muscle cells, Ca^{2+} is released at the calcium release units (CRUs), or sites of junctions between the SR and T tubules (dyads or triads), which contain the ryanodine receptors (RyRs or feet). If mitochondria are located in close proximity of CRUs, they are expected to see short-lived but high concentration pulses of Ca^{2+}. Our measurements indicate that diffusion distances between CRUs and mitochondria are extremely short in rat left (LV) and right ventricular (RV) myocardium.

METHODS

Left and right ventricles of adult (4–6 wk old) Sprague-Dawley rats were fixed in glutaraldehyde and osmium and stained *en bloc* in uranyl acetate. The following distances were measured: *Near* **(NFD)** and *far* **(FFD)** *feet distances,* are the smallest dis-

[d] Address for correspondence: Dr C. Franzini-Armstrong, Department of Cell and Developmental Biology, University of Pennsylvania Medical School, 245 Anatomy-Chemistry Building, 36th St and Hamilton Walk, Philadelphia, Pennsylvania 19104-6058. Phone: 215-898-3345; fax: 215-573-2170.

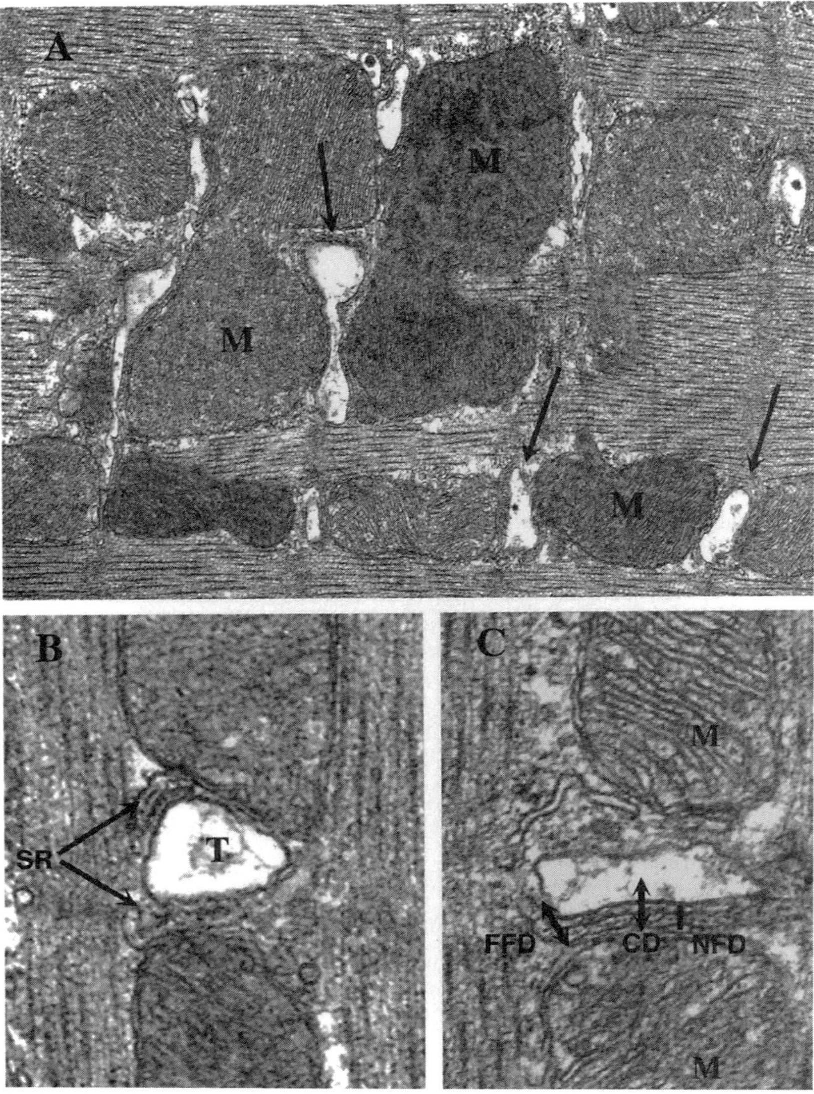

FIGURE 1. Mouse cardiac muscle: Left ventricle fibers, thin longitudinal section. **(A)** Mitochondria (M) in in close proximity to the CRUs *(arrow)*. **(B)** Two SR elements are apposed to a T tubule profile (T) to form a triad. **(C)** The three distances measured are indicated (see text).

tances between the mitochondrial membrane and the nearest and farthest feet (RyRs) within an adjacent CRU. *Center distance* (CD) is the smallest mitochondria to center of T tubule distance. (*N*=100 measurements from 3 rats).

RESULTS

Mitochondria are densely packed in continuous rows between the myofibrils and CRUs are mostly nestled between the ends of two elongated, longitudinally oriented mitochondria (FIG. 1). Most of the mitochondrial profiles (122 over 194 or 63%) are in close proximity of a CRU and over 90% CRUs are in close proximity to a mitochondrion. The actual contacts between the two organelles are probably more frequent than this number, since many are not in the plane of section (FIG 1,C). Near and far feet distances are an average of 33 and 188 nm (TABLE 1). The center of the T tubule, approximately equidistant from all the channels in the CRU, is also in close proximity to the mitochondria (138–160 nm).

DISCUSSION

During activation of muscle fibers, Ca^{2+} release from CRUs is the sum of individual events that result in a spatially delimited short-lasting Ca^{2+} spikes or "sparks".[8] In cardiac muscle of the rat, we find that practically all mitochondria are very closely apposed to CRUs, which transiently exposes them to a relatively high concentration of Ca^{2+} within a few msec of Ca^{2+} release from the SR. Contrary to previous reports,[9] our preliminary data using Ca^{2+} dyes (unpublished observation) also show that mitochondria sequester Ca^{2+} on a beat-to-beat basis at low frequency stimulation. It is not yet known whether Ca^{2+} uptake by mitochondria affects relaxation in cardiac muscle. In red skeletal muscle fibers which, like cardiac muscle, have a high content of mitochondria, the rate of relaxation is affected by these organelles.[7]

The above considerations suggest that the distribution of mitochondria within the muscle cell may have a significance that has not yet been fully appreciated. For example, what might be the effect of two vastly different distributions of mitochondria that are found in two different very fast muscles: the flight muscle of the dragonfly and the sound-producing muscle of the toadfish swimbladder? In the former, mitochondria are quite intimately associated with CRUs between the myofibrils, while in the latter they are segregated in the fiber core, away from myofibrils and CRUs.

TABLE 1. Distances between Mitochondria and Adjacent Calcium Release Unit

	Near Feet Distance (NFD) (nm)	Far Feet Distance (FFD) (nm)	Center Distance (CD) (nm)
Left ventricle (LV)	37.3 ± 19.8	187.6 ± 63.7	138.6 ± 53.8
Right ventricle (RV)	35.9 ± 9.8	178.9 ± 74.5	157.6 ± 44.8

NOTE: NFD and FFD are the distances between the mitochondrial outer membrane and the nearest and farthest feet in the adjacent calcium release unit. The center distance (CD) measures the distance between the center of a T tubule and the nearest mitochondrial membrane. The values shown are averages ± 1 SD from 100 measurements in 3 different hearts.

REFERENCES

1. GUNTER, K. K. & T. E. GUNTER. 1994. Transport of calcium by mitochondria. J. Bioenerg. Biomembr **26** (5): 471–485.
2. CARAFOLI, E. 1987. Intracellular calcium homeostasis. Ann. Rev. Biochem. **56:** 395–493.
3. CROMPTON, N. *et al.* 1976. A kinetic study of the energy-linked influx of Ca^{2+} into the heart mitochondria. Eur J. Biochem. **69:** 429–434.
4. RUTTER, G. A. *et al.* 1993. Stimulated Ca^{2+} influx raises mitochondrial free Ca^{2+} to supramicromolar levels in pancreatic-cell line. J. Biol. Chem. **268:** 22385–22390.
5. HAJNOCZKY, G. *et al.* 1995. Decoding of cytosolic calcium oscillations in mitochondria. Cell **82:** 415–424.
6. CHACON, E. *et al.* 1996. Mitochondria free calcium transients during excitation-contraction coupling in rabbit cardiac myocytes. FEBS Lett. **382:** 31–36.
7. GILLIS, J. M. 1997. Inhibition of mitochondrial calcium uptake slows down relaxation in mitochondria-rich skeletal muscles. J. Muscle Res. Cell Motil. **18:** 473–483.
8. CHENG, H., W. J. LEDERER & M. B. CANNELL. 1993. Calcium sparks: Elementary events underlying excitation-contraction coupling in heart muscle. Science **262:** 740–744.
9. MIYATA, H. *et al.* 1991. Measurement of mitochondrial free Ca^{2+} concentration in living single cardiac myocytes. Am. J. Phys. **261:** H1123–H1134.

Modeling Short-Term Interval-Force Relations in Cardiac Muscle

J. JEREMY RICE,[a] M. SALEET JAFRI, AND RAIMOND L. WINSLOW

Department of Biomedical Engineering, The Johns Hopkins University, 720 Rutland Avenue, Baltimore, Maryland 21205, USA

Short-term interval-force (I-F) relations describe the dependence of contraction strength for short (≤ 3-s) interbeat intervals that fall in the physiological range for active mammals. Two phenomena that characterize short-term I-F relations are restitution and post-extrasystolic potentiation, in which changes in stimulation interval produce large and well-characterized changes in output force.[1] Existing biophysically detailed cell cardiac models (Luo-Rudy and OxsoftHeart) fail to reproduce short-term I-F relations.[2] We propose a model of the single cardiac cell that incorporates more detailed descriptions of calcium handling mechanisms and myofilaments based on recent experimental findings and accurately reproduces I-F relations.

METHODS

Our model of a single guinea pig ventricular cell incorporates most membrane currents from the Luo-Rudy Phase II model to produce action potentials (APs). The model also incorporates novel Ca handling mechanisms to reproduce recent experimental findings.[3] The first mechanism is adaptation of the ryanodine receptor (RyR), where an incremental increase in [Ca] transiently increases RyR open probability. The second mechanism is L-type channel Ca-mediated inactivation in which Ca binding to the channel produces a switch to a model where transitions to open states are extremely rare. The third mechanism is a restricted subspace into which the RyR and L-type channels empty, and within which the local [Ca] can rise to a much higher level than the bulk myoplasmic [Ca]. The fourth mechanism is a formulation of the SERCA pump with separate forward and reverse rates, each with different binding constants, and with low cooperativity in both directions (~1.4 forward and ~1 reverse).[4] Isometric force is predicted by a model that incorporates multiple cooperative mechanisms thought to exist in cardiac myofilaments. These cooperative mechanisms contribute in different ways to allow the model to reproduce experimentally determined steady-state F-Ca relations and dynamic twitches.[2]

The simulation protocol is based on the experimental work of Wier and Yue[1] and is shown schematically in FIGURE 1(A). A priming period of 30 sec with fixed stimulus interval of 1,500 msec brings the model to steady state and ensures a constant SR Ca load. The extrasystolic interval (ESI) is then varied between 236.6 and 2842.1 msec in 236.6 msec increments. The post-extrasystolic interval (PESI) is fixed at 3,000 msec. It must be emphasized that the model simulation shown here involves only changes in

[a] Address for correspondence: John Jeremy Rice, Department of Biomedical Engineering, The Johns Hopkins University, 720 Rutland Avenue, Baltimore, Maryland 21205. Phone: 410-502-5091; fax: 410-614-0166; e-mail: jrice@bme.jhu.edu

A. Pacing protocol for restitution/post-extrasystolic potentiation

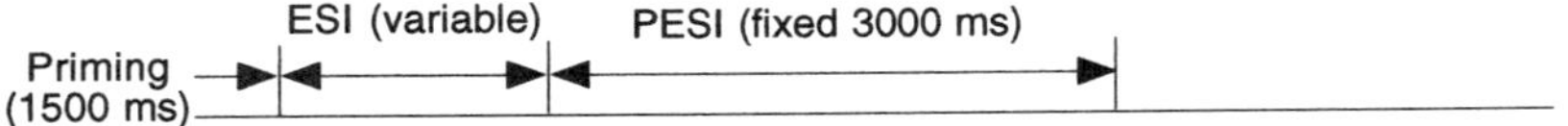

B. Myoplamic Calcium Transients

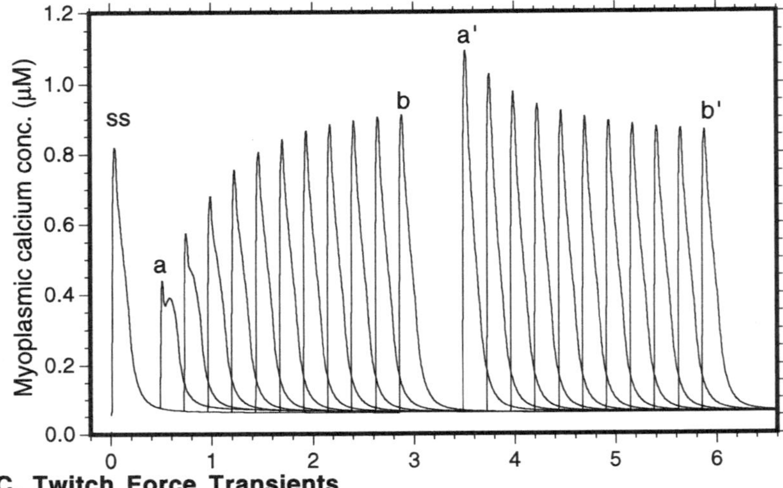

C. Twitch Force Transients

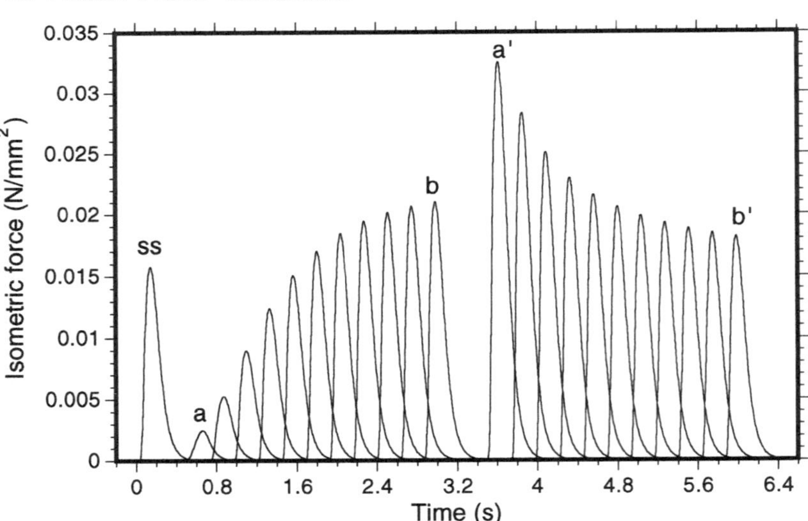

FIGURE 1. Simulation protocol and results. See text for details.

stimulus pattern, and no model parameters are varied to alter restitution/post-extrasystolic potentiation behavior.

RESULTS

Panels B and C of FIGURE 1 show simulation results for myoplasmic Ca concentration ($[Ca]_i$) and isometric twitch force, respectively. The last priming beat (labeled **ss**) is shown to demonstrate the steady state output level. These data show restitution behavior, as seen by the exponential rise (τ = 745 msec) in peak twitch force as ESI increases. There also is an exponential rise in peak force onset (positive dF/dt, not shown) with a similar time constant, consistent with experimental results. The post-extrasystolic beats show inverse behavior in that a small, unrestituted extrasystolic beat leads to a potentiated post-extrasystolic beat (see **a** and **a′**). Likewise, as extrasystolic force rises with restitution, the post-extrasystolic force declines. As seen in the experimental data, the decline of force and rate of force onset are fit well by exponentials with time constants similar to those of restitution. Note that the relative changes in peak $[Ca]_i$ are smaller than the corresponding changes in peak force, as seen in experimental data. This effect shows the important contribution of the myofilaments with high apparent cooperativity.

The restitution and post-extrasystolic potentiation behavior can be explained by an interplay of two features: RyR adaptation and SR Ca loading. Restitution can be explained by the slow recovery of the RyRs from the adapted state. This effect is shown in FIGURE 2(A), where RyR open probabilities are plotted for the same sequence as in FIGURE 1. As ESI increases, the peak open probability increases from 0.27 for the shortest ESI **(a)** to 0.85 for the longest ESI **(b).**

In contrast, the peak open probability is a constant value of 0.87 for each of the post-extrasystolic beats. In this case, SR release of Ca depends mainly on the SR load, as shown in FIGURE 2(B). The upper traces show the network SR (uptake pool) Ca concentration ($[Ca]_{NSR}$), while the lower traces show the junctional SR (release pool) Ca concentration ($[Ca]_{JSR}$). For the shortest ESI **(a)** there is a relatively small decrease in $[Ca]_{JSR}$, which recovers to a higher value. The small release occurs because most of the RyRs are in the adapted state, and *not* because of a slow transfer from NSR to JSR. In fact, NSR and JSR are tightly coupled so that their concentrations are nearly equal, except during a release when $[Ca]_{JSR}$ is slightly lower. FIGURE 2(B) shows that potentiation at **a′** occurs because $[Ca]_{JSR}$ recovers to a level higher than the steady state value during the priming period at **ss.** The small release **(a)** leaves more residual Ca in SR to help potentiate the next beat. Moreover, augmented transarcolemmal influx further increases SR load. First, the small SR release **(a)** produces less Ca-induced inactivation of L-Type channels. Second, the AP for **a** (not shown) has reduced amplitude because the time-dependent K^+ membrane current has not fully recovered at **(a).** Here the peak membrane potential is closer to the optimum voltage for influx through the L-Type Ca channel (near 0 mV) so that the low amplitude AP favors Ca influx. The SERCA pump formulation is important because the low forward cooperatively (~1.4) produces significant SR Ca loading, even for the small $[Ca]_i$ transient at the shortest ESI (see **a** in FIG. 1,B).

CONCLUSIONS

By incorporating detailed descriptions of Ca handling and force generation, we have produced a model that can reproduce short-term I-F relations. The model suggests

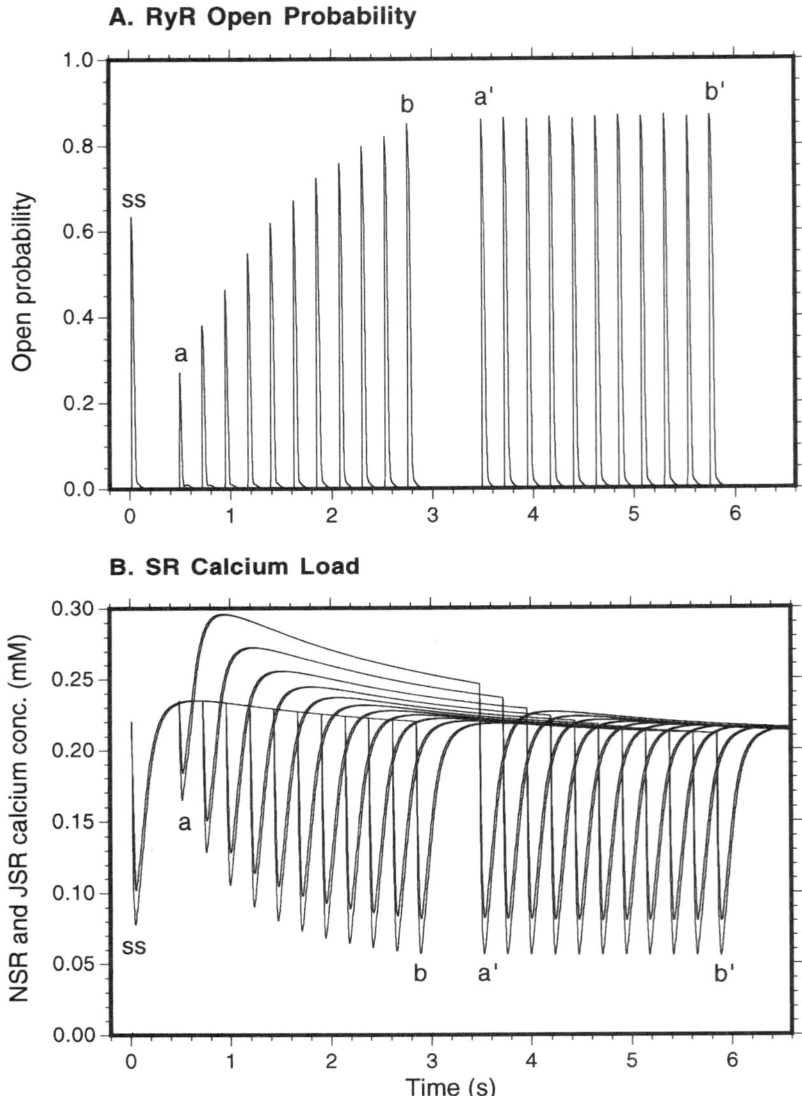

FIGURE 2. RyR adaptation and SR Ca loading. See text for details.

that restitution and post-extrasystolic potentiation behavior can be explained by an interplay of RyR adaptation and Ca SR loading. Restitution results directly from a slow recovery of the RyRs from the adapted state. For a small extrasystole, potentiation occurs because more Ca remains in SR and transarcolemmal influx increases due to reduced Ca-induced inactivation of L-Type channels and reduced AP amplitude.

REFERENCES

1. Wier, W. G. & D. T. Yue. 1986. Intracellular calcium transients underlying short-term force-interval relationship in ferret ventricular myocardium. J. Physiol. **376:** 507–530.
2. Rice, J. J. 1997. Modeling Calcium Handling, Force Generation, and Length Effects in Cardiac Cells. Ph.D. thesis, The Johns Hopkins University, Baltimore, MD.
3. Jafri, M. S., J. R. Rice & R. L. Winslow. 1998. Cardiac Ca^{2+} dynamics: The roles of ryanodine receptor adaptation and sarcoplasmic reticulum load. Biophys. J. **74:** 1149–1168.
4. Shannon, T. S., K. S. Ginsberg & D. M. Bers. 1998. Reverse mode of the SR Ca pump limits SR Ca uptake in permeabilized and voltage clamped myocytes. Ann. N.Y. Acad. Sci This volume.

Reverse Mode of the Sarcoplasmic Reticulum Ca Pump Limits Sarcoplasmic Reticulum Ca Uptake in Permeabilized and Voltage-Clamped Myocytes

THOMAS R. SHANNON, KENNETH S. GINSBURG, AND DONALD M. BERS[a]

Department of Physiology, Loyola University Chicago, Maywood, Illinois 60153, USA

Typical cardiac Ca transients in myocytes reach a resting free cytosolic [Ca] ($[Ca]_c$) of ≈100 nM. Decline in $[Ca]_c$ is largely due to the activity of the SR Ca pump (FIG. 1). Ca transport is often described by the classic Hill equation plus a non–pump-mediated leak flux (e.g., via the SR Ca release channel). For a SR Ca pump K_m of 0.2–0.6 μM Ca, the resting Ca leak flux at steady state would be quite large (≈1/5 of the V_{max} of the pump). However, Bassani and Bers measured a steady state unidirectional Ca leak flux in isolated intact myocytes that was about 100 times smaller.[1]

We hypothesize that accumulated intra-SR free [Ca] ($[Ca]_{SR}$) limits both total SR [Ca] and $[Ca]_c$ decline at rest by causing a flux of Ca from the SR to the cytosol mediated by the SR Ca pump (FIG. 1). Such a reverse flux through the pump has been demonstrated in SR membrane vesicles.[2,3,5,6] We term this transport from the SR *backflux*. In this model (FIG. 1), $[Ca]_{SR}$ would build up until the thermodynamic gradient for Ca across the SR membrane becomes sufficient to counter the free energy available in the form of ATP in the cytosol (ΔG_{ATP}). The ΔG_{ATP} acts to drive the pump in the forward direction. Backflux through the pump would produce ATP from ADP + P_i, which is the reversal of the reaction concomitant with the forward pump flux. The reversal of the pump at steady state would therefore conserve cellular energy and be more efficient than a pump-leak balance.

This hypothesis was first tested in digitonin-permeabilized rabbit myocytes in a cuvette using indo-1, with an ATP regeneration system and no precipitating anions. Sequential addition of Ca to the cuvette produced a progressively slower Ca uptake into the SR as the intra-SR Ca content progressively increased. The first Ca pulse could be fit reasonably well with the classic Hill equation:

$$V = \frac{V_{max}}{1 + (K_m/[Ca]_c)^n} \tag{1}$$

Note that this equation accounts only for unidirectional Ca influx and has no term to account for accumulation of $[Ca]_{SR}$. It is not surprising then that uptake curves from subsequent Ca pulses progressively deviated downward from this fit.

[a] Address for correspondence: Donald M. Bers, Department of Physiology, Loyola University Medical Center, 2160 South First Avenue, Maywood, Illinois 60153. Phone: 708-216-1018; fax: 708-216-6308; e-mail: dbers@luc.edu

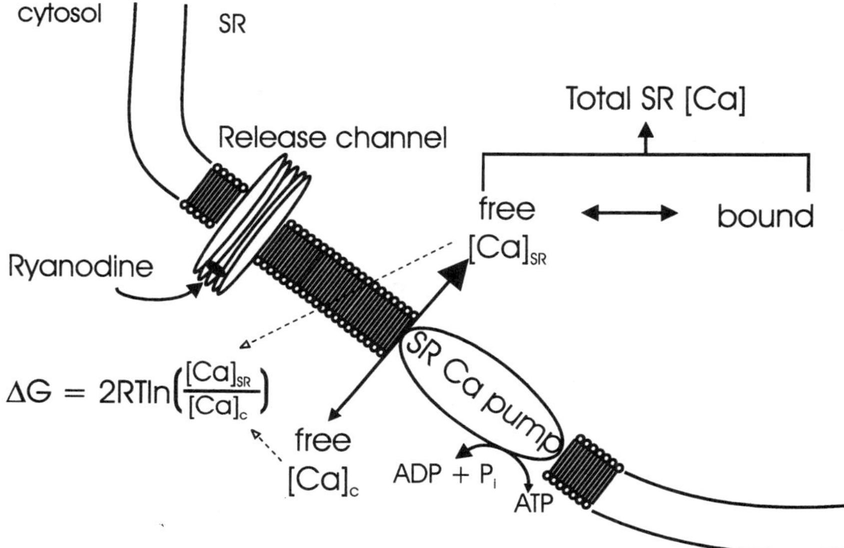

FIGURE 1. Does the Ca pump reverse at resting $[Ca]_c$? The figure depicts the process by which Ca is accumulated within the sarcoplasmic reticulum (SR). As cytosolic Ca declines, Ca is transported into the SR and a free [Ca] gradient is established between the SR and the cytosol. Only a small, non–SR pump-dependent leak from the SR is present. As the free energy (ΔG) of the gradient approaches the ΔG of energetic phosphates within the cytosol (e.g., ATP), SR Ca pump-mediated influx slows. Finally a steady state between Ca influx and efflux through the pump is established, and no net transport takes place.

Ca uptakes from sequential pulses were next fit to the Hill equation plus a component to account for leak flux:

$$V = \frac{V_{max}}{1 + (K_m/[Ca]_c)^n} + k([Ca]_{SR} - [Ca]_c) \tag{2}$$

This equation now accounts for a balance of fluxes across the membrane, a unidirectional influx mediated by the Ca pump, and a unidirectional efflux mediated by leak back across the membrane. SR Ca leak was measured after thapsigargin addition. $[Ca]_{SR}$ was calculated from total SR Ca using Ca buffering parameters that have been previously characterized in our laboratory.[4] Fits to this equation were very poor.

Analysis was next performed using an equation that accounted for pump-mediated flux in both directions:

$$V = \frac{V_{maxf}([Ca]_c/K_{mf}) + V_{maxr}([Ca]_{SR}/K_{mr})}{1 + (K_{mf}/[Ca]_c)^{nf} + (K_{mr}/[Ca]_{SR})^{nr}} + k([Ca]_{SR} - [Ca]_c) \tag{3}$$

Where the parameters for SR Ca flux in both directions are K_{mf}, K_{mr}, V_{maxf} and V_{maxr}. This equation described the uptake data at increasing SR Ca loads very well.

This same slowing of SR Ca transport occurs in voltage-clamped myocytes when loaded progressively by I_{Ca} pulses. Ca transients were measured using K_5-indo-1 and Na-free solution within the patch pipette and with 0Na solution outside to inhibit Na/Ca exchange. The data were fit with the three equations as described above. The best description of the data by far was obtained using Equation 3.

We conclude that SR Ca accumulation at rest is limited not by leak from the SR, but by backflux through the SR Ca pump.

ACKNOWLEDGMENTS

The authors wish to thank Mrs. Christina Hovance, Mr. Steve Scaglione, and Ms. Sarah Wimbiscus for their careful technical work in isolating the myocytes for some of the experiments performed.

REFERENCES

1. Bassani, R. A. & Bers, D. M. 1995. Rate of diastolic Ca release from the sarcoplasmic reticulum of intact rabbit and rat ventricular myocytes. Biophys. J. **68:** 2015–2022.
2. Feher, J. J. & F. N. Briggs. 1984. Unidirectional calcium and nucleotide fluxes in sarcoplasmic reticulum. II. Experimental results. Biophys. J. **45:** 1135–1144.
3. Makinose, M. 1971. Calcium efflux dependent formation of ATP from ADP and orthophosphate by the membranes of the sarcoplasmic vesicles. FEBS Lett. **12:** 269–270.
4. Shannon, T.R. and D.M. Bers. 1997. Assessment of intra-SR free [Ca] and buffering in rat heart. Biophys. J. **73:** 1524–1531.
5. Takenaka, H., P. N. Adler & A. M. Katz. 1982. Calcium fluxes across the membrane of sarcoplasmic reticulum vesicles. J. Biol. Chem. **257:** 12649–12656.
6. Weber, A., R. Herz & I. Reis. 1966. Study of the kinetics of calcium transport by isolated fragmented sarcoplasmic reticulum. Biochem. Z. **345:** 329–369.

A Critical Role for L-type Ca^{2+} Current in the Regulation of Ca^{2+} Release from the Sarcoplasmic Reticulum in Human Ventricular Myocytes from Dilated Cardiomyopathy

K. R. SIPIDO,[a] T. STANKOVICOVA, J. VANHAECKE, W. FLAMENG,[b] AND F. VERDONCK[c]

Laboratory of Experimental Cardiology, and [b] Division of Cardiac Surgery, University of Leuven, B-3000 Leuven, Belgium
[c]Interdisciplinary Research Center, University of Leuven/Kortrijk, Kortrijk, Belgium

Failing human cardiac muscle is characterized by the lack of a positive inotropic response to increased frequency of stimulation, often accompanied by a rise in diastolic tension at these higher frequencies.[1] It has been proposed that a decrease in Ca^{2+} uptake into the sarcoplasmic reticulum (SR), due to decreased expression of the Ca^{2+}-ATPase, is responsible for these abnormalities.[2] A decrease in SR Ca^{2+} uptake would impair the increase in SR Ca^{2+} load necessary for a positive frequency response and would slow the removal of Ca^{2+} from the cytoplasm. Other factors may also contribute to the negative cascade. In the present study we have studied Ca^{2+} release from the SR at different frequencies and the role of L-type Ca^{2+} current in the regulation of Ca^{2+} release from the SR in failing human cardiac muscle.

METHODS

Single ventricular myocytes were isolated enzymatically from a segment of the left ventricular wall removed from the hearts of transplant recipients with terminal heart failure due to dilated cardiomyopathy ($N_{hearts} = 6$, $N_{cells} = 16$). Membrane potentials and currents were recorded during whole-cell patch clamp; $[Ca^{2+}]_i$ was monitored with fluorescent $[Ca^{2+}]_i$ indicators. The pipette solution contained: (in mM) K-aspartate 120, KCl 20, K-HEPES 10, MgATP 5, $MgCl_2$ 0.5 (free $[Mg^{2+}]$ 0.8), NaCl 10, fluo-3 0.06 (or fluo-3 0.03 and fura-red 0.07); pH 7.20. The external solution contained: (in mM) NaCl 130, KCl 5.4, Na-HEPES 11.8, $MgCl_2$ 0.5, $CaCl_2$ 1.8, glucose 6; pH 7.35; T=36°C. With these solutions a junction potential of +10 mV occurred, which was not corrected for in the data presented. Ca^{2+} release was estimated from the rapid increase in $[Ca^{2+}]_i$ in the first 25 msec after depolarization. Data are presented as mean±SEM. The experimental setup, recording, and calibration procedures were described before.[3]

[a] Address for correspondence: Karin R. Sipido, M.D., Ph.D., Laboratory of Experimental Cardiology, K.U.L., Campus Gasthuisberg O/N 7th floor, Herestraat 49, B-3000 Leuven, Belgium. Phone: 32-16-347153; fax:32-16-345844; e-mail: Karin.Sipido@med.kuleuven.ac.be

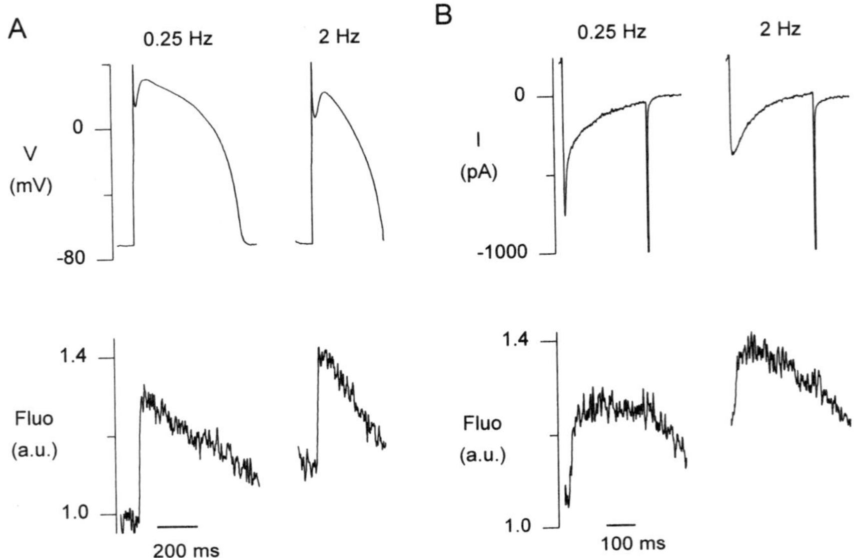

FIGURE 1. **(A)** Action potentials (membrane voltage, V) and $[Ca^{2+}]_i$ transients, shown as normalized fluorescence in arbitrary units (Fluo, a.u.) during steady state stimulation in current clamp mode at the indicated frequencies. **(B)** In the same cell membrane, currents and $[Ca^{2+}]_i$ transients, shown as normalized fluorescence, were recorded during stimulation with 225-ms voltage clamp pulses to 0 mV at the indicated frequencies. Holding voltage was –70 mV; just before recording, a brief (25-ms) prepulse to –45 mV inactivated the Na^+ current. Records were obtained in the presence of 2.5 mM 4-aminopyridine to suppress the transient outward current.

RESULTS

Ca^{2+} release was recorded during stimulated action potentials at different frequencies (0.03, 0.25, 0.5, 1, and 2 Hz). In all cells, Ca^{2+} release was largest at frequencies of 0.25 or 0.5 Hz, and declined steeply at 1 and 2 Hz (average $\Delta[Ca^{2+}]_i$ at 25 msec for a stimulation rate of 2 Hz was 54±6 % of maximal release), together with a pronounced rise in diastolic $[Ca^{2+}]_i$ (by 37±5%). This is illustrated by an example in FIGURE 1(A), showing the action potentials and $[Ca^{2+}]_i$ transients during steady-state stimulation at 0.25 and 2 Hz. With increasing frequency of stimulation the action potential duration decreased (APD_{90} was 511±50 msec at 0.25 Hz, and 340±20 msec at 2 Hz); the plateau voltage also decreased (from 33±3 to 23±2 mV), as evident in FIGURE 1(A). We investigated whether changes in Ca^{2+} current were involved in the change in action potential configuration and whether they contributed to the negative cascade.

Cells were stimulated in voltage-clamp mode by square pulses, and L-type Ca^{2+} current (I_{CaL}) and Ca^{2+} release were studied at different frequencies of stimulation. From a holding voltage of –70 mV, a 25 msec prepulse was given to inactivate the Na^+ current, followed by a step to 0 mV to activate I_{CaL}. A typical result is shown in FIGURE 1(B), from the same cell as in FIGURE 1(A). At 2 Hz the inward Ca^{2+} current was only 0.47 of the current at 0.25 Hz. At 2 Hz, the amplitude of the $[Ca^{2+}]_i$ transient was also reduced, and resting $[Ca^{2+}]_i$ was elevated. Frequency-dependent modulation of I_{CaL} was

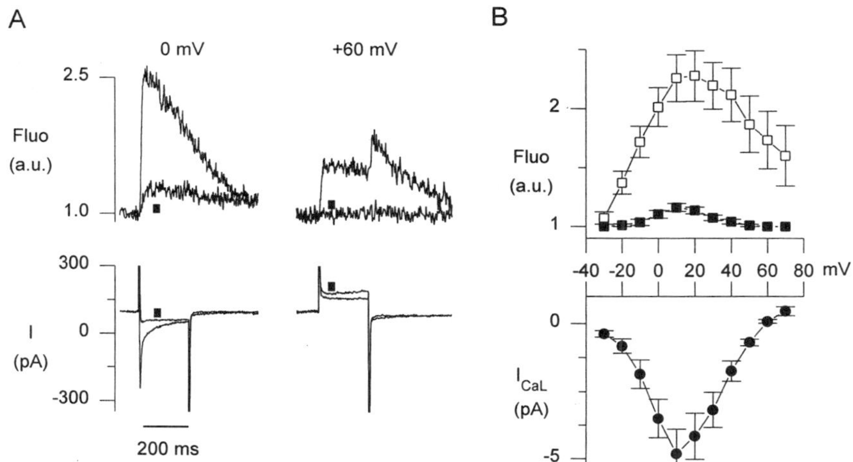

FIGURE 2. **(A)** Membrane currents and $[Ca^{2+}]_i$ transients, shown as normalized fluorescence (Fluo, in arbitray units), were recorded during a depolarizing pulse from –45 mV to the indicated potential; each record was preceded by six conditioning pulses from –70 to +60 mV (for 300 ms, repeated at 1 Hz) to load the SR with Ca^{2+}. After application of 20 μM nifedipine (records marked by *solid squares*), Ca^{2+} release was suppressed nearly completely. **(B, top)** Voltage dependence of Ca^{2+} release, measured as the increase in fluorescence at 25 ms after the depolarizing step, in control conditions *(open squares)* and after addition of 20 μM nifedipine *(solid squares);* the small remaining $[Ca^{2+}]_i$ transient is due to incomplete block of I_{CaL}. **(Bottom)** Voltage dependence of I_{CaL}, measured as the density of the peak nifedipine-sensitive current. Pooled data of seven cells.

studied in eight cells. The inhibition varied between 5 and 71%, and was associated with a reduction in Ca^{2+} release; the largest inhibition corresponded to the largest decrease in action potential plateau voltage.

We examined the role of I_{CaL} as trigger for Ca^{2+} release by studying the voltage dependence of release and the effect of Ca^{2+} channel block. FIGURE 2 illustrates a typical result. A large $[Ca^{2+}]_i$ transient was seen during a step to 0 mV which activated a large I_{CaL}, while at +60 mV Ca^{2+} release during the depolarizing step was small, but a tail transient was seen on repolarization. FIGURE 2(B, top) shows the voltage dependence of Ca^{2+} release during the depolarizing steps (open squares), which is a mirror image of the voltage dependence of I_{CaL}, shown in the bottom panel (solid circles). Nifedipine, 20 μM, nearly completely suppressed Ca^{2+} release [records marked by solid squares in FIG. 2(A), and in the top panel of FIG. 2(B)]. The small remaining transient is due to incomplete block of I_{CaL}; small inward currents could be detected and the voltage dependence is bell-shaped. Ca^{2+} release triggered by Na/Ca exchange could be detected in only 2/11 cells, and only after depolarizing to potentials >+40 mV; this release typically was preceded by a delay of more than 50 msec (results not shown).

DISCUSSION

Cells from patients with dilated cardiomyopathy exhibit a decrease in Ca^{2+} release with increasing frequency of stimulation, together with an increase in diastolic $[Ca^{2+}]_i$.

These findings can explain the existence of a negative force-frequency relation in the failing heart; the increase in diastolic $[Ca^{2+}]_i$ will contribute to diastolic dysfunction.

We observed a frequency-dependent decrease in I_{CaL}. One possible mechanism of this frequency-dependent inhibition of I_{CaL} is the increase in diastolic $[Ca^{2+}]_i$ at higher frequencies, which will lead to $[Ca^{2+}]_i$-dependent inactivation. The observed decrease in I_{CaL} will contribute to the negative cascade as it will decrease the trigger for Ca^{2+} release, as well as Ca^{2+} loading of the SR. The importance of I_{CaL} as trigger for release is clear from the voltage-clamp study showing a direct relation between I_{CaL} and Ca^{2+} release, and confirms earlier findings.[4] We could not find evidence that reverse mode Na/Ca exchange is important as trigger for Ca^{2+} release.

We conclude that I_{CaL} has a critical role as trigger for Ca^{2+} release from the sarcoplasmic reticulum in dilated cardiomyopathy; frequency-dependent inhibition of I_{CaL}, presumably linked to the slow removal of Ca^{2+} by the SR Ca^{2+} pump, can contribute to the negative cascade of the failing heart.

REFERENCES

1. Mulieri, L. A. *et al.* 1992. Altered myocardial force-frequency relation in human heart failure. Circulation **85:** 1743–1750.
2. Hasenfuss, G. *et al.* 1994. Relation between myocardial function and expression of sarcoplasmic reticulum Ca^{2+}-ATPase in failing and nonfailing human myocardium. Circ.Res. **75:** 434–442.
3. Mubagwa, K. *et al.* 1997. Monensin-induced reversal of positive force-frequency relationship in cardiac muscle. J. Mol. Cell. Cardiol. **29:** 977–989.
4. Beuckelmann, D.J. *et al.* 1992. Intracellular calcium handling in isolated ventricular myocytes from patients with terminal heart failure. Circulation **85:** 1046–1055.

Efficiency of L-type Ca^{2+} Current Compared to Reverse Mode Na/Ca Exchange or T-type Ca^{2+} Current as Trigger for Ca^{2+} Release from the Sarcoplasmic Reticulum

KARIN R. SIPIDO[a]

Laboratory of Experimental Cardiology, University of Leuven, B-3000 Leuven, Belgium

In ventricular myocytes, L-type Ca^{2+} channels or dihydropyridine receptors, are closely associated with the Ca^{2+} release channels of the sarcoplasmic reticulum (SR).[1] Ca^{2+} influx through the L-type channel and the increase in local $[Ca^{2+}]$ opens the nearby SR release channels.[2,3] However, since the Ca^{2+} release channel of the SR opens in response to an increase in $[Ca^{2+}]_{cyt}$, any transsarcolemmal Ca^{2+} influx is a potential trigger for release. It has been proposed that Ca^{2+} entry through Na/Ca exchange (reverse mode) would contribute to the trigger for Ca^{2+} release.[4,5] We have studied the characteristics of reverse-mode Na/Ca exchange and of T-type Ca^{2+} current as trigger for Ca^{2+} release, and compared these to L-type Ca^{2+} current as trigger.

METHODS AND RESULTS

Single guinea pig ventricular myocytes were studied in whole-cell voltage clamp mode with fluo-3 and fura-red, as $[Ca^{2+}]_i$ indicators. To study reverse mode Na/Ca exchange as trigger for release, we used a K^+ aspartate-based pipette solution containing 20 mM Na^+, and an external Tyrode's solution with 1.8 mM Ca^{2+}, T=36°C. Conditioning pulses to +60 mV ensured comparable Ca^{2+} loading of the SR, Ca^{2+} release was measured during depolarizing pulses from a holding potential of –45 mV to –40 up to +70 mV. In the presence of L-type Ca^{2+} current, I_{CaL}, $[Ca^{2+}]_i$ transients typically had an early and rapid rising phase reflecting Ca^{2+} release (ryanodine-sensitive), and the delay to the maximal Ca^{2+} release, measured as the delay to the maximal derivative of the $[Ca^{2+}]_i$ transient was 8±1 ms (mean±SD, N=6) at +10 mV (Fig. 1A,a). At more positive voltages, Ca^{2+} release declined (Fig. 1B,a). After block of I_{CaL} (nisoldipine 20 µmol/L), Ca^{2+} entry through Na/Ca exchange was the only Ca^{2+} entry pathway. At +10 mV, the early rapid rise of $[Ca^{2+}]_i$ was blocked, and a slower $[Ca^{2+}]_i$ transient (still due to Ca^{2+} release as it was ryanodine sensitive) was now preceded by a significant delay (Fig. 1A,b); the average time to peak Ca^{2+} release was 90±35 ms at +10 mV. At +70 mV, Ca^{2+} release was only slightly affected by Ca^{2+} channel block (Fig. 1B,b compared to 1B,a), and the average time to peak release was 24±4 ms, about 20 times less than previously reported at room temperature.[9] We calculated the Ca^{2+} influx preceding the triggered Ca^{2+} release through both pathways, by integrating the L-type Ca^{2+} current (nisoldipine-sensitive current) and the outward Na/Ca exchange current (current

[a] Address for correspondence: Karin R. Sipido, M.D., Ph.D., Laboratory of Experimental Cardiology, K.U.L., Campus Gasthuisberg O/N 7th floor, Herestraat 49, B-3000 Leuven, Belgium. Phone: 32-16-347153; fax: 32-16-345844; e-mail: Karin.Sipido@med.kuleuven.ac.be

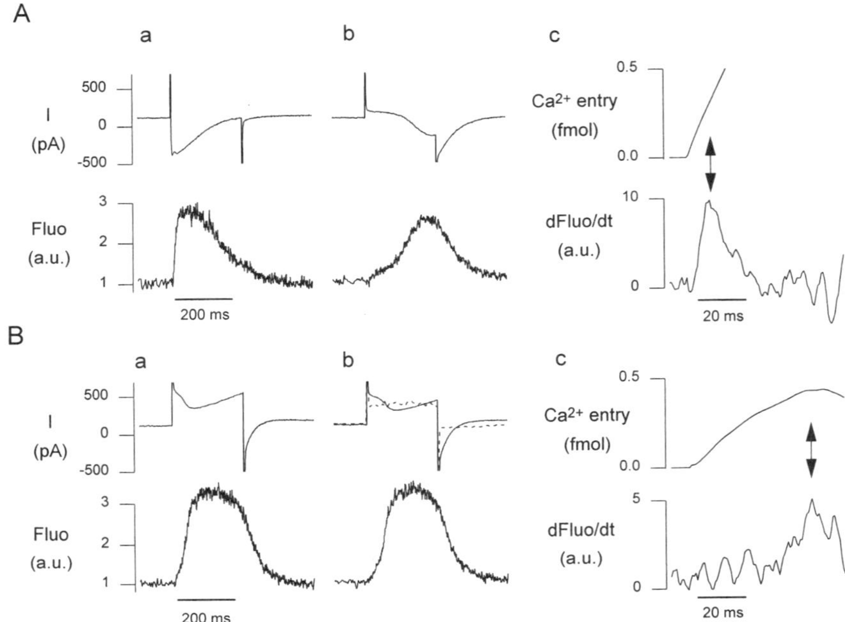

FIGURE 1. **(A, a)** Current and $[Ca^{2+}]_i$ transient, shown as the change in fluorescence (normalized to baseline values, arbitray units) during a depolarizing step from –45 to +10 mV; the record was preceded by six conditioning steps to +60 mV to load the SR. **(b)** During a similar voltage protocol but after block of I_{CaL} (20 μM nisoldipine); a caffeine test had shown that the Ca^{2+} load of the SR was not significantly altered. **(c, top)** Ca^{2+} influx for **(A,a)** was calculated by integrating the nisoldipine-sensitive current, and dividing by valence and Faraday's constant; **(bottom)** the derivative of the fluorescence record in **(A,a)** shows that the peak Ca^{2+} release rate is at 8 ms after the onset of depolarization, marked by the *arrow*. **(B,a)** Current and $[Ca^{2+}]_i$ transient during a step from –45 to +60 mV, same conditioning protocol as in **A.** **(B, b)** After block of I_{CaL}, dashed current record is in the presence of 5 mM $NiCl_2$ to block Na/Ca exchange. **(c, top)** Ca^{2+} influx for **(B,b)** was calculated from the outward Na/Ca exchange current; **(bottom)** the derivative of the fluorescence record in **(B,b)** shows that the peak Ca^{2+} release rate is at more than 40 ms after the onset of depolarization, marked by the *arrow*.

blocked by 2 mM $NiCl_2$ in the presence of nisoldipine). Such data are shown for I_{CaL} during a step to +10 mV (FIG. 1A,c), and for the Na/Ca exchanger during a step to +70 mV (FIG. 1B,c). The trigger efficiency was calculated as the ratio between Ca^{2+} release (estimated as peak dFluo/dt) and the preceding Ca^{2+} influx, i.e., the integral up to the time of peak dFluo/dt, indicated by the arrows in FIGURE 1. In a total of six cells, this value was on average approximately five times higher for L-type Ca^{2+} current (measured for the step to +10 mV) than for reverse-mode Na/Ca exchange (at +70 mV after block of I_{CaL}).

To study T-type current as trigger for Ca^{2+} release, we used internal and external K^+- and Na^+-free solutions to record Ca^{2+} currents uncontaminated by Na^+, K^+ or Na/Ca exchange currents; fura-2 was the $[Ca^{2+}]_i$ indicator, T=23°C.[6] After switching to the Na^+-free solution, conditioning pulses from –90 to 0 mV were repeated every 10 s to en-

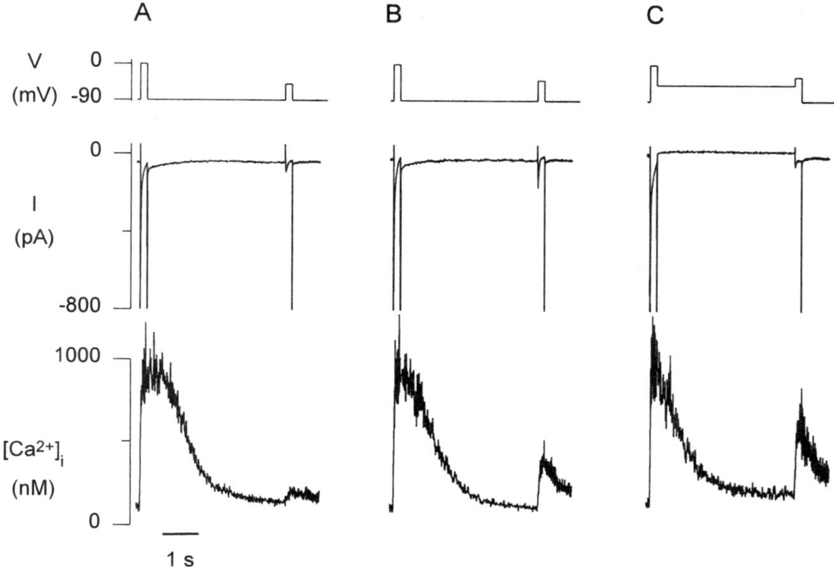

FIGURE 2. **(A)** Current and $[Ca^{2+}]_i$ transient during the last conditioning step to 0 mV, and during the test step from –90 to –50 mV, illustrating the T-type current and the small $[Ca^{2+}]_i$ transient associated with it. **(B)** During a step from –90 to –40 mV more T-type current and Ca^{2+} release are activated. **(C)** During a step from –50 to –30 mV, Ca^{2+} current through L-type Ca^{2+} channels evokes a Ca^{2+} release larger than for T-type current despite the fact that the current amplitude is less. The $[Ca^{2+}]_i$ transient during the last conditioning step to 0 mV is comparable for all three panels, indicating that the loading status of the sarcoplasmic reticulum was comparable.

sure adequate Ca^{2+} loading of the SR. We examined whether T-type current could trigger Ca^{2+} release during steps from –90 to –50 mV, where no L-type current is activated. T-type currents at –50 mV were small, and very little release was observed (FIG. 2A). For steps to –40 mV, a larger current was seen, with more Ca^{2+} release (FIG. 2B). However, during a step from –50 mV to –30 mV, activating L-type current only, even more Ca^{2+} was released, despite the fact that the peak current was comparable to the one evoked during the step from –90 to –50 mV, and was much smaller than during the step from –90 to –40 mV (FIG. 2C; note that for all three steps the $[Ca^{2+}]_i$ transient during the step to 0 mV is comparable, indicating comparable loading of the SR). These results indicate that although T-type current can trigger release, it is less efficient than L-type current. Similar results were obtained in five other cells.

DISCUSSION

We confirmed that aside from the L-type Ca^{2+} current, Ca^{2+} influx through other pathways is capable of triggering Ca^{2+} release. However, our findings also indicate that for a similar amount of Ca^{2+} influx on the whole-cell level, more Ca^{2+} release is triggered by the L-type Ca^{2+} current, in line with previous observations on reverse-mode Na/Ca exchange at romm temperature.[9] Differences in trigger efficiency most likely are related to differences in the local Ca^{2+} influx near the Ca^{2+} release channel. For the Na/Ca exchanger the influx per exchanger molecule is three orders of magnitude less than for the L-type Ca^{2+} channel, and modeling of the increase in local [Ca^{2+}] is clearly in favor of the Ca^{2+} channel.[7] For the T-type channel, the single channel flux may not be the limiting factor, since the conductance in 10 mM $CaCl_2$ was only 4–5 pS vs. 6.9 pS for L-type channels in similar conditions.[8] However, T-type channels inactivate very rapidly, reducing the possibility to reach the necessary local [Ca^{2+}]. At present the location of T-type channels is unknown.

In conclusion, L-type Ca^{2+} current has the highest efficiency as trigger for Ca^{2+} release, most likely related to a high molecular Ca^{2+} entry rate for L-type Ca^{2+} channels and to close association with Ca^{2+} release channels.

BIBLIOGRAPHY

1. Carl, S. L. *et al.* 1995. Immunolocalization of sarcolemmal dihydropyridine receptor and sarcoplasmic reticular triadin and ryanodine receptor in rabbit ventricle and atrium. J. Cell Biol. **129:** 672–682.
2. Lopez-Lopez, J. R. *et al.* 1995. Local calcium transients triggered by single L-type calcium channel currents in cardiac cells. Science **268:** 1042–1045.
3. Cannell, M. B. *et al.* 1995. The control of calcium release in heart muscle. Science **268:** 1045–1049.
4. Leblanc, N. *et al.* 1990. Sodium current-induced release of calcium from cardiac sarcoplasmic reticulum. Science **248:** 372–376.
5. Kohmoto, O. *et al.* 1994. Relation between reverse sodium-calcium exchange and sarcoplasmic reticulum calcium release in guinea pig ventricular cells. Circ. Res. **74:** 550–554.
6. Sipido, K. R. *et al.* 1995. Inhibition and rapid recovery of I_{Ca} during calcium release from the sarcoplasmic reticulum in guinea-pig ventricular myocytes. Circ. Res. **76:** 102–109.
7. Langer, G. A. *et al.* 1996. Calcium concentration and movement in the diadic cleft space of the cardiac ventricular cell. Biophys. J. **70:** 1169–1182.
8. Balke, C. W. *et al.* 1992. Macroscopic and unitary properties of physiological ion flux through T-type Ca^2 channels in guinea-pig heart cells. J. Physiol. (Lond) **456:** 247–265.
9. Sham, J. S. K. *et al.* 1995. Functional coupling of Ca^{2+} channels and ryanodine receptors in cardiac myocytes. Proc. Natl. Acad. Sci. USA **92:** 121–125.

EJSR/JSR: Three-Dimensional Geometry of an Ionic Charge with Fuse[a]

J. R. SOMMER,[b] T. HIGH, P. INGRAM,[c] D. KOPF, R. NASSAR,[d] AND I. TAYLOR

Department of Pathology, Duke University and Veterans Administration Medical Centers, Durham, North Carolina 27710, USA
[c]Research Triangle Institute, Research Triangle Park, North Carolina 27709, USA
[d]Department of Pediatrics, Duke University Medical Center, Durham, North Carolina 27710, USA

In 1969 we discovered in avian cardiac muscle both the absence of transverse tubules and the presence of a novel organelle (extended junctional sarcoplasmic reticulum, EJSR) that was a morphological and probable functional homologue[1] of junctional SR (JSR), but lacked plasmalemmal contact. EJSR and JSR both intercalate into free SR. EJSR forms intricate retes throughout Z/I regions by continuous and discontinuous (in the form of patches) extension of plasmalemmal JSR.[cf.1] JSR both stores and releases calcium and forms structure-function complexes with surface plasmalemma at peripheral couplings (PC) and with plasmalemma of transverse tubules at interior couplings (IC). Couplings are the instruments of translating muscle excitation into contraction. For phylogenetic continuity, a subset of EJSR exists in mammalian hearts (i.e., corbular SR,CSR)[1]; its prominence in mammalian conduction fibers, which lack transverse tubules and interior couplings, may explain the retention of calcium-induced calcium release (CICR) even after such cells had been stripped of peripheral couplings.[2]

The fundamental significance of EJSR is its structural and presumed functional homology with JSR in combination with the absence of plasmalemmal contact. Whereas JSR of IC gets the signal for calcium release via transverse tubules through an action potential that initiates CICR across a distance of ~0.025 μm at couplings, the comparable distance for EJSR to get its message is up to 4.00 μm! Thus, and without transverse tubules, EJSR in avians functions most likely as the structural matrix for both, signal propagation over long distances and for calcium release (both mediated by CICR[3–5]). These two separate, if related, JSR functions are achieved not by a qualitative differentiation, *sui generis,* but by quantitative extension of an already existing mechanism, albeit obscured in a single JSR at a coupling for lack of need at short distances. What remain to be sorted out are the safeguards guiding graded activation/inactivation so as to avert all-or-none calcium cascades.[3,5]

Molecular biologic efforts complementing prior morphologic evidence have now established that excitation-contraction coupling in striated muscle is a controlled cascade of steps initiated by the action potential, mediated through voltage sensors in the plasmalemma, and followed by CICR from the JSR at couplings via calcium release channels in junctional processes (JP).[6] Whereas in striated muscle in general the transverse tubular system synchronizes global contraction, in avian hearts an alternative mecha-

[a] This research was supported by National Institutes of Health Grant R01-12486-27 and the Veterans Administration Research Service.

[b] Address for correspondence: J. R. Sommer, Department of Pathology, Duke University and Veterans Administration Medical Centers, Box 3548, Durham, North Carolina 27710. Phone: 919-286-0411 (ext. 6501); fax: 919-286-6818; e-mail, somme001@acpub.duke.edu

nism must operate, aided by a small cell diameter (~4 μm). A speculative quasi-saltatory CICR along strings of JP that populate the JSR/EJSR surfaces at close quarters, like a powder fuse, might afford global cardiac contraction, provided that points of calcium release (i.e., the JP) on rapidly replenishable calcium stores are near each other over the distances to be negotiated. This is apparently so, as the serial sections and their exploitation in the form of three-dimensional stereo images show, thus, supplementing and confirming earlier morphometries.[1,11] Similar matrix-bound vectorial "ionic fuses" may exist elsewhere in other cells for communicating specific messages over distance.

The quantitative data were obtained from two sets of measurements from 15 serial sections of known thickness through the Z/I region of a single finch cardiac myocyte (FIGS. 1, A,B,C), by direct measurements of JSR and EJSR dimensions and by mea-

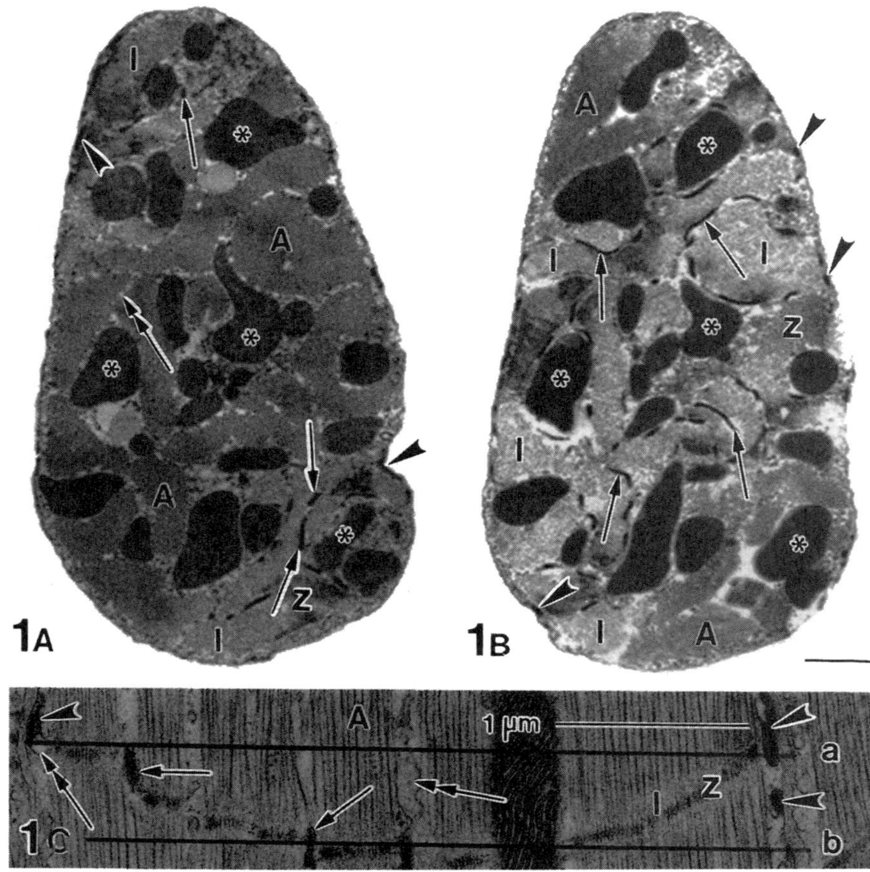

FIGURE 1. **(A** and **B)** Printout of 2 of 15 digitized serial transverse EM images of a single finch cardiac myocyte at the approximate levels through an arched Z/I region as suggested in **C (a,b).** JSR of peripheral couplings *(arrowheads),* EJSR *(arrows),* free SR *(double arrows).* A,I,Z (A, I, Z band, respectively), mitochondria *(asterisks). Bar* = ~1 μm.

surements from three-dimensional stereo and movie renditions (FIG. 2).[7] The measurements have been reported previously.[8,9] The data are reliable geometric parameters suitable to test attempts at modeling CICR theoretically.[6,10] They show directly that (1) EJSR intercalated into free SR forms a visible, continuous rete of known spatial dimensions throughout the Z/I region, a region that harbors the thin filaments and calcium-sensitive regulatory proteins; and (2) that the numerous discontinuous EJSR patches, ~0.2 µm apart, are structural homologues of the JSR of PC and IC irrespective of plasmalemmal contact. Preliminary studies on the JSR of mouse cardiac myocytes suggest similar geometries, albeit contaminated by transverse tubules.

ACKNOWLEDGMENTS

We are grateful to Drs. Neal Shepherd and Gerhard Meissner for seminal discussions.

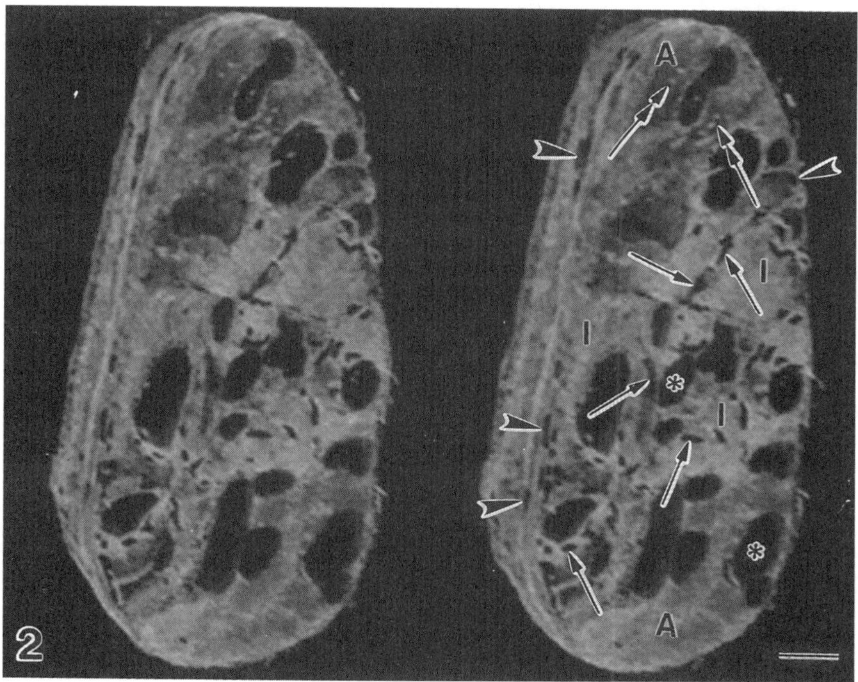

FIGURE 2. Stereo image of one emphasized level of 15 transverse EM sections through a single finch cardiac myocyte closer to the apogee of an arched Z/I region as shown in FIG. 1. Its slanted plane is rendered slightly opaque and contains mainly EJSR *(arrows),* I band proteins (I), Z line material, and mitochondria rendered transparent *(asterisks).* JSR (peripheral couplings, *arrowheads*), free SR *(double arrows),* A (A band). *Bar* = 1 µm.

REFERENCES

1. Sommer, J. *et al.* 1991. To excite a heart: a bird's view. Acta Physiol. Scand. **142** (Suppl. 599): 5–21.
2. Sommer, J. R., E. Bossen & A. Fabiato. 1982. Junctional sarcoplasmic reticulum in excitation-contraction-coupling. Presented at the Fortieth Annual Proceedings Electron Microscopy Society of America. Washington, DC, August 9–13, 1982.
3. Anderson, P. A. W. *et al.* 1976. Cardiac muscle: an attempt to relate structure to function. J. Mol. Cell. Cardiol. **8:** 123–143.
4. Sommer, J. R. & R. A. Waugh. 1976. The ultrastructure of the mammalian cardiac muscle cell, with special emphasis on the tubular membrane systems. A review. Am. J. Pathol. **82:** 192–232.
5. Fabiato, A. 1985. Calcium-induced release of calcium from the sarcoplasmic reticulum. J. Gen. Physiol. **85:** 189–320.
6. Stern, M.D. 1992. Theory of excitation-contraction coupling in cardiac muscle. Biophys. J. **63:** 497–517.
7. Kopf, D.A. *et al.* 1995. Interactive elemental image acquisition and processing. *In* Microbeam Analysis. J. Friel, Ed.: 317–318. VCH Publishers. New York.
8. Sommer, J. R. *et al.* 1997. Avian extended junctional SR: 3-D geometry rendered in stereo. Microsc. Microanal. **3** (Suppl.): 247–248.
9. Sommer, J. R. *et al.* 1997. JSR and EJSR in the finch heart: morphometry by serial sections. Microsc. Microanal. **3** (Suppl.): 249–250.
10. Cannell, M. B. & C. Soeller. 1997. Numerical analysis of ryanodine receptor activation by L-type channel activity in the cardiac muscle dyad. Biophys. J. **73:** 112–122.
11. Sommer, J. R. T. High & I. Taylor. 1995. The geometry of the EJSR Z-rete in avian cardiac muscle. *In* Proceedings of Microscopy and Microanalysis. G. W. Bailey, M. H. Ellisman, R. A. Hennigar, & N. J. Zaluzec, Eds.: 940–941. Jones and Begell Publishing New York.

Cardiac Sarcoplasmic Reticulum Membrane Lipid Asymmetries[a]

ROGER J. BICK, W. BARRY VAN WINKLE, AND GEORGE E. TAFFET[b]

University of Texas at Houston Medical School and Baylor College of Medicine, Houston, Texas, 77030, USA

The phospholipid head groups and fatty acyl chains comprising the skeletal muscle sarcoplasmic reticulum (SSR) membrane are asymmetrically distributed across the bilayer and in distinct protein-associated versus bulk pools. This spatial orientation of specific lipids modifies SSR function.[1,2] Phosphatidylethanolamine (PE) activates delipidated SSR Ca-ATPase[3] and PE and phosphatidylserine (PS) are strategically situated to allow conformational changes of the SSR Ca-ATPase.[2] Since the cardiac sarcoplasmic reticulum (CSR) Ca-ATPase carries out similar transport functions to those shown by SSR, albeit more slowly, we hypothesized that CSR phospholipid requirements and distribution could be similar. We describe the asymmetric nature of the CSR membrane, compared to SSR, and detail the protein-associated lipids.

MATERIALS AND METHODS

Sarcoplasmic Reticulum Isolation

Canine left ventricle was used in all preparations and following a standard differential centrifugation protocol, an aliquot was oxalate-loaded.[4] Fast twitch skeletal muscle SR was prepared from rabbits by the method of Van Winkle and colleagues.[5]

Inner versus Outer Layer Phospholipids

SR vesicles were incubated with phospholipase A2 and the formation of lysophospholipids (LPL) was followed by thin layer chromatography.[6] Digestion of the outer monolayer resulted in an increasing amount of LPLs, a halt in production, then again an increase. This break in LPL production was taken as the point beyond which the inner membrane became leaky, no longer protected against digestion by the outer monolayer.

[a] This work was supported in part by National Institutes of Health Grants AG 13251 and HL 13870.

[b] Address for correspondence: George E. Taffet, M.D., Huffington Center on Aging, Baylor College of Medicine, One Baylor Plaza, Houston, Texas 77030-3498. Phone: 713-798-5804; fax: 713-798-6688.

Protein-Associated Phospholipids

SR membranes were mixed with increasing amounts of the detergent $C_{12}E_8$ (octaethylene glycol monododecyl ether) and the protein and associated membrane lipids were recovered by centrifugation as detailed in Bick and colleagues.[2] Both the protein pellet and supernatant were extracted and examined for lipid content and type

RESULTS

When the CSR outer monolayer is compared to the inner monolayer, a striking asymmetry in the distribution of phospholipids is apparent (TABLE 1). PE is primarily in the outer leaflet and PS in the inner leaflet. Phosphatidylcholine (PC) is distributed equally between the leaflets. However, the asymmetric distribution of PE is less striking in CSR than SSR (p<0.05).

TABLE 2 details the amounts and types of phospholipid found in native preparations and after "stripping" by detergent. The native skeletal and cardiac membranes are similar, but following detergent the pattern changes dramatically. SSR shows a loss of PC, but with only a minor removal of PE by detergent. This suggests the close proximity of PE to the Ca-ATPase protein. CSR tends to retain a phospholipid content not greatly different from the native membranes; the amount of PS remaining with the protein is approximately twice that of the native fraction. This difference did not attain statistical significance. For both CSR and SSR the retained PE was enriched in plasmalogen content, with the PC retained in the CSR after detergent stripping also being highly enriched in plasmalogen content.

CONCLUSIONS

Membrane lipids are not distributed randomly in either CSR or SSR. PE is located primarily in the outer leaflet of both CSR and SSR. PS is found primarily in the inner leaflet. Detergent stripping results in a protein-associated lipid fraction that is enriched in plasmalogenic species in both CSR and SSR and in aminophospholipids (PE and PS) in SSR. The CSR proteins showed little phospholipid head-group specificity. Because the non-random distribution of membrane lipids in SSR modifies SSR Ca-ATPase function, it is likely that the asymmetrically distributed lipids of CSR modify CSR Ca-ATPase function, an important consideration for studies using membrane recon-

TABLE 1. Inner Versus Outer Leaflet Phospholipids (%)

	CSR ($N = 7$)	SSR ($N = 7$)
Inner PE	27 ± 2.2	20 ± 1.5*
Outer PE	73 ± 3.2	80 ± 2.0
Inner PC	54 ± 3.8	52 ± 2.8
Outer PC	46 ± 3.1	48 ± 2.0
Inner PS	76 ± 4.4	84 ± 1.3
Outer PS	24 ± 3.3	16 ± 4.9

*$p < 0.05$ versus CSR. Data are shown as means ± SEM.

TABLE 2. Amounts and Types of Phospholipids Found in Native Preparations and after Detergent "Stripping"

		Native CSR	Stripped CSR	Native SSR	Stripped SSR
Phospholipids of native and detergent-treated SR (%)	PE	28±4	23±3	16±2	38±2*
	PC	53±3	59±4	67±5	38±6*
	PS	10±4	17±3	7±2	24±5*
Plasmalogen content of native and protein associated phospholipids (%)	PE	64±2	77±3**	63±2	96±2**
	PC	58±3	100±4**	24±1	22±3
	PS	52±3	38±2**	46±4	39±6
	N =6				

$^{**}p < 0.01$; $^{*}p < 0.05$ versus native membranes.

stitution. The lesser head-group specificity of CSR may simply reflect the competing lipid requirements of other CSR proteins, necessary for calcium transport or other functions.

REFERENCES

1. Bick, R.J., *et al.* 1987. Phospholipid fatty acyl chain asymmetry in the membrane bilayer of isolated skeletal muscle sarcoplasmic reticulum. Biochemistry **26:** 4831–4836.
2. Bick, R.J., *et al.* 1991. Unsaturated aminophospholipids are preferentially retained by the fast skeletal muscle CaATPase during detergent solubilization. Arch. Biochem. Biophys. **286:** 346–352.
3. Hidalgo, C., *et al.* 1982. Uncoupling of Ca^{2+} transport in sarcoplasmic reticulum as a result of labeling lipid amino groups and inhibition of Ca^{2+}ATPase activity by modification of lysine residues of the Ca^{2+}ATPase polypeptide. J. Biol. Chem. **254:** 4224–2432.
4. Jones, L.R., *et al.* 1979. Separation of vesicles of cardiac sarcolemma from vesicles of cardiac sarcoplasmic reticulum. Comparative biochemical analysis of component activities. J. Biol. Chem. **254:** 530–539.
5. Van Winkle, W.B., *et al.* 1981. Substrate utilization by cardiac and skeletal muscle sarcoplasmic reticulum. J. Biol. Chem. **256:** 2268–2274.
6. Herbette, L., *et al.* 1984. Phospholipid asymmetry in the isolated sarcoplasmic reticulum membrane. Arch. Biochem. Biophys. **234:** 235–242.

Measurement of Sarcoplasmic Reticulum Ca Content and Sarcolemmal Fluxes during the Transient Stimulation of the Systolic Ca Transient Produced by Caffeine

A. W. TRAFFORD,[a] M. E. DÍAZ, AND D. A. EISNER

Department of Veterinary Preclinical Sciences, University of Liverpool, Liverpool L69 3BX, United Kingdom

In mammalian cardiac muscle, the bulk of the calcium ions that activate contraction come from the sarcoplasmic reticulum (SR). Calcium release is initiated by the process of calcium-induced Ca release (CICR). In this mechanism the entry of a small amount of calcium into the cell via the sarcolemmal L-type Ca channel triggers the opening of the SR Ca release channels or ryanodine receptors (RyR) and thence allows the release of a larger amount of calcium from the SR. There has been considerable recent interest in the effects of modulation of CICR on excitation-contraction coupling. For example, the gain of CICR has been suggested to be increased by phosphorylation.[1] Similarly it has been suggested that the compound cyclic ADP ribose (cADP-Ribose) may stimulate CICR and thence increase the systolic Ca transient.[2]

We have, however, previously reported that stimulation of CICR with caffeine only produces a transient increase of the systolic transient.[3] The transient nature of the response was suggested to result from a decrease of SR Ca content due to the enhanced Ca release stimulating Ca extrusion from the cell. In this work we have attempted to confirm this hypothesis by measuring SR Ca content and the accompanying sarcolemmal Ca fluxes directly.

The experiments were performed on isolated rat ventricular myocytes. Cells were voltage-clamped using the perforated patch technique[4] with amphotericin-B. The switch clamp facility of the Axoclamp-2B (Axon Instruments, Foster City, CA, USA) amplifier was used at rates of 1–4 kHz in order to avoid problems due to access resistance. The resting membrane potential was held at –40 mV, and 100 ms depolarizing voltage clamp pulses to 0 mV were applied at 0.33 Hz. Electrodes were fabricated from borosilicate glass and had resistances of 1–3 MΩ when filled with (mM): KCH_3O_3S, 125; KCl, 20; NaCl, 10; HEPES, 10; $MgCl_2$, 5; titrated to pH 7.2 with KOH. Amphotericin-B was prepared as a stock solution in DMSO (60 mg/ml) and added to a final concentration of 240 μg/ml. Cells were bathed in a control solution of the following composition (mM): NaCl, 135; glucose, 11; HEPES, 10; KCl, 4; $MgCl_2$, 1.2; $CaCl_2$, 1; pH 7.4 with NaOH. To avoid interference from outward currents all experiments were performed in the presence of 5 mM 4-aminopyridine and 0.1 mM $BaCl_2$. All experiments were performed at 23°C.

In the experiment illustrated in FIGURE 1, the addition of caffeine (100 μM) resulted in a transient increase of the systolic Ca transient. After a few stimuli in caffeine the magnitude of the Ca transient was identical to that in control. On removal of caffeine

[a] Phone: 44-151-794-4228; fax: 44-151-794-5347; e-mail: trafford@liv.ac.uk

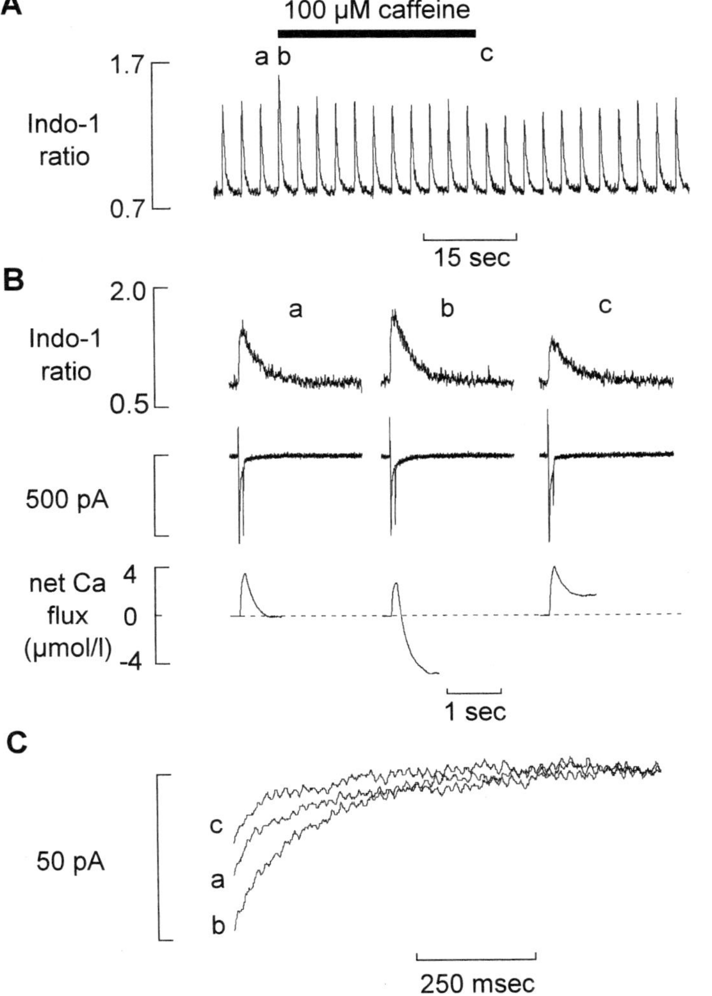

FIGURE 1. The effects of a low concentration of caffeine on $[Ca^{2+}]_i$ and sarcolemmal Ca fluxes. **(A)** Time course of effects on Ca transient. Caffeine (100 μM) was applied for the period shown. **(B)** Specimen records of (from top to bottom): $[Ca^{2+}]_i$, current, cumulative integral from the pulses indicated on **A.** **(C)** Expanded versions of the current tails.

there was a transient decrease of the Ca transient.[3] The Ca transients are shown in more detail in FIGURE 1(B), which also shows membrane current records. The calcium current on depolarization is slightly decreased during the first pulse in caffeine. On repolarization the inward Na-Ca exchange tail current[5] is stimulated by the larger systolic Ca transient on this pulse. The lower traces show the calculated cumulative sarcolemmal Ca fluxes. In the control pulse the Ca entry during the L-type Ca current (initial upward deflection) is exactly balanced by the efflux via Na-Ca exchange on repolarization (downward deflection) such that there is no net Ca flux confirming that the cell is in a steady-state for calcium content. On the first pulse in caffeine (b) there is a decrease of the Ca entry accompanied by a larger increase of Ca efflux. The net result is a loss of calcium of about 4 μmol/l. In the steady-state in caffeine (c) cell Ca balance is again restored.

Experiments such as that illustrated in FIGURE 1 suggest that, in caffeine the cell loses calcium. This will presumably result in a decrease of SR Ca content and it is possible to measure the SR Ca content directly to confirm this.[6] In FIGURE 2, 10 mM caffeine was initially applied to release the SR Ca content. This produced an increase of resting $[Ca^{2+}]_i$, which then decays to control levels as the Ca is pumped out of the cell largely by Na-Ca exchange. The Na-Ca exchange current can be seen in FIGURE 1(B) and the Ca content of the SR can be measured from the cumulative integral of this current (lower panel) as described previously.[6,7] As shown in FIGURE 2(A), after removing the high concentration of caffeine, the cell was stimulated. A low (here 200 μM) concentration of caffeine was then added resulting in a transient increase of systolic $[Ca^{2+}]_i$. The subsequent measurement of SR Ca content shows that exposure to the low caffeine concentration had indeed decreased the SR content. That these effects are reversible is shown in the right hand panel.

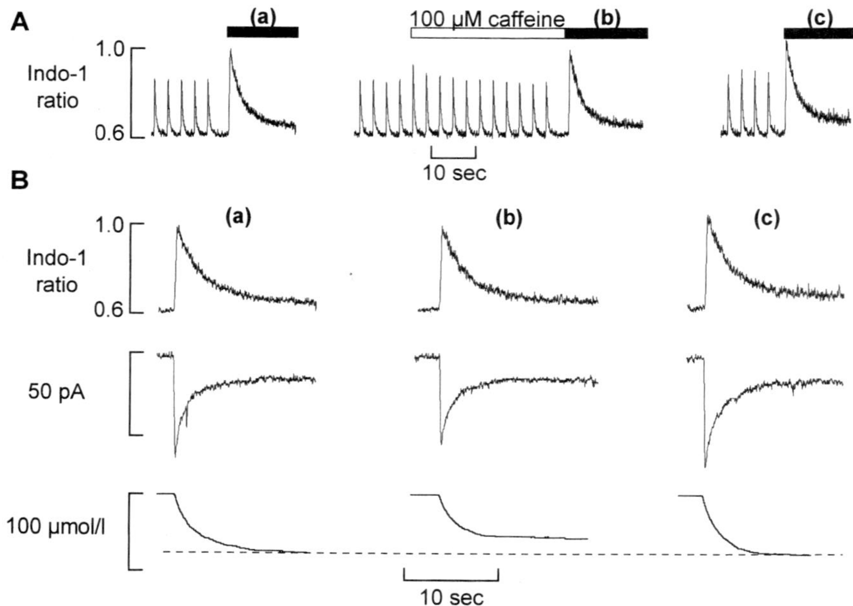

FIGURE 2. The effects of a low concentration of caffeine on $[Ca^{2+}]_i$ and SR Ca content. **(A)** Continuous record of $[Ca^{2+}]_i$. Caffeine (10 mM) was applied as shown by the *solid bars*. 100 μM caffeine was applied in the **middle panel** as shown by the *open bar*. **(B)** Measurement of SR Ca content. The traces show: **top,** $[Ca^{2+}]_i$; **middle,** current; **bottom,** cumulative integral of current. The records were obtained from the caffeine applications in **A.**

The above results show that stimulation of CICR produces only a transient increase of systolic Ca transient. As discussed previously,[3] for the cell to be in a steady state the amount of Ca that enters the cell on depolarization (largely via the Ca current) must be pumped out of the cell before the next depolarization. Assuming that the properties of the Ca pumping mechanisms are not changed then, in order to balance a given Ca entry, the magnitude of the Ca transient must be constant. When caffeine is first applied, the stimulation of CICR results in an increased systolic Ca transient, which therefore means that Ca efflux will transiently be greater than Ca entry. In the steady state, however, the systolic Ca transient comes back to control levels (the decrease of SR Ca content exactly compensates for the stimulation of CICR). These results are presumably relevant to other factors that affect CICR. Our hypothesis is that such factors cannot produce maintained effects on the magnitude of the systolic Ca transient and that any such effects must be due to other mechanisms.

REFERENCES

1. duBell, W.H., W.J. Lederer & T.B. Rogers. 1996. Dynamic modulation of excitation-contraction coupling by protein phosphases in rat ventricular myocytes. J.Physiol.(Lond.) **493:** 793–800.
2. Rakovic, S. A. Galione, G.A. Ashamu, B.V.L. Potter & D.A. Terrar. 1996. A specific cyclic ADP-ribose antagonist inhibits cardiac excitation-contraction coupling. Cur. Biology **6:** 989–996.
3. O'Neill S.C. & D.A. Eisner. 1990. A mechanism for the effects of caffeine on Ca release during diastole and systole in isolated rat ventricular myocytes. J.Physiol.(Lond.) **430:** 519–536.
4. Horn, R. & A. Marty. 1988. Muscarinic activation of ionic currents measured by a new whole-cell recording method. J.Gen.Physiol. **92:** 145–159.
5. Fedida, D., D. Noble, Y. Shimoni, & A.J. Spindler. 1987. Inward current related to contraction in guinea-pig ventricular myocytes. J.Physiol.(Lond.) **385:** 565–589.
6. Varro, A., N. Negretti, S.B. Hester, & D.A. Eisner. 1993. An estimate of the calcium content of the sarcoplasmic reticulum in rat ventricular myocytes. Pflug.Arch. **423:** 158–160.
7. Negretti, N., A. Varro & D.A. Eisner. 1995. Estimate of net calcium fluxes and sarcoplasmic reticulum calcium content during systole in rat ventricular myocytes. J.Physiol.(Lond.) **486:** 581–591.

Regulation of Alternative Splicing of the SERCA2 Pre-mRNA in Muscle

FRANK WUYTACK,[a] LUDO VAN DEN BOSCH, MARK VER HEYEN, FAWZIA BABA-AÏSSA, LUC RAEYMAEKERS, AND RIK CASTEELS

Katholieke Universiteit Leuven, Laboratorium voor Fysiologie, Campus Gasthuisberg, Herestraat 49, B-3000 Leuven, Belgium

THE SERCA2 mRNA DIVERSITY

The Ca^{2+}-transport ATPase isoform expressed in the sarcoplasmic reticulum of cardiac muscle, slow-twitch skeletal muscle, and partially smooth muscle (i.e., SERCA2a) represents a splice variant of the ubiquitously expressed SERCA2b isoform. We here summarize some of our findings on how alternative splicing is controlled at the 3′-end of transcripts derived from the sarco/endoplasmic reticulum Ca^{2+}-transport ATPase gene 2 (SERCA2). At this site, transcripts remain either unspliced, but polyadenylated at one of two different positions, pA_u or pA_d generating species denoted as "class 2" or "class 3" mRNA, respectively; or use two potential 5′-donor splice sites 5′D1 or 5′ D2, which splice to a common downstream acceptor 3′A in a mutually exclusive fashion to generate "class 1" or "class 4" transcripts, respectively (FIG. 1). Class 1 transcripts encode the SERCA2a protein, which is expressed abundantly in cardiac and slow-twitch skeletal muscle cells, much less in smooth muscle and some neuronal cells, but not or only at low levels elsewhere. Class 2–4 transcripts differ from each other only at their 5′-untranslated region, and all three encode the SERCA2b protein. Interestingly, transcripts of class 4 are found exclusively in the neuronal cells, although the significance of this finding has not yet been elucidated.

THE *CIS*-ACTIVE SERCA2 TRANSCRIPT ELEMENTS

It is clear from the sequence that polyadenylation at pA_u or splicing from 5′D1 to 3′A are mutually exclusive processes. A possible explanation for the splicing of SERCA2 transcripts in muscle versus polyadenylation in non-muscle cells could be that there exists a competition between both processing modes, with the splicing being favored in muscle. We found however the situation to be more complicated since destruction of pA_u did not by itself induce splicing in non-muscle cells.[1] The sequences of the optional processing sites 5′D1, 5′D2, and pA_u deviate considerably from consensus (i.e., specify weak sites) and we found this to be a prerequisite for allowing alternative processing. Indeed, making 5′D1 consensus elicited constitutive muscle splicing even in non-muscle cells, making 5′D2 consensus induced neuronal splicing in fibroblasts and myocytes and furthermore prevented the muscle splicing in the latter. Muscle splicing is also strongly suppressed when pA_u is replaced by a strong synthetic polyadenylation site (SPA). The sequence of the common optional acceptor site

[a] Phone: 32-16-345936; fax: 32-16-345991; e-mail: frank.wuytack@med.kuleuven.ac.be

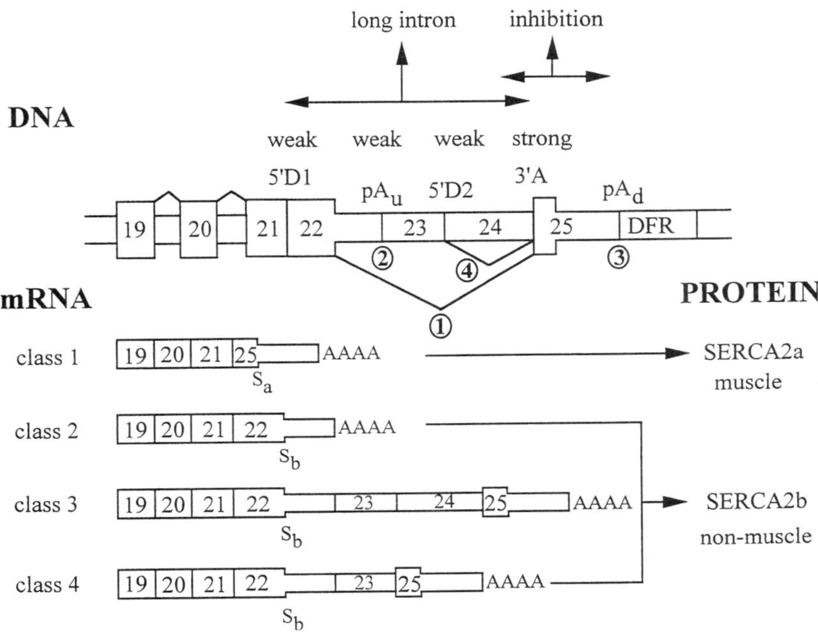

FIGURE 1. Schematic illustration of the prerequisites for regulated expression of the SERCA2 isoforms. The genomic structure of the 3′ end of SERCA2 is shown as well as the prerequisites necessary to obtain regulated processing of the SERCA2 pre mRNA. The 3′ ends of the four different SERCA2 transcripts generated due to alternative processing and the protein isoforms translated from these messengers are also indicated. Exons 22, 23, and 24 are optional and can act as introns (spliced out). 5′D1 is a splice donor site used in muscle (and exceptionally also in neurons). 5′D2 is a donor splice site exclusively used in brain. 3′A is a splice acceptor site common to muscle and neurons. pA_u and pA_d are two alternative polyadenylation sites. S_a and S_b represent STOP translation sites for SERCA2a and SERCA2b, respectively. Class 1 mRNA is found in muscle, whereas class 2 and 3 are present in non-muscle/non-neuronal cells. Class 4 is restricted to neurons.

3′A is however close to consensus and replacing it by a weaker site prevents muscle and neuronal specific splicing. A further necessary condition for muscle splicing is that the optional intron that is spliced out in muscle (removal of exons 22–24) is sufficiently long. Indeed, deleting parts of this sequence induced in non muscle a level of splicing roughly proportional to the length of the removed stretch. Replacing the deleted fragment with an heterologous sequence again suppressed splicing, thus pointing to a pure distance effect and ruling out the presence in the deleted stretch of regulatory *cis*-active sequences.[2] Negative *cis*-active elements, that upon their removal elicit splicing, were however found in two regions of the transcript: in a zone stretching over the entire exon 25 and in the last 237 nt of exon 24. Swapping exon 25 with exon 3 from the rabbit β globin or with an unrelated λ phage sequence, elicited class 1 in fibroblasts or in undifferentiated BC_3H1 myoblasts. A similar result was obtained when parts of exon 25 were removed. Hence the 3′ end of exon 24 must not only contain interaction sites involved in making the decision to splice or not to splice, but furthermore in an as yet unknown way directs splicing either to muscle (class 1) or neuronal mode (class 4).[3]

TRANS-ACTING FACTORS

Our experiments gave also some hints with respect to the *trans*-acting factors responsible for blocking the optional splicing in non-muscle/non-neuronal cells. The expression of myogenin (a member of the helix-loop-helix transcription factors) in fibroblasts represents a sufficient condition for eliciting ectopic muscle-type splicing in these cells. However myogenin expression cannot be a necessary condition since cardiac muscle and neuronal cells do not express this transcription factor but do splice the transcripts. The *trans*-acting factors involved in alternative SERCA splicing also differ from those that regulate alternative splicing of the IgM heavy chain in B-cells versus plasma cells, in spite of the fact that the alternatively spliced parts of the IgM and SERCA2 transcripts show a similar architecture. Indeed, whereas IgM transcripts are spliced in B cells, they are polyadenylated in plasma cells and a number of constructs with a similar layout of splice sites behave in the same way. These observations have been explained in terms of a change in general splicing activity upon maturation of B cells. However, the SERCA2 transcripts, which also present a similar gene layout, do not behave as such. SR proteins like ASF/SF2, SC-35, 9G8, represent a family of proteins known to modulate alternative splicing when two or more optional splice donor sites are involved. However, we could neither detect significant changes in the levels of these proteins between myoblasts and myocytes, nor could we find any effects of overexpressing ASF on SERCA2 transcript processing. All these observations strongly sug-

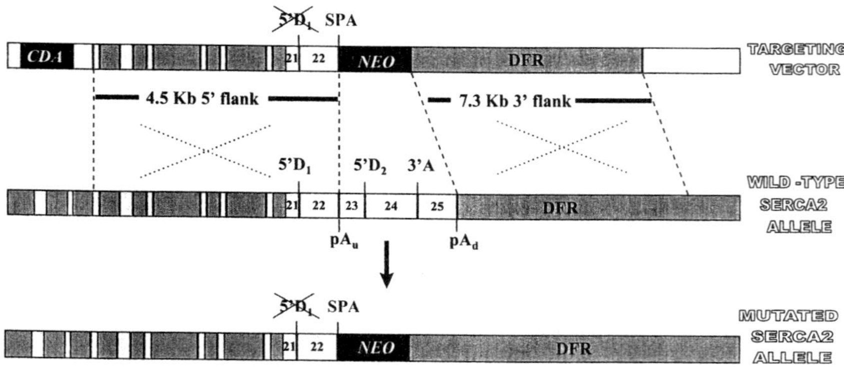

FIGURE 2. Strategies to mutagenize the SERCA2 gene, abolishing splicing to the muscle-specific SERCA2a isoform. A schematic representation of the 3′ end of the SERCA2 gene from exon 13 onwards to the downstream flanking region (DFR) is given in the **middle,** with the relevant transcript processing sites indicated **below. Above,** the targeting vector with the corrupted 5′ donor splice site 5′D1 (silent mutation), the synthetic polyadenylation site (SPA), and the absence of the exons 23–25. Neo indicates a neomycine resistance cassette, which in the transgenic will replace the latter exons and allows a positive selection, while CDA (cytosine deaminase) indicates the negative selectable marker. After homologous recombination the modified gene represented at the **bottom line** should be obtained that allows only the expression of the class 2 mRNA coding for the "housekeeping" nonmuscle SERCA2b isoform.

gest that the regulation of alternative SERCA2 splicing requires muscle-specific *trans*-acting factors rather than general factors.[4]

A GENE-TARGETED MOUSE MODEL UNABLE TO EXPRESS SERCA2A

Our knowledge on the structural requirements of the SERCA2 transcripts necessary to obtain regulated splicing in muscle prompted us to develop a gene-targeted mouse model that would be unable to express the SERCA2a splice variant, but would instead express the housekeeping SERCA2b isoform in all tissues, including in muscle. The SERCA2 gene was modified by corrupting the 5′D1, introducing a SPA site in place of pA_u and removing exon 25 (FIG. 2). It is hoped that this mouse will help us to unravel the physiological significance of the SERCA2a/2b isoform diversity.

REFERENCES

1. VAN DEN BOSCH, L., J. EGGERMONT, H. DE SMEDT, L. MERTENS, F. WUYTACK & R. CASTEELS. 1994. Regulation of splicing is responsible for the expression of the muscle-specific 2a isoform of the sarco/endoplasmic-reticulum Ca^{2+}-ATPase. Biochem. J. **302:** 559–566.
2. MERTENS, L., L. VAN DEN BOSCH, H. VERBOOMEN, F. WUYTACK, H. DE SMEDT & J. EGGERMONT. 1995. Sequence and spatial requirements for regulated muscle-specific processing of the sarco/endoplasmic reticulum Ca^{2+}-ATPase 2 gene transcript. J. Biol. Chem. **270:** 11004–11011.
3. VAN DEN BOSCH, L., L. MERTENS, S. GIJSBERS, M. VER HEYEN, F. WUYTACK & J. EGGERMONT. 1997. Sequence elements surrounding the acceptor site suppress alternative splicing of the sarco/endoplamic reticulum Ca^{2+}-ATPase 2 gene transcript. Biochem. J. **322:** 885–891.
4. VAN DEN BOSCH, L., L. MERTENS, Y. CAVALOC, M. PETERSON, F. WUYTACK & J. EGGERMONT. 1996. Alternative processing of the sarco/endoplasmic reticulum Ca^{2+}-ATPase transcripts during muscle differentiation is a specifically regulated process. Biochem. J. **317:** 647–651.

The Sarcoplasmic Reticulum Ca^{2+}-ATPase Is Depressed in Stunned Myocardium after Ischemia-Reperfusion, but Remains Functionally Coupled to Sarcoplasmic Reticulum–Bound Glycolytic Enzymes[a]

KAI Y. XU,[b] KOENRAAD VANDEGAER, AND LEWIS C. BECKER

Department of Medicine, Division of Cardiology, The Johns Hopkins Medical Institutions, Baltimore, Maryland 21224, USA

Dysfunction of cardiac sarcoplasmic reticulum (SR) Ca^{2+}-ATPase (Ca pump) contributes to intracellular calcium overload during global ischemia.[1] Following reperfusion after brief myocardial ischemia, contractile function often does not return to normal, despite the absence of necrosis. This phenomenon is known as "myocardial stunning." Dysfunction of the SR Ca pump has been reported in stunned myocardium and may contribute to the persistent depression of function.[2] Studies of isolated normal SR vesicles have shown that the chain of glycolytic enzymes from pyruvate kinase (PK) to aldolase, including enolase, phosphoglyceromutase, glyceraldehyde 3-phosphate dehydrogenase, and phosphoglycerate kinase, is bound to SR and that glycolytically derived ATP is functionally coupled to the Ca^{2+}-ATPase.[3] Glycolytic ATP has been shown to play an important role in the functional recovery of the reperfused heart by supporting the SR Ca^{2+}-ATPase pump, thereby helping to achieve Ca^{2+} homeostasis during reperfusion.[4,5] The purpose of this study was to determine whether functional coupling between SR-bound glycolytic enzymes and the SR Ca^{2+}-ATPase remains intact following ischemia-reperfusion and whether any uncoupling may contribute to reduced SR Ca pump function in stunned myocardium. The binding of the key glycolytic enzyme PK to SR membrane following ischemia-reperfusion was also examined.

METHODS

New Zealand White rabbits (4–5 lb) were anesthetized with sodium pentobarbital. The hearts were quickly excised and perfused with a modified-Krebs-Henseleit buffer at constant pressure (80 mm Hg), with a latex balloon in the left ventricle connected to a pressure transducer. The intra-ventricular balloon was emptied of fluid during the ischemic period. Recorded average pressures at baseline were: 109.5±10.4 mmHg (left-ventricular developed pressure) and 13.5±3.4 (end-diastolic pressure). Following 20

[a] This work was supported by National Institutes of Health Grants HL33360, HL52315, and HL52175.

[b] Address for correspondence: Asthma & Allergy Center, 1A-2, 5501 Hopkins Bayview Circle, Baltimore, Maryland 21224. Phone: 410-550-2021; fax: 410-550-2448; e-mail: kxu@welchlink.welch.jhu.edu

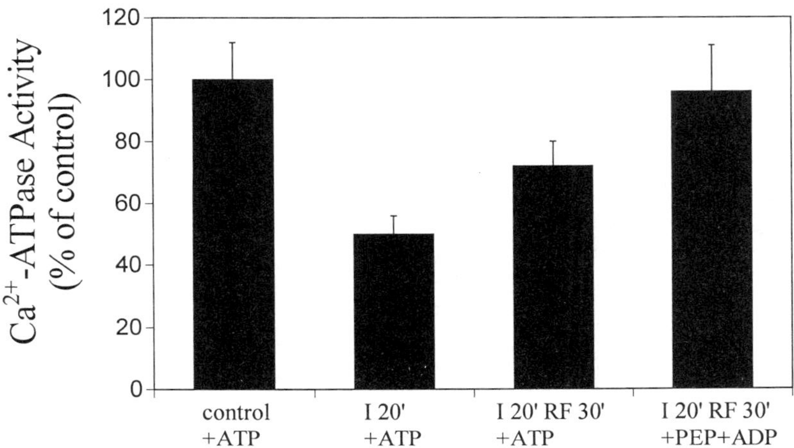

FIGURE 1. Cardiac SR Ca^{2+}-ATPase activity after 20 min ischemia, with and without 30 min reperfusion. Results indicate that enzyme activity is significantly depressed after 20 min ischemia and begins to recover by 30 min reperfusion. However, endogenous ATP generated by the glycolytic enzyme, PK, supports the function of the SR Ca^{2+}-ATPase more efficiently than does exogenous ATP. The data represent the mean of three independent experiments.

min zero-flow ischemia and 0 or 30 min reperfusion at room temperature, hearts were removed from the perfusion apparatus and cardiac SR vesicles were isolated as previously described.[3] Ca^{2+}-ATPase activity was assayed in the isolated SR vesicles by a modification of the method of Kyte.[6] The enzymatic activity was defined as the thapsigargin-sensitive hydrolysis of Mg^{2+}-ATP (1 mM) in the presence of Ca^{2+} (10 μM).

^{45}Ca uptake was initiated by the addition of SR vesicles (0.6 mg/ml) to the reaction mixture for 20 min at 37°C. The mixture contained ^{45}Ca (1 μCi/ml), Ca^{2+} (10 μM), P^1,P^5-di(adenosine-5′)pentaphosphate (0.4 mM), oligomycin (4 μg/ml), ruthenium red (30 nM), Mg^{2+} (4 mM), and either glycolytic substrates specific for PK [phosphoenolpyruvate (PEP, 2 mM) and ADP (1 mM)], or exogenous ATP (1 mM). The reaction was stopped by pelleting the samples at 14,000 rpm for 10 min, and the pellet was then dissolved in 0.5 ml of 10% SDS solution. An aliquot was taken from each sample, and the radioactivity was determined by a β-scintillation counter. The results were expressed as thapsigargin-sensitive ^{45}Ca uptake.

Immunogold labeling was performed by adsorbing SR vesicles on copper grids and incubating the grids with the primary antibody (anti-PK) diluted 1:250 in PBS. Following 30 min of incubation at room temperature, the grids were washed with PBS and then incubated for 30 min with a secondary antibody (donkey anti-goat IgG) conjugated to 12 nm colloidal gold diluted 1:40 in PBS. Following the labeling, all grids were contrasted with lead citrate and examined on a Zeiss 10A TEM operating at 80 kV. The apparent immunogold labeling density was determined by counting all of the gold particles on the surface of the SR vesicles in electron micrographs printed at a final magnification of ×154,000–308,000. Labeling density was expressed as the number of gold particles per μm^2 of SR surface area. The data were corrected for background labeling.

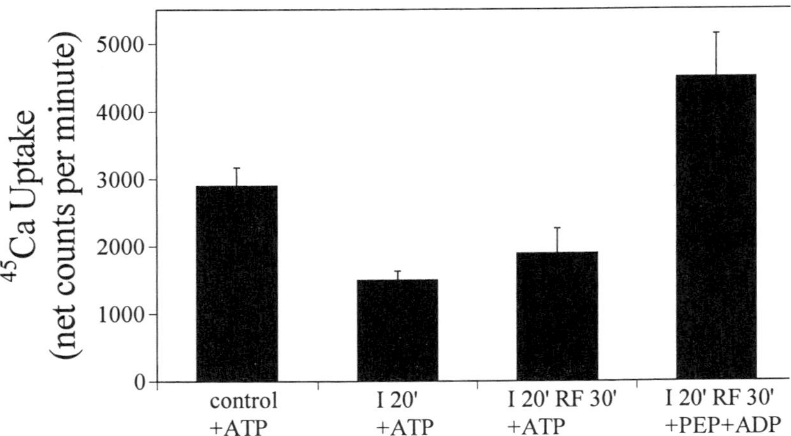

FIGURE 2. ^{45}Ca uptake by cardiac SR vesicles 20 min after addition of phosphoenolpyruvate plus ADP (1 mM) or ATP (1 mM). The data represent the mean ± SD from three separate experiments. The results show that SR ^{45}Ca uptake is depressed after 20 min ischemia, and begins to recover by 30 min reperfusion. However, ATP produced endogenously from PEP and ADP supported twofold more ^{45}Ca uptake in these reperfused SR vesicles than did exogenously supplied ATP under the same experimental conditions.

RESULTS AND CONCLUSIONS

Cardiac SR Ca^{2+}-ATPase activity was decreased to 56% of baseline after 20 min of ischemia (FIG. 1). Following 30 min reperfusion, Ca^{2+}-ATPase activity recovered to 73% of the baseline value in the presence of 1 mM exogenous ATP (FIG. 1). In contrast, when phosphoenolpyruvate (PEP, 4 mM) and ADP (1 mM), the substrates for pyruvate kinase, were added to SR from reperfused hearts, 96% of baseline enzyme activity was recorded (FIG. 1). Similarly, ATP produced endogenously from PEP and ADP supported twofold more ^{45}Ca uptake in these reperfused SR than did exogenously supplied ATP (FIG. 2). Electron microscopic double-immunogold labeling studies showed that Ca^{2+}-ATPase and PK were anatomically co-localized on SR from ischemic-reperfused hearts (data not shown). Furthermore, single-immunogold labeling studies revealed that the apparent labeling densities of PK were 1,216±306, 1,263±70, and 1,200±302/μm^2 for a control heart (20 min baseline flow), ischemic heart (20 min ischemia), and reperfused heart (20 min ischemia and 30 min reperfusion), respectively, indicating that no significant loss of PK binding to cardiac SR occurred under these ischemic conditions, with or without reperfusion. These results demonstrate that following ischemia-reperfusion, cardiac SR Ca^{2+}-ATPase activity and SR Ca transport are significantly reduced. However, binding of PK to SR remains intact, as does functional coupling between ATP generated by SR-bound PK and the Ca^{2+}-ATPase. Glycolytic ATP generated by PK continues to support the activity of functionally depressed SR Ca^{2+}-ATPase more efficiently than does a similar concentration of exogenous ATP. Given the significant depression of SR Ca pump function found in stunned hearts, glycolytic ATP may play an even more important role in SR Ca^{2+} active transport after ischemia-reperfusion than under normal conditions.

REFERENCES

1. KRAUSE, S. & M.L. HESS. ML. 1984. Characterization of cardiac sarcoplasmic reticulum dysfunction during short-term, normothermic, global ischemia. Circ. Res. **55:** 176–184.
2. KRAUSE, S.M., W.E. JACOBUS & L.C. BECKER. 1989. Alterations in cardiac sarcoplasmic reticulum calcium transport in the post-ischemic "stunned" myocardium. Circ. Res. **65:** 526–530.
3. XU, K.Y., J.L. ZWEIER & L.C. BECKER. 1995. Functional coupling between glycolysis and sarcoplasmic reticulum Ca^{2+} transport. Circ. Res. **77:** 88–97.
4. JEREMY, R.W., G. AMBROSIO, M.M. PIKE, W.E. JACOBUS & L.C. BECKER. 1993. The functional recovery of post-ischemic myocardium requires glycolysis during early reperfusion. J. Mol. Cell. Cardiol. **25:** 261–276.
5. JEREMY, R.W., Y. KORETSUNE, E. MARBAN & L.C. BECKER. 1992. Relation between glycolysis and calcium homeostasis in postischemic myocardium. Circ. Res. **70:** 1180–1190.
6. KYTE, J. 1971. Purification of the sodium- and potassium-dependent adenosine triphosphatase from canine renal medulla. J. Biol. Chem. **246:** 4157–4165.

Pharmacology of the Cardiac Sarcoplasmic Reticulum Calcium ATPase-Phospholamban Interaction

ROBERT G. JOHNSON, JR.[a]

Department of Pharmacology, Merck Research Laboratories, West Point, Pennsylvania 19486, USA

ABSTRACT: Accumulating evidence points to the critical role of phospholamban (PLB) regulation of the cardiac sarcoplasmic reticulum (SR) calcium ATPase in influencing the kinetics of calcium handling within the cardiac myocyte under normal and pathological conditions. Based on the data, it has been hypothesized that PLB inhibitors (e.g., calcium ATPase stimulators) would be of potential importance as positive lusitropes and inotropes in the treatment of heart failure. Experiments measuring tension transients in saponin-permeabilized cardiac muscles from genetically engineered mice under a variety of SR calcium loading conditions provide evidence of the functional alterations that can be achieved by manipulation of the degree of PLB inhibition of the calcium pump. Testing of the above hypothesis will ultimately require a selective, high-affinity, membrane-permeable small molecule stimulator of the cardiac calcium pump. Screening for cardiac calcium pump activators has produced a series of agents exerting apparently different mechanisms of action; some may be tools to help to elucidate the nature of the PLB–calcium ATPase interaction(s). The rationale for PLB as a drug target, the optimal profile of a PLB inhibitor, and the properties of several low-molecular-weight compounds will be explored.

The intensive research efforts over the past 20 years directed towards the cardiac sarcoplasmic reticulum proteins have resulted in an unparalleled understanding of the central role that these proteins serve in regulation of calcium fluxes within the heart. Indeed, greater resources and attention have been focused historically on understanding the mechanisms of calcium action at the level of the myofilaments. Despite this bias, the evidence that has accumulated from the laboratories of many of the participants in this volume (particularly during the past five years) has enabled an accurate and integrated understanding of the relationship of the calcium uptake, storage, and release at the level of the sarcoplasmic reticulum (SR) and how the magnitude of the vectoral fluxes at the subcelluar level translates into muscle dynamics and ultimately ventricular function. Based on years of investigation, the unique roles of each of the major SR proteins are firmly established and assigned, their relative contributions to calcium entry and efflux documented, and their physiological regulations broadly outlined.

Just one of the examples of the application of recently available techniques to investigation of the SR is the generation of PLB knockout and overexpression mice that have permitted conclusions concerning the relative importance of PLB in regulating the myocardial contractility and to assess the magnitude of its contribution to the beta adrenergic effects on the heart (for review see Ref. 1). It has been possible to unify mol-

[a]Present address: Robert G. Johnson, Jr., M.D., Ph.D., Chiron Corporation, 4560 Horton Street, Emeryville, California 94608. Phone: 510-923-4034; fax: 510-923-7460; e-mail: robert_g_johnson@cc.chiron.com

ecular events (the degree of binding of PLB to the calcium ATPase) with subcellular events (rate of calcium fluxes into and out of the SR) with whole organ physiology (inotropy and lusitropy).

Many of the details of the precise short-term regulation of the SR proteins still remain to be elucidated. For example, the precise manner in which PLB interacts with the cardiac SR calcium-ATPase (SERCA2), the exact mechanism by which calcium is pumped through the calcium ATPase against an enormous concentration gradient along the fine tuning of the calcium release channel regulation are unknown. While the details are being unraveled, the field has begun to address the next higher level of questions: how are the SR proteins regulated under pathological conditions? and is the abnormal regulation contributing to or attempting to reverse the underlying deficit in calcium handling? is there an appropriate target for pharmaceutical development within the cardiac SR that would serve to correct derangements in calcium handling? and if so, what are the mechanism(s) that must be considered in order to achieve the established goals?

While there are theoretically several potential drug targets within the cardiac SR, we have chosen to concentrate on the calcium ATPase–PLB interaction for the reasons given below and to approach the inhibition with a search strategy to discover small-molecular-weight compounds that block the SERCA2-PLB interaction. (This is not to denigrate other approaches that also have validity.) What follows is the raison d'être for the investigation into the calcium ATPase–PLB complex as a target for altering the heart failure phenotype and a status report on the findings to date.

THE BASES FOR THE INTEREST IN SR CARDIAC PROTEINS AS DRUG TARGETS

Heart failure is the clinical syndrome against which pharmacological therapy based on cardiac SR proteins may have benefit. The marketplace is sufficiently saturated with so-termed preload and afterload reducers for symptomatic relief of the symptoms of heart failure. Despite the availability of these preload/afterload-reducing therapeutic agents, there is no effective, safe, oral chronic cardiotonic therapy for treating systolic and diastolic dysfunction in heart failure. And it can be effectively argued that safe and effective positive inotropes and lusitropes are needed. The clinical need in terms of incidence and prevalence of heart failure and cost to the health care system is staggering.

Congestive heart failure (CHF) is the fastest-growing therapeutic target group within the cardiovascular area and is associated with significant morbidity and mortality and substantial economic costs. With the aging population, the incidence and prevalence is rising (doubling every decade after age 45). Congestive heart failure has become the single largest hospital-based diagnostic category in the United States: it has been projected that in 1997 one million patient discharges were assigned to CHF as their primary diagnostic related group (DRG); there are currently 3.5 million patients with CHF.[2] Worldwide, of course, the incidence and prevalence are even greater. And one can speculate that as a greater degree of myocardial salvage increases with acute interventional therapy and other life-threatening diseases no longer represent an immediate risk to certain elderly patients, the incidence should continue to increase. Because the contractility of the heart is compromised in heart failure, a logical therapy would be to improve the efficiency of the contraction-relaxation cycle. Therefore, the objective has been to identify appropriate molecular target(s), focusing in our case upon the cardiac SR, where pharmacological intervention may result in activity as mild inotropes and particularly lusitropes.

Drugs with a direct effect on the heart have historically displayed multiple drawbacks relating to issues of efficacy, precise mechanism of action, and adverse effects. How can the performance of a failing heart be improved through a cardiotonic action without a detrimental effect?

THE ROLE OF THE CARDIAC SR IN REGULATION OF CARDIAC CALCIUM HOMEOSTASIS

In order to understand the importance of the calcium ATPase–PLB interaction in cardiac myocyte homeostasis, it is necessary to review the contribution of calcium transients to the excitation-contractile coupling mechanisms (FIG. 1). During a normal cardiac cycle, depolarization of the sarcolemma due to opening primarily of potassium channels ultimately results in calcium channel opening. The entry of calcium into the myocyte in close proximity to the foot processes of the SR (described by Franzini-Armstrong *et al.,* this volume) triggers calcium release from the SR through the calcium release channel (so-called calcium-induced calcium release). Calcium diffuses to the myofilaments, where it activates the calcium-sensitive myofibrillar proteins, and contraction is initiated. As the calcium within the myoplasm rises, the calcium pump turnover

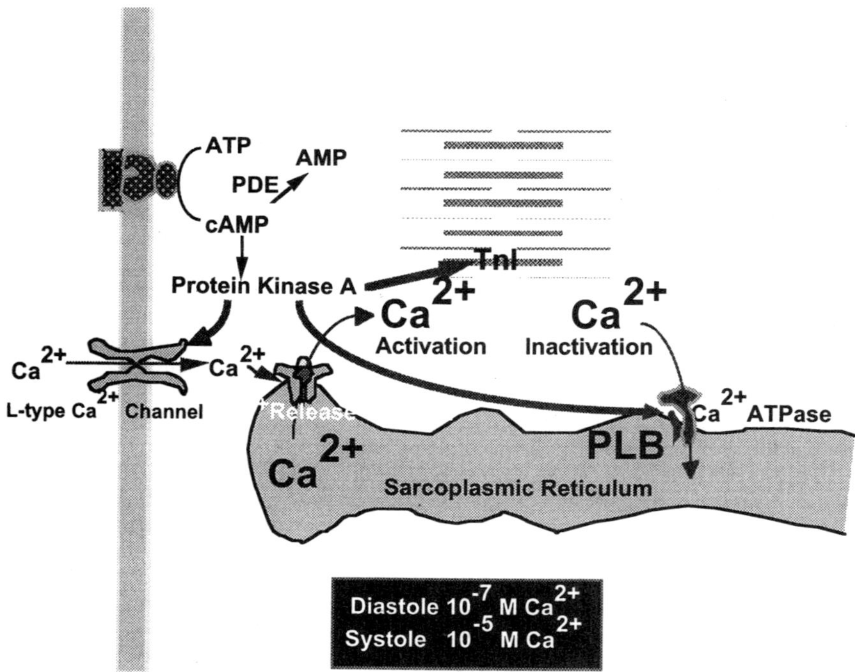

FIGURE 1. Schematic diagram of the calcium pathway within the heart to illustrate the central role of the sarcoplasmic reticulum in excitation-contractile coupling.

increases commensurate with its K_m for calcium. As the calcium concentration within the myoplasm falls, the myofilaments and therefore the muscle fibers relax. There are many critical features of the SR function within this calcium cycle, but two interrelated properties of these deserve emphasis: the contractility of the muscle is dependent upon the absolute amount of calcium delivered to and removed from the fibers as well as the rate of the rate of appearance and removal. Based upon the architecture of the muscle, there is also a spacial as well as a temporal contribution.

Cardiac muscle differs from skeletal muscle in that every cell contracts with every cardiac cycle. (In skeletal muscle increased demand is met primarily by recruitment of additional muscle fibers). One of the ways that the cardiac myocyte balances output and demand is through the beta adrenergic pathway. During times of increased demand the beta receptors within the heart are stimulated to increase cardiac output. One result is to increase the heart rate (positive chronotropy) Another is to increase the inotropy and lusitropy of the heart. This occurs when the beta receptors in the sarcolemma are activated, which ultimately results in activation of adenylate cyclase and increased levels of cAMP. The increase in the cyclic AMP levels serves several functions: to activate protein kinase A (PKA), which phosphorylates the calcium channel (to increase calcium influx); to activate troponin T (to decrease the calcium sensitivity and enhance relaxation during fast heart rates); and finally (and probably most importantly) to phosphorylate PLB. This phosphorylation serves to disinhibit the calcium ATPase and therefore to permit it to fully activate. Activation of the pump functionally results in more rapid influx of calcium into the SR and therefore faster relaxation (dominant effect); and since more calcium is pumped per unit time, there is more calcium within the intra-SR space available for release, resulting in enhanced contractility. The signal is terminated when the cAMP falls and phosphorylated PLB (PLB-P) falls to basal levels. A phosphatase associated with the SR serves to regulate the degree of PLB phosphorylation and itself is controlled by a variety of factors.

The enormous influence that PLB has upon the function of the SERCA2 can perhaps be best illustrated by studying the uptake of calcium into isolated cardiac SR. A representative experiment is noted in FIGURE 2, where isolated canine SR is incubated in varying calcium buffers, and the rate of ^{45}calcium uptake into the vesicles is measured by taking aliquots and filtering the samples. Under basal conditions, the PLB is not phosphorylated and therefore acts as an inhibitor of the calcium ATPase. When canine SR is incubated at pCa 6.75, there is a measurable but low rate of ^{45}calcium uptake. This is due to the low substrate availability and the inhibitory effect of PLB. When PLB is phosphorylated or an antibody directed against PLB (in the particular case shown a monoclonal antibody (mAb) directed against the N-terminal portion of PLB) is added to the incubation mixture at the beginning, a remarkable result occurs. The uptake is stimulated almost two orders of magnitude. The calcium dependence of the calcium uptake is now shifted to the left. For example, at pCa 7 in the presence of PLB bound to the pump there is little turnover of the ATPase. However, when the PLB antibody is added (as a surrogate for PLB phosphorylation), the uptake is stimulated almost two orders of magnitude. Under both conditions (presence or absence of Mab 1D11) the pump is maximally activated at high calcium concentrations (i.e., the V_{max} is the same). There is a clear calcium dependence of activation of the pump as the calcium is increased (data not shown) with a V_{max} at approximately pCa 5.5.

Note that diastolic calcium is around 100 nM (pCa 7), and systolic calcium approaches 10 μM (pCa5). So the functional effect of phosphorylating PLB is to shift the calcium dependence curve to the left; i.e., the phosphorylation of PLB results in an apparent increase in the K_m of SERCA2 for calcium.

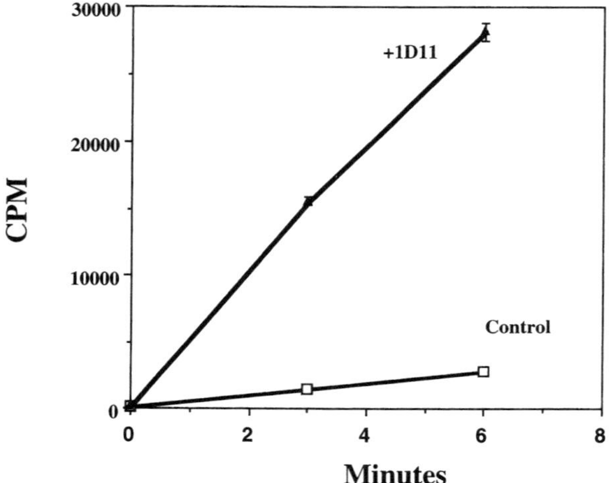

FIGURE 2. Uptake of 45calcium (UPCAL) into cardiac SR. Canine cardiac SR (100 µg/ml) is incubated in a buffered calcium solution (175 µl) at pCa 7.0 containing 45 CaCl2 (1.5 µl/ml). Uptake is initiated by adding 3.16 mM ATP and 15 mM creatine phosphate using 96-well microtiter plates at room temperature. Initiation of uptake occurs simultaneously in all wells using a Quadra 96 pipetting system. At the times indicated, 50 µl from each well is simultaneously vacuum filtered on a 0.45 µm HA Millipore filter, washed, dried, and counted in a Packard Topcount Scintillation Counter. The values represent the mean of 20 determinations.

So the calcium ATPase–PLB complex is a highly regulated, sensitive, and centrally situated element in the calcium regulatory pathway, an important criteria to be met as a target for calcium regulation.

There are four main questions that need to be adequately answered prior to definitively deciding that inhibition of the calcium ATPase–PLB interaction is a worthy goal. First, what is the evidence that the complex is an appropriate target for pharmaceutical intervention in congestive heart failure? Second, what are the theoretical mechanisms through which manipulation of the complex would yield beneficial results? Third, what are the potential drawbacks of these approaches? And finally, what is the evidence that any low-molecular-weight entity can under the appropriate conditions provide the desired effect?

DATA SUPPORTING THE SERCA2-PLB COMPLEX AS AN IMPORTANT AND VIABLE DRUG TARGET FOR HEART FAILURE

A variety of hard and soft data supports the hypothesis that the calcium ATPase-PLB complex is a drug target in congestive heart failure. What follows is a summary of existing evidence that is consistent with the hypotheses. In cases where the data and/or interpretation are inconsistent or controversial, the issues are summarized. In the final analysis, it is only when an appropriate inhibitor is adequately tested in the clinic that the rationale will or will not be borne out. A brief summary is listed in TABLE 1.

TABLE 1. Why Is the Calcium ATPase-PLB Complex of Interest as a Drug Target?

- PLB as an inhibitor of the cardiac calcium ATPase is the primary regulator of inotropy and lusitrophy in the heart
- PLB is at the end of the cyclic AMP–stimulated phosphorylation cascade pathway (limits adverse events)
- PLB is highly cardiac specific
- PLB is highly conserved across species

1. The Calcium Fluxes in Myocytes from Failed Hearts Are Abnormal

One of the hallmarks of congestive heart failure at the cellular level is the abnormal calcium transients measured in isolated ventricular strips or myocytes. First described in human ventricular strips using aqueorin[2,3] and then later in isolated myocytes using calcium-sensitive dyes,[4] the measured calcium transients in general are slow and with diminished amplitude. The calcium transients correlate with the measured force generation, which is also blunted and slow—e.g., the force generation is submaximal, with slow kinetics of time to peak contraction and time to half-relaxation. It has not been determined whether this abnormality is a primary cause of heart failure (HF) or whether it is a compensatory phenotypic alteration to preserve function (for example, by decreasing energy expenditure). But it is clear that one possible mechanism of the abnormal calcium transients may be the decreased calcium pump activity, which would explain the inability of the SR to adequately remove the calcium from the cytosol (thereby impacting diastole) and why less calcium is available for release (impacting systole).

2. Clinical Data Supports a PLB/SERCA2 Mismatch

Recent clinical data in which the protein levels of SERCA2 and PLB were measured in samples obtained from normal and failed hearts showed that while both the calcium pump and PLB expression were down-regulated in the hearts of patients with heart failure, the down-regulation of the calcium pump is much greater.[5] The net result is that the ratio of calcium ATPase to PLB is lower in failed than in normal hearts (relative PLB overexpression). Is there any physiological insight that can be used to ascertain whether a SERCA2/PLB mismatch is of functional consequence? The elegant data concerning the PLB knockout (KO) mice has already been documented (Chu *et al.*, this volume and REFS. 6,7). Absence of PLB results in a hyperdynamic heart. What about more subtle differences? A portion of the answer arises from the use of animal models in investigating the effect of thyroid hormone on cardiac function. Under hypothyroid conditions in which cardiac phenotype is described as hyodynamic there is down-regulation of SERCA2 and up-regulation of PLB.[8,9] Under hyperthyroid conditions, the reverse is observed: the protein expression of PLB decreases and that of the calcium ATPase increases.[10] The hyperthyroid heart is often described as "hyperdynamic." The alterations in these two SR proteins are not the only phenotypic changes that would be observed in the human heart under hyper/hypothyroid conditions. But based on the animal data, the alterations in these two proteins may be sufficient to explain the majority of the changes in cardiac dynamics as a function of the thyroid status. And these hormone-induced alterations in the SERCA2-PLB ratios may be a paradigm for SERCA2-PLB mismatches in congestive heart failure.

3. Studies of SR Function in Situ *Demonstrate a Direct Correlation between Gene Dosage of PLB and Can Result in a Heart Failure Phenotype*

Due to the importance of determining the phenotype of altered calcium ATPase/PLB ratios with regard to cardiac contractility, we have studied SR function *in situ* in a permealized cardiac muscle preparation (Wiedmann *et al.*, this volume). In this preparation, the sarcolemma is permealized with a mild detergent, but the SR is left intact. Thus, this preparation is more physiological than isolated SR, where the spacial orientation is disrupted and vesicles are formed. Here the geometry between the sarcolemma and the SR is maintained, and the SR is in its native configuration. The effect of PLB gene dosage on calcium uptake into SR within the mouse permeabilized ventricular muscle was compared in wild-type (PLB = 1x), PLB knockout mice (PLB = 0), and PLB overexpression mice (PLB = 4X).

This data represents the first example of the successful adaptation of skinned muscle technology to mouse cardiac muscle and also illustrates the dramatic phenotypic response of alterations in the SERCA2-PLB ratio. Since the experiments were performed in the range of diastolic calciums, the data supports the hypothesis that an increase in the PLB/calcium ATPase ratio as reported in failing hearts can contribute to diastolic dysfunction.

Recent generalized somatic cardiac gene transfer studies are also consistent with this notion. When PLB was overexpressed in rat hearts (2.8-fold) using a recombinant adenoviral vectors, the rats, when compared with control hearts, demonstrated lower peak left ventricular pressures, decreased peak rates of pressure rise and fall, and significant increases in the time constant of left ventricular relaxation.[11] In isolated cells there was a corresponding increase in resting calcium, decrease in calcium release, and prolonged calcium relaxation phase. The decrease in systolic pressure, increase in diastolic pressure, and large increase in the time constant for isovolumic relaxation were noted to recapitulate many of the pathophysiologic abnormalities observed in heart failure. And most strikingly, when isoproterenol was given to these hearts, the maximal stimulation produced decreases in the isovolumic relaxation and increases in LVSP similar to those seen in the controls, suggesting that the intrinsic SERCA2 activity is the same in the PLB-transfected and control-transfected hearts and that the abnormalities are specifically due to the result of PLB-mediated inhibition of the SR ATPase.

4. Basal P-PLB Levels May Be Abnormally Low in Heart Failure Due to Lowered Cyclic AMP Levels

Since in the face of markedly increased exposure to catecholamines the beta adrenergic receptors down-regulate and uncouple from their effector molecules, the basal cyclic AMP levels have been reported to be lower in heart failure. If this is truly the case, then, even under basal conditions, a lower percentage of PLB may be in the dephosphorylated state, contributing to negative inotropy and lusitropy. The effect may be exacerbated by increased phosphatase activity and, of course, an abnormal ratio, described above.

5. PLB Is Highly Cardiac Specific and Highly Conserved across Species

One of the genuinely appealing aspects of this target is its cardiac specificity. The protein is expressed almost exclusively in the heart (>99%). Such specificity for a drug target cannot be overestimated or underappreciated. Small amounts (nonstoichiometric with respect to the calcium ATPase) are found in some vascular smooth muscle and tiny amounts in some fast-twitch skeletal muscle.[12] The role of PLB in these other muscle types has not been established; PLB has not been definitively shown to regulate the calcium pump in these tissues. PLB is a highly conserved protein across species.

6. PLB Is at the End of the Pathway Cascade and Therefore SERCA2-PLB Targeting May Provide Specificity and Limit Adverse Events

While the inhibition of upstream events is considered an advantage in many systems, in this case it may be reasoned that distal inhibition is advantageous. The primary regulator of the PLB phosphorylation status is protein kinase A, whose activity is regulated by cAMP. Elevation of cAMP would be predicted to activate a wide variety of mechanisms, some of which may be beneficial, others detrimental. For example, phosphodiesterase (PDE) inhibitors administered to patients with heart failure results in dramatic short-term improvement, through mechanisms that in part may relate to the enhanced phosphorylation of PLB. However, other detrimental actions, including proarrythmic effects and increased mortality, have limited their usefulness. In this case, increases in cAMP in nonmyocyte cells and elevations in cGMP may provide the negative actions. These concerns would not be dictated by a SERCA2-PLB target.

POTENTIAL MECHANISMS FOR ALTERING THE CALCIUM ATPASE–PLB INTERACTION

There are two general methods for altering the calcium ATPase–PLB interaction. The first is to increase the proportion of PLB that is excluded from binding to the calcium pump. The second is to decrease the total pool of PLB available. They are not mutually exclusive. The schemata in FIGURE 1 can be used for reference. The potential mechanisms are also summarized in TABLE 2.

1. Decrease the Relative Proportion of PLB That Binds to the Calcium ATPase

Physiologically, this occurs with elevated calcium or by increasing the phosphorylation of PLB. Increasing the cytosolic calcium to regulate PLB is not rational. Decreasing the relative portion that binds to PLB can be achieved through increasing the

TABLE 2. Potential Mechanisms for Altering the Calcium ATPase–PLB Interaction

- Increase the amount of P-PLB
    - Decrease the P-PLB phosphatase activity
        - Phosphatase inhibitor
    - Increase PKA activity (increase cAMP)
        - Beta-receptor activation
        - PDE inhibition
    - Increase calcium calmodulin–dependent kinase activity
- Increase the amount of expressed SERCA2
    - Stimulate promoter
    - Gene therapy
- Decrease the amount of expressed PLB
    - Block promoter region of PLB gene antisense

PKA activity (through elevated cAMP). Due to the generic influence of myocyte cAMP levels this is not an approach in favor, although more specific PDE inhibitors may limit the effect to the myocyte, and combination therapy (with a beta-adrenergic blocker, for example) may provide synergy and limit the downside actions. Another approach would be to inhibit the P-PLB phosphatase activity. The cardiac SR contains a significant amount of serine/threonine phosphatase,[13,14] which is responsible for recycling the PLB back to the dephosphorylated form This is a type I phosphatase whose specificity is not significantly different from other phosphatases in its class, the specificity being defined more by its spacial distribution. Targeting of the attachment site on the SR is a theoretical but as yet untested target.

Finally, a low-molecular-weight compound that interferes with the SERCA2-PLB interaction would be of utility. Stretching the definition of low, a prototype of a low-molecular-weight entity is the 1D11 monoclonal antibody that binds to the N-terminal region of the cardiac ATPase and results in its activation.

2. Alter the Ratio of Expressed Calcium ATPase and/or PLB

Based on the data reviewed here, it appears reasonable that increasing the amount of expressed cardiac calcium pump in failed hearts and/or decreasing the amount of PLB should improve the inotropy and lusitropy of the heart. As reported by Dillman, Inesi, and others in this volume, increased expression of the ATPase in isolated cells or within a normal heart results in increased calcium uptake and enhanced contractile effect. Therefore either direct introduction of the gene into the myocardium or identification of promoter molecular activation should improve cardiac function. An intellectually similar but more difficult approach would be to down-regulate PLB through promoter manipulation or antisense. A thyroid hormone analog with properties that primarily effect only the transcription of SERCA2 and PLB and would be acceptable for clinical trials would be desirable, but has not been forthcoming.[15]

POSSIBLE LIMITATIONS OF A SERCA2-PLB INHIBITOR

There are a variety of factors that must be acknowledged that may serve to limit the effectiveness of this mechanism. (TABLE 3). The first set of factors relates to the unknown regulatory mechanisms. For example, is the level of PLB phosphorylation al-

TABLE 3. Difficulties with Identifying and Developing a Calcium ATPase Activator–PLB Inhibitor

- Must disrupt a protein-protein interaction
  - Few examples of low-molecular-weight compounds
  - Affinity of calcium ATPase–PLB interaction is unknown
  - Binding site(s) of interaction are unknown
    - No high resolution structural data
- In heart failure, is the PLB already highly phosphorylated?
- Will a calcium ATPase activator–PLB inhibitor induce counterregulatory mechanisms to negate the effect?
- Will a calcium ATPase activator–PLB inhibitor "whip" a dying heart?
  - Increase mortality? morbidity?

ready high in the failing heart? Although based on the above arguments this likelihood is low, it has not been adequately tested in human heart failure. Another potential pitfall is whether inhibiting the interaction may induce counterregulatory mechanisms that negate the effect. For example, PLB expression may become even more up-regulated. And finally, will the increased energy expenditure involved with the pump stimulation, although a small percentage of the overall cellular consumption, be sufficient to affect morbidity and even mortality?

The Approach to Finding Low-Molecular-Weight Entities as Inhibitors of the SERCA2-PLB Interaction

Unfortunately, there is a disturbing lack of high-quality, high-resolution structural data of the SERCA2 or PLB and virtually none of the complex. This stems from the difficulty in forming high-quality crystals of either protein, the size of SERCA2 (for NOR studies), and the transmembrane nature of both. There are encouraging developments in the field relating to electron microscopy and solution nuclear magnetic resonance, but the resolution still is nonoptimal.[16–18] Structure-function studies have provided new and provocative findings as to the nature of the site of interaction through the work on site-directed mutagenesis; however, peptides directed against the regions of putative binding have failed to date to affect the interaction. So the approaches by this laboratory and others have been rather pedantic: set up high-volume screens using cardiac SR at low calcium concentrations where the stimulatory capacity is greatest and test for agents that significantly increase the rate of uptake of ^{45}calcium. Fortunately, the counterscreen for an assay of this sort is straightforward: skeletal muscle SR. The SERCA1 pump is related to the SERCA2 isoform, but no PLB is present.

EXAMPLES OF LOW-MOLECULAR-WEIGHT ACTIVATORS OF THE SERCA2-PLB COMPLEX

One of challenges of this field is to properly designate the syntax of positive findings. The goal is to stimulate the SERCA2 activity through dysinhibition of the PLB binding. At this junction, the binding of a small compound could be either to the SERCA2 or to PLB, although binding to PLB would be preferable given the tissue specificity. Since the sites of binding of the protein-protein interaction are not established, nor is the precise understanding of how exactly PLB limits the SERCA2 turnover (nor, for that matter, the role of pentamer vs. monomer PLB states), any molecules that may provide some insight into potential mechanisms would be of great interest to the field.

One of first compounds to be identified was quercitin.[19] This compound had previously been shown to inhibit skeletal muscle SR calcium ATPase activity and ^{45}calcium uptake.[19] However, in cardiac muscle a biphasic effect was observed (FIG. 3). At low quercitin concentrations (<25 μM) a stimulation of the calcium ATPase was observed, while at high concentrations inhibition was measured with a dose dependence similar to that seen with skeletal SR. Only inhibition was confirmed in skeletal muscle SR or when the PLB inhibition of cardiac SR was removed through the use of mAb 1D11 or small amounts of detergent. Interestingly, the maximal antibody and quercitin stimulation were identical; and when submaximal antibody concentrations were used, stimulation was additive with quercitin. The steady state formation of the phosphoenzyme from ATP or Pi was increased at low concentrations of quercitin, but decreased at high concentrations. The central observation was that quercitin, even under conditions

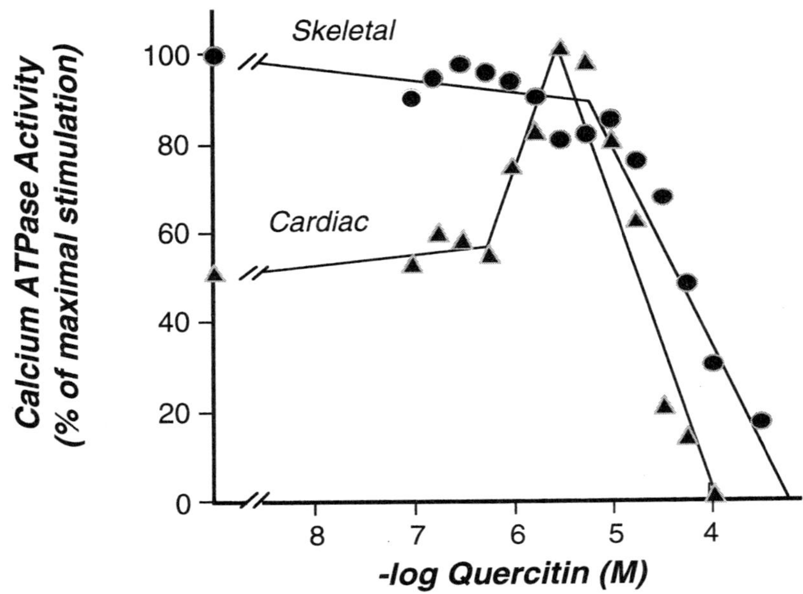

FIGURE 3. The effect of quercitin on cardiac and skeletal SR SERCA2 ATPase activity. The calcium-stimulated ATP hydrolysis at pCa 6.75, 0.5 mM ATP, and 5% Me2SO (room temperature) was assayed by the generation of Pi.

where it was measured to be stimulatory, was a competitive inhibitor of ATP at its catalytic site. There was no evidence of a direct PLB interaction. The data suggests that quercitin interacts with the catalytic site nucleotide binding site and that this by some mechanism unmasks PLB's inhibition of SERCA2. It can be postulated that PLB may interact at or near the nucleotide binding site. A structure-function relationship revealed that even closely related alkaloids failed to produce a stimulatory or inhibitory effect.[19]

Subsequently, other compounds have been shown to produce a "quercitin-like" effect. One of these was tannin[20]; representative data is shown by Coll *et al.* (this volume). In contrast to tannin, ellagic acid addition stimulated the ATPase and ^{45}calcium uptake in cardiac SR at low concentrations, but the inhibitory effects were observed at much higher concentrations (>100 times the IC_{50}).

An additional outcome of this data is the recruitment model advanced by McKenna *et al.*[19] that attempts to better explain the turnover of SERCA2 in the presence of PLB.

SUMMARY

There is a strong rationale for regarding the SERCA2-PLB complex as a therapeutic target for heart failure. A series of compounds are beginning to be identified that demonstrate that low-molecular-weight compounds can stimulate the SERCA2 activity. Future work is necessary to identify more potent stimulators and those with novel structures while at the same time obtaining additional insight into the properties of the SERCA2-PLB interaction. In addition, other approaches such as gene therapy may shortly contribute.

REFERENCES

1. KOSS, K. L. & E. G. KRANIAS. 1996. Phospholamban: A prominent regulator of myocardial contractility. Circ. Res. **79:** 1059–1063.
2. RICH, M. W. 1997. Epidemiology, pathophysiology, and etiology of congestive heart failure in older adults. J. Am. Geriatr. Soc. **45:** 968–974.
3. GWATHMEY J. K., L., R. MACKINNON, F. J. SCHOEN, M. D. FELDMAN, W. GROSSMAN & J. P. MORGAN. 1987. Abnormal intracellular calcium handling in myocardium from patients with end-stage heart failure. Circ. Res. **61**(1): 70–76.
4. D. J., M. NABAUER, C. KRUGER & E. ERDMANN. 1995. Altered diastolic [Ca2+]i handling in human ventricular myocytes from patients with terminal heart failure. Am. Heart J. **129**(4): 684–689.
5. MEYER, M. W., W. SCHILLINGER, B. PIESKE, C. HOLUVARASCH, C. HEILMANN, H. POSIVAL, G. KUWAJIMA, K. MIKOSHIBA, H. JUST & G. HASENFUSS. 1995. Alterations of sarcoplasmic reticulum proteins in failing dilated cardiomyopathy. Circulation **92:** 778–784.
6. LUO, W., I. L. GRUPP, J. HARRER, S. PONNIAH, G. GRUPP, J. J. DUFFY, T. DOETSCHMAN & E. G. KRANIAS. 1994. Targeted ablation of the phospholamban gene is associated with markedly enhanced myocardial contractility and loss of beta-agonist stimulation. Circ. Res. **75:** 401–409.
7. HOIT, B. D., S. F. KHOURY, E. G. KRANIAS, N. BALL & R. WALSH. 1995. In vivo echocardiographic detection of enhanced left ventricular function in gene-targeted mice with phospholamban deficiency. Circ. Res. **77:** 632–637.
8. NAGAI, R., A. ZARAIN-HERZBERG, C. J. BRANDL, J. FUJII, M. TADA, D. H. MACLENNAN, N. R. ALPERT & M. PERIASAMY. 1989. Regulation of myocardial Ca^{2+}-ATPase and phospholamban mRNA expression in response to pressure overload and thyroid hormone. Proc. Natl. Acad. Sci. (USA) **86:** 2966–2970.
9. KISS, E., G. JAKAB, E. G. KRANIAS & I. EDES. 1994. Thyroid hormone-induced alterations in phospholamban protein expression: Regulatory effects on sarcoplasmic reticulum Ca^{2+} transport and myocardial relaxation. Circ. Res. **75:** 245–251.
10. KHOURY, S. F., B. D. HOIT, V. DAVE, C. M. PAWLOSKI-DAHM, Y. SHAO, M. GABEL, M. PERIASAMY & R. A. WALSH. 1996. Effects of thyroid hormone on left ventricular performance and regulation of contractile and Ca(2+)-cycling proteins in the baboon. Implications for the force-frequency and relaxation frequency relationships. Circ. Res. **79**(4): 727–735.
11. HAJJAR, R. J., U. T. MATSUI, J. L. GUERRERO, K. H. LEE, J. K. GWATHMEY, G. W. DEC, M. J. SEMIGRAN & A. ROSENZWEIG. 1998. Modulation of ventricular function through gene transfer in vivo. Proc. Natl. Acad. (USA) 28: 5251–5256.
12. BRIGGS, F. N., K. F. LEE, A. W. WECHSLER & L. R. JONES. 1992. Phospholamban expressed in slow-twitch and chronically stimulated fast-twitch muscle minimally affects calcium affinity of sarcoplasmic reticulum Ca^{2+}-ATPase. J. Biol. Chem. **267:** 26056–26061.
13. MACDOUGALL, L. K., L. R. JONES & P. COHEN. 1991. Identification of the major protein phosphatases in mammalian cardiac muscle which dephosphorylate phospholamban. Eur. J. Biochem. **196:** 725–734.
14. AHMAD, Z., J. GREEN, H. SUBUHI & A. M. WATANABE. 1989. Autonomic regulation of type 1 protein in cardiac muscle. J. Biol. Chem. **264:** 3859–3863.
15. MORKIN, E., G. D. PENNOCK, T. E. RAYA, J. J. BAHL & S. GOLDMAN. 1996. Development of a thyroid hormone analogue for the treatment of congestive heart failure. Thyroid **6**(5): 521–526.
16. MASLENNIKOV, I. V., A. G. SOBOL, J. ANAGLI, P. JAMES, T. VORHERR, A. V. ARSENIEV & E. CARAFOLI. 1995. The secondary structure of phospholamban: A two dimensional study. Biochem. Biophys. Res. Commun. **217:** 1200–1207.
17. MORTISHIRE-SMITH, R. J., S. M. PITZENBERGER, C. J. BURKE, C. R. MIDDAUGH, V. M.

GARSKY & R. G. JOHNSON. 1995. Solution structure of the cytoplasmic domain of phospholamban: Phosphorylation leads to a local perturbation in secondary structure. Biochemistry **34:** 7603–7613.

18. STOKES, D. L. 1997. Keeping calcium in its place: Ca^{2+}-ATPase and phospholamban. Curr. Opin. Struct. Biol. **7:** 550–556.
19. MCKENNA, E., J. S. SMITH, K. E. COLL, E. K. MAZACK, E. J. MAYER, J. ANTANAVAGE, R. T. WIEDMANN & R. G. JOHNSON, JR. 1996. Dissociation of phospholamban regulation of cardiac sarcoplasmic reticulum Ca^{2+} ATPase by quercitin. J. Biol. Chem. **271:** 24517–24525.
20. CHIESI, M. & R. SCHWALLER. 1994. Reversal of phospholamban-induced inhibition of cardiac sarcoplasmic reticulum Ca(2+)-ATPase by tannin. Biochem. Biophys. Res. Commun. **202:** 1668–1673.

Index of Contributors